Surgical Errors and Safeguards

Contributors

Alexander Brunschwig, M.D.

Vincent J. Collins, M.D.

Edward L. Compere, M.D.

Max Cutler, M.D.

David O. Dale, M.D.

Osman Gialloreto, M.D.

Arnold S. Jackson, M.D.

Aaron E. Kanter, M.D.

Jules Laberge, M.D.

Francis L. Lederer, M.D.

S. A. Mackler, M.D.

José H. Mateos, M.D.

Gertrude Novak, M.D.

Neal Owens, M.D.

Frederic J. Pollock, M.D.

Harry C. Rolnick, M.D.

E. A. Rovenstine, M.D.

Emanuel M. Skolnik, M.D.

Paul B. Szanto, M.D.

Max Thorek, M.D.

Philip Thorek, M.D.

Arthur Vineberg, M.D.

Harold C. Voris, M.D.

James W. Watts, M.D.

SURGICAL ERRORS
AND SAFEGUARDS

MAX THOREK

M.D., LL.D., SC.D., F.I.C.S., F.B.C.S., F.P.C.S. (Hon.),
D.C.M., F.R.S.M.

*Professor of Surgery, Cook County Graduate School of Medicine;
Surgeon-in-Chief, American Hospital of Chicago; Founder and
Secretary General of the International College of Surgeons; For-
merly Attending Surgeon, Cook County Hospital, and Consulting
Surgeon, Municipal Tuberculosis Sanitarium; Honorary Fellow,
Surgical Society of Rome, Italy; Honorary Fellow, Piedmont
Surgical Society; Fellow, Mexican Academy of Surgery; Honorary
Fellow, Peruvian Academy of Surgery; Fellow (Honoris Causa),
Royal Surgical Society of Bulgaria; Fellow, National Academy of
Medicine, Colombia; Corresponding Member, Société de Chirur-
giens de Paris; Fellow (Honoris Causa), Vienna Medical Society;
Honorary Fellow, Tusco-Umbrian Surgical Society*

Fifth Edition

455 Illustrations, Many Colored

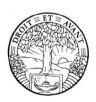

J. B. LIPPINCOTT COMPANY
Philadelphia · Montreal

To the Memory

of

MAX THOREK
1880–1960

Surgeon — Author — Humanitarian

Preface to the Fifth Edition

Since the appearance of the previous editions of this volume, the advances in every field of surgery have been so numerous and so rapid that it is no longer feasible for one man to attempt to cover the surgical spectrum. Therefore, this edition has been completely rewritten with the assistance of 22 collaborating authors who have contributed chapters in the fields of their specialized interests. New to this edition are two fields now covered in detail: anesthesiology and cardiac surgery. Both of these have made giant strides in the last decade.

The steady progress of surgery has brought a closer approach to perfection in method and surgical technic and has diminished the errors of diagnosis. However, there are variations in the levels of surgical competence, and mistakes are made even by the most skilled. This book attempts to warn and to guide—mainly the younger surgeons and those of limited experience—by lighting the danger signals and noting the pitfalls. Future progress depends upon analysis of past performances, recognition of mistakes and, finally, correction and improved technics. If this book can contribute at any level in this chain of progression, my father would feel satisfied that his efforts and those of his collaborators have been worthwhile. It was to the improvement of surgical practice that he devoted his life, and this volume should stand as his last and most helpful effort.

PHILIP THOREK, M.D.

Preface to the First Edition

No person is so perfect in knowledge and experience that error in opinion or action is impossible. In the art of surgery, error is more likely to occur than in almost any other line of human endeavor, and it is in this field that it should be most carefully guarded against, since incorrect judgment, improper technic, and a lack of knowledge of surgical safeguards may result in a serious handicap for the rest of the life of the patient, or may even result in the sacrifice of that life. For the surgeon, perfection in diagnostic skill is of equal, if not of more, importance than operative skill.

No surgeon, no matter how skillful or proficient he may be, should ever consider himself beyond the possibility of error or accident. The individuality of the patient is such a complicated mass of varying factors, that, no matter how wise the surgeon, he cannot always gauge the human equation by any known tests, yet this personal equation may entirely change the outcome of a brilliantly planned and faultlessly executed operation. Surgical procedure cannot be standardized, applied at random and the result invariably predicted. To remove a gallbladder or drain a pelvic abscess is not the same operation in any two individuals, for no two patients are alike, physically, psychologically or surgically.

The surgeon must acknowledge that, no matter how often he may have performed the simplest surgical operation, he must, on each new occasion, mentally review the possibility of error and, during the course of the procedure, he must be wary of meeting some new and unexpected peril. It is always well to keep the danger signposts in the mental vision and it is for the purpose of erecting these signposts and danger signals that this book is written. So far as is known, there is no American work dealing with the subject. There are scattered descriptions of possible accidents and mishaps in different surgical procedures and our surgical textbooks tell us what to do and how to do it, but it is seldom that they tell us what not to do, how to avoid complications and technical errors or how to act when face to face with some of the abnormal circumstances which constantly present themselves during the course of a surgical operation.

It is a duty incumbent upon those who have had considerable experience and have, themselves, passed through the painful ordeal of learning what is erroneous and dangerous in surgery, to record and pass on such acquired knowledge for the benefit of the inexperienced. While it is human to err, it is inhuman not to try, if possible, to protect those who entrust their lives into our hands from avoidable failures and danger.

The author feels that a personal experience of over twenty-five years in the practice and clinical teaching of general surgery justifies him in acting, without presumption or vanity, as a mentor to those who are entering on the perilous paths of surgical practice which he has trodden. Indeed, it is because of his own mistakes and the dangers which he himself has met that the author is filled with the keen desire to impress their possibility on others, so that they may benefit from his failures and disappointments.

Although many of the matters included in this volume have been gathered from the experience of others, as recorded in their writings and from constant scientific intercourse with some of the world's greatest contemporary surgeons, the chief contributions are the author's personal experiences—things which he has actually lived through.

Although the era of the furor operandi has passed, one still has almost daily evidence of the disastrous effects of major surgical procedures, attempted lightly by young, or even inexperienced older surgeons. The author would in no way dampen the ardor of the neophyte, or check his ambition to acquire skill. Still, it is well to suppress the feelings of cocksureness and egoistic pride (to which the writer, unfortunately, was no stranger) which impel the novitiates to undertake risks they know not of, and which often lead to disastrous results.

If this book helps to fulfil this purpose and to incite conservatism, the author will feel more than compensated for his efforts in writing it.

The author wishes to express herewith his profound appreciation to the authors who so graciously permitted him to reproduce some of their illustrations and to the publishers, the J. B. Lippincott Company, for their aid and counsel in making the volume worth while.

MAX THOREK

The American Hospital of Chicago

Contents

MAX THOREK, M.D.

1 Errors and Safeguards in General

As the reader will realize at once, as soon as he examines this book, the general scheme has been changed quite considerably from that of the earlier editions. Elsewhere I have spoken of the valuable aid and assistance that I have received from my colleagues who so graciously have given of their time, skill and knowledge to contribute separate chapters. Many points of importance apply chiefly, or even solely, to the individual fields of these specialists.

However, there are many other items equally as important which apply to all fields of surgery alike. Also, there are precautions applying both generally and specifically which my co-authors have covered in their respective chapters, but which, I feel, will certainly bear restatement, without justifying charges of repetitiousness. Items in these latter two categories I propose to cover in this first chapter.

GENERAL CONSIDERATIONS

The primary object of surgery, as of all other branches of the medical arts, is to cure disease and to restore the patient promptly to health and efficiency. Hence, when a surgeon is faced with a situation where removing tissue or organs seems indicated, the problem arises of whether or not some other way may be found to produce the desired end-results. Good surgery is curative rather than destructive; to keep this constantly in mind may help to stay the surgeon's hand when he is tempted to perform some brilliant feat that might redound to his own credit but do the patient more harm than good in the long run.

It might truly be said that *no surgery is the best surgery* in far more instances than many of us are inclined to believe. The best surgeon is the one who adopts the most conservative attitude consistent with existing conditions.

He spares his patient the ordeal of an operation as long as there remains any reasonable hope that the desired end may be attained by less drastic measures. Yet, when the need for operative intervention has been clearly manifested, he must have the courage to be as radical as need be and not hesitate even to sacrifice important bodily structures if, by so doing, he is convinced that he can assure the removal of imminent danger and the ultimate restoration of the patient to a relatively useful, normal existence.

It must also be remembered that the words "operation" and "surgery" are not necessarily synonymous. Operative intervention must be employed only when all other methods have failed, or have clearly shown that they will fail, to obtain the desired objectives. It is far more to a surgeon's credit to withhold the knife when and until those natural or non-operative processes commonly designated "medical treatment" have had the fullest opportunity to do their work.

THE QUALITIES OF A SURGEON

Certain qualities are demanded of him who undertakes to become a surgeon. The patient must be protected, whenever possible, from the dangers inherent in any surgical procedure. When surgery becomes unavoidable, the conscientious surgeon is fully aware that he is undertaking a fearsome task, in that he may be risking the very life of a fellow creature.

Nor are the pitfalls in his way always limited to the patient or his disease. They may also lie in the mental equipment of the surgeon himself; as such they might be listed somewhat as follows:

1. Failure to obtain a correct and complete history

2. Failure to make a thorough and comprehensive physical examination

3. Too great haste to operate

4. Too great dependence on mechanical diagnostic aids (e.g., roentgenograms)

5. Faulty interpretation of observed signs and symptoms

6. Failure to give due weight to the operative mortality for a given procedure, both over-all and with respect to each step of that particular procedure.

Some 18 years ago, O'Donnell summed up the problem succinctly when he said, in effect, that we must, for example, balance the dangers of draining an abscessed appendix or gallbladder against the chance of spreading peritonitis by removing the organ. Or again, drainage for intestinal obstruction must be compared with resection and anastomosis. We must be able to judge when an operation should be done in more than one stage. In making such decisions, not only must we consider the patient and his individual ability to withstand the trauma involved, but also, if possible, we must have a correct estimate of our own capabilities and of the conditions under which we must work. We must not put ourselves in the untenable position of subjecting a good-risk patient to so prolonged and extensive a procedure that he will be unable to withstand postoperative complications if they should arise. We must always bear in mind that *the first duty of the surgeon is to do his patient no harm.* (Italics mine.)

SURGICAL JUDGMENT

This is the one indispensable quality of the good surgeon and can be based only on a thorough familiarity with pathologic anatomy and the conditions which influence it. On such judgment will depend every decision on when and how to operate, in view of all the considerations involved.

Operative Technic. When, in the surgeon's opinion, operation is clearly indicated, three points must be considered for the protection of the patient. These involve not only his chances of recovery but also avoidance of complications. They are (1) conservatism consistent with efficiency; (2) simplicity of technic (i.e., restriction to what is absolutely necessary); (3) operative skill. This includes gentleness, dexterity and speed.

THE UNFORGIVABLE SINS

These are two in number. The first is to operate when it is not necessary. The second is to undertake a procedure for which the surgeon lacks sufficient technical skill.

It is all too well known that such errors are inexcusably common in these days of increasingly frequent and unrestricted operative interventions. Nevertheless, this does not obviate the moral obligation of the surgeon both to the patient and to himself. There *may* arise an occasion when a surgeon feels that he is called on to undertake some operation with which he is unfamiliar. If the situation makes it imperative, then he is morally bound to do the best he can under the circumstances. Aside from such occasions—and they arise much oftener in popular fiction than in real life—it is wholly unwarranted for any surgeon to experiment with the future usefulness, or even the life, of a fellow human being by undertaking any procedure without having the necessary skill and experience.

The Needless Operation. Every surgeon, at some time in his career, is faced with a situation where pressure of one sort or another is brought to bear upon him to operate when his surgical judgment dictates otherwise. These temptations are too diverse and numerous to list in detail. A few examples will serve to illustrate.

There is the patient with an obscure ailment who has heard of some brilliant new technic which he believes might fit his own needs and demands its application. A similar situation obtains in the case of the vain and silly person who has little wrong with him beyond being cursed with "more money than brains," who would like to be able to brag to his friends about what had been done to him and by whom. These two types might almost—though not quite—be dismissed for exactly what they are worth, were it not for the fact that some surgeons *have* yielded to this sort of pressure, with neither benefit to the patient nor credit to themselves.

Graver are the emotional pressures within the surgeon's own mind when some situation arises where none of the tried-and-true methods seems to be applicable, but some unfamiliar technic—even if it has been used successfully elsewhere—appears to promise relief for a puzzling condition. Also, sometimes there is the impulse to "swap horses in midstream," to abandon a carefully planned course of action in favor of something which has not been adequately prepared for, because some unforeseen situation becomes obvious during the course of treatment. Not that either of these paths *necessarily* leads to disaster; rather, such impulses should be scrutinized very narrowly from all possible angles before the decision is made to follow them.

Dexterity. Some years ago, Sir Hugh Devine had this to say: "No matter how much knowledge the surgeon may possess, if he is unskilful he will not be able to make his knowledge available for the cure of his patients. Indeed, lack of dexterity may account for almost as much postoperative morbidity . . . and mortality as . . . lack of knowledge; for the delicate endothelial tissues and rich sympathetic nerve supply of the abdominal cavity are often profoundly injured by the unskilful operator, who, unconscious of the damage he does, causes much shock. . . . The properly equipped abdominal surgeon must, therefore, systematically train his fingers to be gentle and dextrous." The same applies, in essence, to all other surgeons as well.

Haste. In addition to needless and clumsy operations, there are also those performed in too much of a hurry. The literature yields all too many examples of tragedy following operations performed in the ofttimes mistaken conviction that only instantaneous action would save the patient's life. This is especially apt to occur in dealing with such obvious emergencies as foreign bodies in the esophagus or the trachea, or a strangulated hernia. Yet, it is almost certainly true that many more hospital deaths are due to such errors than ever get into print. Any surgeon would be understandably reluctant to admit his guilt in such a case, even were he prompted to do so in the hope that it might save others from similar burdens on their consciences.

Haste is not limited to decisions as to when and how to operate. It can also take its toll at any and every step of the operation itself. Again, perusal of the literature will yield appalling evidence of the results of incomplete inspection of the parts being dealt with and of insecure or inadequate closure of operative wounds. How often have ureters been mis-

taken for tubes and tied off during removal of an ovarian cyst or some other pelvic operation? How often has a solitary kidney been removed without the surgeon apprising himself of the fact that there was no other? How often has the omission of an extra row of sutures resulted in the breakdown of an anastomosis and subsequent fatal peritonitis? The number of *reported* cases gives us only a hint of the true situation.

The New Technic. Once upon a time, each and every standard operation that we know today was new and untried. Some of them were introduced with much fanfare; others gradually came into general use almost unnoticed. Similarly, other procedures have been introduced, either spectacularly or quietly, but have not met the test of time and have fallen into deserved disuse.

The same process is going on today. Certain operative procedures receive great publicity and sometimes are even used to promulgate the interests of publicity-seeking individuals or groups. It is true that some of these procedures have intrinsic merit, but all too often only in the hands of those who devised them. Others are published only after the most thorough and conscientious study and practice on the part of their advocates. In either instance, it does not necessarily follow that facility in the technic can easily be acquired by outsiders, or that they can be successfully performed by young and relatively inexperienced men, regardless of how anxious they may be to bring themselves into prominence by the execution of some seemingly brilliant new operation.

It is a matter of the gravest concern to those who value the honor of surgery that far too many operations are carried out in this spirit by men unfamiliar with the basic technics involved. Still more tragic is the inevitable corollary that it is the unsuspecting patient who pays the penalty.

Again, the prominence given in the lay press to some new surgical method may lead the public to seek its application in preference to older technics. This, in turn, brings us back to the matter of external pressures upon the surgeon, defying his better judgment.

Expedition. While haste has been and always must be condemned, nevertheless, it is true that, consistent with the nature of the work being done, speed is imperative in all operations. This may easily be understood when we consider that the longer the operation takes, the longer must be the anesthesia, the longer are the tissues exposed to cooling, manipulation and operative trauma and, consequently, the greater the risk of shock.

Even so, adequacy at each step of the operation must never be sacrificed to mere speed for its own sake. The only justifiable speed is that which derives from confidence and sure knowledge. Conservatism must be tempered with boldness. Timidity, while it may render the patient safer than in the hands of the overconfident, is, to quote Bickham, "generally an agony to the operator himself" and nearly always a confession of ignorance; yet boldness which comes from a combination of ignorance and recklessness "cannot be too sweepingly condemned."

INDICATIONS FOR SURGERY

These fall into a number of categories. First is that which roughly parallels the classification of "surgical risks" as given on page 9.

Group 1. Here we find those patients so desperately ill that surgery offers only a faint hope of relief. In this group the mortality rate is necessarily high.

Group 2. These are the patients in whom the indications are fairly clear and who show no gross contraindications for surgical therapy. Examples might include patients with myomatous uterus or with chronic cholecystitis with cholelithiasis.

Group 3. In this group the indications are not always clear, but other forms of therapy have failed to effect a cure. Signs and symptoms are present which may or may not be due to disease amenable to cure by surgery. It is in this group that so much of success or failure depends on surgical judgment, in choice of procedure and estimation of the over-all surgical risk.

Preoperative estimation of the patient's vital capacity and of the condition of his various bodily functions has assumed increasing importance in recent years. The great improvement in surgical prognosis and the reduction of operative mortality and postoperative morbidity bear witness to the increasing emphasis on the imperatives of pre- and postoperative care. Without minimizing the importance of correct surgical technic, we now have come to realize that the era of brilliant operations has given place to one in which surgery is judged more by its ultimate results than by its execution.

The multiple-stage operation can represent a real lifeguard. In certain types of procedures, more particularly indicated elsewhere in this book, multiple-stage operations are to be preferred, but they demand courage, judgment and eternal vigilance. Not only do conditions within the patient himself have a bearing but also every factor affecting him, such as the hospital facilities available and the skill and experience of both the surgeon and his team.

The Bad Surgical Risk. In the first group noted above, we find patients in such grave condition that some simple procedure such as drainage of the gallbladder under local anesthesia would tax their vital capacity to the limit and should be undertaken only to preserve life itself. There are even situations when a ruptured appendix should not be removed. Even after the abdomen has been opened, an acutely inflamed appendix (whether ruptured or not) may be found so bound down by adhesions or encased in omentum and loops of bowel that removal might be fatal. On the other hand, if such an appendix is not disturbed and the abdomen is closed over it, the inflammation may subside and 6 months later it may be removed safely.

As stated some time ago by Brandeis, except in the case of malignancy, the old idea of a condition being "operable" or "inoperable" no longer satisfies the contemporary view regarding estimation of operative risks. In many instances, the "poor risk" may be rendered a comparatively "good risk" by various means now at our command of ameliorating the collateral adverse factors in his over-all status.

Inflammatory Lesions. Here we are faced with two sets of alternatives. The inflammation may resolve spontaneously under conservative medical measures, so that either the patient is spared all need for surgery or surgery can be postponed until a more propitious time. There may also be a choice between a mere palliative operation, which entails minimal risk but retains the prospect of further surgery later, and a more radical procedure having a greater chance of effecting a permanent cure but carrying greater risk for the patient. Here again, surgical judgment is all-important in balancing the various factors for and against each alternative.

Malignant Disease. Here the indications are nearly always plain. The most radical procedure that the patient can be expected to withstand should be performed. Only so can we even hope for anything resembling permanent cure.

Putting these two situations in another way, we might say that in inflammatory lesions, we may try to make the operation fit the patient; but in malignancy, if possible, we must make the patient fit the operation.

Surgery in the Aged. Even in a healthy person of advanced years there will nearly always be found an increased susceptibility to fatigue and a decrease in reserve power to withstand the rigors of surgery. If possible, these must be determined and allowed for in advance. In addition, such patients usually suffer from certain conditions which are practically synonymous with old age. Some of these are obvious, and appropriate preoperative measures can be instituted to counteract their effects to some extent. Others are the composite end-result of whatever diseases may have afflicted the patient in the past, e.g., syphilis or tuberculosis. Mild forms of heart disease or kidney impairment may become troublesome only under the extra load of an operative procedure.

Additional Aids. Various other aids to estimating and improving the over-all surgical risk need little more than to be mentioned briefly. *Saline, serum and whole blood* given before, during and after the operation frequently tip the scale in the patient's favor, provided that the heart and the kidneys are able to handle them. *Diathermy* is often a useful means of supplying the internal heat so essential for keeping the functions of the vital organs, especially the liver, at their best, both before and during the operation.

Diabetes. Here the risk is far less today than before the introduction of insulin and of the various forms of local anesthesia. Under suitable management, the diabetic can be subjected to most surgical procedures with little additional danger (Fig. 1). It must be remembered, however, that certain changes in the system are still present—the diabetic is still

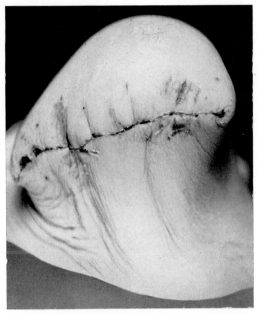

FIG. 1. Supracondylar leg amputation for diabetic gangrene, 14th postoperative day. No. 24 cotton interrupted sutures used throughout; no drain. (Dr. Philip Thorek's case.)

a diabetic, insulin or no—and results can be painfully unexpected in some instances (Fig. 2). Some forms of inhalation anesthesia are strictly contraindicated.

Pregnancy. Here we find our best judgment taxed to the utmost. In a doubtful situation, the possibility of pregnancy can markedly alter the nature of the risk. An abortion superimposed upon an operative procedure may render doubtful an otherwise safe situation.

Sugar and salt reserves must be estimated accurately before operation and brought up to normal levels if they are not so already.

Hepatic capacity must also be fully known. Elective surgery should be avoided or postponed if the patient is found to have low physiologic hepatic reserves.

Fear. Many surgeons are prone to underestimate the importance of the patient's mental attitude before surgery. If a neurotic individual is convinced that he is going to die on the operating table, he quite probably will do exactly that, regardless! The surgeon with a pleasant, confident manner and a ready smile has a more valuable instrument at hand

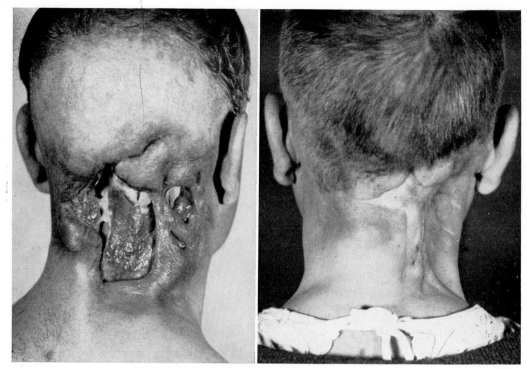

FIG. 2. (*Left*) Extensive destruction of tissues following carbuncle in a patient suffering from diabetes. (*Right*) Same patient following insulin therapy and plastic reconstruction.

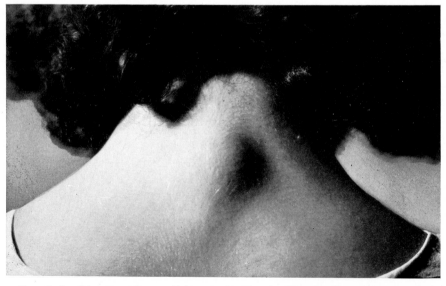

FIG. 3. In this case, the condition was variously diagnosed as osteoma, chondroma, etc. The simple, chronic, inflammatory nature of the tumefaction was not revealed until the *occupation* of the patient (acrobat) was brought out.

than any other he could have in his armamentarium.

Latent Conditions. A latent *infection* may flare up when the natural defenses of the body are lowered by surgery. Any *endocrine imbalance* can have unexpected and untoward effects if not recognized and corrected beforehand. Under certain conditions, the same is true if a persistent or hyperactive *thymus* gland is present. When metabolism is markedly disturbed, it is important to know whether or not the *thyroid* secretion is abnormal, especially when planning an abdominal operation.

THE PATIENT'S HISTORY

The "snapshot" diagnosis and the inadequate history go hand in hand. Both are equally inexcusable.

History taking is the first and, in many ways, the most important single step in diagnosis. A good history is both complete and explicit. It is amazing how frequently some seemingly insignificant, even irrelevant, detail may provide the one missing link in a diagnostic chain. I can think of no more pertinent example of this point than was demonstrated in a case reported in earlier editions of this work. The patient, a young woman, had a swelling over the seventh cervical vertebra, for which half a dozen possible explanations presented themselves to the group which was examining her (Fig. 3). None seemed to be satisfactory. At last, a single, stray question, "What is your occupation?" brought out the fact that she was an acrobat, and that the lower cervical region was subjected to constant friction. The diagnosis then became obvious—simple hypertrophy of the segmentary and subcutaneous structures as a result of pressure and friction.

Two other divergent cases also come to mind. In one, lead poisoning successfully mimicked appendicitis until, again, the patient's occupation, this time that of painter, was shown (Fig. 4). In the other, a mass just below the knee of a man of 50 was diagnosed as sarcoma and the leg was amputated, without awaiting the results of biopsy and, more importantly as it turned out, of a Wassermann test. To the chagrin of all concerned, the biopsy revealed a granuloma, and sections from the amputation specimen confirmed the final diagnosis of gumma. This also demonstrates once more that it pays to wait when no real urgency exists.

A still more spectacular and farfetched instance serves to demonstrate another point about history taking. As Sir William Osler once said, the examiner will find that it often pays to be a good listener; if he listens carefully enough, the patient may furnish his own diagnosis. Again I quote from the earlier edition.

A Negro woman, aged 27, was shot by her "boy friend." One bullet grazed her right forearm, then entered the upper right abdominal quadrant and emerged through an opening in the region of the left hypochondrium. Another bullet entered the left side opposite the anterosuperior spinous process of the ilium and emerged on the opposite side a little above the crest of the right ilium.

Bladder examination revealed free blood, leading to a diagnosis of ruptured bladder.

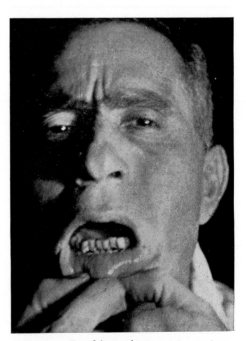

FIG. 4. In this patient, acute gastroenteritis led to an erroneous diagnosis of acute appendicitis. A blue line along the gum, as shown here, suggested the true cause—lead poisoning.

Further, an increased pulse rate, together with extreme tenderness over the right and left hypochondria, suggested the possibility of injury to the liver. The patient was prepared for surgery, but while listening to a discussion in her presence of the differential diagnosis of the blood in the bladder, she suddenly exclaimed: "Don't worry, Doctah, about this hyah blood! Ah's been treated foh kidney stones foh a long time befoh mah boy frien' shot me and Ah's allas passin' blood!"

On the strength of this statement, 200 cc. of boric-acid solution was injected into her bladder and was retained; when the solution was siphoned off, it was entirely free of blood. Further examination disclosed that all the pain was due to edema, the result of damage to the superficial structures, and that there had been no intra-abdominal injuries of any kind!

Osler's old dictum was never better demonstrated than in the above anecdote.

It is surprising how often the history, when carefully and expertly taken, will be all that is needed to lead to a correct diagnosis. It must be remembered, however, that many patients will complain of only one symptom, though they actually have several others. A few even have no real complaint but simply fear that they may be suffering from some dreaded malady. It is important, therefore, to elicit the pertinent facts by friendly conversation and judicious questioning.

Before beginning to record the history, it is well to get a general idea of the entire story, so that, for the record, the details may be presented in logical sequence. Many apparently irrelevant items will be obtained from the *family history,* yet they should be investigated because they may contain information suggestive of the correct diagnosis. Data regarding the patient's health throughout his life prior to the present illness should be carefully obtained and can be especially useful when the diagnosis is uncertain or a lesion to explain his symptoms is not readily discernible. Occasionally, also, data from the past history may *exclude* certain possibilities. Naturally, the history of the *present illness* must be very complete and should include progress of symptoms, history of trauma and the like, as well as all routine information.

THE SURGICAL EXAMINATION

This should include, first, the physical examination, then the reports of all laboratory and special tests. Naturally, follow-up examinations, when needed, must also be included in the reports.

Any surgeon who subjects a patient to any major procedure without adequate preoperative examination of his blood, heart and excretions, without determining if foci of infection exist and without remedying such deficiencies as are found, as far as it is possible to do so, is guilty of exposing that patient to unnecessary risks and, by so doing, is failing in his duty to the patient.

However, after all these admonitions have been taken to heart, there is still a certain margin for error. This lies in those items which may be beyond the surgeon's control, or at least, may so appear. These are conditions lying within the patient himself which are capable of causing even the most brilliantly planned and faultlessly executed procedure to fail and are the situations which call forth from the laity the cynical comment, "The operation was a success but the patient died!" The history, through no assignable fault, may be incomplete. The patient may deliberately misrepresent his symptoms or withhold essential information. Or, occasionally, some condition may remain concealed until the operation is actually under way or even until after it is completed. Untoward results can then be a greater surprise to the surgeon than to anyone else.

The degree of the patient's own resistance is by no means always easy to ascertain. We have no sure way of determining it. The frail-looking individual may come through an operation that would kill someone who looks far more robust.

EVALUATING THE SURGICAL RISK

In these pages we have already covered some aspects of this subject. However, we have said little about estimation of the risk as a whole in relation to such items as anesthesia, premedication and the like.

Classification of Risks. We use the terms "good risk" or "poor risk" rather loosely. A more exact classification might be somewhat as follows:

Good Risk—a patient in whom nothing is found that would adversely affect his chances for recovery

Fair Risk—a patient in whom one or more adverse factors are present but none of these appears seriously to affect his chances for recovery

Poor Risk—a patient in whom (1) there exists one or more seriously adverse factors or (2) one so gravely ill that death is likely unless the progress of his malady is quickly reversed.

In this system of classification, it will be noted that all unfavorable conditions and diseases, *including the one for which the operation is proposed,* are considered together. In other words, the *severity of the operation* is not taken into account.

Risk Due to Anesthetic. In earlier editions, I cited the case of a boy who was subjected to tonsillectomy. The surgeon was competent. The patient demonstrated no contraindications. The operation was done under ether anesthesia, and there was little hemorrhage. Everything seemed to go normally until 3 hours after he was returned to his bed. He then developed hyperpyrexia, which resisted all attempts at relief, and died 9 hours after the operation. Necropsy revealed no cause for death except a slight hemorrhage into the pons cerebelli.

Here was a denouement which no surgeon could foresee, yet the parents doubtless blamed the surgeon. We can only assume that this was a case of changes produced in the organism by the anesthetic.

Changes of this sort may take the form of a sudden, severe drop in blood pressure (as in spinal anesthesia) or of the production of cardiac insufficiency. Even slight surgical shock may combine with the effects of an anesthetic to turn the scale against the patient (see Chap. 2).

Premedication. The choice of premedication is almost as important as the anesthetic itself. Rightly used, it permits deeper anesthesia with a lower concentration of the agent. It reduces the metabolic rate, which, in turn, reduces reflex irritability and, with it, resistance to the anesthetic. As noted elsewhere, patients between the ages of 6 and 18 require the most premedication, while infants and the aged require the least. Patients of advanced years, especially if weak and cachectic, tolerate any premedication poorly.

The use of *hypothermia*, which recently has received considerable publicity, especially in the lay press, might be thought to belong in this section. However, we personally feel that these methods are relatively too new and unproved to merit inclusion here.

PREOPERATIVE CONSIDERATIONS

PREOPERATIVE PREPARATIONS

Shock. Again and again throughout this book the reader will find reference to operative shock. The mention of it here is for the special purpose of pointing out that *all operations,* bar none, impose some degree of shock on the patient's system. The more extensive the operation, naturally, the greater the degree of shock that must be expected. This situation must be met head-on, by bringing the patient, preoperatively, to the highest possible condition of bodily resistance to such surgical shock.

Age of Patient. Also in connection with operative shock, the question of the patient's age is important. This is especially true in those who are being considered for thyroid or gallstone operations or appendectomy. While persons under the age of 40 endure major surgery rather well as a rule, in the succeeding decades, the proportions of deaths from operative shock mounts up very rapidly. For example, in the surgical treatment of simple goiter, the operative mortality is only about one half of 1 per cent in patients under 40, whereas it is between 20 and 25 per cent in those over 60.

Vital Resources of Patient. Every person reacts differently to surgery. The same person may react differently to the same procedure at different times because of differences in his vital resources. To illustrate, I recall a case cited in earlier editions, of a woman, aged 40, who was operated on for fibromyoma of the uterus. Though the operation was severe, she made an uneventful recovery. Before leaving the hospital, she requested that I repair a laceration of the perineum. I acquiesced, arguing that there was no reason to fear a simple perineoplasty in a patient who had so well withstood a supravaginal hysterectomy. Three weeks after the major procedure, the repair was undertaken, the operation lasting only about 30 minutes. Everything appeared to go well, but she never rallied, and death occurred on the third postoperative day, in spite of every effort to save her life. A thoroughgoing necropsy demonstrated no cause for her demise. Therefore, I must conclude that the second ordeal, though seemingly slight, was simply too much for her powers of resistance.

Gastro-intestinal Tract. If it has been shown that the patient's metabolism is unbalanced, or that the intestinal flora are abnormal, these conditions must be corrected as far as possible before surgery is undertaken. Reduction of pathogenic bacteria in the intestines is of especial importance when an anastomosis in this area is to be done.

In my own practice, I look especially for foci of infection and take every precaution to remedy such infections. This markedly reduces the chance of postoperative parotitis or pneumonia.

As far back as 1920, Kellogg, of the Battle Creek Sanitarium, pointed out that patients who come to the operating table with coated tongue, foul breath and other symptoms of intestinal poisoning are much more likely to suffer shock, renal failure, acidosis, anemia, peritonitis or other complications leading to prolonged and stormy convalescence than those who show a clean tongue and an inoffensive breath.

The colon should be thoroughly cleansed and kept clean for some time before the operation is scheduled. A bland, nontoxic diet should be given, avoiding meat (see below).

Catharsis, however, depletes the fluids necessary to the system, as well as causing distention and irritation to the bowel. Further, it predisposes to abdominal inflation and "gas pains," thereby interfering with peristalsis. Drastic preoperative purging, so common in the past, seems to me to be quite needless, if the bowel has been put into a clean condition and has been working satisfactorily for some time. However, it should be added that, *under emergency conditions*, if the patient has eaten within 6 hours, the *stomach* should be emptied before any operation.

Preoperative diet should be planned so as to provide adequate amounts of glycogen. Further, it should be light and nutritive, providing little bulk, easily assimilated and thoroughly cooked.

Hemocoagulants and Transfusion. In situations where extensive bleeding is to be expected during the operation, preoperative administration of hemocoagulants should almost always be ordered. The use and the value of these preparations has been both demonstrated and publicized in the recent past in the care of President Eisenhower. Calcium preparations and vitamin K are also of value here. Preoperative blood transfusions (see Chap. 3) and, in the case of biliary disorders, the administration of bile salts should also be considered.

Urine. If the urine is highly acid, the simple expedient of administering small doses of bicarbonate of soda for some days prior to operation is still useful. However, in some situations where this is inadvisable (as with gastric ulcer), other special preparations now on the market may be used profitably instead. In either case, such treatment will serve to bring the reaction to a more normal level.

Other Dangers. In addition to trauma and shock, every operation entails a certain amount of hemorrhage, and, in spite of all possible care and caution, there is always some danger of infection (*vide* succeeding chapters). Further, it has been pointed out that the variations in tonus and the sudden fluctuations in blood pressure that occur under narcosis or anesthesia subject the circulatory system to a singularly heavy burden. Respiration is likewise heavily taxed. Metabolism, as already mentioned, is often adversely affected. In addition, such mechanical factors as elevation of the diaphragm from some operating-table positions and postoperative intestinal atony must be considered in estimating the probable effects of any nonemergency operation. The effects of *fear* have been mentioned elsewhere; occasionally it is known to influence blood pressure and it may have other unpleasant results.

SEPTICEMIA

Serious blood-stream infections may accompany or follow such apparently simple affections as furuncles, small abscesses, sore throat, otitis and the like. Septicemia may also follow any operation, and the cause remain obscure or unrecognized. Various terms are applied to such infections: "microgenetic," if they follow small local disturbances; "cryptogenic," if the immediate cause is not discoverable; "masked," if, as sometimes happens in children, they are concealed by some secondary focus of infection.

Surgical interventions during such occult infections can precipitate a generalized septicemia, particularly when the surgery opens a path for the pathogenic micro-organisms into the blood stream during a virulent phase of the infection. The danger is greatest when the infection is staphylococcic.

Therefore, it is of the utmost importance that any surgical intervention be avoided in patients suffering from sore throat, furunculosis, anthrax or even so "mild" a condition as acne. Only the most dire emergency should contravert this rule.

Latent infections may also flare up following a surgical intervention. In doubtful situations, the diagnostic acumen of the surgeon is put to the severest test; under such conditions, the decision for or against operation at that particular time often determines the ultimate survival of the patient. Fortunately, present tendencies are toward a "wait-and-see" attitude until the inflammation can be contained. When such an infection results in the formation of pus, this should be evacuated with the least possible surgical trauma.

Management. Today, three main means of combating septicemia are at hand. They are (1) preventive and/or therapeutic measures; (2) surgery aimed at frustrating the spread of infection into the general circulation through thrombosed veins; (3) chemotherapy. All of these means are designed to support and maintain the natural defense mechanisms of the body itself. The use of vaccines as a fourth measure should be considered only if the type of micro-organisms involved can be accurately determined and should never be resorted to if the infection is severe, as results are uncertain in any case.

Intravenous therapy of any type should also be avoided, especially in patients possibly already made sensitive by prior serotherapy. Small immunogenic blood transfusions may be useful, but it is dangerous to inject a large quantity of blood, since it may provoke infarctions or pulmonary complications.

PREPARING THE OPERATIVE SITE

Obviously, the rules for preparing the site of incision vary according to the operation to be performed, but at least one point should be observed in preparing for any invasion of the trunk. The *umbilical pit* is a prolific source of wound infections. It is difficult to sterilize effectually; leaving it open is an error. After the usual surgical preparation of the skin, some half-strength tincture of iodine should be dropped into it and the whole sealed over with collodion.

OPERATIVE CONSIDERATIONS

Again we come to a field of thought which is covered rather particularly in each of the chapters that follow, but, again, we feel that repetition should not invoke a charge of repetitiousness. Precautions bearing on the operation itself fall into various categories, including asepsis, physical precautions, sedation, prevention of hemorrhage and other misfunctionings of the circulation, and various factors having to do with opening and closing of the operative wound.

ASEPSIS

It should not be necessary to mention the need for the strictest precautions regarding asepsis in everything connected with any surgical procedure. Every surgeon is, or should be, fully alive to the imperatives for avoiding every source of infection; yet, even in the past few months, we have seen in the public press an increasing number of accounts of tragedies occurring in some of the best-equipped and supposedly most modern hospitals, the direct result of the sort of infection we thought had long since been barred forever from such institutions!

There is no one explanation for these misfortunes, but at least a considerable share of the blame seems to rest on overdependence on the antibiotics and the new therapeutic chemicals. We, like the mariners of old, have listened too long and too well to their siren song and have believed that they could protect from all evils whatsoever. NOT SO by any means!

While it is true that these "wonder drugs" have been of the most far-reaching significance in combating infections of many kinds, it is certainly *not* true that they can replace or even undo the damage resulting from neglect of plain, ordinary, old-fashioned cleanliness, in the broadest therapeutic sense of that word. For this reason, if for no other, I take the liberty of calling attention here to several points that I believe are most apt to be ignored in this connection.

Gloves and Gowns. No surgeon should glove his own hands. He should be gloved by the sterile nurse, whose hands have already been aseptically gloved. Short-sleeved gowns which leave a portion of the forearms bare have no place on the operating surgeon. In short, the skin of those working about the operating table should never be allowed to come in contact, even indirectly, with any part of an unprotected wound. This is especially important in the case of bone and joint surfaces, of muscle wounds and of free fascial flaps, all of which are particularly liable to infection.

Insufficient scrubbing, especially of the thumb and the index and middle fingers of the right hand, can cause trouble, particularly if the further sin of using punctured or torn gloves has also been committed. As a further insurance of surgical asepsis, I have found it advantageous, after scrubbing, to submerge the finger tips for a few minutes in a 1:1,000 solution of Metaphen or some similar antiseptic of known potency before gloving. This reduces the danger of direct contact if a glove happens to be torn during the operation.

Operating Room Air. A considerable number of writers have cited instances of infection in what should have been perfectly clean operative wounds, which were traceable to contamination in the air of the operating room, often originating with some member of the surgical team. For example, a common cold or a chronic throat or sinus infection in someone in the room (even though masked) can spell disaster for the operative patient. This is especially apt to happen when the operation is long and complicated, involving much drain on the patient's resources and prolonged exposure of the wound to the air.

Since the introduction of air sterilization by ultraviolet radiation, the decrease in the incidence of such infections has been dramatic. In series after series, such decreases as 32 per cent to 0.35 per cent and 9.0 per cent to 0.22 per cent have been reported regularly.

In some types of procedures, the incidence of infection has dropped to zero!

Foreign-body Irritants. In a previous edition of this book, I quoted from Ramsey and Douglass to the effect that introduction into the tissues of such foreign substances as talc or lycopodium powder can cause an irritant reaction and produce inflammation of a granulomatous type. These lesions are not necessarily dangerous unless they destroy important tissues or cause adhesions or contracting scars. These writers stated that many physicians and surgeons seemed to be unaware that these substances might be introduced into the body on gloves or suppositories, on tubing or rubber drains or by absorption when used as dusting powder. It is also well to see that there is no free powder on the *insides* of sterile gloves, as a tear at the finger tip could release such powder into the operative wound.

They added that rectal or vaginal suppositories that had been stored in powdered talc or lycopodium should be freed of the material before use. When such suppositories have been used, it might be well to keep in mind the possibility that nonhealing granulomatous lesions could develop from this source.

PHYSICAL PRECAUTIONS

When a patient is under general anesthesia, he is unable to react to the untoward effects of pressure on the superficial nerves. Consequently, especially during protracted procedures, it is entirely possible for a nerve to become paralyzed because one of the patient's limbs has been restrained in such a position as to compress a nerve. Such pressure paralysis may be very persistent or even permanent.

Some years ago, I had occasion to observe a young woman who had undergone abdominal surgery elsewhere some 2 months earlier. There had been sharp pains along the course of the long thoracic nerve on the right side shortly after she was returned to her bed. Later, she was unable to raise her right arm, and there was protrusion ("winging") of the scapula, as shown in Figure 5. This appears to be rather typical of the pressure paralyses produced by carelessness in positioning of the patient during operation.

Other examples have been found involving "foot drop" following simple cholecystectomy and "wrist drop" after operations for inguinal hernia. Again, these were most likely the result of carelessness.

One patient walked with a brace for 3 months and did not fully recover for another 3 months because, apparently, a too tight leg strap produced pressure paralysis of the superficial peroneal nerve. Bed covers tucked in too tightly, causing hyperextension of the feet during recovery from the anesthetic, could have the same effect.

If the patient's elbow is allowed to extend beyond the edge of the table, it may be leaned upon by some member of the operating team. It is also possible that the rigid band used to fasten the diaphragm of the blood pressure stethoscope to the patient's arm can press on the nerves. Either of these situations may result in weeks of needless idleness for the patient before he recovers the use of his hand. The same may be true if his hands or fingers are pinched or otherwise injured when his position is being changed on the table, causing brachial-plexus palsy. The abominable practice of tucking the patient's hands under his buttocks, to get them out of the way, has led to more than a few instances of unpleasant and embarrassing aftereffects.

The moral is obvious. Avoid pressure on all vulnerable parts of the patient's body while he is on the operating table and also after he is returned, unconscious, to his bed, and you will help to avoid medical and legal complications afterward.

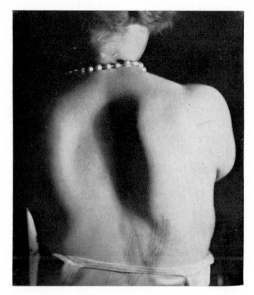

FIG. 5. "Winged scapula," indicating compression paralysis of the long thoracic nerve, resulting from carelessness in positioning this patient on the operating table during surgery 2 months previously.

SEDATION

Morphine has its legitimate uses, but it can also dig pitfalls for the unwary. Many addicts claim to trace their habit to the therapeutic use of the hypodermic needle. Prescribe morphine only when conditions definitely demand it and do not allow the patient to know what he is receiving. Also, keep constantly in mind that morphine may mask the very symptoms the surgeon needs to see; it has no place in the treatment of any acute illness attended by abdominal pain until a firm diagnosis has been established. Morphine can render the surgeon as well as the patient somnolent!

HEMORRHAGE

Loss of blood during any operation should be kept to the absolute minimum. This may be accomplished by the most careful hemostasis at each step of the procedure. Artery forceps should be narrow. Preferably, arteries should be tied when first picked up, but, if the situation makes this impossible, they may be left in position for a time with an artery forceps attached.

Saline Infusion and Blood Transfusion. In recent years the general use of blood transfusion before, during and after operation has somewhat changed the picture with regard to the dangers from bleeding. But the use of saline infusion is still valuable to correct a marked fall in blood pressure (hypodermoclysis or venoclysis). The giving of subcutaneous saline now seems to be inferior to a slow continuous flow into a vein in such conditions as shock, dehydration from vomiting, oliguria and many forms of toxemia. The exact amount of fluid the patient is receiving is known and the results generally more closely approach a physiologic norm. On the other hand, massive doses of intravenous saline make no sense unless there has been a corresponding loss of body fluids. Further, it is not suggested that the continuous intravenous infusion should entirely supersede the 4-hourly rectal saline infusion or the continuous rectal drip. These are completely satisfactory in many instances.

Where continuous intravenous saline is being used in the treatment of shock, it may be useful to add an ampule of Coramine to each pint of the solution. Adrenalin in an amount of 5 min. 1/1,000 per pint may also be added.

CONTRAINDICATIONS. These are few but definite. They include (1) any condition indicating a failing heart, such as dyspnea on exertion, uncompensated valvular disease or any other cardiac weakness making an increase in the bulk of circulating fluid inadvisable; (2) pulmonary congestion; (3) hypertension; and (4) Bright's disease.

Some years ago, Hamilton Bailey laid down what I call some "golden rules" on the administration of continuous intravenous saline:

1. When in doubt as to whether the poor pulse is due to cardiac weakness or to another cause, I have many times placed the patient on continuous intravenous saline and Coramine, and waited for an hour or more to see if the blood pressure improves. If it does so, the flow is reduced to 30 drops per minute and the patient is again visited after a lapse of an hour or so.

2. Unless there are definite indications to the contrary there is seldom need to continue the flow after the third day. A good working rule is to remove the needle or cannula at the end of 72 hours, and, if necessary, to reinsert it into another vein after six or twelve hours.

3. Especially after 48 hours watch the bases of the lungs for signs of edema.

4. If the flow stops, do not disassemble any part of the apparatus without due thought of the possibility of air embolism. Rather remove the needle or cannula, and if necessary reinsert it into another vein.

5. For various reasons the interceptor may become filled with saline and the fall of the drops is obscured. This is a constant source of trouble. There is no need to disassemble the apparatus—the interceptor can be cleared by passing a long hollow needle through the tube into the interceptor.

6. In some cases redness and tenderness develop along the course of the vein. This is hardly ever anything more than a chemical phlebitis, which soon settles down after the flow into that vein has been discontinued.

7. A 5 per cent glucose solution in six pints of saline contains about 180 Gm. of glucose, so at the usual rate of flow the patient is receiving 720 calories in the 24 hours. This may be increased if no other source of nourishment can be utilized by the patient.

INCISION AND CLOSURE

Only a few points need be mentioned here regarding the operative wound itself, since this subject is covered much more fully in the chapters which follow.

A sharp, clean cut through the soft tissues in any area of the body will heal better and more quickly than a jagged, irregular incision, since in the latter instance, hollows and pockets (dead spaces) are sure to be left after closure. Similarly, an incision which runs parallel to the underlying muscle fibers will heal best.

Moderate reddening of stitch holes does not necessarily mean impending trouble; therefore, removal of sutures is not always demanded.

In my personal experience, cotton for suturing materials has proved to be most satisfactory. In my own work and in numerous cases under my direct observation, it appears to retain its tensile strength in the tissues better than catgut, linen or silk. Further, it is easy to sterilize and is inexpensive. I use it routinely and find that it promotes rapid, dry healing and can even be buried safely in infected wounds without resulting sinus formation.

Blood Clots. These unexpected complications, occurring often some days after the operation, can turn a smooth convalescence into a dismal tragedy. Pulmonary embolism, especially, may come as a complete surprise. Various operative precautions may help to avert these accidents:

1. Avoid bruising or puncturing deep epigastric vessels.

2. Avoid muscle splitting whenever possible.

3. When working in the area of the broad ligament, control bleeding by use of isolated ligatures rather than over-and-over sutures.

4. Avoid transfixion of veins by a suture, since the suture becomes, in effect, a foreign body in the lumen.

5. When using retractors, avoid impinging on iliac vessels or the inferior vena cava.

6. Avoid use of cutting needles in suturing tissues.

7. Use the finest suture material possible and limit the size and the number of knots.

Other Considerations

There are numerous small points that all too often are neglected, any one of which, though apparently insignificant, can lead to serious trouble.

Make sure that *drainage tubes* are fastened securely both to the skin with sutures and to the outside dressing as well. Be sure that all retention apparatus, for example, a Levine tube for continuous suction drainage, is in proper running order. If liquid should flow, see personally that it actually is flowing.

Cleansing and debridement of superficial injuries should be adequate and thorough. If the presence of foreign material is indicated or suspected, be sure that *all* of it has been removed before closure and dressing. This is especially important in dealing with the frequent minor injuries of children, such as cut scalps, embedded splinters and the like. Much prolonged and wholly needless expense and suffering have resulted from inattention to such points.

These are but a sampling of the sort of minor but important items that must be given due attention, right along with all the seemingly much larger precautions covered elsewhere in this book, if our lifework is to be as valuable and rewarding as we wish it to be and know it must be if we are to merit the confidence of our fellow men.

POSTOPERATIVE CONSIDERATIONS

General Precautions

Oxygen. During and after certain procedures the administration of oxygen, either employing a tent or *via* the mask of Boothby and Lovelace, can constitute a real lifeguard.

Fluids. Their postoperative use entails accurate observation of the fluid balance and of the percentage of chlorides in the urine, together with amounts of sugar, if present. Sugar tolerance is reduced in the operative patient. The smaller the percentage of injected fluid eliminated, the higher the operative mor-

tality rate. The same holds true of excessively high or low salt elimination.

Obesity. Certain complications are practically implicit in the obese patient. Chance of wound infection is greatly increased. Fatty degeneration of vital organs is probable. Respiration may be impeded. Fat embolism is not uncommon following operations on those who are markedly overweight.

Anemias and Other Blood Deficiencies. In the anemic patient, both the quantity and the quality of the blood are altered. In forecasting the effect of anemia on the surgical prognosis, the platelet count is of more importance than the determination of red or white cells because of their more intimate association with clot formation. Moreover, anemia is inevitably increased by the unavoidable loss of whole blood during operation. These dangers are better met today with improved methods of blood transfusion, but even here certain dangers are inherent (see Chap. 3). Also, the *viscosity* of the blood almost always is increased by operation. This is usually accompanied by an increase in the protein substances present. How far this can affect surgical results we do not know, but some toxic or other effects may be expected in such a departure from the normal. This could be serious in some cases.

Bolognesi referred to what he termed the *"colloidal lability"* of the blood serum, which occurs whenever normal relationships between albumin and globulin constituents of the blood are changed, as is likely to occur as a result of surgery. He observed that this situation had been found in fatalities following surgery and was much more marked than in patients who recovered.

Hemophilia. This is a condition too familiar to need enlargement here. In its victims (always males) postoperative hemorrhage can be fatal. Routine preoperative determination of clotting time will alert us to the situation and permit the use of whatever preventive or precautionary measures are indicated.

Thrombosis and Embolism. These may be guarded against to some extent. Although, as previously mentioned, they may come as a "bolt from the blue" (and are more common in females) in a patient who appears to be

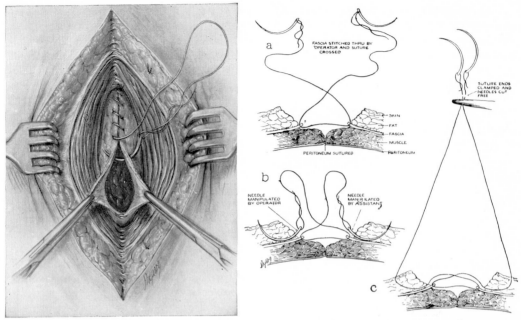

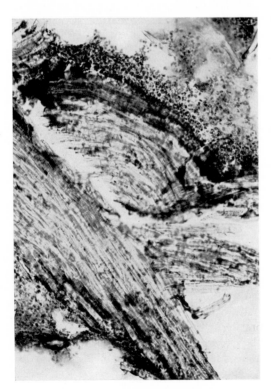

FIG. 6 (*Left*). Author's method of closing abdominal wound. First step: peritoneum being closed. Continuous or interrupted sutures with cotton or catgut may be used. (See Fig. 7.)

FIG. 7 (*Right*). Author's method of wound closure (*cont.*). (a) Fascia stitched with through-and-through sutures, crossed. (b) One needle manipulated by surgeon, one by assistant. (c) Suture ends clamped and needles cut free.

well on into convalescence, today decreased use of Fowler's position has lessened this danger somewhat. Nevertheless, precautions are still very much in order (see p. 18).

To date, we have few ways of combating these tragedies effectively or even of foretelling them. Embolism occurs in the excellent-risk patient equally as often as in the bad risk.

Wound Infections

Any consideration of postoperative complications in the broadest sense turns naturally, first of all, to the subject of wound infection. The causes have been discussed thoroughly in many places; the consensus appears to group these under a number of general headings.

FIG. 8. Shows anchoring cotton suture removed from common duct on 12th postoperative day. Note leukocytic response around suture but without infiltration into suture structure proper. (Dr. Philip Thorek's case.)

Sutures. Despite much progress in the choice and the manufacture of catgut, absolute sterilization of this material has not yet been attained. The basic ingredient from which it is made, being organic, is intrinsically septic, swarming with bacterial flora capable of forming spores and rendering themselves highly resistant to destruction. Though the use of iodized catgut has enjoyed a certain degree of popularity, many forms of postoperative infections, such as stitch abscess, adhesive peritonitis and even tetanus, have been ascribed, probably with some justice, to the use of catgut.

If it is recalled how much suture material the system is sometimes expected to absorb in the course of postoperative healing, the origin of much trouble in this area will, I think, be better understood. Many modern surgeons, in a thoroughly commendable effort to ensure against bursting of wounds, postoperative hemorrhage resulting from slippage of ligatures and similar catastrophes, have a tendency to use more suture material than is strictly necessary; hence the intrusion of the opposite horn of the dilemma. Leukocytosis is increased, there is enormous congestion both active and passive, and liquifaction of repair products invites invasion by different groups of malevolent bacteria. My own observations, both in experimental work and in the hospital, bear out these contentions.

For these reasons, therefore, I have attempted to limit myself to the fewest possible sutures, especially in abdominal work (where the error of excessive quantities is most tempting), usually using one for the peritoneum and one additional for the overlying layers (Figs. 6 and 7). I further restrict myself, as far as possible, to nonabsorbable suture materials (Fig. 8). As indicated elsewhere, my preference is for cotton, though other types of nonabsorbable sutures will probably do as well in the hands of those who prefer them.

Allergic Reaction. Referring again to catgut sutures, there is another point that should be borne in mind. Acting as an antigen, catgut may provoke a local reaction. Studies have shown that a patient already in a hyperallergic state, due to other prior treatment, has a special "catgut sensitivity." The formation of adhesions and even possible intestinal occlusion may result. Therefore, in such persons, if at all possible, the type of allergy should be determined and steps taken to desensitize them beforehand.

Trauma. Injury of the neighboring tissues during operative procedures is another prime cause of postoperative infection. Avoid harsh or protracted pulling on the wound with retractors. Do not use mass ligatures on subcutaneous tissues. Avoid devitalization of fat, fascia, muscle and skin by careless or excessive use of artery forceps. See that laparotomy sponges are not too hot. These and other similar precautions will eliminate many complications of this type.

Delayed Suture. On occasion it is advisable to be in no great haste to suture an operative wound. It may be wiser to leave an antiseptic dressing upon the open wound for 24 hours or even longer, after which it will be found in better condition for suture and repair. Then, if no infection is apparent, the temporary dressing is removed and the superficial portions of the wound closed. In case of infected wounds, irrigation with one of the chemotherapeutic solutions may be of value. This should be done immediately after closing the peritoneum.

PULMONARY AND OTHER POSTOPERATIVE COMPLICATIONS

Besides hemorrhage (see p. 19), shock (q.v.) and infection, many postoperative deaths and disabilities are due to pulmonary and associated difficulties. *Pneumonia* seems to be more apt to follow major procedures than the simpler operations such as herniorrhaphy. This indicates *trauma* as the exciting factor. Certain abdominal operations in which there is prolonged manipulation of delicate structures are especially liable.

Aspiration Pneumonia. This may be avoided by aspirating the stomach following gastric operations. If vomiting is persistent, constant lavage (Levine) may prove to be valuable in this area. Keep the tracheobronchial tract clear!

Chilling. Simpler than most other precautions, yet too often ignored, is the avoidance of chilling of the patient's body. Merely by making sure that the patient is not exposed to drafts can, in my experience, eliminate more cases of postoperative pneumonia than all other steps together. Unnecesary exposure of the body surface, use of cold solutions, leaving the patient in a cold, drafty corridor, even putting him into a cold bed to recover from the anesthetic, are all reprehensible.

In the recovery room, fresh air is important, but there should never be a draft, even a warm one, that is allowed to reach the patient. The use of electric blankets simplifies warming the bed and avoids the danger of burns or scalds from hot-water bottles.

Hypostatic Pneumonia. It is believed that hypostatic postoperative pneumonia is due to circulatory stasis in the lungs with a superimposed infection. Postoperatively, there is a definite fall in blood pressure. The use of digitalis routinely may be of value in avoiding this complication. Diminished lung action, resulting from pain or too tight bandages, as well as injudicious use of sedatives (which allay the reflex excitability of the air passages, thereby favoring retention of aspirated material) also may contribute their quota of cases.

Preventive Measures. In my experience, certain measures have proved to be helpful in obviating postoperative lung complications. These include (1) avoiding protracted use of the Trendelenburg position; (2) oral hygiene following operation; (3) use of deep breathing exercises several times daily.

Pulmonary Collapse. This is a not uncommon postoperative complication, often mistaken for "ether pneumonia." It may follow any type of operation. It usually may be avoided by frequently changing the patient's position and the routine use of deep-breathing exercises as suggested above. It may be either prevented or, if already present, relieved by frequent inhalations of oxygen 90 per cent with carbon dioxide.

Thrombosis. Closely akin to the pulmonary affections are those of the circulatory system (Fig. 9). When thrombosis may be anticipated (e.g., following removal of a gangrenous appendix), it has been recommended that an injection of 10 cc. of 3.8 per cent sodium citrate be given daily for 6 days, and that knee-bending and deep-breathing exercises be done 3 times a day. However, if thrombosis

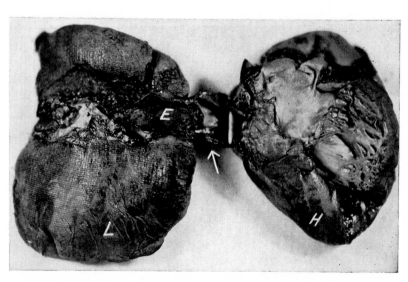

Fig. 9. Fatal pulmonary embolism. This patient, aged 30, was recoving normally from an operation for an ovarian cystoma. Without warning, while she was sitting up on the 16th postoperative day, characteristic embolism symptoms appeared, and death occurred 1 hour later. (L) Lung. (H) Heart. (E) Embolus plugging pulmonary vessel. The arrow indicates the pulmonary artery.

actually has developed, the legs should be kept at rest, preferably elevated on an inclined plane.

Hemorrhage. It is important to distinguish between the symptoms of shock and of postoperative hemorrhage, as antishock treatment, if applied when the true condition is internal bleeding, will generally only aggravate the trouble.

Flatulence. This can cause much misery for the patient. Oil of cajeput, 1 min., has been found to be definitely helpful in this connection. A rectal tube may be passed; if this does not serve, and there are no contraindications, a small enema may be given.

Hiccup. This occurs frequently after upper abdominal operations and in uremic patients. If persistent, it can be exhausting. Morphine sometimes helps, but inhalation of air with an excess of carbon dioxide is considered to be better. As a last resort, injecting the phrenic nerve with alcohol may be considered.

Retention of Urine. This is a somewhat common complication, especially following operations for strangulated hernia or those done under spinal anesthesia. Every effort should be made to have the patient pass his urine naturally. The various familiar nursing procedures are useful here. If these fail, a hot fomentation to the hypogastrium and administration of potassium acetate (parasympathetic stimulant and diuretic) may be useful. Hypodermic Prostigmin (if not contraindicated, as in bowel resection or appendectomy) sometimes has served well in this situation. Failing all of these, a catheter must be passed. Use every aseptic precaution in doing this.

Burns. Since electric pads and blankets have become generally available, there is no longer any possible excuse for using hot-water bottles. An unconscious patient or a nurse at a distance can be equally unaware that a burn is being sustained. Why take chances? A properly prepared recovery bed, warmed in advance, and *no hot-water bottles* will eliminate burns and accumulating malpractice suits.

Causes of Postoperative Deaths

This subject is covered rather thoroughly in most of the several chapters which follow. I merely propose to summarize here.

"Liver Death." There is no operative procedure which the liver does not resent in some manner. There is no type of anesthesia which does not affect it. Postoperative hepatic insufficiency may be serious, even if not fatal. It may activate some latent condition; the result may then be merely to change one set of symptoms for another. Other causes may also contribute. Even with the most careful preoperative testing, unpleasantly surprising results may follow any operation if the liver is prompted to misbehave.

Death Due to Anesthetic. Here we are in an area so intimately associated with other phases of care that the choice of anesthetic and prognostication of its effects cannot possibly be considered alone. Death directly attributable to the anesthetic may result from a pre-existing myocardial degeneration, degeneration of hepatic or renal cells, alterations in the blood or a dozen and one other shortcomings of the organism, natural or acquired. Again, as elsewhere, surgical judgment is indispensable to success.

Further, death attributed to the anesthetic may not be due to this factor alone. The patient may simply die *sooner* of some cardiac condition of which he would have died eventually in any event. Some workers believe that the mortality among heart patients is no more than 5 per cent higher than normal. The "bad-risk cardiac" is the one with arteriosclerotic coronary disease (with or without angina), syphilitic heart disease, aortitis, myocardial degeneration accompanied by auricular fibrillation or heart block of any type or degree.

SURGICAL FAILURE FROM MECHANICAL CAUSES

INSTRUMENTS

Designs and Materials. In the earlier editions of this book, I devoted considerable space to the troubles caused by instruments of poor design and/or inferior materials and to my recommendations for some possible ways of eliminating these troubles. I still feel that too little attention is being paid to the quality and the fitness of the instruments provided by industry for the use of the surgeon. That commercial interests are permitted to originate and popularize many surgical supplies is generally an excellent arrangement.

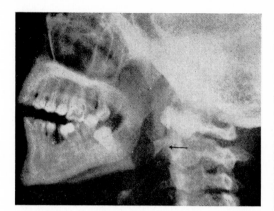

Fig. 10. Fragment of needle used for procaine injection lodged in pharyngeal wall. Attempts at removal at time of accident and twice later failed. Exact localization by roentgenogram is helpful in such situations.

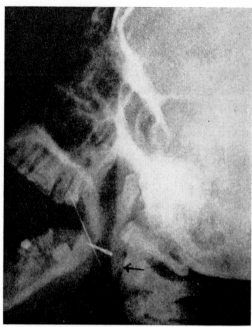

Fig. 11. Same patient as in Figure 10. This shows guides used in final successful attempt at removal.

Nevertheless, it seems also to be true that the medical profession would do well to establish some sort of governing body with direct power to oversee the industry as a whole.

The manufacturer who undertakes to provide surgical instruments for use under circumstances where the entire future life and usefulness of a human being are at stake should have a conscience not hardened by commercialism. He is normally responsible, right along with the surgeon himself, if, by reason of the failure of one of his products, a life is wrecked or lost.

Further, a surgeon's skill can be adversely influenced if, for any reason, he lacks complete confidence in the tools and the materials that he is using. Even one accident due to mechanical failure, in a moment of stress, could for a long time, or even forever, reduce that surgeon's fitness for his job.

A Bureau of Standards? A group formed within the framework of one of the major surgical organizations should draw up and demand compliance with a standard set of tests covering the entire field of commercial instruments and supplies. It could certify each manufacturer who met such standards and make known to the profession a list of those so approved. All complaints against any manufacturer, whether certified or not, could be handled by it, with removal from the certified list or published censure of the offender, where indicated. In this way, the quality of an item could be judged by more than the mere name and reputation of the maker or the persuasive patter of the salesman.

I do not profess to know how such tests should be set up or of what they should consist. That is a field as specialized as my own. However, I do know that certain specific points should be covered.

Tempering. Good tempering of steel is even more important than good steel *per se*. Since I am given to understand that good tempering is, in some instances at least, a matter of luck, it may not necessarily follow that the most expensive instrument is sure to be the best.

Specific Adaptations of Instruments. Although the individual will choose those instruments and types of instruments which he has learned by experience best suit his own particular needs, certain general rules apply to nearly all of these.

Pedicle clamps should be strong and well ribbed to avoid slipping. *Chisels* and *osteotomes* should be of steel in preference to

FIG. 12. Tonsil snare which proved to be a delusion as well!

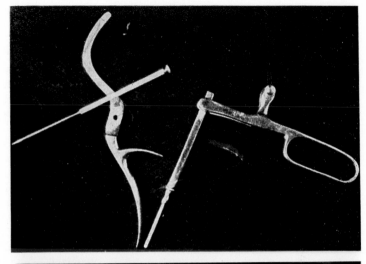

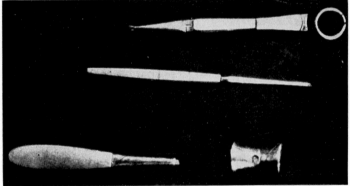

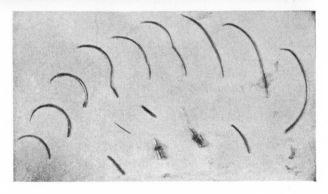

FIG. 13. Instruments (*top*) and needles (*bottom*) broken during operation.

nickel- or chrome-plated, since the latter are prone to chip in use. *Mallets* constructed entirely of steel are most durable and most easily sterilized. *Intestinal clamps* cause less trauma if sheathed in rubber.

Any instrument intended to *manipulate bony fragments* must be of the sturdiest construction and have jaws wide enough to conform to the diameter of the bone. *Metal plates* for use in orthopedic surgery should be so designed that the screws will not loosen, with consequent loss of fixation, infection and collection of fluid about the metal.

Electrical equipment should be as simple as possible. Electrodes must be completely insulated to avoid burns.

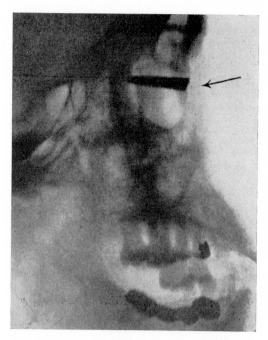

FIG. 14. Roentgenogram showing broken blade of turbinectomy scissors which could not be removed. Fatal meningitis followed.

Needles are more subject to damage by rust than from any other cause (Figs. 10 and 11). Breakage due to interior rusting is particularly to be feared in the case of spinal-puncture needles. The safest material here is one of the high quality, rustproof alloy steels.

Defective Instruments. Little need be said about the things that can happen to and because of instruments that fail. The accompanying illustrations tell their own story and are well worth careful persual (Figs. 12 and 13). However, one point I do wish to stress is that instruments that can be "taken apart" are dangerous. They often *fall apart* when least expected. Those that are fixed with a screw are as efficient and as easily cleaned. The same is true of artery forceps with spring catches, which may fail to hold when subjected to tension and lacerate the tissues.

Sterilization of Instruments. A point germane to the same subject is sterilization. High temperatures often affect the temper of steel, making it brittle. Needles become less elastic. Knives lose their edge. All instruments that must be subjected to sterilization by either heat or chemicals should be retested periodically.

FOREIGN BODIES

Although, understandably, there are relatively few such incidents reported in the literature, it is fairly well established that a considerable number of cases of "things left behind" during surgery do occur each year. It is also obvious that such accidents may not only cause immediate failure but also can necessitate reoperation later and/or lead to a whole string of corollary troubles, including law suits and chronic invalidism or even death for the patient (Figs. 14 and 15).

Occasionally, it appears that foreign objects left in the abdomen after laparotomy are unavoidable. Far more often they are the result of sheer carelessness. Gauze sponges or pads head the list of such objects; next in frequency are artery forceps.

Under emergency conditions—when a patient is moribund on the table or when life itself depends on speed at every step—it is at least understandable that strict counts of sponges or instruments might not be possible. Unless we know all the circumstances, it is unjust to condemn any surgeon who leaves a foreign object in his patient's body.

There may also be conditions, physical, legal or some other, that would suggest avoiding revelation of such an error, even if the surgeon became aware of it. The offending object may become encysted or quiescent. Its presence may cause the patient no serious inconvenience. It may be eliminated spontaneously.

Or, again, it may be discovered accidentally during some subsequent operation by another surgeon, who may not even know who was responsible or may keep such knowledge to himself for ethical reasons. Statistics based on reported cases are probably misleading. Yet it seems to me that such incidents *should* be reported as often as possible because of the valuable aid these reports can give to others forced to deal with the same problem later on.

INCIDENCE

From what published statistics are available, it appears that women are more apt, by some 13 per cent, to be the victims than men when soft objects such as sponges are involved. Of these, about 80 per cent are gyne- cologic patients. Some of the foreign objects have remained undiscovered for as long as 12 years. In one series, some one tenth of the total was discovered accidentally at necropsy, and another one fifth was eliminated sponta- neously. In another series, dating back to the end of the 19th century, forceps were by far the most frequent finding, but one patient even turned up a pair of spectacles! While most such cases involve the abdomen or the chest, Haberer reported removing one piece of gauze from the cranial cavity. Those who wish to pursue this subject further are re- ferred to the illuminating volume, *Foreign Bodies Left in the Abdomen,* published in 1940 by Crossen and Crossen.

About 1 case in 4 appears to involve in- struments or pieces of instruments (Fig. 16). The seriousness of this situation is demon- strated by the fact that some 40 per cent of these patients die!

Instruments or needles that break during use are a fertile source of such foreign ob- jects. If the pieces are small, they can easily be overlooked. Again, the illustrations speak for themselves (Fig. 17).

Symptoms

Lost sponges or instruments (Fig. 18) may be missed before or after the closure of the operative wound or they may show up only as the probable source of postoperative in- flammation, acute or subacute. They may cause a persisting sinus. Deep suppuration may require secondary operation, or a mass may be the only sign, indicating aseptic encapsulation. Any of these latter conditions may show up only weeks, months or even years later.

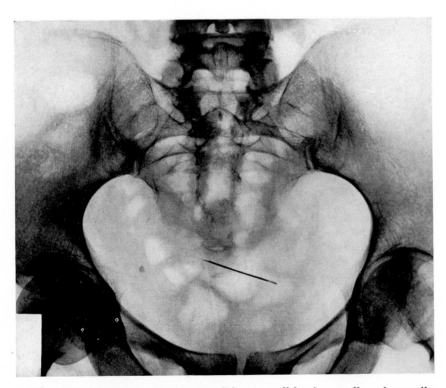

Fig. 15. This patient, a seamstress, did not recall having swallowed a needle but was in the habit of holding needles in her mouth. She had undergone several gynecologic procedures without obtaining relief for a variety of abdominal symptoms. When a roentgenogram finally revealed its presence, removal of this needle from the terminal ileum was followed by full recovery.

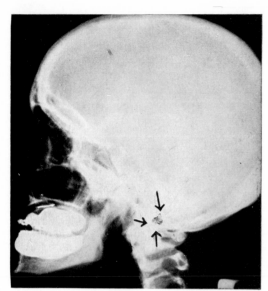

FIG. 16. Portion of a chisel discovered in the mastoid region 10 years after an operation for mastoiditis.

HOW IT HAPPENS

It may be well to call attention to some of the ways that slips have occurred in order to suggest how they may be avoided. It is amaz-ing what small things—what slight inatten-tions—may break a link in the chain of security, regardless of how systematic the prior planning may have been.

Sponge counts may appear to be correct even though they are not. Someone may have picked up an extra sponge and failed to report it. A sponge may be torn in two, deliberately or accidentally, and part of it left behind.

On the other hand, through an inadver-tence, a report of "sponge missing" may result from one having been dropped on the floor, lost in a fold of the drapes or carried from the room, resulting in a long, dangerous and futile search for it within the operative site. The one is as bad as the other!

All soiled sponges and used small instru-ments should be placed in a spot definitely provided beforehand. The use of "stick sponges" (small sponges in forceps) is a valid safety measure, though these, too, can be dangerous if they slip out of the holder and pass unobserved, especially in the haste of some emergency. Particular care in this respect is needed when ordinary forceps are used as sponge holders, for once a sponge has slipped away, there is nothing to indicate that it was ever present.

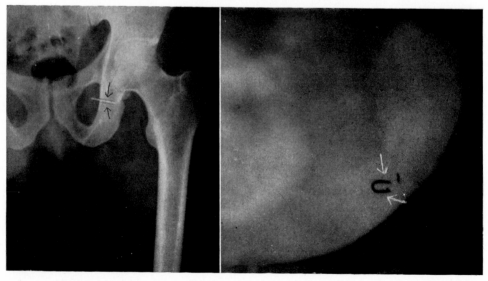

FIG. 17. "Silent" objects (i.e., those which cause no symptoms) should be left alone. It is an error to subject such patients to surgery for their removal. (*Left*) Needle broken during injection of sciatic nerve. Numerous attempts at removal failed. (*Right*) Silver wire suture used in repairing inguinal hernia, 15 years in situ.

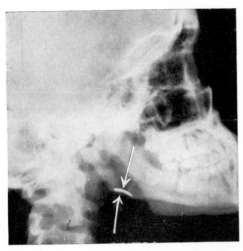

FIG. 18. Blade of tonsillectomy knife broken and left behind. A thin object of this sort, with its edge toward the camera, can easily be overlooked in studying a roentgenogram.

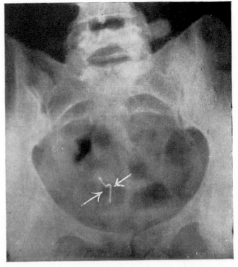

FIG. 19. Part of contraceptive device broken off and left behind during removal. Endometritis resulted.

LOCATIONS

Female Genital Tract. In addition to foreign objects left following gynecologic operations, there is a whole class of things, usually contraceptive or abortifacient devices (Fig. 19), that find their way *via* the genital tract into other parts of the abdomen. Flexible bougies and soft rubber catheters lead this list. They furnish a striking indication of the tragic dangers of abortion. They also give valuable information as to the pathology, the diagnosis and the treatment of intraperitoneal foreign bodies in general. The length of time the object has been in the abdomen is an important factor in relation to the extent of the pathologic changes and resulting symptoms.

In every case where a foreign object is known or suspected to be in the abdomen, a critical examination is necessary. Hasty assumption that such an object was left behind at some previous operation could be quite wrong. Wounds in this area heal rapidly, sometimes leaving very little indication of the track of entry. The woman who has attempted an abortion on herself, or has had one done illegally, will usually try to deny it and take every opportunity to lay the blame somewhere else. A previous abdominal operation could be used quite effectively in this direction, with great injustice to the surgeon and the hospital involved.

Uterine and vaginal operations are out of sight during normal after-care. Drains or packing can easily be overlooked. Keep a conspicuous record of all such materials, with the date for their removal, where it will be checked over daily. The deep situation also adds to the difficulty in discovering pieces of gauze or loose parts of packing that may be left behind. All parts of a pack must be securely fastened together. Especially avoid overlooking pieces of gauze used for sponging in this area or left behind temporarily to control oozing.

Urinary System. Urethral and bladder maladies lead to some bizarre mishaps. Some of these originate with the patient himself, who tries to introduce some foreign object into the urethra and allows it to become lost in the bladder.

Other incidents happen during surgery. Kidney operations ordinarily are carried out through the lumbar incision, but even though the operative field is then extraperitoneal, any foreign object left in the area actually lies in close proximity to the colon. Hence, it may ulcerate through into the intestinal canal and be expelled per rectum. More often, however, the tendency seems to be toward the outside,

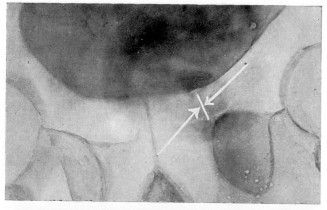

FIG. 20. Needle broken during injection in nonsurgical treatment of hernia. This was subsequently removed during a radical operation for hernia.

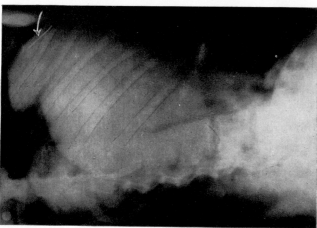

FIG. 21. Needle broken off under breast during hypodermoclysis.

with a persisting sinus in the lumbar region.

Abdominal Wall. In this area there are two classes of surgical invasion, those such as herniorrhaphy (Fig. 20) or lipectomy, which involve the wall itself, and those required for access to the interior. If a foreign object is left behind here, obviously it will be extraperitoneal.

Breast. Large spaces are often left following breast operations, and prolonged drainage may be needed. These conditions favor loss of such articles as drainage tubes. The situation is aggravated by the depth of the pleural cavity, the natural movements of the chest wall and inevitable efforts to avoid discomfort for the patient (Figs. 21 and 22).

Otolaryngeal Area. In operations about the nose, the mouth or the throat, concentration of attention on technical details during the procedure and on making the patient comfortable later may draw attention away from foreign objects left behind. These can cause a great deal of disturbance (see Fig. 21).

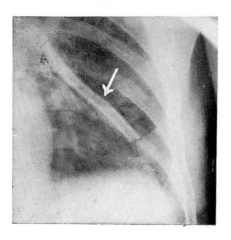

FIG. 22. Drainage tube lost in the chest during an empyema operation. (Discovered 3 years later.)

Goiter operations constitute a large part of neck surgery. As in any extensive operation on a relatively large surface, they may supply hiding places for sponges, small drains and the like.

Spine. During spinal puncture for diagnosis or for spinal anesthesia, needles sometimes break (Figs. 23 and 24). Such fragments are the most frequent foreign objects left in this area. Though such an accident, at first glance, may seem to be fairly simple to remedy, experience proves that it may be quite otherwise. Here also sponges or drains can go astray.

Extremities. Though the upper extremity would seem to offer little opportunity for sponges to be lost, yet such accidents have occurred even here. In working about the thigh and the hip joint, the operative wounds are so much larger than in the arm that they are often the sites for lost objects.

Gastro-intestinal Tract—Swallowed Articles. There is abundant evidence that swallowed articles of various kinds may work out of the intestines and be found in the peritoneal cavity later, exactly as though they had been left after an abdominal or a pelvic operation. This calls for a somewhat detailed examination of this phase of the subject in order to determine what types of objects may behave in this way.

In seeking to discriminate between swallowed foreign objects and objects left after surgery, the swallowed objects may be classified as follows (Crossen):

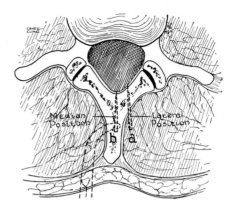

Fig. 23. Shows two possible positions for needle broken during spinal therapy. (Lahey Clinic)

1. Those which might be mistaken for foreign objects left at operation.

2. Those which complicate the problem of x-ray visibility.

3. Those which complicate treatment.

Swallowed articles may include soft materials such as various types of gauze, tapes, sewing threads and ligature materials. Metallic objects include needles (both household and surgical) and various household and hospital dressing-room tools and appliances which simulate small or broken surgical instruments.

In the case of gauze or cloth passed by rectum, extracted from an abscess or found at operation, it is often extremely difficult to determine how it entered the system in the

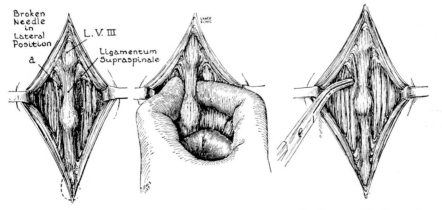

Fig. 24. Diagram showing a method of removing a broken needle from the spine. See also Figure 23.

first place. Consequently, when any such item is encountered, it must be subjected to the most critical examination, the same as any other important pathologic specimen.

Needles and pins are used in such quantities, both in the operating room and during postoperative care, that they may easily become the subject of litigation for alleged retention in abdominal operations, in spite of the fact that they are used as frequently in the home.

Most articles lost during operations in the upper respiratory tract are swallowed and find their way into the stomach. When an object slips away and disappears down the esophagus, the surgeon is confronted with the problem of what to do next.

Treatment for a swallowed foreign body, in the absence of perforation, should always be conservative, until it has been definitely shown that the object will not be eliminated naturally, or until it is plain that there is, or is about to be, perforation. Careful x-ray examination of the abdomen should be made daily so that the progress of the object through the gastro-intestinal tract may be watched.

It has been demonstrated that foreign bodies will usually pass through the digestive tract within 7 days from the time of ingestion. Therefore, serious consideration should be given to surgical intervention if the object remains in one place in the *viscerae* (not necessarily in relation to bony landmarks) for a week or longer. Of course, if abdominal symptoms develop sooner, laparotomy should be performed without delay.

It is important that stools be strained to confirm the elimination of the foreign body if it does appear to be passing naturally. Ambulation is not contraindicated, but rest is desirable.

MALINGERING

Every doctor encounters at some time in his career the individual who, to escape work, danger or responsibility, to arouse sympathy or attract attention, to satisfy some sexual perversity, or in the hope of "getting something for nothing," will allege some sort of illness or physical problem or will seek to mask or alter the true state of affairs when there really is something wrong with him. Deliberate, self-inflicted injuries fall into the same category. Therefore, it is of the utmost importance to investigate with all possible care every case in which it is claimed that a foreign body has been left behind at operation in order to eliminate the possibility of falling afoul of one of these impostors.

PRECAUTIONARY MEASURES

Measures to avoid leaving instruments and other foreign objects in the body present some difficulties not encountered in the special case of sponges. Instruments are necessarily numerous—their numbers cannot be predicted accurately nor their removal made automatic, as with sponges.

The following list of precautions represents the end-results of much study and experience in many places by many people:

1. Eliminate *small* instruments.

2. Make and record a complete preoperative count of all instruments to be used.

3. See that all needles are either in their original boxes or attached to sutures.

4. Examine the operative field thoroughly before wound closure.

5. Count all instruments before wound closure.

6. Count and inspect again immediately when the operation is completed.

Habit plays a definite part in the procedures of many surgeons. In spite of the obvious danger of using small instruments, too many surgeons still continue to use numerous small hemostats and the like in abdominal surgery simply because they have become accustomed to doing so. It is far better to change to long instruments entirely, especially for abdominal work and to do it now—today—for, truly, tomorrow may be too late!

The *human element* can also play its part in even the best regulated operating room. Counts of sponges and instruments may be inaccurate, even when carried out by two people. It goes without saying that the conscientious surgeon will always satisfy himself personally that everything has been checked on and indicated to be corect *before* an operative wound is closed.

As hemostats seem to be the most likely candidates for disappearance, they should receive special attention. In every suspicious case the abdomen should be studied roentgenologically before the patient is discharged from the hospital.

I have mentioned elsewhere the method I have used successfully for many years, that of attaching a metal ring to the end of each laparotomy sponge, not only to make it more conspicuous but also so that it will show up unmistakably in a roentgenogram.

As mentioned earlier in this chapter, *drains* are especially vexatious about getting themselves lost. A further word of caution seems to be in order here. When a drain is looked for and not found, the question immediately arises as to whether it has been removed and thrown away accidentally or whether it has slipped inside the body and disappeared. Insistence on full records of all drains and packing in the daily orders for each patient will eliminate much of this problem. Also, it should be borne in mind that ordinary red rubber tubing is much more clearly visible in roentgenograms, even in the small sizes, than either black or amber tubing. For this reason, if no other, it should be used in preference to either of the others, if at all possible, so that if it does become lost, at least the roentgenogram can be relied on to help answer the vital question of where it went.

MINOR SURGERY

Finally, a word about "minor surgery." *To me, there is no such thing!*

Every operation carries with it the risk of unexpected complications, no matter how "simple" the procedure may appear to be. Lives have been lost following the opening of a furuncle. Uterine curettage has claimed many victims. The sooner the surgeon learns to look on *every* operative procedure as seriously worthy of his best technic, the sooner

will his wisdom be favorably reflected in his mortality and morbidity rates.

The pernicious practice, now, fortunately, fast disappearing, of doing "minor" operations in the office, is to be condemned unreservedly. All such procedures should be undertaken only in a well-equipped hospital.

BIBLIOGRAPHY

Boone, D. W., and Davito, S. J.: The surgical tolerance of the cardiac patient; a review of 143 cases, J. Am. Osteopath. A. **57**:239-244, 1957.

Donigiewicz, S. B.: Preoperative examination and preparation of problem patients, Canad. Anaesth. Soc. J. **5**:75-90, 1958.

Dunlop, D. M., and Duncan, L. J.: The surgery of the diabetic, J. Roy. Coll. Surgeons Edinburgh **3**:81-90, 1957.

Finochietto, R.: Talco y granulomas, tétonos, olvidos, Sem. med. **111**:843, 1957.

Goode, J. V.: Pitfalls of general surgery, Am. Surgeon **23**:1075-1080, 1957.

Gordon, J. R.: Anesthetic preparation and premedication for emergency patients, Postgrad. Med. **22**:572-577, 1957.

Kovács, K., Kovács, G., Kovács, B., and Petri, G.: Effect of preoperative psychic anxiety on the antidiuretic activity of the serum, Orv. Hetil. **98**:1294-1296, 1957.

Krakovskii, N. I.: Errors and defects in surgical practice, Vestnik khir. **78**:104-108, 1957.

McDonald, S., and Timbury, M. C.: Unusual outbreak of staphylococcal postoperative wound infection, Lancet **273**:863-864, 1957.

Meleney, F. L., and Foman, J. J.: Ways and means of preventing and minimizing surgical infections, Am. Surgeon **23**:883-890, 1957.

Sheldon, J. M., and Patterson, R.: Surgical risk in the allergic patient, Univ. Michigan M. Bull. **23**:330-334, 1957.

Tôn-Thât-Tûng: Surgery in opium addicts, Zentralbl. Chir. **82**:1305-1309, 1957.

E. A. ROVENSTINE, M.D., and VINCENT J. COLLINS, M.D.

2 Anesthesiology

INTRODUCTION

ROLE OF THE ANESTHESIOLOGIST

The basic safeguard in anesthesia practice is the presence of a physician anesthesiologist. The role of the anesthesiologist is that of a consultant. He is the medical internist in the operating room and advises the surgeon concerning physiologic dysfunction, pharmacologic needs and the treatment of medical complications that arise in the patient during the course of anesthesia and surgery.

Every surgical patient must be visited by the anesthesiologist at least the day before operation. At this time there should be a complete assessment of the patient with three distinct objectives in mind, namely, (1) determination of physical condition, (2) choice of anesthetic technic and agent, (3) estimation of operative risk.

OPERATIVE RISK

It is evident that operative risk involves many variables which cannot be pinpointed. Such variables fall into three categories: (1) those relating to the patient, (2) factors related to the surgical procedure and operating condition and (3) considerations of the anesthesia.

TABLE 1. CLASSIFICATION OF PHYSICAL STATES

Class 1. No organic pathologic conditions or a pathologic process which is localized and does not cause any systemic disturbance or abnormality.

EXAMPLES. This includes patients suffering from fractures, unless shock, blood loss, emboli or systemic signs of injury are present. It includes congenital deformities unless they are causing systemic disturbance. Infections that are localized and do not cause fever, many osseous deformities and uncomplicated hernias are included. Any type of operation may fall into this class, since only the patient's physical condition is considered.

Class 2. A moderate but definite systemic disturbance caused either by the condition that is to be treated by surgical intervention or which is due to other existing pathologic processes.

Class 3. Severe systemic disturbance from any other cause or causes. It is not possible to state an absolute measure of severity, as this is a matter of clinical judgment. The following examples are given as suggestions to help demonstrate the difference between this class and Class 2.

EXAMPLES. Complicated or severe diabetes; heart disease—functional capacity IIb; combinations of heart disease and respiratory diseases or others that impair normal functions severely.

Class 4. Extreme systemic disorders which have already become an eminent threat to life regardless of the type of treatment and because of their duration or nature have already caused irreversible damage to the organism. This class is intended to include only patients who are in an extremely poor physical state. (There may not be much occasion to use this classification, but it should serve a purpose in separating the patient in very poor condition from others.)

EXAMPLE. Severe trauma with irreparable damage.

Emergency Surgery. An emergency operation is arbitrarily defined as a surgical procedure which, in the surgeon's opinion, should be performed without delay.

Class 5. Emergencies that would otherwise be graded Class 1 or Class 2.

Class 6. Emergencies that would otherwise be graded Class 3 or Class 4.

In this entire picture we must realize that only the patient is the *constant factor*. The patient is presented to the surgical team "as is." Both the surgeon and the anesthesiologist have a role in treating the patient. In any case, the patient cannot take a poor operation or a poor anesthetic. Only the physicians concerned provide poor surgery or administer a bad anesthetic. As a result of such considerations, patients have been graded for surgical procedures into several classes of physical condition, termed *physical status* (Saklad). This has been adopted by a committee of the American Society of Anesthesiologists as a system providing uniformity of patient classification.

PHYSICAL STATUS

A distinction is noted here between the total operative risk and the physical status of the patient. This idea is perhaps novel and therefore needs further explanation. It refers to the medical condition of the patient and the over-all efficiency and function of his organ systems. It is concerned with the fitness of the patient in general and the reserve of the systems specifically to withstand stress. It is known in the athletic world as the contestant who is in the "pink" of condition as the result of training. Many patients can have their various physiologic mechanisms improved and brought to the point of optimal efficiency by appropriate and interested medical therapy or conditioning. They will be better prepared to survive the insults of anesthesia and surgery.

In determining the physical status, reliance must be placed on the examination and the reports of the internist. Not only should diseases and disabilities be noted, but also the anesthesiologist should learn whether the internist believes that any derangements can be corrected or whether functional preparation is optimal. If no further improvement can be reasonably expected, the patient can be considered to be medically prepared. Specific points which the anesthesiologist now should determine for himself, which have a bearing on the conduct of safe anesthesia, include the following:

1. Physical habitus and weight of patient. Obese individuals and short, thick-necked patients are a great risk because of the possibility of airway obstruction.

2. Dental hygiene is evaluated and the presence of dentures noted.

3. Habits: use of alcohol, drug addiction and use of drugs, and smoking. For example, when smoking is excessive, postoperative pulmonary complications are increased sixfold. The alcoholic requires a longer period for induction, has a resistance to the effects of anesthetic agents, and is prone to go through an excitement phase, with the possibility of vomiting and ventricular fibrillation.

4. Allergies—drug reactions; avoid their use.

5. Previous operations and anesthetics should be listed.

6. Medication: *cortisone therapy*—if taken within 6 months, patient must be placed on hydrocortisone preoperatively and continued for 8 hours postoperatively. *Antihypertensive therapy*—many such drugs potentiate anesthetics and lead to persistent hypertension. Examination of the patient is also necessary; blood pressure should always be taken by the anesthesiologist the day before operation. The quality of the pulse should be assessed. Posture and mechanics of breathing should be checked. Patency of nasal passages is important. A simple bedside test of breath-holding (Sebarese's Test) will provide information about the pulmocardiac reserve. Thus, a subject unable to hold his breath longer than 15 to 20 seconds has a diminished reserve, and if the breath-holding is less than 20 seconds, function is compromised.

SURGICAL FACTORS

In the estimation of operative risk, the magnitude of the surgical procedure and the skill of the operating surgeon must be considered. Variations in these features can play a prominent role in increasing or decreasing the chances of the patient's survival. These chances and the morbidity and mortality associated with various procedures are best known to the surgeon. He must acquaint his teammate, the anesthesiologist, with the plan of surgery. Part of the risk involved is the actual operating conditions. Thus, the excellence of physical facilities and equipment and the expertness of the nursing personnel all play a part in patient safety.

ANESTHESIA FACTORS

The anesthetic and the administrator enter into the determination of risk. When either the skill or the experience of the anesthesiologist is deficient, the hazards will be increased proportionately. The improper choice of either anesthetic technic or agent enhances total risk. By relating the surgical needs to the physical state of the patient, the anesthesiologist can arrive at the proper selection of an anesthetic method which, in his hands, is going to be safe and adequate.

In the interests of safety it seems to be necessary to make one plea—a plea for physiologic anesthesia. This does not necessarily mean smooth anesthesia, nor should smooth anesthesia be the only goal in administering an anesthetic. The goal should be to maintain a good physiologic state. However, too often anesthetists have been desirous of making things appear good and in doing so have compromised body function. Many surgeons have fostered this attitude, and in some clinics it has become routine to induce anesthesia in *all* patients with intravenous thiopental. It is erroneous to attempt to prevent excitement by this technic if it is achieved at the price of good physiology. The patient is depressed and the blood pressure lowered. In many instances anesthetists have sacrificed principles for expediency. This is both an abuse of a drug and an abuse of our patients. It is recommended that more anesthetists develop their ability to administer an inhalation anesthetic. By this we mean carrying out an induction with an inhalant that is rapid and smooth and physiologic. One must become an expert in talking a patient to sleep, calm him with suggestions and, in a sense, develop powers of hypnosis. A preoperative visit with the patient is mandatory, and a postoperative observation is essential. This is the psychology of anesthesia.

PRINCIPLES IN CHOICE OF ANESTHESIA

The choice of anesthesia should be based on individualization of every case that is presented for evaluation. In general, the goal of anesthesia is to provide a painless operation. Four factors must be considered in determining a technic and an agent: (1) safety to the patient; (2) convenience for the surgeon; (3) comfort of the patient; (4) ability of the anesthesiologist.

Whatever agents or technics are used, they must be safe for the patient. To submit the patient to unnecessary risk and to jeopardize his life by untried and toxic agents, or to administer excessive doses or unnecessary agents, subverts the moral responsibility of any anesthesiologist.

Having provided a painless state that is safe, one should also aim at providing good working conditions for the surgeon. If such conditions are provided, obviously the surgeon can complete his surgery expeditiously and hence contribute to the greater welfare and subsequent rapid convalescence of the patient. These conditions must not be achieved at the price of safety. It is also desirable to provide the maximum of mental comfort to the patient. However, all things being equal, it is preferable to use safe methods that will expedite the surgery. To achieve this goal it may be necessary to sacrifice comfort.

Despite the above important factors, it is often necessary to consider the ability of the anesthesiologist in determining the anesthetic agent or technic. Thus, there are anesthesiologists who are quite expert in managing many problems with a specific agent, e.g., ether; on the other hand, some anesthesiologists might be equally facile with the use of spinal anesthetic technics. To demand of such men that they change their technics to one with which they are less familiar obviously jeopardizes the patient's well-being. It is preferable that the man who is quite competent with a given technic, and perhaps unfamiliar or inexperienced with a technic which is more advisable on pharmacologic and physiologic grounds, continue to use that with which he is most skilled.

Nevertheless, routine use of anesthetics which is based on personal preference is to be abhorred. It is not a matter of like or dislike. Today, with well-trained anesthesiologists it is a matter of choice, based on physiologic or pharmacologic considerations. Each drug has its indications, its contraindications and its field of usefulness. For example, in diabetes, ether is contraindicated because it upsets acid-base balance, depletes liver glycogen and causes hyperglycemia. Again, to administer cyclopropane to an asthmatic is not sound practice; cyclopropane is a parasympathomimetic drug and may cause bronchoconstriction which, when superimposed upon the asthmatic state, may be hazardous. In this situation, *ether* is preferable. When shock or hemorrhage or prolonged surgery is anticipated, *cyclopropane* is the pre-eminent choice. These illustrations do not mean that the other drugs cannot be employed with some measure of success. But it does mean that, in the overall picture, the pharmacologic characteristics of some agents are more satisfactory and are associated with minimal stress.

SAFETY PRACTICES IN PREMEDICATION

Precautions in Premedication. Careful, safe anesthesia begins with proper medication. The objective is a *calm* and acquiescent patient in basal state. Objectives in preanesthetic medicine include lessening of apprehension; decrease in the amounts of anesthesia and, hence, lowered toxicity; protection against untoward reflexes; prevention of undesirable effects such as secretions and excitement. Three approaches are available: (1) the classic mode, utilizing narcotics; (2) predominant use of barbiturates; (3) use of tranquilizers.

Since each approach has a specific target in the nervous system, it is preferable that each approach be applied according to circumstances. Thus, *the narcotics* provide a general depression of the central nervous system and, by an over-all lessening of stimulating influences, provide a basal state. *The barbiturates* primarily depress cortical activity and are useful in worried, emotionally upset subjects. *The tranquilizers* selectively depress subcortical centers and, hence, are effective in states of agitation. Logically, medication should be directed at suppressing specific segments of the central nervous system, which seem to be overactive under the given circumstances.

Dangers exist in using any medication. This is inherent in the chemical and pharmacologic nature of the drugs and in the individual sensitivity of each nervous system. Therefore, an emphasis on precautions and contraindications in the use of the various preanesthetic medications is in order.

The first precaution in administering depressant drugs concerns the route employed. Generally the subcutaneous or intramuscular route is preferred in surgery. However, in any condition of impending or overt shock, or appreciable blood loss (over 500 cc.), the peripheral circulation will be impaired and absorption inadequate or delayed. Therefore, drugs should be administered in half the usual dose and by the intravenous route.

MORPHINE

Morphine is a classic and dependable premedicant and analgesic. It cannot be abused. The average effective adult dose to achieve generalized suppression of the central nervous system is 10 mg. This is likewise the dose which affords over 75 per cent reduction in the pain experience. Morphine is the analgesic *par excellence* for the relief of somatic-type pain and pain arising from integumentary structures. Since morphine is vagomimetic, it may aggravate the pain of smooth muscle spasm. Thus, when used in biliary colic it is generally inadequate, unless given in doses large enough to induce unconsciousness. However, the addition of an anticholinergic agent, such as atropine or scopolamine, in a dose ratio of 1 part to 25 parts of morphine will result in remarkable relief and counteract any pharmacologic spasm.

Contraindications. Among major contraindications to the use of morphine one can properly list situations of respiratory depression, bronchospastic diseases, increased intracranial pressure and poor circulatory status.

The effects of morphine on the cardiovascular system should also be appreciated. A summary includes: depression of the vasoconstrictor center; decreased peripheral circulation (Papper); diminished circulatory compensation to postural changes (Dripps); and decreased cardiac output. These changes are, of course, more evident with large doses and are revealed when a stress is placed on the subject.

The Geriatric Patient. The older patient does not tolerate the usual doses of morphine. No more than 5 mg. should be given to the 70-year-old patient. Thereafter, it is recommended that the dose be decreased by 1 mg. for each decade of life. Confusion and un-cooperative behavior are seen after ordinary morphine dosage in these patients. An analogue of morphine, *Dilaudid,* is recommended for the older patient. The dose is 1 to 2 mg. every 4 to 6 hours. On a weight basis, this is more potent than morphine, and pain is relieved without producing sleep or clouding of consciousness.

MEPERIDINE

This agent was originally introduced as a spasmolytic, but the analgesic properties were readily apparent. Pain of all types is relieved but that originating in viscera is particularly obtunded. Thus, following gastro-intestinal and urinary tract surgery, the results are most gratifying. However, it should be noted that the action on the biliary tract is similar to that of morphine, and that there is a spasmogenic effect. Gaensler has shown that a single therapeutic dose raises the biliary tract pressure to about 4 times the normal pressure.

The average recommended doses are: children—1 mg. per pound; adults (15 to 50)—between 100 and 150 mg. These doses do not produce sleep, and because of this lack, repeated administrations are frequently carried out. Sleep is not an index of pain relief. Important considerations in the use of meperidine are the following: (1) unpredictable respiratory depression sometimes occurs; (2) hypotension and syncope are an expected result of its use. Since this agent has significant vagolytic activity, it is known to convert conduction blocks of the heart from a 6 or 8 to 1, to a 4 or 2 to 1 block. This puts an added burden on the myocardium by virtue of the increased ventricular rate. Thus, meperidine is relatively contraindicated in auricular arrhythmias.

BARBITURATES

These are a useful and versatile group of agents in anesthesia. A range of effects from mild sedation to deep unconsciousness can be produced. Selection should be careful. The long-acting members of this group are handled by the kidney and, hence, are undesirable in renal disease. The short-acting congeners are detoxified by hepatic mechanisms and are contraindicated in liver disease. Most short-acting drugs are vagomimetic, hence produce some increase in bronchomotor tone. Avoidance of pentobarbital and secobarbital in asthma and related bronchospastic states is desirable. Recent studies also demonstrate the prolonged impairment in mental activity and efficiency by barbiturates in general. Hangover is marked with pentobarbital particularly.

Amobarbital. This may be better classified as an intermediate-acting barbiturate; however, it has little influence on bronchomotor tone and may be used in asthmatics. It is also not accompanied by extensive hangover. The cerebrovascular resistance is actually lowered by therapeutic doses, and it has merit in eclamptic and convulsive states. Of importance to the abdominal surgeon is the fact that the

overnight gastric secretion is usually unchanged or reduced following amobarbital, in contrast with the situation following pentobarbital. The conclusion from these observations is that amobarbital is to be preferred for sedation in patients scheduled for gastric surgery.

TRANQUILIZERS

Subcortical centers are the special targets of the tranquilizers. Suppressive action is particularly on the arousal mechanism of the reticular activating system. The consequence is a calm, acquiescent subject. Their utility is evident in anxiety and agitated states and in preparing alcoholics for anesthesia.

Certain precautions must be exercised. Anesthetic agents are potentiated; therefore, the doses of these should be reduced. This is especially true of the barbiturates and other agents requiring detoxication.

Cardiovascular effects are also pronounced, and lowering of the blood pressure is a constant accompaniment of tranquilizer use. Contraindications include shock, hypotension, jaundice and spinal anesthesia.

In this regard, patients should be questioned concerning their use of antihypertensive drugs, such as reserpine. When anesthetics are subsequently administered, circulatory depression occurs. It is recommended that reserpine be withheld for 2 weeks prior to surgery.

ANTICHOLINERGIC AGENTS

Every patient undergoing anesthesia should be premedicated with an anticholinergic agent. Advantages include (1) reduction in salivary secretions; (2) reduction in secretions of the respiratory tract; (3) prevention of bronchospasm and laryngospasm; (4) suppression of untoward cardiovascular vagal reflexes; (5) decrease in excess motility of gastro-intestinal tract; (6) counteraction of the respiratory depression of narcotics.

Of the naturally occurring and of the synthetic preparations available, it appears that scopolamine is most effective and the preferred agent. It is an all-purpose agent. The antisecretory effect is maximal, and at the same time the vagal blocking action is equally as good as with atropine. Occasionally, levohyoscine (levo- form of atropine, i.e., Bella-foline) may be used when better vagolysis is desired for short periods. For prolonged anti-cholinergic action, Antrenyl is indicated.

One must be judicious in ordering these drugs in the presence of heart disease, specifi-cally in rapid auricular action or conduction block. There may be an increase in ventricular rate, with failure. In cases of glaucoma, there may be some increase in intra-ocular tension, although systemic belladonna drugs generally do not introduce a problem. Nevertheless, there should be no interruption in glaucoma therapy; and the intra-operative instillation of pilocarpine (1 to 2%) in patients over 40 years of age with a predetermined increase in tension is perhaps desirable.

INDICATIONS AND CONTRAINDI-CATIONS FOR ANESTHETIC AGENTS

There is no ideal anesthetic agent. Every anesthetic agent has its place and utility. Each agent has its particular merits. An ideal agent is probably not attainable and may not be desirable. According to the patient's condition and surgical circumstances, an agent may be desirable and advantageous. Under other cir-cumstances the same agent might be highly undesirable.

Therefore, it is necessary to exploit the pharmacologic effect of each substance ac-cording to the needs of the moment. By ap-propriate selection of an anesthetic agent, many complications are judiciously avoided. Selection thus becomes one of the major principles leading toward greater patient safety.

Of the general anesthetic agents, two are outstanding. First, this is related to the fact that they are quite potent and capable of a wide range of use by themselves and, second, to the fact that each possesses opposite effects on the autonomic nervous system. These agents are *cyclopropane* and *ether*. Because they are all-purpose agents and to some extent anesthetic workhorses, a brief review of their pharmacologic actions and a summary of in-dications and contraindications based on such actions is appropriate.

ETHER

Most of the apparent effects of this agent can be ascribed to its stimulation of the sympathetic nervous system. There is a re-lease of epinephrine; hyperglycemia and acidemia result. Liver glycogen is depleted and carbohydrate metabolism is impaired; hence, it is a poor agent in diabetics. A trend toward exhaustion of the sympatho-adrenal axis makes this agent a poor choice in conditions of extreme stress, in patients of extreme adrenal insufficiency, in most disturbed endo-crine states and, of course, in circulatory stress.

Considering the respiratory system, admin-istration of ether is accompanied by local irri-tation, marked decrease in ciliary movement and increased salivary and mucus secretions. Bronchiolar muscles are relaxed and, in light planes of anesthesia, there is a 15 to 25 per cent increase in minute ventilation. Thus, ether is salutary in asthma, in emphysema and in other bronchospastic conditions.

Although the effects of ether on the cardio-circulatory apparatus appear to be good, nevertheless, this is superficial and due to epinephrine. Actually, there is direct myo-cardial depression (Brewster). It is relatively contraindicated in infectious pulmonary dis-eases and in tuberculosis.

CYCLOPROPANE

This is a potent, rapid-acting and readily eliminated gas and can be administered with abundant oxygen. On the cardiac mechanism, cyclopropane has some desirable properties. There is an improved myocardial action due to a positive inotropic effect, with strength-ened contraction. Hence, this drug is indicated in patients with myocardial insufficiency and failure. Because there is depression of the sino-atrial node and slowing of the cardiac rate, this agent allows for a longer diastolic pause. Such an action is desirable in patients with rheumatic heart disease. On the other hand, rhythms of ventricular origin are enhanced, and multifocal ventricular tachycardia may be perpetuated.

The peripheral circulation is maintained in excellent condition with little depression of the capillary units. Hence, the drug is indi-cated in cases of hemorrhage, trauma, shock, prolonged surgery or the poor-risk patient.

The entity of cyclopropane hypertension, erroneously called "cyclo shock," can be ascribed to a combination of factors. These include carbon dioxide accumulation, with subsequent peripheral vascular dilation, and electrolyte upset with depressed sodium level. Such hypotension is usually self-limited and innocuous, but it can be—and preferably is—corrected by administration of small doses of a vasopressor. Peripheral action of Neo-Synephrine in dilute solutions (1:100,000) has been found to be especially effective. The administration of half normal saline solution (500 cc.) tends to prevent hypotension.

Cyclopropane, like ether, is flammable. Therefore, it is contraindicated when open sources of ignition are present. Administration of epinephrine to patients anesthetized with cyclopropane at present is considered to be a hazardous procedure.

Nitrous Oxide

Very few body functions are altered by this agent in the presence of adequate oxygen content. However, the drug is impotent, and basal narcosis and hypnosis are necessary. As a supplement to intravenous meperidine or thiopental, it is an excellent anesthetic. It is recommended that one extend the maximum of its potential by administering mixtures of 75 per cent with 25 per cent oxygen. It is especially tolerated when properly administered to elderly poor-risk patients and can be combined with regional technics to good advantage.

Thiopental

This agent is finally attaining its proper place as an anesthetic adjunct. However, its safety depends on realizing that it is not an anesthetic and does not alleviate pain. Far from being a short-acting drug, it is detoxified at the rate of only 15 per cent per hour, and the depressant effects may persist for 15 or more hours. In addition, there are certain pharmacologic effects that must be appreciated. It causes depression of myocardial contractility and decreases tone of peripheral vessels. Hypotension occurs even with small doses, and the cardiac output is diminished. Because of its parasympathomimetic activity, bronchomotor tone is enhanced, and, therefore, it is contraindicated in asthma, emphy-

sema and bronchospastic disorders. Reliance on this agent to secure smooth anesthesia is a poor substitute for proficiency with other agents and technics. The price in poor physiology is too much to pay for ease of induction.

TECHNICAL CONSIDERATIONS

Preparation of Equipment

All equipment pertaining to anesthetic procedures must be kept in optimal working condition. Responsibility rests with the user. The anesthesiologist is a craftsman, and his results are dependent on the state of his tools. The usability of a particular item may mean the difference between life and death. Details of maintenance are contained in appropriate texts. Brief reference in terms of safe practice will be made to a few.

Cylinders of all compressed gases should be handled with care. Grease and oils must be eliminated from contact with outlets. Attention should be paid to the color code which designates each medical gas. Since 1955, a system of noninterchangeability between the yoke on anesthetic gas machines and the cylinder's valve post has been employed. This is the Pin-Index Safety System. Each gas has a combination of pins and holes. Two pins project from the yoke assembly of the anesthetic appliance, and these are positioned so as to meet corresponding holes in the body of the cylinder. Ten such combinations are available. Unless the correct cylinder is attached, the pins and holes will not match. Thus, it is impossible to attach a nitrous oxide cylinder to the oxygen yoke. Such a system eliminates the error of accidental substitution of one gas for another.

All parts of an anesthetic appliance should be kept clean. Sticky valves pose one of the greatest hazards in the use of the circle-type anesthesia system. Such valves raise the resistance to gas flow and increase the effort of breathing, sometimes profoundly. This hazard does not exist with the to-and-fro anesthesia system.

The avoidance of carbon dioxide excess is dependent on fresh absorbent. Attention to the recording of hours of use of canisters is a detail which cannot be neglected.

Sterilization technics for anesthesia equipment have undergone considerable investigation. Autoclaving has been found to be most satisfactory. Spinal anesthetic ampules should be preferentially sterilized by autoclaving. Present evidence indicates that the content of ampules containing spinal drugs can be contaminated through microscopic defects in glassware. It is also thought that some percolation can occur through more porous glassware. One-time autoclaving of the spinal drugs does not affect potency to a measurable extent.

Cleansing of equipment, such as masks, tubing, airways and endotracheal catheters, is mandatory. This should be both mechanical and bacteriologic. It is recommended particularly that endotracheal airways should be scrubbed thoroughly, especially with some solution containing hexachlorophene.

AIRWAY

A good airway is a prerequisite to any inhalation or general anesthesia. It should not only be clear and patent but also adequate. A restricted airway impedes gaseous exchange. A well-known axiom is that noisy respiration is obstructed respiration. In elderly edentulous patients, where there is relaxation of the pharynx, an endotracheal airway is indicated. An endotracheal airway is also indicated in situations where an abnormal posture is to be assumed or when the chest is to be opened. This airway is also a life-saving device.

Compensated or aided respiration is valuable. The technic consists of the assisting of inspiration by graded manual pressure on the breathing bag. By this means a patient's effort is diminished and fatigue lessened.

Positions interfering with either respiration or circulation are to be condemned. The head-down position is deleterious to the circulation in most cardiac patients. The causes of dyspnea do not disappear during anesthesia—only the patient's complaint disappears. Yet orthopneic patients are often seen in a steep head-down position, or in Trendelenburg position, indicating both a lack of common sense and a lack of comprehension of physiologic factors on the part of the operator.

Another situation seen on the operating table, which the anesthetist must guard against, is that of the "tired assistant," who rests on the patient's chest. This is intolerable.

FLUID THERAPY

This is a controversial issue, particularly in the cardiac patient, but the safest rule is to replace whatever is lost. During surgery it is obvious that blood is going to be lost. Therefore, the vascular fluid balance should be maintained by giving blood. One should not compromise because the patient has a cardiac problem. Blood should be started early and administered slowly. This is a far better arrangement than suddenly to find a situation where a large volume is needed in a short period, as when circulation is rapidly deteriorating from hemorrhage. Altschule has shown that quite large amounts of fluid can be given over a period of several hours without causing any circulatory or cardiac disturbance. In the person without cardiac disease, saline or glucose, administered at rates of 20 cc. or less per minute, results in no significant changes in cardiovascular function. At greater speeds, prolonged rise in venous pressure and other changes may occur. The administration of fluids at 10 cc. per minute or less to cardiac patients results in little change in the cardiovascular function (Altschule).

Measurement of blood loss during extensive surgery is a useful safeguard. It is recommended that every surgical specialty in a given institution determine the average losses for common operations. These figures will serve as an index to expected blood loss in milligrams per sponge or pack. This estimate, together with the volume of blood suctioned, will furnish a rough minimal guide to better replacement. More accurate figures may be obtained by application of a method of measurement in all major surgery. Two methods are recommended: (1) gravimetric determination—by weighing sponges, and (2) serial blood volume determinations—by using red blood cells tagged with radioactive chromium together with the scintillation counter (Alpert).

Transfusion of a large volume of blood may be followed by persistent oozing, which may be both at the operative site and generalized. Such oozing may occur after "massive transfusions." This is defined as an amount of blood equal to the patient's own blood volume. In adults it represents about 5 liters or 10 units of whole blood. However, such oozing occurs after the administration of smaller amounts, but rarely when less than half the patient's volume is replaced. The mechanism of the coagulation defect is uncertain, but is probably related to several factors. These include the effects of excess citrate; platelet deficiency if old, stored blood is administered; reduced levels of accelerator globulin; fibrinogen deficiency; and the presence of fibrinolysin. To combat the oozing, three measures are recommended: (1) administration of 1 Gm. of calcium chloride (10 cc. of 10% solution) for every 2 to 3 units of blood administered; (2) the use of fresh whole blood; and (3) administration of antihemophilic globulin.

HAZARDS RELATED TO POSITION

Two categories of complications result from inattention to proper positioning. These are physiologic and anatomic. The influence of posture on physiology is well-known. Generally the head-up position favors respiration, while the head-down position favors circulation. The supine horizontal position is the one most conducive to maximal physiologic function. On assuming the erect position or a steep head-down position, gravity produces circulatory and respiratory changes. Compensatory cardiovascular and respiratory reflexes are initiated to re-establish a steady state.

In the narcoticized individual these reflexes are depressed. Furthermore, many operative positions are uncomfortable and not only interfere with physiology but also, by pressure, induce ischemic tissue changes. A summary of the effects of malpositioning follows.

PHYSIOLOGIC COMPLICATIONS

1. **Hypotension.** This occurs especially in obese patients when supine or in head-down position. A common operating-room error is to use steep head-down or Trendelenburg position. In this position the pulse is slowed, cardiac stroke output is decreased, and in patients with myocardial disease, acute dilation may occur. Extreme lithotomy position also precipitates bradycardia and decreases minute output. Move all patients gently.

2. **Respiratory Distress.** This is provoked by any position which interferes with respiration. Thus, the lateral, prone and jackknife positions impair movements of chest and diaphragm. Hypoxia is the result. Restricting braces and adhesive supports are hazardous. Modern anesthesiology and excellent relaxation make unnecessary such positions as the Trendelenburg, or the use of flexion bars. Deep anesthesia must be avoided. An endotracheal airway should be provided for all unusual positions, i.e., any position wherein it would be difficult for the anesthetist to have immediate access to airway. Assisted respiration is recommended throughout.

ANATOMIC COMPLICATIONS

1. **Brachial Plexus Palsy.** This error is related to extreme abduction and extension of the arm for purposes of an infusion. This position places tension on the cords of the plexus in the following manner. The nerves of the plexus are fixed at the transverse processes and at the axillary fascia in the arm; between these points the nerves are compressed between the first rib and the clavicle; if the arm is externally rotated and extended, then the nerves must wind around the head of the humerus.

The errors in positioning include: (1) unnecessary abduction of arms (only a natural position should be permitted); (2) external rotation of arm (internal rotation is recommended); (3) poorly adjusted shoulder braces (these should be over acromioclavicular prominence); (4) suspension of body by wrist straps (such straps are not needed).

2. **Peroneal Nerve Palsy.** This is due to poor padding in the lithotomy and lateral positions. Pressure on the leg just below the knee on the head of the fibula must be avoided.

3. **Radial or Ulnar Nerve Paralysis.** This is due to the elbow being allowed to hang over the side of the table and rest against the metal edge. If the upper arm is allowed to hang over the edge of the table, pressure paralysis may occur.

4. **Ocular Complications.** Hypotony with ocular pain, blurring of vision and increased intraocular tension are due to pressure on the eyeballs by the mask or the Bailey head-rest.

5. Skin. There may be contact dermatitis from a dirty face mask and ulceration of the nose from mask pressure.

6. Neurovascular Syndrome. This results from hyperabduction of the arms, with obliteration of pulse and atrophic changes due to compression of subclavian vessels (and nerves) between the clavicle and the first rib. The vascular symptoms are coincidental with the nerve palsies.

EXPLOSIONS AND FIRE HAZARDS

An explosion in the operating room is a rare but tragic event—tragic because of its preventability. The over-all incidence is placed between 1 per 100,000 and 1 per 1,000,000 anesthetics given. Most of the common inhalation anesthetic agents are flammable. It is sometimes considered that ether is not a great hazard, but this is indeed erroneous and no further reference is warranted. Chloroform, Trilene and many of the newer halogenated compounds are nonflammable. Nitrous oxide is nonflammable but supports combustion. Any of the flammable agents are apt to be present in explosive concentrations during an anesthetic procedure.

The conditions necessary for an explosion are three: (1) a flammable mixture; (2) adequate oxygen supply; (3) an ignition source.

Of these factors, only the third is controllable, and measures should be directed toward eliminating any source of ignition. Sources in the operating room can be listed as (1) open flames—smoking, alcohol lamp; (2) electric sparks—x-ray apparatus, suction machines, open switches, cauteries, surgical lamps, endoscopic equipment; (3) static electricity—may be generated on personnel, on clothing and on equipment.

Co-operation of all personnel is needed to eliminate the hazard. It is not enough to recognize the problem and leave the solution to others. Each person concerned with the operating room is *responsible*. Strive for isoelectric conditions in the operating theater to avoid static charges. Insulated bodies should be prohibited. All electrical equipment must be checked frequently. All anesthetic equipment should be kept in leakproof, efficient working condition.

Precautions necessary to avoid an explosion include the following:

1. Grounding. Proper floors are necessary. Ground the equipment with drag chains and/or conductive casters. Soapy solutions should not be used to clean the floors. Intercoupling is an adjunct. The best policy is for the anesthetist to maintain contact with the patient, the anesthesia machine and the operating table. Lastly, all regular personnel should be urged to wear conductive rubber-soled shoes. Other shoe devices of less expensive nature merely represent second-rate solutions. They may be used by transient personnel.

2. Sparkproof equipment.

3. No flammable anesthetic should be permitted when cautery is used. A surgeon should forego this luxury if an explosive agent is more beneficial to the patient's physiology.

4. *No smoking* in the operating theater. This needs emphasis.

5. A relative humidity of 60 per cent is desirable. Adequate circulation of room air will dissipate explosive anesthetic mixtures.

CONTROL OF COMPLICATIONS

VOMITING AND ASPIRATION

There have been more anesthesia deaths from vomiting and aspiration than from any other cause. The over-all incidence of frank vomiting may be placed at about 22 per cent (Moore). Women vomit twice as frequently as men. Different anesthetics are associated with different rates; thus, ether has the highest, while Pentothal-nitrous oxide anesthesia and regional technics are associated with the lowest rates. However, it must be appreciated that regional technics are not devoid of vomiting as a complication.

Recent studies also emphasize the problem of regurgitation or silent vomiting. In these studies, dyes (carmine red, Evans blue) were placed in the stomachs of anesthetized patients via a Levine tube. At the conclusion of the anesthesia and the surgery, the pharynges as well as the tracheas were inspected. The incidence of dye appearance in the pharynx was found to be from 14 to 20 per cent. More importantly, about one half of these patients had aspirated, as evidenced by presence of dye in the tracheas.

Thus, the seriousness and the insidiousness of this complication is obvious.

Prevention. Careful preoperative preparation is the first consideration. An empty stomach is always a prerequisite. A patient should have nothing for at least 6 hours before surgery and be without solid food for at least 12 hours. A nasogastric tube may be helpful at times. However, the physician must keep in mind the fact that this often stimulates secretions and air swallowing. Tubes with balloons for tamponade against the cardia have some utility.

Many drugs have been employed to reduce the activity of the emetic center. Dramamine is effective in minor surgical procedures where emotions and physical motion have a significant role. In major surgery, chlorpromazine in doses of 25 to 50 mg. will reduce the incidence of vomiting by 50 per cent.

Narcotics, if employed, should be in minimal effective doses and given at least 1 hour before the induction of anesthesia. Anesthesia should be smooth, rapid and physiologic. Positions should not be extreme. No more than an 8° head-down position is needed for pelvic surgery. Hypoxia is a major inciting factor in causing vomiting.

Airways should not be inserted when the gag reflex is active. Mucous secretions should be removed at the end of a surgical procedure by pharyngeal and tracheolaryngeal cleansing under vision.

Treatment. When vomiting occurs, the patient must be inclined on the operating table about 8 to 10°. This will place the trachea on an incline and encourage gravity drainage. Adequate high-volume flow suction must be available and employed. A metal suction-tip can often be inserted between the jaws behind the molar teeth. If not, a 16-F or 18-F catheter can be inserted through the nose. As soon as possible, the pharynx should be inspected under vision by laryngoscopy.

When aspiration is evident, tracheal suction is mandatory. This can be accomplished by catheterization. However, it is recommended that bronchoscopy be performed, that sterile saline, 10 to 30 cc., be introduced into the trachea and that the tracheobronchial passages be lavaged. This will dilute the acidic gastric secretions and minimize chemical pneumonitis.

HYPOXIA

Avoiding this is difficult to accomplish because of several variables in the mechanisms of body oxygenation. These include the ventilation factor, the transport component, the cardiocirculatory system and the tissue enzyme mechanisms. Features of each of these variables may be outlined as follows:

1. *Ventilation Factor.* Provision for an adequate concentration of oxygen in the breathing mixture is primary. This must be conducted to the alveoli. Patent and adequate air passages must be present. No obstruction is permissible. Moreover, the air must be moved in and out of the alveoli, and this requires an efferent respiratory apparatus with intact mechanical thoracic cage and unimpaired muscular action.

2. *Transport Factor.* Blood is the "middle man" in bringing oxygen to the tissues. The volume must be adequate. Hypovolemia must be corrected before surgery, and there must be a full complement of hemoglobin. Anemias are a major hazard in the performance of safe anesthesia. As a general guide, no elective surgery should be performed on patients with a hemoglobin under 10 Gm. per 100 cc.

3. *Cardiocirculatory System.* To propel the oxygen-carrying red cells, cardiac action and an intact circulatory system are obviously necessary. Correction of myocardial insufficiency should never be neglected. A good endocrine and vitamin balance goes far to maintain the peripheral circulatory apparatus in optimal state.

4. *Tissue Uptake.* Peripheral edema interferes with transfer of oxygen from the blood to the tissues. Stagnation of circulation must be avoided. Hypotension should be corrected, and even the technic of planned pharmacologic hypotension must not be applied indiscriminately. Thiamine is concerned with glucose utilization in heart muscles and other tissues. In its absence tachycardias are more easily developed. Thus, vitamin supplements are indicated, especially in the aged.

It is hardly necessary to remind the competent anesthetist that oxygen under proper tension must be provided. This allows of no modification. Furthermore, the oxygen must be brought into contact with the alveolar membrane. Since all anesthetics are depressants, it is incumbent upon the anesthetist to complement spontaneous respiration or to control respiration when apnea occurs.

Specific Errors Leading to Hypoxia. These may be outlined as follows:

1. Inadequate supply of oxygen in breathing mixtures:

A. Empty tanks of oxygen. Prevent by checking beforehand and providing a reserve unit.

B. Faulty flowmeters. Test all meters every month.

C. Leaks allowing ingress of air. Do not use defective rubber goods or faulty connections.

D. Dilution with atmospheric air.

2. Obstruction:

A. Tongue falling back into pharynx. Use pharyngeal airway and position head properly.

B. Foreign bodies in air passages, such as loose teeth, chewing gum, tobacco or peanuts (in children). Check mouths of all patients before beginning anesthesia.

C. Secretions. Remove as they appear; prevent by prior administration of anticholinergic drugs.

D. Vomitus. Patients must fast preoperatively; suction any gastric contents; seal off air passages as previously discussed.

E. Laryngospasm. This is alarming and dangerous. Prevent by not stimulating pharynx of partially narcotized patients; do not insert airways in lightly anesthetized patients; avoid use of parasympathomimetic drugs in sensitive patients; administer adequate doses of belladonna drugs. Avoid excess carbon dioxide or hypoxia; check for dust in absorbents.

F. Bronchospasm. This is noted by gradual increase in resistance to respiration and to manual inflation of lungs. Eliminate pharmacologic causes; administer bronchodilators. Do not select Pentothal sodium or cyclopropane for patients with asthma or severe emphysema. Treat myocardial failure.

3. Respiratory paralysis:

A. Overdoses of anesthetic agents.

B. Use of relaxants with residual hypoventilatory effects. The avoidance of this error is self-evident.

4. Inadequate circulation:

A. Anemias. Treat preoperatively.

B. Hypovolemia. This should be treated by blood administration preoperatively.

C. Hemorrhage must be treated progressively during surgery.

RESPIRATORY ACIDOSIS

This condition may be defined as an increase in the carbon dioxide tension of the blood. It is well known that oxygen is supplied by pulmonary ventilation, but it is less appreciated that the pulmonary system is the principal means for the elimination of the waste products of tissue metabolism. As a consequence, respiratory acidosis is fairly commonplace today in many anesthesia clinics. This is unnecessary, and a knowledge of the fundamentals of gas exchange is essential to the control of carbon dioxide levels. Three principles are involved.

First, there is the capillary-alveolar equilibrium established between the gases in the alveoli and the gases in the blood. This is governed by the laws of diffusion and partial pressure. Under the conditions usually encountered in the operating room, we can state that the partial pressure of carbon dioxide in the peripheral arterial blood is determined solely by the partial pressure of carbon dioxide in the alveolar air.

Second, the alveolar gas equation considers that a greater quantity of air than the dead-space volume must be moved into the lungs to induce gas exchange properly. Effective alveolar ventilation is thus equal to the tidal volume minus the dead-space air. Alveolar carbon dioxide is then directly determined by the patient's alveolar ventilation.

Third, by application of the principles relating pressure changes to volume changes we can state that the amount of gas entering or leaving the lungs depends on changes in the differential pressure across the lungs-thorax system. This is termed compliance.

In summary, it is evident that blood carbon dioxide can be regulated by controlling the pressure across the lungs. During anesthesia this is the responsibility of the anesthesiologist. Despite the ease with which the anesthetist can accomplish elimination of carbon dioxide, respiratory acidosis continues to be reported frequently. To overcome the hazard we must emphasize a fundamental anesthesia concept, that is, to avoid *hypoventilation* by assisted and controlled respiration. Related to the need for adequate assisted ventilation is the recognition of the enemies of good ventilation (Maloney).

I. Depressant Drugs. These all diminish ventilation. The barbiturates, the narcotics and all anesthetic agents are offenders. The slowly eliminated drugs are particularly insidious, especially in the postoperative period, and the fact that thiopental is detoxified at a rate of only 15 per cent per hour must be thoroughly realized.

2. Relaxant Drugs. These produce hypoventilation by impairing the muscular component of the respiratory mechanism. Avoid their unnecessary use, avoid overdoses and compensate for residual hypoventilatory effects.

3. Mechanical Impedence is a major deterrent to good ventilation. Consideration must be given to such factors as posture, tired surgical assistants leaning on the patient's chest, pneumothorax, large intraperitoneal packs and excessive strong retraction on the subcostal margin.

In conclusion, blood carbon dioxide or respiratory acidosis is related to inadequate effective alveolar ventilation. All other factors have only an indirect bearing on arterial concentrations of this gas in so far as they influence alveolar ventilation. The avoidance of this undesirable condition is accomplished by proper manual or mechanical means. By manual compression of the breathing bag over the period of a half dozen breaths, one can convert respiratory acidosis to normality.

SPINAL ANESTHESIA

This form of anesthesia when used for surgery of the abdomen and lower portions of the body provides advantages lacking in other technics. It is important to realize that every anesthetic places stress on a patient's physiology. It is considered that with spinal anesthesia, as compared with other technics, such stress is minimal. In fact, in comparable types of operations, the mortality with spinal is lower than with general anesthesia. In *An Analysis of Operating Room Deaths,* by Todd and Beecher, this contention has been supported.

PRECAUTIONS IN THE USE OF SPINAL ANESTHESIA

Careful selection of patients for this form of anesthesia is the first line of safety. Contraindications include pre-existing neurologic disease, such as central nervous system syphilis or poliomyelitis; patients with chronic backache or recurrent headaches; a history of pernicious anemia; any evidence of neuromuscular disability; or difficulty with bowel and bladder function. The patient's attitude is also important. Anyone who has developed a fear of the spinal technic or whose previous experience may have been bad is a poor candidate. Un-co-operative patients should not be given spinal anesthesia. The presence of many skin diseases in the area of spinal puncture and markedly distorted spinal vertebral anatomy further preclude spinal anesthesia.

The second line of safety concerns the technic. This must be meticulous. (1) Agents should be sterilized by autoclaving. Chemical sterilization by immersion in antiseptic solutions is fraught with danger due to percolation of such solutions into the ampule of anesthetic, so is not recommended. (2) Equipment must be properly autoclaved. (3) The procedure should be accomplished under sterile conditions. Thus, the operator should scrub as for a surgical procedure and wear sterile gloves; the area of spinal puncture should be prepared as for an operation. (4) In performing spinal tap, the use of the Sise introducer is recommended. Such a device allows the introduction of the spinal needle without having the needle itself touch the skin. Experience indicates that this step will lower the incidence of headache, meningismus, meningitis and local infections. (5) In addition, small needles such as gauge 22 or 24 are desirable. Headache is directly proportional to the size of the needle employed.

A third line of safety concerns the drugs employed. These should be secured from a reliable pharmaceutical firm. Accepted doses for given levels of anesthesia should not be exceeded. It is sound policy to administer only that amount which will furnish adequate anesthesia of sufficient duration. Besides the dose, attention to concentration is important. For example, laboratory evidence and clinical experience point to the fact that with *procaine* a concentration greater than 5 per cent is undesirable and unnecessary. In animal investigations, concentrations above 10 per cent will cause some demyelinization, while 17 per cent will invariably cause such changes.

When an operation is to take a long time, it is recommended that large doses of agents be avoided and that "continuous" technic be employed. One can use an agent of relatively low toxicity, like procaine, and administer frequent small doses. A safe guide in this connection is never to administer more than 1 mg. per minute after the initial anesthetizing dose.

Indications for Spinal Anesthesia

Anesthesia by this route is particularly adaptable for abdominal surgery, in which it supplies excellent relaxation. This is attained at a much smaller price than that exacted by a general agent or by general anesthesia plus a relaxant. The dangers of relaxants are evident, considered in terms of detoxication, prolonged hypoventilation and possible mortality (Beecher). However, it must be remembered that with high spinal levels, oxygen supplements and vasopressor therapy are necessary parts of the technic.

Patients in the age group of 15 to 100 years have been good subjects for spinal anesthesia. Younger children are not ideal candidates but can be handled well by experienced anesthesiologists. The geriatric patient is a particularly fit candidate. In this group, avoidance of central cerebral depression and drugs which cloud the consciousness are desirable.

In general, it is advantageous to select spinal anesthesia for persons with myocardial disease or pulmonary affections. Spinal anesthesia is preferable in patients suffering from low intestinal obstruction, obesity or diseases of the kidneys and the liver. In these conditions the undesirable effects of general anesthesia outweigh any disadvantages of the spinal route.

Complications of Spinal Anesthesia

It is recognized that there are certain hazards peculiar to spinal anesthesia. Three of these are prominent and require comment.

Hypotension. This is frequently encountered during spinal anesthesia. Diagnosis is established by finding a lowered blood pressure with a normal or slow pulse. Thus, it has to be definitely differentiated from shock. The chief influence is the level of anesthesia. It has been demonstrated that the umbilical level (T9 to T10) is the critical level, and when the anesthesia progresses above this, there is an increase in the incidence and severity of the hypotension. However, this is not invariable. It appears that the spinal anesthesia merely causes a loss of capacity for reflex compensation, while secondary factors, such as blood loss and surgical manipulation, actually provoke the fall in pressure.

During spinal anesthesia careful hemostasis is essential; surgical manipulations must be gentle and tissues handled delicately. This anesthetic technic is designed for good surgeons. Furthermore, the following precautions should be taken to avoid the development and the consequences of low pressure:

1. Prophylactic vasopressor at time of administration of spinal anesthetic.

2. Administration of oxygen in all spinal anesthetics with levels above T-9.

3. Establishment of an intravenous route for administration of drugs and fluids.

4. Selective vasopressor therapy by intravenous administration of dilute vasopressor solutions. Dilute solutions are more controllable and allow one to titrate a dose against a response. Single large doses precipitate "overshoot," tachyphylaxis and post-therapy depressor responses.

5. Seventy-five per cent of hypotensions are due to predominant loss of arteriolar tone. Phenylephrine, diluted 1:100,000, is effective in overcoming this failure. On the other hand, about 25 per cent of cases, especially the aged, have a predominant *decrease* in cardiac output. A significant fall in diastolic pressure is observed in this circumstance, and the treatment is with ephedrine.

Headache. The incidence of headache following spinal anesthesia has been placed at 10 per cent. This is an acceptable incidence under ordinary circumstances. However, this can be reduced to no greater than 1 or 2 per cent by observing the following rules: (1) hydration of patient preoperatively; (2) proper sedation; (3) avoidance of "fanfare" in carrying out the procedure, with careful omission of the word "headache"; (4) use of the Sise introducer to diminish chances of contamination of deep structures, epidural and subdural spaces; (5) use of small-gauge needles, that is, 22 or 24 gauge; (6) early ambulation to minimize the occurrence of headache by restoring to normal cerebrospinal-fluid dynamics.

Neurologc Sequelae. Although neurologic sequelae of a permanent nature are rare, they do occur. It must be realized that these same complications appear following general anesthesia. Thus a cause-and-effect relationship is not automatic and exclusive. Many other possibilities must be kept in mind. A recent long-term study of patients showed no persistent paralysis following spinal anesthesia and further indicated that meticulous attention to details probably eliminates the occurrence of minor sequelae.

Spinal anesthesia is a valuable modality in the armamentarium of the anesthesiologist. It must not be abused; otherwise patients will be deprived of a safe and useful means of pain relief, and surgeons will be deprived of a superior method of furnishing good surgical conditions. No physician should condemn this technic on the basis of an infrequent neurologic complication. Vociferous and biased statements have been made in the past. This is unscientific. It may be reasonably concluded that spinal anesthesia has assumed a proper, useful and safe place in anesthesia practice.

REGIONAL ANESTHESIA

Reactions to agents employed in regional anesthesia are quite frequent. Many are mild and self-limited, but fatalities do occur. Most often the mild reactions are ignored or considered to be inconsequential; this attitude is foolhardy. The mild reactions should be considered to be warning signals, as evidence of an untoward response that may be the precursor of a more severe type reaction which can jeopardize the patient. Tetracaine (Pontocaine), administered topically, showed a 2 per cent incidence in reactions, and half of these (1%) were severe (Beck and Rand).

Mechanism of Toxic Reactions

In considering toxic reactions, it should be emphasized that they are almost entirely due to the absorption of the drug into the blood stream. The labeling of untoward reactions as due to idiosyncrasy or hypersensitivity is a snare and a delusion. Less than 1 per cent of reactions may be considered as being allergic in nature or due to idiosyncrasy (Dripps *et al.*).

Therefore, toxicity is directly proportional to the blood level of the agent, and this, in turn, is related to the ratio of absorption over disposition.

It can be concluded from this that the factors influencing toxicity are either *technical*, influencing the absorption, or *clinical*, influencing the destruction or elimination of the drug.

Technical Factors Influencing Toxicity

The different local anesthetic agents vary as to their potency and their toxicity. These usually parallel each other; thus, as potency increases, toxicity also increases. For comparative purposes, procaine is taken as a standard and is designated as having a toxicity of 1. On this basis, piperocaine is 3 times as toxic, cocaine 4 times, tetracaine 12 to 20 times, and dibucaine 20 times (H. Braun).

The concentration of the agent used varies with the procedure. To block a large nerve trunk requires a more concentrated agent. Similarly, to block motor nerves requires a stronger solution of agent in contrast with sensory fibers which can be blocked with a solution only one tenth as strong. Whatever the requirements, one should employ the weakest concentration which will produce the desired result. Generally, a 0.5 to 1.0 per cent solution of procaine is used for infiltration anesthesia, a 1 per cent solution is used for field block, and a 1.5 to 2 per cent solution is used for conduction or "trunk block." Toxicity increases geometrically with concentration; this is not a simple arithmetical relation. For example, 120 cc. of a 1 per cent solution of procaine will kill a rat in 20 minutes, while only 40 cc. of a 2 per cent solution will produce the same lethal effect; that is, with weak solution 1.2 Gm. of procaine is lethal, while only 0.8 Gm. of procaine kills when employed in concentrated form (Kay and Blalock).

Whatever the concentration and the purpose of anesthetic procedure, one should be guided by the average total dose considered to be safe. For each drug there is a total dose which should not be exceeded.

Though the type of drug, the amount and the concentration are all safe, one variable remains which may cause a local anesthetic reaction. This is the technical facility of the anesthetist. Failure to aspirate after placement of a needle and improper placement of a needle account for many disasters. Also of tremendous importance is the *rate* of injection. A rapid rate of injection enhances absorption and raises the blood level of the agent, sometimes to a toxic point.

The environmental temperature also plays an important role in increasing the incidence of reactions. Higher temperatures increase absorption and diffusion of the injected drugs.

CLINICAL FACTORS INFLUENCING TOXICITY

The condition of the patient alters susceptibility to the development of a reaction. This is brought about either through changes in the rapidity of absorption or through variation in the disposition of the drug. Hyperpyrexia, for example, increases absorption. Debility, shock, starvation, old age, low metabolism and vitamin C deficiency all diminish the patient's ability to detoxify local anesthetics. Richards (quoted by Melrose *et al.*) recommends that all poor-risk patients who are about to receive a local anesthetic should be given an infusion of dextrose with ascorbic acid. The various anesthetic procedures influence toxicity differently. An injection into a highly vascular area naturally carries a greater risk of producing a high blood level of the agent. In topical anesthetization it is important that the patient does not swallow the excess anesthetic solution, since absorption through the gastric mucosa may be extremely rapid.

CLASSIFICATION OF TOXIC REACTIONS

This is based on the underlying derangement in physiology which is induced by the anesthetic agent. The dominant manifestation is emphasized for diagnostic purposes. In general, it is conceded on pharmacologic grounds that in all reactions there is initial stimulation followed by depression. However, the stimulation may predominate and persist. In any event, the clinical picture at the moment of treatment should govern the type of treatment. The following classification is clinically useful:

1. Central Nervous System Stimulation. Stimulation may be considered as falling into three grades of severity. In the mild form, the patient is inebriated; he is talkative, pugnacious, unreasonable; he may feel dizzy, and movements are often not co-ordinated; the face may be flushed, and the blood pressure is frequently elevated, with a rapid pulse. In the moderate grade of stimulation, the patient is restless; he complains of headache and may have blurring of vision; nausea and vomiting are frequent; muscular twitchings may be in evidence; the blood pressure remains elevated, but the pulse is usually slow, full and bounding—this is apparently evidence of hypoxia as well as medullary stimulation. In the severe form of stimulation, the patient shows all the preceding signs, but the muscular twitchings progress to frank convulsions, asphyxia and death. The development of convulsions sometimes may be so rapid that the other premonitory features are absent or overlooked.

TREATMENT. The aim in treatment of central nervous system stimulation is to modify or stop the convulsion and to supply an abundance of oxygen to combat asphyxia. During the convulsion the respiratory muscles are ineffective. Practical steps include: (1) administration of thiopental sodium intravenously, administration of curare intravenously; (2) providing an adequate airway, preferably endotracheal; (3) artificial respiration.

2. Central Nervous System Depression. Depression of the central nervous system is frequently of a downward descending type beginning with the cortical centers and progressing to the medulla. Manifestations include drowsiness, analgesia, unresponsiveness and loss of consciousness; muscular relaxation and flaccidity develop. The skin is pale and moist. This situation is accompanied by a fall in blood pressure and a weak, thready, rapid pulse. Respirations become shallow and slow, and death is due to persistent hypotension and respiratory failure.

At times the depression of the medullary centers seems to predominate without noticeable changes in the sensorium. Almost immediately, under these circumstances, respiration becomes inadequate and is closely followed by central vasomotor collapse.

TREATMENT. The aim in treatment of central depression is to maintain the vital functions. This is accomplished by supplying oxygen and by the use of vasopressors. Oxygen administration should be started immediately, utilizing an artificial airway and artificial respiration. An infusion should be started and vasopressors given intravenously. The vasopressors of choice are those which possess some central action; they include ephedrine and desoxyephedrine (Methedrine).

3. Peripheral Cardiovascular Collapse (Syncope). Collapse due to the peripheral action of procaine may be brought about by the direct action of the local anesthetic on the heart. In the case of procaine there is reduction of myocardial irritability, and frequently bradycardia is quickly noted. Cardiac output decreases, and the situation may progress to cardiac arrest. With respect to cocaine, ventricular tachycardia is frequent and is usually followed by fibrillation.

Peripheral collapse may also develop through the action of procaine, predominantly on the vascular bed. Procaine in this respect is known to be a potent vasodilator. The hypotension which ensues may result in cardiac arrest.

TREATMENT. The aim of treatment is to maintain the oxygen system of the body. This includes artificial respiration, administration of fluids and intravenous vasopressors. The choice of vasopressors under circumstances of peripheral vascular collapse includes Neo-Synephrine, methoxamine and norepinephrine. When cardiac arrest supervenes, artificial circulation should be established by cardiac massage.

4. Allergic Reactions. Allergic reactions are considered to be those typically based on immunologic sensitization. Such altered reactivity is usually denoted by cutaneous or mucosal manifestations and by respiratory difficulties and anaphylaxis. The former includes urticaria, rashes and angioneurotic edema; the latter includes bronchospasm, wheezing and status asthmaticus, often accompanied by anaphylactoid shock.

It should be noted that idiosyncrasy is a very loose term denoting abnormal reactions. As such it is similar to allergy. Such reactions are very rare. The reports of fatalities in the literature which are labeled "idiosyncrasy" are, in all probability, simple cases of overdose. The term "hypersensitivity" is used to denote reactions of the expected pattern which occur following minimal doses.

TREATMENT. In allergic states treatment revolves around the use of epinephrine and the administration of antihistaminics. Benedryl is an effective parenteral antihistaminic. The dose is 10 to 50 mg. of a 1 per cent solution. Aminophylline is valuable; in cases of severe angioneurotic edema and of asthmalike attacks, sodium or potassium iodide given intravenously will cause the mucosal edema to subside.

The Use of Epinephrine

Epinephrine, by causing vasoconstriction in dilute solutions, inhibits absorption and thereby prolongs activity of local anesthetics. The proper concentration of epinephrine is related to the concentration of the local anesthetic. Thus, for 0.5 per cent procaine the epinephrine dilution is $1:500,000$; for 1.0 per cent procaine the dilution is $1:250,000$ and for 2.0 per cent procaine it is $1:100,000$. This is accomplished by adding 0.4 cc. of $1:1,000$ solution of epinephrine to 200 cc. of 0.5 per cent procaine, to 100 cc. of 1 per cent and to 50 cc. of 2 per cent solution. Such dilutions give maximal vasoconstriction and minimal reactions. The addition of epinephrine to anesthetic solutions is the most widely used method for increasing potency; but it should be remembered that with increased potency there is increased toxicity. It has been demonstrated that by the addition of epinephrine to procaine solutions there is an increase in toxicity.

Epinephrine similarly increases the toxicity of piperocaine. However, when it is added to tetracaine and dibucaine there is a *decrease* in toxicity.

Toxic reactions due to the epinephrine can occur. Hence, it is important to adhere strictly to the recommended dilutions. The inaccurate method of adding a "few drops" or minims is dangerous and should be replaced by a careful measurement with a syringe of the desired amount. The reactions that may result from the epinephrine are anxiety, palpitation, tachycardia and rise in blood pressure; pulmonary edema and ventricular fibrillation may follow.

SOME PROBLEMS IN ANESTHETIC MANAGEMENT

Certain conditions existing in surgical patients present challenges in their management. An awareness of these dangers and a knowledge of their proper care, together with some skill in management, go far in safeguarding the patient.

The Full Stomach

Recent intake of food lays the background for vomiting and aspiration. Following accidents, the occurrence of a severe illness or the use of sedative drugs, the gastro-intestinal movements are inhibited. Hence, food is retained for long periods. Furthermore, a full stomach is more sensitive to the effects of anesthesia, and vomiting is more frequent.

For elective surgery, patients should fast for 12 hours prior to the beginning of anesthesia. *For urgent surgery,* at least a 6-hour waiting period is desirable if solid food has been ingested. *For emergency surgery,* the following procedures can be instituted:

1. Insert large-bore gastric tube and lavage stomach. This will remove much of the liquid contents, but large food particles will remain. If intake has been entirely liquid, this will be quite adequate.

2. Induce vomiting (often provoked by attempts at inserting the lavage tube). The administration of apomorphine will cause vomiting and is employed when the condition of the patient is not precarious.

3. Administration of regional anesthesia when abdominal surgery is planned. Spinal anesthesia with minimal doses of depressant drugs is preferred. However, this is not complete assurance against aspiration of regurgitated material.

4. Endotracheal intubation in the conscious state. This will establish an airway while the patient is in fuller possession of his protective reflexes; if a cuff is inflated, the respiratory tract can be sealed off from the alimentary tract. Then, general anesthesia can be induced with the greatest measure of security.

INTESTINAL OBSTRUCTION

Low obstructions do not present a major problem and can generally be handled by means of spinal anesthesia. However, high intestinal obstruction is a major challenge to anesthetists and presents a grave risk. The administration of any type anesthesia is usually accompanied by reverse peristalsis, relaxation of the cardiac sphincter and regurgitation of fecal-like material. The last may be in overwhelming quantities. The following safeguards in management are presented: (1) availability of excellent *high-volume flow* suction; (2) presence of bronchoscope in the operating room; (3) use of slight head-down position. The slope of the trachea with the horizontal is approximately 8°; (4) preliminary lavage; (5) placement of naso-gastric tube of large bore; (6) endotracheal intubation in the conscious state under topical anesthesia, the sealing off of the pulmonary system and the institution of general anesthesia.

SHOCK AND CIRCULATORY FAILURE

In general, surgery should be delayed until a blood pressure of 50 mm. Hg. systolic is attained. Sometimes this is not possible and is dependent on arrest of large-vessel bleeding—the surgery may be crucial in stabilizing circulation and saving life. Military experience indicates the value of obtaining measurable pressure—subsequent anesthesia and surgery are better tolerated. However, no attempt should be made to restore pressure to normal levels.

At least one patent intravenous route must be established for administration of fluids, but two are preferable. Anything smaller than a 16-gauge needle is of limited value. In the face of active bleeding, blood transfusions must be given. These should be rapid. When hemorrhage is occurring, 500 ml. can be given in 5 minutes without danger. One must not temporize. Two precautions are noted. First, if blood is pumped into a patient, a dual blood-administration set is recommended, with a ball-valve trap. This will help avoid air embolism. Second, one person should be assigned full responsibility for managing fluid therapy.

The anesthetic of choice in hemorrhagic or traumatic shock is cyclopropane. All other agents are essentially abettors of the shock state. Spinal anesthesia is contraindicated. Cyclopropane has a salutary effect on peripheral circulation and on the myocardium; it helps to maintain peripheral resistance, protects against capillary stagnation and enhances cardiac stroke output.

CARE IN THE IMMEDIATE POSTOPERATIVE PERIOD

The postanesthetic and immediate postoperative period, in the past, has been a most dangerous time—more so than the actual operation. This hazard has been changed by the advent of the recovery room. Here the vigilant care of the operating room is continued, and any threats to the unconscious or depressed patient are subject to early detection and prompt treatment. Experience has shown that the greatest danger to the surgical patient coincides with the first hour after anesthesia and operation.

Recovery Units

Two types of recovery units may be recognized. The first is the postoperative recovery ward in which patients are managed both during recovery from anesthesia and the subsequent readjustments to the surgery. The postanesthesia recovery unit, called PAR, is the second and more common. Here patients are observed and treated during the postanesthesia hours and through the acute phase of surgical adjustment. At this time all care and measures are provided which are designed to revivify the patient and to promote a maximum of vital physiologic function. It is a time when the patient is incapable of adequate spontaneous or rational self-care. He must be maintained under the close observation of the anesthesiologist, of specially trained nurses and of the surgeon. The time spent in a PAR unit usually ranges from 1 to 12 hours. The average time is almost 3 hours. For individual cases one may say that the time spent in recovery approximates the time spent in surgery.

Inherent in the definition and requirements are to be found the *advantages* of the unit. These are threefold—prevention of morbidity, economy of time and personnel and economy of equipment. The PAR unit saves lives, time and money.

Operation of PAR Unit

Selection of Patients. It is neither intended nor necessary to send all patients to the recovery unit at the conclusion of surgery. The individual requirements of each patient must be considered. After most minor operations performed under carefully administered anesthesia, either the patient will be awake or the regional anesthetic will have worn off. If the patient is also in good condition, he can be returned to his hospital floor. Certain criteria will be used to arrive at any decision. These include the presence of an airway, the presence of cyanosis or pallor, the state of the circulation, the type of anesthesia and the presence of shock.

The anesthesiologist who is cognizant of how well the anesthetic and the surgical procedures have been tolerated can expertly assess the need for observation and care in the immediate postoperative period. After consultation with the surgeon, it may be found that PAR care is unnecessary.

PAR Patient Management. Immediately on admission to the unit, the time is noted, and a check of vital signs is made. These include blood pressure, pulse and both rate and depth of respiration. Thereafter, observations are made at least every 5 minutes for the first one half hour, or oftener, if indicated.

As situations arise requiring specific medications, these are administered accordingly under the direction of the physician. Generally, the need for oxygen, sedation, analgesics, vasopressors, digitalis and antiarrhythmic drugs (arrhythmias related to anesthesia) will be determined and ordered by the anesthesiologist. Fluid therapy and blood replacement are continued or begun according to the order sheet. Careful check is made to ensure the flow of fluids in an intravenous system.

Patients are postured according to circumstances. A patient who is still narcotized or unconscious may be placed in the semilateral "coma position" as a prophylactic measure against aspiration. This is approximately the Sims' position. The uppermost leg is flexed at right angles, and the upper arm is extended. The patient should lie on the arm in which intravenous fluids are administered so that movements of the patient will be less likely to dislodge the needle. A small sheet-roll should be placed under the armpit and shoulder to avoid venous obstruction. Most important, the head must be positioned to secure a free airway and to promote drainage of mucus and vomitus from the mouth. This is the sniffing position. This position may be undesirable if the patient is actually vomiting. Experience indicates that more efficient pharyngeal suction can be performed in the supine position and bronchoscopy is facilitated. A small pillow placed under one or the other shoulder will allow the operator to turn the patient's head completely to the opposite side and yet provide more advantageous control of the respiratory passages. Furthermore, the semisupine position does not interfere with ventilation, as occurs to some extent in lateral positions.

Transportation. This is accomplished by means of specially designed stretcher carts or by stretcher beds. Transfer from the operating room to the recovery unit is accomplished by the operating-room personnel. Every patient assigned to PAR must be accompanied by a nurse and one physician. When any anesthetic or surgical complication has occurred, or following prolonged or extensive surgery, the participating anesthetist should also accompany the patient.

Certain precautions must be observed. These include the use of restraint straps, the placement of guardrails, proper positioning and the use of the cart infusion bracket. The accompanying physician must be adequately instructed and experienced in the care of the patient's head and airway.

Return of a recovered patient to his room is the responsibility of the recovery unit. The same special beds or carts are utilized, and the same standard precautions are observed. Since the patient is now conscious, he need not be accompanied by a physician. The PAR orderly and a student nurse are sufficient for management. An inflexible rule is that all female patients must be attended by a female aide or nurse.

Whenever a patient, unconscious or not, is moved, adequate help should be available so that the patient is not jarred or "bounced." This causes profound blood pressure changes which are not always realized. A minimum of 4 people is necessary. The anesthetist supports the head on his forearms, while his hands are placed under the shoulders for a bracing effect. Merely supporting the head is fraught with the danger of jerking or snapping the head and causing damage to the cervical vertebrae. A student nurse or female aide supports the legs. Two people on opposite sides of the patient firmly grasp the body drawsheet and "set" themselves for lifting. The anesthetist should now direct the procedure, and any prearranged signal system may be used. Besides minimizing physiologic disturbances in patients, the above recommendations will also prevent back and hip injuries in the nurses and the doctors.

Criteria for Recovery. A common error is to send a patient back to his room too soon. He must not be returned to his hospital room until certain criteria indicating recovery are met. *First,* a patient should be "reacted." This term designates the patient who responds to noxious stimuli. He must possess his gag or pharyngeal reflex, be capable of coughing on proper stimulation and respond to painful stimuli. Briefly, this patient has recovered his protective reflexes. *Second,* the patient should be conscious. A conscious patient is one who responds to verbal commands such as "Open your eyes!" He is also oriented to places and his condition. However, most patients may not recall any of their experiences in the PAR, since the amnesic effect of the anesthetic drugs will have been in operation.

PROBLEMS IN THE IMMEDIATE POSTOPERATIVE PERIOD

The various problems and complications which occur in patients recovering from anesthesia and surgery, who are treated in the PAR, fall into 6 categories: (1) control of pain; (2) correction of respiratory derangements; (3) correction of circulatory collapse; (4) control of cardiac dysfunction; (5) control of neuromuscular aberration; and (6) control of gastro-intestinal problems.

CONTROL OF PAIN

Each of the two recognized aspects of pain is a basis for a method of control. One method deals with the psychic aspect and utilizes pharmacologic tools such as analgesics, opiates and other central blocking agents. The other method deals with the physiologic aspect, blocking the pain impulses before they reach the central nervous system. In the first method, the central blocking agents raise the pain threshold but, more important, they change the pattern of reaction. The patient may perceive pain as a sensation, but it no longer bothers him. Specifically, morphine is the most commonly used agent, but it is needless to state that it is abused.

Too often postoperative orders direct the automatic administration of an opiate to a patient on the assumption that pain must be present. This is fallacious. In the majority of instances the only actual need is to provide comfort. Simple measures, such as fixing a pillow, proper positioning or adjustment of a nasal tube, will serve the purpose. Sometimes a sedative is all that is required. Beecher has studied pain in traumatized individuals. On careful analysis of war-wounded patients, he found that only 25 per cent of injured men actually complained of pain and asked for relief. All others obtained relief or comfort by simple measures. Furthermore, it is of note that in the average adult male, maximum pain relief is achieved by 8 to 10 mg. of morphine. Larger doses are accompanied by so little additional benefit that they represent a distinct hazard. One may say that all too frequently morphine and opiates have been administered routinely and have been prescribed for a situation rather than actually because of pain.

In tense or emotionally disturbed patients, the use of subcortical blocking agents, in doses of 10 to 25 mg., has been found to be effective —a course which has proved to be dramatic in tension and anxiety states and in relieving alcoholics. Another agent employed to achieve pain relief and comfort, especially in burned patients, is intravenous-drip procaine, 1 per cent solution. Intravenous alcohol is also an asset in certain conditions, including, in general, pain relief by pharmacologic means, which is achieved both by reducing the intensity of the perception of the pain-sense modality and by alteration of the realization and the pattern of response.

The second mode for attacking pain is by blocking the conduction of the pain from the source or point of application of the stimulus to the central nervous system. In most instances, nerve block is applied as a last resort —if thought of at all. Specifically, it should be applied following major surgery, when the administration of depressants may represent an excessive risk. Thus, in the geriatric patient and in the patient with diaphragmatic irritation and splinting from bile peritonitis or gastric perforation, intercostal nerve blocks are indicated.

CORRECTION OF RESPIRATORY DERANGEMENTS

Among the derangements encountered are respiratory depression, apnea, obstruction, bronchospasm, aspiration and atelectasis. The goal in each instance is to correct the difficulty and provide oxygen as soon as possible. Thus, in apnea and respiratory depression from drugs, artificial oxygenation with bag and mask should be instituted immediately. The depression is combated with the narcotic antagonists, such as normorphine or nordromoran. In cases of overdose, these will dramatically terminate the effects of morphine, meperidine and others in a matter of 2 to 3 minutes. The dose varies from 1 to 5 mg., and the administrator should use fractional doses until the proper response is obtained. An excessive dose of normorphine will itself produce depression.

Obstruction is relieved by airways including endotracheal tubes. If mucus or vomitus with aspiration is the problem, two procedures are employed. The first is T.B.T., or tracheobronchial toilet. This utilizes a simple rubber catheter with a proper droop. It is inserted through a patient's nostril into the hypopharynx and, with the patient sticking his tongue out, may then be introduced further into the trachea. The tussic squeezing by the patient at this point is more important than any actual suction of material by the catheter. The second procedure, bronchoscopy, is used by the anesthesiologist when large volumes of vomitus are regurgitated and aspirated. It is recommended, under the circumstances, that 5 to 10 cc. of normal saline be used to lavage the trachea. This is directed at diluting the acidity of the vomitus and allaying the occurrence of chemical pneumonitis.

Restrictive dressings often cause insufficient ventilation. Situations commonly encountered are those resulting from the encircling bandages after radical mastectomy, the tight binders applied after upper abdominal surgery and body plaster casts. Tracheal obstruction can be due to dressings applied after head and neck operations. Care in the application of all dressings is the best safeguard. Such care will be used once the consequences of inept wound dressings are known.

A comment is necessary on the use of so-called analeptic drugs in drug depression. Such agents as Metrazol, caffeine, picrotoxin and Coramine are stimulants, not true antagonists. They increase oxygen needs and do more harm than good. Their status in treating drug depression has been carefully evaluated by the Council on Pharmacy and Chemistry of the American Medical Association and has been found wanting. In our experience, they are of no value when needed most and should be abandoned. Bronchospasm is relieved by atropine, ephedrine or aminophylline.

CORRECTION OF CIRCULATORY COLLAPSE

Shock and hypotension are presented daily in an active surgical theater. The first is treated by a combination of blood, fluids, expanders, oxygen, pain relief and hydrocortisone. If, despite these measures, the systolic pressure remains at levels below 80 mm. Hg., a vasopressor drug is given cautiously intravenously in extremely dilute solutions. The agent of choice is norepinephrine diluted to 8 μg. per ml. or 8 mg. per 1,000 cc.

One must be alert to unrecognized or inadequately treated blood loss. Bleeding concealed by poor pressure dressings and the accumulation of blood in major cavities when drains become obstructed are frequent hazards. A high degree of suspicion on the part of the anesthesiologist is the best safeguard.

On the other hand, hypotension is to be distinguished from shock by the presence of a slow pulse. It may occur after spinal anesthesia and cyclopropane anesthesia. It is self-limited. In most instances little or no treatment is required, for no serious after-effects have been determined. However, on the principle of maintaining an approximately normal physiologic state, a systolic tension of 100 mm. Hg. is desired. To this end, a drip solution of Neo-Synephrine, in dilution of 1:100,000 mg. per 100 cc., is employed.

The hypotension associated with pain relief by meperidine should be recognized. This narcotic is a circulatory depressant in the postanesthesia period and may confuse the physiologic situation. It is treated by an antagonist or by a vasopressor. To guard against side-effects administer doses within a range of 25 to 75 mg. and repeat if necessary.

Control of Cardiac Dysfunction

Three principal complications are encountered: those related to the patient with coronary artery disease, those associated with myocardial insufficiency, and the problem of arrhythmias.

Concerning coronary artery disease, it is recognized that there is a significantly enhanced risk, and that the incidence of severe cardiac complications and mortality associated with the operative and postoperative period is about 10 times greater than in the patient without cardiac disease. It is our routine to administer to anginal and coronary-insufficiency patients a dose of Peritrate (10 to 20 mg., 1 hour, intramuscularly). We recommend the same dose in the immediate postoperative period. Other recommended drugs are papaverine, nitroglycerine, oxygen and analgesics.

For patients who evidence myocardial insufficiency or failure, either during operation or in the PAR, we recommend that ouabain or acetylstrophanthin be administered in 2 doses of 0.6 mg. approximately 15 minutes apart. The onset of action is about 5 minutes, and peak action takes place in about 15 minutes. The duration of effect is only 4 hours.

Control of Neuromuscular Aberrations

We are interested here primarily in convulsions on the one hand and excitement on the other. The first are relatively rare and can be controlled by the administration of relaxant drugs (our preference), though small doses of barbiturates have been used in the past. Oxygen must always be administered and assistance to respiration furnished. Emergence excitement is frequent and is seen in alcoholics and in tense anxious patients. The use of chlorpromazine in this situation has already been mentioned. Another drug useful for controlling disorientation, especially in older patients during recovery, is apomorphine. It is properly a cortical sedative in doses of 1 to 2 mg. Larger doses produce emesis.

Persistent Relaxant Effect

Residual muscular paralysis must be considered to exist in varying degrees at the completion of operations involving the use of muscle relaxants during the anesthesia. This is not often significant but can go unrecognized. It occurs after all types of relaxants. If there is any suspicion of persistent pharmacologic effects, pulmonary ventilation must be assisted, oxygen administered and hypoxia prevented. Antagonists to the blocking agents may be employed. If succinylcholine hypopnea exists, then artificial respiration must be continued until spontaneous respiration is adequate. Measurement of spontaneous tidal volume can be carried out by means of the ventilometer. Fresh whole blood, calcium chloride, alkalinizing solutions and Cholase will help to neutralize the succinylcholine. However, avoidance of overdose and adherence to contraindications are preferable safeguards.

CONTROL OF GASTRO-INTESTINAL PROBLEMS

Vomiting is the bane of the postanesthetic period. This may be overt and readily noted. More insidious is silent regurgitation. In either case, aspiration is the harmful feature. It has been shown that gastric contents may appear in the trachea. Fortunately, with good anesthesia in experienced hands, the incidence is low. Furthermore, a series of drugs is now available, the members of which minimize both the incidence and the severity of the vomiting. The outstanding drug in this regard is, again, chlorpromazine.

Distention is a frequent intruder in the recovery period. Patients who swallow are particularly disturbing. Sometimes there can be enough gastric distention to cause vagal overactivity with cardiac manifestations. A Levine tube corrects the situation, but more important than treatment is the recognition of the problem.

BIBLIOGRAPHY

Anscombe, A. R.: Pulmonary Complications of Abdominal Surgery, Chicago, Yearbook Pub., 1957.

Coakley, A. S., *et al.*: The place of chlorpromazine in anesthesia and surgery, Current Res. in Anesth. & Analg. **35**:101, 1956.

Collins, V. J.: Principles and Practice of Anesthesiology, Philadelphia, Lea & Febiger, 1953.

————: Evaluation of thiopental anesthesia, Bull. New York Acad. Med. **31**:438, 1955.

————: Recovery room in care of surgical patient, New York State J. Med. **55**:782, 1955.

Dripps, R. D., and Vandam, L. D.: Long-term follow-up of patients who received 10,098 spinal anesthetics, J.A.M.A. **156**:1486, 1954.

Etsten, B. E., and Li, T. H.: Hemodynamic changes during thiopental anesthesia in humans, J. Clin. Invest. **24**:500, 1955.

Etsten, B. E., *et al.*: Appraisal of coronary patient as operative risk, New York State J. Med. **54**:2065, 1954.

Slocum, H. C.: Problems of overtreatment of surgical patients with depressant drugs, J.A.M.A. **156**:1523, 1954.

Rovenstine, E. A., and Wertheim, H. M.: Present status of therapeutic regional anesthesia, New York State J. Med. **42**:123, 1942.

Todd, D., and Beecher, H. K.: Study of the deaths associated with anesthesia, Ann. Surg. **140**:2, 1954.

Wyant, G. M., and Drobkin, A. B.: Antisialogogue drugs in man, Anesthesia **12**:203, 1957.

PAUL B. SZANTO, M.D., AND GERTRUDE NOVAK, M.D.

3 Blood Transfusion

Blood transfusion is not a surgical operation in the usually accepted meaning of that term. However, it is so frequently employed in connection with surgical operations that it is often considered as an integral part of these procedures. As such, it becomes subject to the same liability to error and the same necessity for safeguarding as the primary operation itself. So a consideration of blood transfusion properly takes its place in a work limited to *surgical errors and safeguards.*

SELECTION OF BLOOD FOR TRANSFUSION

Since the selection of blood for transfusion immediately offers opportunity for error, an understanding of the fundamentals of blood grouping is essential.

The 7 Blood Group Systems

At present 7 blood group systems are known. This grouping is based on the recognized types of antigens found on the red blood cells.

An *antigen* is any substance which, when introduced parenterally, stimulates the formation of a specifically reacting substance known as an *antibody.* According to the available evidence, antibodies are *modified gamma globulin molecules.* This modification in the structure—the so-called "active patch"—enables this molecule to fit—like a key into a hole—to that specific antigen which has stimulated its formation. The antigens present on the surface of the red blood cells are named *agglutinogens* because *clumping,* i.e., agglutination, occurs when a contact with the specific antibody is made. However, if this agglutination occurs in the presence of complement, then hemolysis takes place. The same antigens are also named "hemagglutinogens." These antigens are inherited, appear early in fetal existence and remain unaltered throughout life. Based on the various antigens, 7 systems, regulated by 7 different pairs of chromosomes, can be distinguished:

1. ABO system
2. Rh system
3. MN system
4. P system
5. Le (Lewis) system
6. K (Kell) system
7. Lu (Luther) system

ABO System. Landsteiner, in 1901, distinguished 3 blood groups by crossmatching the red blood cells and the serum of a great number of individuals. A year later, a fourth group was described by Decastello and Sturli. The 4 groups have been named O, A, B and AB. Originally it was thought that only 2 antigens occur, namely, A and B. The fact that the red blood cells of Group O also contain a corresponding antigen has been recognized only recently.

The presence of antigens A and/or B in the red blood cells of an individual is revealed by the use of sera containing *anti-A* or *anti-B* antibodies. The serum of a person of Group A contains anti-B antibodies, that of a person of Group B contains anti-A antibodies. These antibodies are designated as *iso-agglutinins.* Serum of an individual belonging to Group O contains both anti-A and anti-B antibodies, while the serum of a person belonging to Group AB contains neither of these iso-agglutinins.

For the identification of a blood group, known serum containing anti-A antibodies (B serum) and known serum containing anti-B antibodies (A serum) are each mixed on a slide with a drop of diluted blood of the individual to be tested. If the red blood cells are not clumped by either of the sera, then the blood belongs to Group O; if clumping occurs with both sera, then we are dealing with Group AB. Red blood cells of an individual belonging to Group A will be agglutinated by

B serum and, similarly, the red blood cells of a person of Group B by A serum.

For *confirmation,* portions of the serum from the individual are tested against known A and known B red blood cells. In addition, just prior to the blood transfusion, *cross-matching* should be done. This procedure consists of mixing the red blood cells of the recipient with the serum of the donor and vice versa. *Compatibility* is indicated by the complete absence of agglutination.

In the United States 44.0 per cent of the population belongs to Group O, 39.5 per cent to Group A, 11.8 per cent to Group B and 4.2 per cent to Group AB.

SUBTYPES OF A-AGGLUTINOGENS. In 1911, von Dungern and Hirszfeld were able to differentiate between 2 subtypes of A-agglutinogens, now designated as A_1 and A_2. This subdivision was based on the observation that Group B serum, when absorbed by certain Group A red cells, was still able to agglutinate other Group A red cells, as well as AB red cells (A_2 and A_2B subtypes). A third (rare) subtype, A_3, was discovered later. Anti-A_1 antibodies are occasionally found in the serum of A_2 and A_2B individuals. Anti-A_2 and anti-O antibodies are found rarely in sera of A_1 and A_1B individuals.

On the basis of the data cited above, it is evident that with respect to the 4 main blood groups, 2 types of incompatibility can be distinguished: (1) agglutination of the erythrocytes of the donor by the serum of the recipient and (2) agglutination of the erythrocytes of the recipient by the serum of the donor.

The first type of incompatibility is the more serious and absolutely must be avoided. Let us assume that the transfusion consists of 500 ml. (1 unit) of blood, about half of which is plasma and the other half red blood cell mass. If the red blood cells of the donor are incompatible, e.g., transfusion of Group A blood into a Group B blood recipient, then the donor's red blood cells will be clumped, with resulting transfusion reaction. However, if Group O blood is transfused into a Group B recipient, then the red blood cells of the transfused blood will not be hemolyzed. The donor's serum does contain anti-A and anti-B antibodies which, theoretically, could agglutinate

the erythrocytes of the recipient. However, in practice there will be no ill effect because the antibody titer in the donor's blood is likely to be relatively low; so the quantity of antibody injected will be absorbed without damage by the cell volume of the recipient's blood. Therefore, blood of Group O individuals can be used with comparative safety, not only for O recipients, but also for individuals belonging to Groups A, B and AB. On this account, Group O blood has been designated as *universal donor* blood. During World War II, such Group O blood was collected from the civilian population, refrigerated and flown to combat areas.

However, it should be pointed out that the use of Group O blood as universal donor blood may be hazardous if its antibody titer is high (as is found in about 20% of the universal blood donors). In such instances, many red blood cells of the recipient's blood may be clumped and hemolyzed, especially if there were more than 1 unit of blood transfused. We can safeguard against such dangerous accidents by one of two methods: (1) by determination of the anti-A and anti-B titers of the Group O blood, and using as universal donor only that blood which has a low agglutination titer and (2) by neutralization of the anti-A and anti-B antibodies with purified, water-soluble Group A and Group B antigens prior to transfusion, thus preventing agglutination of A or B red cells of the recipient's blood.

However, despite these precautions, serious transfusion reactions have occurred when Group O blood was used as universal donor blood. Therefore, it is an error to use it in this capacity, except when immediate transfusion is essential and no other group-specific blood is available.

In 1926, Landsteiner and Levine demonstrated the presence of group-specific A and B antigens in spermatozoa. Some years later, Witebsky showed by complement-fixation that alcoholic extracts of any bodily organ of a Group A individual contain A antigen and, similarly, any organ of a Group B individual contains B antigen. A and B antigens—though more frequently A—have also been found in the tissues of animals and plants. For example, A antigen has been extracted from the gastric mucosa of hogs, and B antigen from the gastric mucosa of horses. A and B antigens have also been isolated in water-soluble form and used in concentrated solution for the neutralization of anti-A and anti-B antibodies in whole human blood and plasma. About 80 per cent of the members of Groups A, B and AB secrete group-specific substances in their saliva and gastric juice. Such individuals are called *secretors*. This ability to secrete group-specific substances is inherited as a simple mendelian dominant. The following explanation is given for the difference between secretors and nonsecretors. Group-specific substances occur in alcohol-soluble and water-soluble forms. The alcohol-soluble form appears in the red blood cells and in every tissue of the body with the exception of the brain. The water-soluble form is also present in various tissues, but only the glandular organs of the secretors are able to manufacture and secrete these water-soluble antigens so that they appear in the saliva and gastric juice.

After the first year of life, anti-A and anti-B agglutinins occur regularly as natural antibodies. Immune anti-A and anti-B antibodies appear in a woman of Group A or O who is carrying a Group B fetus, or in a woman of Group B who is carrying a Group A fetus. A small percentage of the cases of *erythroblastosis foetalis* is caused by immune anti-A or anti-B antibodies inducing hemolytic reactions in the fetus.

Rh System. In 1940, an antiserum against the red cells of the Rhesus monkey was prepared by Landsteiner and Wiener, by injecting the red cells into rabbits. These investigators also found that this serum agglutinates the red blood cells of 85 per cent of humans belonging to the Caucasian race. Therefore, they assumed that the red blood cells of the individual reacting with this anti-Rhesus serum contain an antigen similar to or identical with the antigen present in the red blood cells of the Rhesus monkey. Human blood which reacts with anti-Rhesus serum is termed *Rh positive;* blood not reacting with the anti-Rhesus serum is termed *Rh negative*. Natural antibodies for the Rh factor occur rarely, if at all, in human blood. They appear in Rh-negative individuals by iso-immunization, either as a result of multiple transfusions of

Rh-positive blood, or in an Rh-negative woman bearing an Rh-positive child. Transfusion of Rh-positive blood into an Rh-negative person who has developed Rh agglutinins will result in a hemolytic reaction.

Subsequent extensive studies showed that the human red blood cells contain a number of Rh factors related to the original Rhesus factor. There are 4 such factors: Rh_0, rh', rh'' and rh^w. The blood originally called "Rh negative" contains 1 of the 2 Hr factors, hr' or hr'', both being weak antigens. Of the various Rh factors, Rh_0 is the closest to the Rhesus factor. It is the most frequent type and also the one with the strongest antigenic property, which gives it the greatest clinical significance.

Hemolytic disease of the newborn (erythroblastosis foetalis) is caused by isosensitization of the expectant mother to a factor present in the red cells of the fetus. The iso-antibodies formed by the mother against this antigen pass through the placenta into the fetal circulation, combining with the red blood cells of the fetus.

As a safeguard against transfusion reactions, the Rh type of the donor and of the recipient should be determined by testing the red cells with anti-Rh serum. All Rh-negative recipients should receive Rh-negative blood to prevent iso-immunization. This is especially important for Rh-negative women in the childbearing age.

MN System. M, N and S are weak antigens occurring in the erythrocytes. Anti-M and anti-N antibodies are seen only occasionally and then only in low titer. Clinically, the incidence of transfusion reactions due to anti-M and anti-N is so rare that typing for these antigens is unnecessary.

P System. Rabbit serum immunized with human erythrocytes will agglutinate 75 per cent of red blood cells of all humans, irrespective of ABO and MN groups. The antigen responsible for this reaction is termed P antigen. Anti-P occurs frequently in P-negative humans. It is a naturally occurring, weak cold agglutinin of no clinical importance.

Le (Lewis) System. Le antigen occurs in the red blood cells of a fifth of the general population. It causes no clinical problems.

K (Kell) System. This system is of no practical significance.

Lu (Luther) System. One out of every 10 persons is estimated to carry this antigen in his red blood cells. Hemolytic transfusion reactions have never been observed as a result of sensitization to this antigen.

THE BLOOD BANK

Nowhere in the whole procedure of blood transfusion is there more chance for error or greater need for safeguards than in the management of the blood bank. Under modern peacetime conditions, no surgeon would consider attempting any major operation unless he had access to an adequate supply of blood for emergency or regular transfusion.

The blood bank should be open during the regular working hours. In addition, emergency service should be provided between 5 P.M. and 8 A.M. daily and for Saturday and Sunday.

For the successful operation of a blood bank, an adequate excess of donors is required to maintain a positive balance. To succeed in the maintenance of such a balance, it should be kept in mind that an average of two donors is required for each unit (500 cc.) of blood given.

If blood which has been removed from the bank is returned later for credit, it can be accepted only if the following requisites have been fulfilled: (1) the container has not been opened; (2) no more than 4 hours have elapsed since the blood was withdrawn from the bank; and (3) the blood must have been under constant refrigeration since its withdrawal from the bank.

Examination of Prospective Donors. Before bleeding, the donor's temperature, pulse rate, blood pressure and hemoglobin level should be determined. The temperature and pulse rate should be normal; the blood pressure should be between 100 and 200 mm. Hg. systolic and less than 100 mm. Hg. diastolic.

In taking the prospective donor's medical history, the following points are of importance:

1. Illness in the past month. Upper respiratory infection, severe acute sinusitis or sore throat may make a donor unacceptable or acceptable only after careful consideration.

2. Surgical operations. In the case of donors who have had surgical operations of any type during the previous 6 months, the entire history should be reappraised.

3. Pregnancy. No pregnant woman can be accepted as a donor, and women less than 12 months post partum should also be excluded.

4. Malaria. Any person who has ever had malaria or received an intensive suppressive therapy against this disease should not be accepted as a blood donor.

5. Viral hepatitis. History of viral hepatitis excludes any person from the list of prospective blood donors, except when the blood is to be used only for plasma fractions.

The following diseases or conditions disqualify a donor: (1) tuberculosis; (2) rheumatic fever; (3) prolonged fevers from any cause; (4) chronic eczema; (5) recurring boils; (6) cardiovascular disease (rheumatic heart disease, coronary heart disease); (7) renal disease; (8) convulsive disorders; (9) history of fainting spells; (10) frequent allergic reactions (asthma, food sensitivity, active hay fever).

An important safeguard is the consideration of previous immunizations. A donor may be accepted only when 2 years have elapsed since the last immunization against rabies, 2 weeks after immune reaction (or when scab comes off) after vaccination for smallpox and 2 weeks after the last injection for typhoid, typhus, yellow fever, diphtheria, tetanus or influenza.

Flight personnel of commercial or military planes who have to participate in flights within 14 days should not be accepted.

The prospective donors should be instructed about the kind of nourishment which they can and should take before donating blood. Fatty foods should be omitted (butter, ice cream, whole milk, eggs, cheese, bacon) for the 4-hour period before donating blood, but some nourishment should be taken, such as fruit juice, tea or coffee without cream, plain cracker or dry toast with jelly, before coming to the blood bank. Just before the donation, on entering the bleeding room, donors should be given some sweetened drink in order to increase the blood-sugar level. Longer fasting decreases the blood sugar and increases the reaction rate.

Donor Reactions. About 5 per cent of donors develop some systemic reaction during or after the bleeding. These reactions may be slight, moderate or severe. They usually begin with pallor and perspiration. The pulse becomes weaker, nausea may develop, and the donor may become dizzy, lose consciousness, develop convulsions or even present the picture of a hyperventilation tetany. *Discontinue the withdrawal of blood at the first symptoms—especially fainting.* The feet should be raised to higher-than-head level, and ammonia should be inhaled.

After a bleeding during which there were no complications, the donor should remain for 15 to 30 minutes in the recovery room and should receive warm or cool refreshments. However, overloading of the stomach should be safeguarded against.

There is so much chance of error in the *collection of citrated whole blood* that a full description of the method is set forth as a safeguarding measure. The apparatus used for the drawing of the blood must be sterile and pyrogen-free. Preferably, the receiving unit should conform to the specifications accepted by the Military Medical Purchase Commission. At present, the vinyl plastic bag is having an increased popularity because it is flexible at low temperature and is unbreakable. The surface character of this bag is similar to the endothelial surface of the blood vessels, and any turbulence, foaming or sludging is avoided. The danger of air embolism is completely absent, and pyrogenic reactions are reduced to 0.6 per cent. Any chance of infection is also markedly reduced. The platelet survival rate is also improved when plastic containers are used.

The receiving set contains 120 cc. of anticoagulant solution (100 ml. of this solution contains 0.48 Gm. citric acid, 1.32 Gm. sodium citrate and 1.47 Gm. dextrose). This so-called A.C.D. solution prolongs the period of red blood cell survival. In the usual receiving sets, 21 days after the bleeding, 70 per cent of the red blood cells are viable. By using the plastic bag it was found that 80 per cent of the red blood cells survive after 21 days and 70 per cent even after 30 days.

The pH of the plasma gradually falls to 6.6 as nonvolatile acids accumulate. The potassium in the plasma rises because of diffusion of the potassium out of the red blood cells, while the sodium level of the plasma falls when there is diffusion of sodium into the cells.

The use of sodium citrate or phosphate-dextrose solution instead of A.C.D. solution would increase the survival of the red blood cells.

The containers of citrated whole blood should have labels (blood group, blood type, Wassermann reaction, expiration date). The expiration date for packed red cells and resuspended red cells should not exceed 10 days even if the cells have been stored continuously at 4° to 6° C.

If the blood is used as plasma, the receiving unit should contain, as an anticoagulant, citrate solution (4 Gm. of trisodium citrate dissolved in 100 ml. of water); 10 ml. of this solution should be added to the receiving unit for every 100 ml. of blood, *before* it is sterilized. The supernatant plasma will be drawn from the bleeding bottle after centrifugation or sedimentation into a "pool bottle."

INDICATIONS FOR TRANSFUSION

The indications for transfusion are numerous, and a detailed enumeration of all of those possible is not intended. However, certain general principles should be established.

A most important safeguard is the distinction to be made between *indications for transfusion of whole blood* and conditions which only require either *the soluble components or the concentrated red blood cells of the whole blood.* Before the therapy is undertaken, it should be determined what and how much is needed.

The routine laboratory procedures, such as determination of hemoglobin, hematocrit, red blood cell count and concentration of blood proteins, may yield an equivocal or sometimes even a misleading result. Thus, in a dehydrated patient, normal laboratory findings may mask an actual deficit of total serum protein and total hemoglobin; on the other hand, hemoglobin, hematocrit and serum protein value may be low in a patient who has been excessively hydrated by the use of large amounts of plasma or plasma expanders. In chronically ill patients with reduced body weight, the blood volume may be markedly decreased while the interstitial (extracellular) fluid is increased. This condition may also be associated with a decrease of the protein content of the body, leading to a delay in wound healing and postoperative complications such as suture breakdown and paralytic ileus.

Determination of Blood Volume

Determination or, at least, *estimation of the blood volume* is of great importance. Every surgeon needs a simple reliable method which can be used before, during and after the operation, which, by measurement of the loss of blood, will aid him in the formulation of a blood-replacement program.

The exact determination of any patient's blood volume is a difficult undertaking, subject to many errors. It may be estimated by determination of the plasma volume or of the red cell volume, or, better still, by the independent determination of each. A simple and relatively accurate method consists of intravenous injection of 5 cc. of radioactive iodinated human serum albumin. Ten minutes after injection, 5 cc. of blood is removed from the other arm and sent to the radioisotope laboratory for analysis with the scintillation counter.

By comparing the total blood volume determined by this method with the hemoglobin and hematocrit values, certain conclusions can be reached which are of practical significance. If *low hemoglobin* is associated with decreased blood volume, it may be interpreted as evidence of chronic bleeding, such as takes place in cancer of the stomach or the intestines or in peptic ulcer. Association of low hemoglobin with normal blood volume occurs in iron deficiencies, while the presence of high blood volume associated with low hemoglobin is an evidence of overhydration. Normal hemoglobin is associated with normal blood volume in normal man but with low blood volume in acute bleeding, and with high blood volume in patients who have been overtransfused with whole blood. *Elevated hemoglobin* is associated with low blood volume in shock and dehydration, with normal blood volume in normal individuals at high altitudes and with high blood volume in cases of polycythemia (primary or secondary).

Indications for Transfusions of Whole Blood

The most important indications for whole-blood transfusions are (1) acute blood loss produced by hemorrhage; (2) hemolytic anemia; (3) aplastic anemia; (4) before operation, if the hemoglobin level is below 10 Gm. per cent; (5) acute leukemia; (6) septicemia; (7) anemia in late pregnancy.

There is no question about the absolute indication for whole-blood transfusion in instances of severe anemia resulting from a single massive or recurrent hemorrhage.

In cases of *congenital or acquired hemolytic anemia,* transfusion with whole blood may result in a dramatic, although only temporary, improvement. However, it should be mentioned that the beneficial effect of blood transfusion is greater in the *congenital* than in the *acquired* type of hemolytic anemia. This is because the transfused red blood cells have a normal survival rate in instances of congenital hemolytic anemia, whereas, in cases of acquired hemolytic anemia, the transfused red blood cells will be destroyed as rapidly as are the patient's own red cells. It is an error to give repeated blood transfusions in cases of hemolytic anemia, if it can be avoided, because of the tendency to form specific antibodies.

In cases of *aplastic anemia,* repeated blood transfusion will be a necessity if hemoglobin concentration is to be maintained at 10 Gm. per cent.

It has been observed that in *acute leukemia* repeated blood transfusion may bring about remissions. Occasionally, 20 or more transfusions, with simultaneous withdrawal of the patient's own blood, will be necessary, that is, an application of the principle of "exchange transfusion" therapy, as advocated for fetal erythroblastosis.

In *septicemia,* especially the chronic variety, severe anemia may develop. The hemoglobin should be maintained at the level of 10 Gm. per cent.

In most chronic anemias the plasma volume is normal; only the red blood cell volume is decreased. In such cases the administration of red blood cells is indicated. The red cells can be administered either as resuspended red cells (in 5% glucose in physiologic saline) or in the form of "packed cells" without the addition of another medium (the small amount of plasma present in the packed cells is sufficient to supply the necessary fluidity to the transfused material).

The great advantage of the use of red cell suspension or packed red cells lies in the fact that overloading of the circulation is avoided, while the oxygen-carrying capacity is increased to normal levels.

In some instances there will be an acute loss of plasma from the circulation, resulting in decrease in the circulating blood volume. The chief causes of acute plasma loss are *burns,* or an *acute obstruction of the small intestine* due to strangulation. In such instances an immediate replacement of blood volume can be achieved either by plasma or by serum albumin.

Platelet Concentrates

In instances of essential thrombocytopenia, administration of platelet concentrates is of great therapeutic value, especially in the stage of acute crisis, preparing the patient for splenectomy.

Fibrinogenopenic disorders occur not uncommonly in the various fields of medicine, surgery and obstetrics. The normal plasma fibrinogen level is 300 mg. per cent. Hemorrhagic diathesis due to fibrinogenopenia develops only if the plasma-fibrinogen level is below 50 mg. per cent.

Fibrinogenopenia may result from deficient production, fibrinolysis and intravascular clotting. Deficient production as a cause of fibrinogenopenia may occur as a congenital or acquired condition. The fibrinogenopenia of severe liver disease and polycythemia are due to decreased fibrinogen production.

Fibrinogenopenia due to fibrinogenolysis or fibrinolysis may occur in patients with carcinoma of the prostate, the bladder, the pancreas or the kidney. These tumors produce kinases* which activate the precursor of fibrinolysin present in plasma.

During pregnancy, the hemostatic mechanism of the blood is disturbed by elevated *prothrombin* activity of plasma and fibrinogen. Thromboplastic material given off from tissues, placenta and amnion transforms prothrombin into thrombin, resulting in the formation of thrombi utilizing and consuming the fibrinogen of the plasma, thus leading to

* Kinase: A colloidal substance, existing in various tissues, which serves to activate the specific enzyme of those tissues.

fibrinogenopenia, thrombocytopenia and hypoprothrombinemia.

In instances of intra-uterine death, the macerated fetus is known to liberate simultaneously substances with thromboplastic and anticoagulant properties. *Abruptio placentae* is the most frequent cause of serious fibrinogenopenia due to intravascular clotting. The management of fibrinogenopenia differs according to its various causes. The purified fibrinogen preparations available today contain 2 Gm. of clottable fibrinogen per unit.

The fibrinogenopenia of primary and secondary polycythemia is treated by venesection and administration of fresh plasma or purified fibrinogen preparations. Fibrinogenopenia due to fibrinolysis, as it occurs in prostatic and bladder carcinoma, is best treated with cortisone, which increases the antifibrinolytic titer of the plasma. In fibrinogenopenia due to intravascular clotting (e.g., during thoracic or prostatic surgical procedures), 1 to 4 units of fibrinogen should be administered within 1 hour. Acute fibrinogenopenic states of pregnancy should be treated by (1) prompt delivery; (2) administration of 20 units of ACTH in 250 ml. of 5 per cent dextrose intravenously (2 ml. per minute); (3) administration of fibrinogen if bleeding continues 1 hour after the start of the ACTH infusion; (4) hysterectomy if the fibrinogen fails to control bleeding.

Plasma Substitutes

During the past decades many substances have been advocated as plasma substitutes. The requirements of a good plasma substitute are as follows: (1) it should have an osmotic pressure similar to that of the plasma protein; (2) it should not leave the circulation rapidly after transfusion; (3) it should not be toxic; (4) it should not cause allergy; (5) it should not be stored in the tissues of the body for a long period of time.

In recent years *dextran* has been advocated in various countries as a plasma substitute fulfilling these requirements. It rapidly restores blood pressure and blood volume in hemorrhagic shock. However, the maintenance of blood pressure is less adequate than with the use of plasma. Dextran is stored in small quantities in the tissues for many weeks. It is especially important to know that dextran has been found in cells of the renal tubules which have been previously damaged by anoxia, and, therefore, great caution should be used in the administration of dextran to patients with renal or hepatic functional impairment. It should also be mentioned that dextran in the plasma causes rouleau* formation which may interfere with the performance of the various compatibility tests. Therefore, blood for blood grouping and typing should be obtained before any administration of dextran.

COMPLICATIONS OF BLOOD TRANSFUSION

Most of the adverse reactions to blood transfusion can and should be prevented. The most common complications are (1) hemolytic transfusion reaction; (2) pyrogenic (fever-producing) reaction; (3) allergic or anaphylactic reaction; (4) circulatory overload; (5) hemorrhagic diathesis following massive whole blood transfusion; (6) contaminated blood; (7) tetany; (8) air embolism; (9) hyperpotassemia; (10) transmission of disease—homologous serum jaundice, syphilis, malaria.

HEMOLYTIC REACTION

The hemolytic reaction to the transfusion of incompatible blood, resulting in excessive hemolysis, occurs as the result of transfusion of either ABO- or Rh-incompatible blood. The severity of the reaction to Rh-incompatible blood usually depends on acquired isosensitization in Rh-negative individuals. This isosensitization develops in 10 to 30 per cent of Rh-negative individuals after repeated (2, 3 or more) transfusions with Rh-positive blood and in 5 per cent of the Rh-negative women bearing Rh-positive children. Hemolytic reaction of less severe degree may occur after administration of blood which is compatible but has been improperly stored and (usually) poorly refrigerated, or blood which has been stored over a long period of time.

Clinically, the symptoms of a hemolytic reaction are lumbar pain, chills, substernal oppression, apprehension, prostration, rapid breathing, occasionally urticaria and a state of shock. During the operation, sometimes the

* *Rouleau* (French—"roll"): rolls of red blood corpuscles.

first sign of incompatibility is a marked hemorrhagic tendency, when the amount of blood oozing from the surgical field may reach serious proportions. The first urine obtained after the reaction will be dark reddish-brown in color, containing a few red blood cells. Serum bilirubin level rises and may reach 5 mg. per cent (indirect bilirubin). The severity of the clinical picture depends on the amount of blood which has been transfused.

The clinical symptoms may be manifested immediately but usually appear only after the patient has received at least 50 cc. of blood. Therefore, the recipient of blood should always be observed constantly during the administration of the first 150 cc., so that the surgeon may notice the early danger signals and interrupt the transfusion. During the entire remaining time of the blood transfusion, the patient should be checked every 10 minutes.

The amount of incompatible blood sufficient to cause fatal hemolytic reaction depends on the titer of iso-antibodies in the blood of the recipient. This titer may be depressed in some diseases, e.g., in leukemia. As a rule, however, transfusion of 300 to 400 cc. of incompatible blood will have severe, and possibly fatal, consequences. Rarely, the patient may die within a few minutes or hours following the onset of the hemolytic reaction. Agglutinated red cell thrombi in the capillaries of the brain, together with shock, are given as explanations of this dramatic outcome.

If hemoglobin is released due to hemolysis of the red cells, the liberated hemoglobin will cause a coloration of the plasma from pink to deep red. The hemoglobin concentration of the plasma varies from a trace (slightly pink color of plasma) to dark red (0.5 to 1.0 Gm. per cent). The intensity of hemoglobinuria does not run parallel with the frequency and the severity of the renal complications. Some patients tolerate hemoglobinuria and hemoglobinemia well without renal shutdown. There is a concomitant increase in indirect plasma bilirubin. The heme† portion of the hemoglobin combines with the serum albumin to form methemalbumin, which is practically pathognomonic for intravascular hemolysis.

† Heme: The nonprotein insoluble iron-pyrrol compound found in hemoglobin, in respiratory pigments and many cells, both animal and vegetable.

Hemoglobin is excreted as a threshold substance when the hemoglobinemia is above 50 to 100 mg. per 100 cc. of plasma. Hemoglobinuria is associated with albuminuria and hemosiderinuria, since the tubular epithelium of the kidney converts hemoglobin into hemosiderin. Renal shutdown and acute nephrosis (hemoglobinuric or lower nephron) may occur.

The patient may soon recover from the immediate hemolytic reaction, but some time later may develop oliguria and anuria, or complete anuria may persist from the beginning. In severe typical cases of lower nephron nephrosis the mortality rate is almost 50 per cent, and death takes place within 4 to 18 days after the onset of the hemolytic reaction. Sudden diuresis is the first indication of beginning recovery of the kidney function.

During the oliguric-anuric phase, the urine is a kind of ultrafiltrate of the plasma; its specific gravity is fixed (1.010) and it contains protein, red blood cells, hemoglobin and hemosiderin. Blood levels of NPN, urea and creatinine will rise, and the serum potassium will be markedly elevated (up to 8 mEq/L.) with resulting signs and symptoms of potassium intoxication (bradycardia, electrocardiographic changes of high and peaked T-waves, a broad QRS complex and disappearance of the P-wave). In the second week the volume of urine increases, but the diuresis may cause further disturbance in concentration of the electrolytes. Terminally, the patient will develop flaccid muscular paralysis, tachycardia and ventricular fibrillation.

At autopsy, in such a case of lower nephron nephrosis, the kidney is enlarged, with pale cortex, dark and dusky medulla and accentuated medullary striations. Microscopically, the glomeruli are bloodless; focal necrosis of the epithelium may affect any segment of the tubules, but mostly the distal portion of Henle's loop and the distal convoluted tubules. Red or brown casts (heme casts) are found in the lumina of Henle's loop, in the distal convoluted tubules and in the collecting tubules. The interstitial tissue is edematous and shows foci of mononuclear cells and thrombophlebitis of the small veins. Some of the tubules will have herniated and ruptured into the veins.

Jaundice, appearing a few days after a hemolytic blood-transfusion reaction, is possibly the result of a combination of the following factors:

1. Hemolysis of the red blood cells, leading to excessive formation of bilirubin. Such a hemolysis may occur not only as a result of the destruction of the incompatible red blood cells but even in the absence of a transfusion reaction of any type. About 30 per cent of infused red blood cells are always destroyed.

2. Hepatocellular damage, due partly to the heme component and partly to the globin (peptones and peptides), both of these breakdown products being injurious to the hepatic cells. Therefore, the jaundice is not a purely hemolytic one but has also a hepatocellular component.

In the event of a transfusion reaction, samples of blood should be saved for immediate checking of the blood groupings, blood typing and crossmatching. For direct proof of an intravascular hemolysis, the demonstration of free hemoglobin and methemalbumin in the plasma is required and/or the presence of hemoglobin in the urine. Methemalbumin remains for several days in plasma; its presence renders the plasma a golden brown color, and it gives a positive reaction with benzidine.

Errors Leading to Hemolytic Reactions. These can be (1) a technical error by the blood bank staff (mistake in selection or crossmatching of the blood); (2) a clerical error, with "mix-up" of the bottles; (3) incompatibility of factors having such a low antibody titer that they were not detected in vitro by the routine laboratory tests.

It is estimated that 1 to 3 reactions per 1,000 transfusions occur because of the administration of incompatible blood. However, this estimate varies from one hospital to another.

In paroxysmal nocturnal hemoglobinuria, transfusions with compatible blood are associated with hemoglobinemia and hemoglobinuria. The cause of this phenomenon is unknown.

Treatment. The treatment recommended for hemolytic reactions consists of (1) immediate interruption of the transfusion; (2) shock treatment by supporting the circulation with plasma or compatible whole blood; and (3) fluid and electrolyte therapy, which is of greatest importance, especially if renal failure with oliguria and anuria develops, with salt retention. Salt intake should be restricted and the electrolyte balance carefully evaluated. Alkalinization of the urine should not be attempted; the possible retention of sodium administered as lactate may cause pulmonary edema.

For the prevention of potassium intoxication, the following measures are recommended: (1) daily administration of glucose solution and (2) administration of cation-exchange resin (50 Gm. potassium-free resin in divided doses). In cases of potassium intoxication, intravenous injection of sodium chloride, glucose and insulin gives only temporary relief; dialysis is the treatment of choice (artificial kidney, intestinal irrigation, "peritoneal lavage").

The diffuse bleeding from surgical wounds developing after the administration of incompatible blood is due to fibrinogen deficiency and, therefore, should be treated by the administration of fibrinogen.

PYROGENIC REACTIONS

Pyrogens are substances capable of provoking febrile reactions during or after parenteral administration. Either they are products or derivatives of bacteria or they are organic or inorganic chemical compounds (denatured proteins).

Pyrogenic reactions are the most common reactions to transfusion therapy. They occur under the best conditions, even if all possible safeguards have been employed. Their frequency varies between 2 and 5 per cent. The reactions are characterized by chills and fever, manifested during or within 1 hour after transfusion. The reaction may be mild or severe with violent chills and high fever. It usually lasts less than 4 hours and will be followed by complete recovery within 24 hours. The absence of hemoglobin, methemalbumin or of elevated indirect bilirubin in the plasma will be helpful in the differential diagnosis between pyrogenic and hemolytic reactions.

ALLERGIC REACTIONS

Allergic and anaphylactic reactions have been estimated as occurring in from 1 to 2 per cent of the total number of units of blood given. They are characterized by urticaria,

angioneurotic edema and asthma. The urticaria appears during or after the transfusion. Angioneurotic edema may affect the glottis. Rash, urticarial wheals, swelling of the mucous membrane and itching sensation may be accompanied by nausea and vomiting. *Treatment* consists of epinephrine (0.3 to 0.5 cc. of a 1:1,000 solution given subcutaneously and, in severe cases, 0.3 cc. given intravenously). Antihistaminic drugs may be indicated; the addition of 50 mg. of diphenylhydramine hydrochloride (Benadryl) to 1 unit of whole blood will prevent an *allergic* transfusion reaction but not that of a *pyrogenic* type.

CIRCULATORY OVERLOAD

Circulatory overload leads to pulmonary congestion and edema. During the transfusion, or immediately afterward, the patient may develop dyspnea, orthopnea, cough, cyanosis and physical signs of pulmonary edema. In thoracic surgical procedures (lobectomy, pneumonectomy) or cases in which the patient has but limited cardiac reserve, it is easy to overload the circulatory system, leading to circulatory failure. Any excessive increase of the blood volume due to rapid rate of transfusion or large amounts of the infused fluid may lead to pulmonary edema.

HEMORRHAGIC DIATHESIS

A hemorrhagic diathesis may occur secondary to the transfusion of whole blood (1) as a part of the hemolytic transfusion reaction; (2) due to the transfusion of blood contaminated with bacteria; (3) after transfusion of *unusually large amounts* of compatible blood.

After transfusion of 5,000 ml. of whole blood, the patient develops thrombocytopenia. Decrease in blood platelets is also observed in infants receiving exchange blood transfusion. It was formerly assumed that the thrombocytopenia was due to the fact that in the stored blood the thrombocytes markedly decreased in number. However, this would not explain the observations that (1) thrombocytopenia may occur even after transfusion of fresh blood and (2) the thrombocyte count may decrease to extremely low levels (5,000/cu.mm.).

It is possible that the thrombocytopenia is the result of the presence of a thrombocytopenigenic substance circulating in the donor's blood. After blood transfusion the recipient may simultaneously develop hypoprothrombinemia and hypofibrinogenemia, these additional factors explaining the emergence of the hemorrhagic diathesis.

CONTAMINATED BLOOD

Transfusion with contaminated blood will cause the development of symptoms and signs of bacteremia. The patient must be treated promptly with the appropriate antibiotics.

TETANY

After multiple transfusions the sodium citrate used as an anticoagulant occasionally may induce symptoms of tetany, especially in infants. Citrate is rapidly metabolized in the liver, but in cases of diffuse liver-cell damage the concentration of citrate may rise in the blood, and ionized calcium will be used up for its neutralization. The intravenous injection of calcium gluconate will safeguard the blood calcium and restore it to the normal level.

AIR EMBOLISM

A few cases of air embolism have been reported—but in extremely rare instances—when blood has been administered by an air-pressure apparatus.

HYPERPOTASSEMIA

The plasma potassium of the stored blood may be considerably elevated after 2 weeks of storage. Transfusion with such blood may cause hyperpotassemia in patients with deranged renal function. Transfusion with such blood is an error which must be avoided. Patients with renal disease in any form should receive only relatively fresh blood, i.e., not older than 1 week.

TRANSMISSION OF DISEASE

A constantly present hazard in blood transfusion is the transmission of disease by whole blood or plasma. The most important disease which may be transmitted is *infectious (viral) hepatitis*. It is difficult to safeguard against this, as we have no exact method of determining whether or not the virus is present, either in the plasma or in the whole blood.

The incidence of post-transfusion hepatitis varies between 0.5 and 1.5 per cent. If pooled plasma is used the incidence is much higher; the larger the pool, the greater the incidence of serum hepatitis. After plasma transfusion from large pools (5,000 units) the incidence has been as high as 12.2 per cent of cases, while from small pools of 10 units the incidence has been about 1.5 per cent.

It should be pointed out that the physical condition of the recipient at the time of transfusion greatly influences not only the incidence but also the severity, and even the mortality, of the hepatitis. The greater morbidity of *serum* hepatitis as compared with *infectious* hepatitis possibly is due to the fact that the recipients are usually severely ill and undernourished. It is also possible that allergic individuals are predisposed to serum hepatitis. The virus of serum hepatitis may also be transmitted by the antihemophilic fraction, human thrombin, or by Fraction IV from postpartum plasma; the virus has never been transmitted by other blood products such as serum albumin or gamma globulin.

The incidence of transfusion hepatitis may be lowered by employment of the following safeguards:

1. Inactivation of the hepatitis virus. Ultraviolet radiation did not fulfill the original expectation, but it has been found that prolonged storage (6 months or more) of liquid plasma at room temperature decreases, if not practically eliminates, the hazards of hepatitis.

2. Exclusion of infected donors. Donors should be carefully screened, not only by obtaining a good clinical history and physical examination, but also by laboratory tests—especially thymol turbidity determination.

3. Selection of raw material for transfusion. This is less dangerous than pooled plasma (i.e., whole blood or single plasma units). Serum albumin can be used if whole blood is not indicated. Gamma globulin, if given at the same time as the transfusion, has no protective effects. It should be remembered that the incubation period of S. H. virus ranges from 1½ to 6 months, while that of I. H. virus ranges from 2 to 6 weeks.

In recent years, the transmission of *syphilis* has been reduced to practically insignificant levels, and safeguards against bacterial diseases are also very effective. Prevention of the transmission of *malaria* still remains difficult because it necessitates a most detailed medical and personal history.

When any type of transfusion reaction takes place, the following general measure should be instituted:

1. The blood bank should be notified concerning the type of reaction.

2. The empty bottle or the unused part of the blood should be returned to the blood bank.

3. Blood should be drawn from the recipient and sent to the blood bank for (1) retyping, (2) crossmatching and (3) centrifuging the blood specimen to find evidence of hemoglobinemia.

4. Two or 3 days after the blood-transfusion reaction took place, a blood sample should be taken to the laboratory for determination of serum bilirubin and blood-urea-nitrogen levels.

5. A urine specimen should be examined immediately after the occurrence of a blood-transfusion reaction and daily thereafter for hemoglobin and red blood cells in the urinary sediment, and later for urobilinogen and bilirubin.

The volume of the daily urinary output must also be checked carefully.

BIBLIOGRAPHY

Cohn, E. J., Oncley, J. L., Strong, L. E., Hughes, W. L., Jr., and Armstrong, S. H., Jr.: Clinical, chemical, and immunological studies on the products of human plasma. I. The characterization of the protein fractions of human plasma, J. Clin. Invest. 23:417, 1944.

Davidsohn, I.: Textbook of Clinical Pathology, ed. by S. E. Miller, pp. 293-373, Baltimore, Williams & Wilkins, 1955.

Lehane, D., Kwantes, C. M. S., Upward, M. G., and Thompson, D. R.: Homologous serum jaundice, Brit. M. J. 2:572, 1949.

Murphy, W. P., Jr., Getz, E. J., and Sprout, M. T.: Hemolysis in blood collected for plasma processing, J.A.M.A. 158:449, 1955.

Neve, R.: Intra-arterial transfusion by the femoral route, Lancet 1:746, 1955.

Rosenthal, N., Bassen, F. A., and Michael, S. R.: Probable transmission of viral hepatitis by ultraviolet-irradiated plasma; report of three cases, J.A.M.A. 144:224, 1950.

Strumia, M. M., Colwell, L. S., and Ellenberger, K.: The preservation of blood for transfusions. I. The effect of plastic containers on red cells, J. Lab. & Clin. Med. 46:225, 1955.

NEAL OWENS, M.D.

4 Plastic Surgery

BASIC PRINCIPLES

GENERAL CONSIDERATIONS

Each plastic surgery patient has a separate and individual problem, and the solution must be suited to the particular case. In effecting this solution, certain factors are of importance to the ultimate outcome, including (1) physical condition of the patient, (2) age, (3) economic considerations such as hospital time and cost and disability time. We know that with staged procedures the over-all result may be far more economical, in the broadest sense of that word. Also, it should be remembered that conservatism is of the utmost importance.

Most operations in plastic surgery are elective. In planning a specific procedure, such items as shock, infection or possible injury to vital organs should take precedence. The surgeon must remember that these factors and their effect on the over-all problem are intimately associated with the fundamental principles of plastic surgery. Further, the plastic surgeon may have the dual responsibility of restoring function and improving the cosmetic effect. This usually results in a patient who is happier and again able to lead a normal life, free of embarrassment and psychic scars.

It is of vital importance that the surgeon should visualize the final results and consider the possibilities of each step. He should have in mind at all times a "blueprint" of his activities and the limitations of each step; he must also possess a background of sufficient experience to know when to stop! One of the axioms of plastic surgery is to "make haste slowly." Experience imbues the surgeon with the knowledge that an attempt to accomplish too much at any given moment frequently leads to unfavorable results, loss of valuable tissue and a much greater loss of time.

One of the frequent errors made by younger surgeons without a broad background of experience is to *attempt to fit a given deformity to some method described in a book*. One must learn early that not all patients lend themselves to repair by textbook methods, since many of them present problems which do not conform to any "standard" method. Another fundamental which is frequently overlooked is the fact that descriptions in the literature with drawings and photographs *frequently fall short* of the potential accomplishment. Good surgery always adheres to the basic principles of anatomy and physiology. Following these principles enables us to proceed with the solution of the particular problem in a direct and forceful manner, thereby making full use of all available structures and tissues.

SPECIFIC CONSIDERATIONS

One of the fundamentals of plastic surgery is the gentle handling of tissues. For example, each bite with a toothed forceps causes microscopic necrosis. Always use fine hemostats which grasp as little unnecessary tissue as possible. Ligatures used in tying bleeding points should be equally fine. Bear in mind at all times the necessity for avoiding trauma, either by clamping, ligating or sponging, or even in pressing tissues with the finger tips, for any of these actions can cause *thrombosis*. This is highly important, for the thrombosis may occur in that one vessel which can determine the viability of a flap.

ANESTHESIA

There are some specific problems in the field of anesthesia which deserve mention as *danger signals*. Where the use of the *electrocautery* is anticipated, always clear this with the anesthetist. When the surgeon is working about the neck, and the anesthetist has inserted an *intratracheal* tube, the surgeon should be very careful of entering the trachea, even though the anesthetic is being given by a closed system.

Remember the danger of using *adrenalin* in

65

the presence of *cyclopropane* anesthesia; cardiac complications could ensue. All members of the surgical team should be constantly alert to the necessity of frequently checking the soda lime; unless this is done, a saturated soda lime canister may go undetected, thereby subjecting the patient to anoxia for a period of time, even to the point of causing cardiac arrest.

Hyperthermia. In geographic areas of extreme heat and humidity, the danger of hyperthermia is constantly present. This is particularly true when surgery must be performed without benefit of air conditioning. Remember that hyperthermia insidiously announces itself only when the patient is already in its throes, and it can be rapidly fatal. The surgeon and the anesthetist may be unaware of what is happening until the operation has been concluded. The patient appears to be perfectly normal; then there is a suggestive quiver or evidence of minor shock and his skin feels warm to the touch. On taking a rectal reading, he may be found to have a temperature of 106° to 108° F., and a drastic emergency stares the surgeon in the face. Measures to be instituted immediately consist of the application of a solution of iced alcohol on large sponges or bath towels, with a cooling fan draft turned directly on the patient so that his body is virtually in an ice pack. Unless he responds to a marked degree almost immediately, also instill an ice water enema. The temperature should fall to approximately 100° to 101° within an hour or less. It is usually necessary to place such a patient under an oxygen tent and, when indicated, to give whole blood.

OPERATIVE PRECAUTIONS

Complete Hemostasis. A *hematoma* can be the plastic surgeon's worst enemy; therefore, complete hemostasis is essential. Beware excessive use of *adrenalin*, for there is always danger of a temporary arrest of bleeding or of oozing which will resume after a wound is closed. Be doubly aware of the dangers of the use of adrenalin in a finger injury or in a large

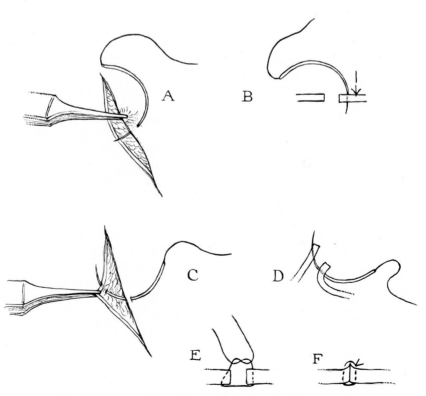

FIG. 25. Manner of suturing skin to obtain slight eversion.

absorptive area. There is a hematoxic element which follows the formation of large clots within tissues. This is demonstrated when one examines the undersurface of a large flap which has been in contact with a hematoma and notes the reaction of the flap tissue. Invariably a thick "rind" will be found which is partially necrotic and subsequently will cause much unnecessary scarring.

Tension. A prime deterrent to wound healing is tension. It should always be avoided. One can frequently overcome wound tension— if the nature of the structures permit—by *undermining*. This should be done whenever necessary. Tension is responsible for breakdown of wound margins, marginal necrosis, poor *scars* of unsatisfactory depth and width and quite frequently for the thick, repulsive

keloidlike cicatrices which, cosmetically, have all the unsatisfactory effects of a true keloid.[7] Tension may also be avoided by other methods chosen on the basis of a careful appraisal of the wound, such as planning *incisions* so as to convert a straight line into the pattern of a Z-plasty. All incisions should be made at a right angle to the plane of the skin to avoid *beveling*.

Sutures. Choice of suture material is of the utmost importance, as has been pointed out by Steffensen.[10] This implies (1) adequate tensile strength in the smallest possible caliber, (2) moderate elasticity, (3) minimal capillarity and (4) an atraumatic needle. Sutures should be placed subcutaneously in a manner which will remove all possible tension from the skin margins. It is important to secure a slight

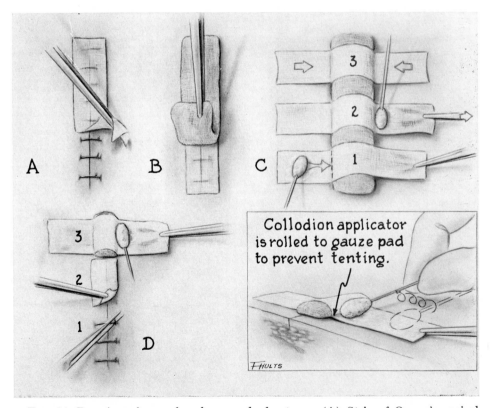

Fig. 26. Dressing of wound and removal of sutures. (A) Strip of Owens' surgical fabric directly over wound to prevent adherence of gauze. (B) Folded gauze over fabric. (C) Application of collodion strips over gauze to exert mild pressure. (D) Removing sutures and supporting wound as sutures are removed to prevent dehiscence.

eversion of wound edges (Fig. 25). All sutures should be carefully placed and tied in a manner to give exact approximation with the least amount of tension on each individual stitch. Otherwise, local necrosis will follow. Be doubly careful to avoid too much tension on *mattress sutures.* When employing *subcutaneous sutures,* use as few as possible and a nonirritating type.

Incision. When placing incisions, it is important to locate them, where possible, parallel with Langer's lines. Straight-line closures are the ideal. Of course, this must always be modified by the requirements of adequate excision and débridement. Always remember that the simplest closures are the best, and scrupulously avoid those of a "tricky" nature, most of which *never work as shown in books!*

Some of the fundamental errors to be avoided are: (1) incisions which cross flexor surfaces, as they invariably cause contracture and frequently produce "fiddlestrings" across areas such as the flexor or extensor surfaces of fingers, the antecubital fossa, the axilla and vertical neck incisions; (2) straight-line scars leading to a free margin, such as the eyelid or the lip, since these almost invariably end in a noticeable notch.

Exact approximation of wound margins is highly important. In the words of Halstead, "gently approximate; do not strangulate." This approximation should result in a slight eversion of wound edges with a few subcutaneous sutures put in with a minimum of tension. All skin sutures should be removed as early as possible, for the earlier a suture is taken out the less scarring and crosshatching there will be. If a wound can be adequately closed by the use of an intradermal suture, a better wound, free of crosshatching, may be anticipated.

Healing. A number of fundamentals must be clearly understood regarding the healing of wounds. A wound usually seals within 48 hours. Those without too much tension will be sufficiently sealed at the end of 24 hours to permit removal of sutures, if properly protected by cross supports of collodion strips (Fig. 26).

Because traditionally sutures were removed from abdominal and other large wounds at the end of 7 days, the concept developed in the minds of many surgeons that wounds were satisfactorily closed within this period. *No greater misconception could exist.* The tensile strength of the healing wound at the end of 7 days is quite unsatisfactory. Even at 14 days, one can separate the average wound with ease by gentle pressure against each margin with 2 fingers! It has been shown physiologically and microscopically that complete and effective healing does not take place short of *4 to 6 weeks.* Collagen fibers, as a rule, can be demonstrated in a wound as much as 30 days old. This suggests that completion of healing is taking place at this period. Clinically, it has been shown that the ideal scar results only when a wound is suitably and adequately supported for a minimum of 4 weeks. The support must be accurate and can best be achieved by the application of collodion cross strips. *For the best cosmetic result, we would recommend support for 5 to 6 weeks.*

In wounds affected by motion of underlying muscles, such as those of the back, the abdomen, the shoulders or the neck, we find ourselves on the horns of a dilemma—to remove sutures early, yet to overcome stress and strain over a long period. It is very difficult to avoid the spreading that results from such strain; one of the best solutions to this problem is the use of subdermal sutures, to remove as much stretch from the wound as possible, along with an intradermal suture, which can be left in for a considerable time. A cosmetically satisfactory scar is virtually impossible to achieve without subjecting the patient to immobilization with a cast.

Cosmetically satisfactory healing is always enhanced by placing incisions, where possible, along natural features and contours, such as the eyebrow, the eyelid wrinkles or in the nasolabial fold. Finally, the importance of matching skin color and texture should be kept in mind when transplanting skin flaps, and it is obvious that hairbearing skin should always be avoided for a lining.

TRAUMATIC INJURIES

GENERAL CONSIDERATIONS

When we consider that the incidence of trauma is increasing in direct proportion to our technologic advances, it is not difficult to conceive that the time may arise when surgical facilities might be unable to cope with the patient load. These increasing accidents, of course, are going hand-in-hand with the increasing output of faster cars, with plane travel and with the production of ever more complex industrial machinery. The cautious, conscientious surgeon will constantly remember that the outcome of any injury may depend on what is done by the first person to see it. Tremendous psychic trauma complicating injuries of the face can be reduced to a great extent by the proper management of these cases.

Plastic surgeons are commonly called upon to manage 3 general types of injuries: (1) craniofacial wounds, (2) burns and (3) compound traumatic injuries to the soft parts of the face and the extremities. Cases involving craniofacial trauma are always of major importance because they may involve severe injuries to the skull and the brain, which may result in death or in persistent deformities from brain damage.

Craniofacial Injuries. A severe injury to the *brain*, of course, takes precedence over all other considerations in treatment except the *arrest of hemorrhage*. Any manipulation of injured parts without first ruling out the existence of cranial damage may be sufficient to cause unnecessary loss of life. If, after ruling out the existence of cranial injuries, distorting fractures of the facial bones are found, it is highly important that these be diagnosed and treated promptly and accurately to avoid permanent disfigurement. Fractures of this nature frequently are treated all too lightly, on the assumption that anyone who sees and diagnoses such an injury is capable of managing it. As a result, distortion of the orbital floor, the eyes and the malar eminence, misfunctioning of the jaw, displaced teeth with malalignment and alveolar and nasal deviation are frequently seen. Once these fractures knit in malalignment, it is often too late to hope for the good results that might possibly have been obtained by skilled treatment directed by an individual with the required training and experience.

Burns. Suffice it to say that many texts have been written on this subject, and it is far too involved to deal with in detail in this limited space. However, it is important to recognize that any burn involving over 5 or 10 per cent of the body's surface area should be regarded as serious and should be cared for by a surgeon who has had special training in this field.

Improper appraisal of a burn in the early hours, when shock is present or impending, may be fatal. This error probably accounts for a considerable proportion of the high mortality which still exists in burn statistics.

A second point of extreme importance in the management of burns is treatment for *shock* and administration of blood; otherwise, poor healing and unnecessary infection may follow. Far too many burns which started as second degree become infected, resulting in a completely denuded surface, thus converting them, for all practical purposes, into third-degree lesions.

Another very important aspect of the treatment of burns consists in removing *eschars* and *sloughs* at the earliest possible moment, in order that the areas where skin has been destroyed may be covered with skin grafts as soon as possible. In certain areas of the body, including the hands, the movable joints and the feet, it is urgent that sloughs be excised promptly in order that coverage may be provided at the earliest possible moment, thus maintaining mobility in the area and avoiding ensuing loss of motion from crippling contractures.

Compound Injuries. Ideally, compound injuries involving the soft parts should be seen as soon as they happen in order to begin treatment during the precontamination stage; only in this way can the damage be converted into a surgically clean wound and disastrous infection avoided. It is far easier to accomplish repair by a suitably staged surgical maneuver (provided that the state of the patient will permit) than to do a hasty "patching up" that allows malalignment and improper union of bones which will have to be treated with subsequent additional surgery. Nevertheless, it is a good general rule not to probe blindly, for important structures may thus be injured which otherwise might not be involved.

Tracheotomy. If the patient is comatose, always suspect blood in the larynx or the trachea causing obstruction. Under these conditions, always consider performing a trache-

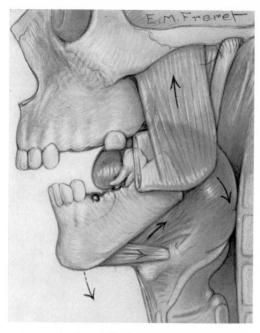

Fig. 27. Retrodisplacement of tongue
due to fracture prolapse.

otomy. Properly done, this can be carried out in a very short time, and the attendant trauma is usually so slight that one cannot afford *not to do it* if it is indicated. Lives have been lost as the result of delays of only minutes in doing a tracheotomy. However, the surgeon should be aware that the simple precaution of having the necessary instruments available may lull him into a false sense of security. When obstruction develops, quickly appraise the situation, and if a tracheotomy is in order, *do it at once!*

SPECIFIC CONSIDERATIONS

Of first importance for a patient suffering craniofacial trauma should be the determination beyond any doubt that there is an adequate *airway*. Fractures of the mandible or the maxilla frequently predispose to blockage of the airway. Mandibular fractures are particularly prone to produce this, since the displacement may be in a direction which permits prolapse of the tongue to block the pharynx completely (Fig. 27). If there is any question, immediately, quickly and with a minimum of added manipulation insert a tracheotomy tube to ensure unhampered respiration.

Evaluation of Injury. It is felt by many that the primary concern of a surgeon in caring for a case of craniofacial trauma should be the use of the *roentgenogram*. In our opinion, in many instances it is more informative to depend on careful palpation of the bony contours of the face, feeling both sides simultaneously for comparison. Not infrequently fractures of the orbital rim, the floor of the orbit, the nose or the zygomatic arch, or transverse fractures of the malar bones, as well as extensive fractures of the mandible, may be located and diagnosed by this simple method. We have seen patients with a transverse fracture of the maxilla which permitted the jaw to be rocked back and forth or sideways, yet it was not diagnosed because it did not show up on the x-ray plate. Roentgenograms are still valuable for determining positively that patients do have fractures and dislocations, but they should not be accepted as negative if they reveal nothing. It is extremely difficult to bring out some fractures of the face due to the dense overlying bones and adjacent sinuses and tissues of varying opacity. However, do not forget that roentgenograms are of extreme value in medicolegal work and therefore should always be taken.

Examination. Be extremely cautious in determining the depth of a wound, making sure that the entire tract is exposed sufficiently to permit examination for foreign bodies. Conserve all viable tissue and then follow through with a skillfully executed débridement. Establish the status of visual acuity when these patients are first seen, as there may be injury to or mechanical compression of the optic nerve, though not immediately evident, gradually ensuing as a result of edema in the surrounding tissue.

A uniform routine of procedure in making such an examination should be followed in every instance. One efficient method begins with simultaneous palpation in the supraorbital rims around both sides. After this, the nose should be palpated carefully to determine malalignment, abnormal convexities of bone, flattening, or deviation or crepitation of the nasal bones. The malar eminences should be felt next and observed visually to determine contour and alignment. The same procedure should be carried out on the upper and the lower jaw, palpating the ramus of the mandible and noting any abnormal movement backward, forward or to the side. With a thumb along the lower molars and the fingers on the rim of the jaw on the outside, the mandible is shucked up and down and backward and forward. In taking roentgenograms, always remember that swelling may distort a normal picture. Double check for the position of the mandible by noting the occlusion of the teeth (Figs. 28 and 29). Remember the possibility of injury to the *facial nerve*; in the initial examination, test all 5 divisions. A very accurate survey can be done by having the patient (1) raise the eyebrows; (2) pucker the eyes; (3) wrinkle the nose; (4) show the teeth and whistle; (5) tighten the platysmal muscles.

A potential danger, which should be borne in mind continually, is *rhinorrhea,* indicating a fracture through the *ethmoids.* In this instance, beware of *meningitis* and initiate prophylactic treatment. Check for *broken teeth* and take steps to avoid aspiration of fragments. If there are missing teeth or fragments, assume the possibility of *aspiration* and x-ray the lungs to rule this out. Occasionally one finds *otorrhea,* which is usually indicative of associated *skull fracture.* A careful neurologic survey should always be carried out in any case of craniofacial trauma. If there is blood in the patient's hair, always look for *scalp lacerations.* These are frequently overlooked. In injuries to the nose, it is important to check the *vestibulae* for possible lacerations, dislocations and fractures of the septal cartilage and septal hematoma.

Hemorrhage. A thorough examination should be made to rule out the presence of hemorrhage, and if there is bleeding, to determine the source exactly. Realizing that trauma to the face can produce hemorrhage deep into the recesses of the nasal cavity and its associated sinuses, one understands that the problem of control might be far from simple.

Adequate control may necessitate packing the nose or some of the associated sinuses. In extreme cases, gelfoam may be useful, but it must be borne in mind that this may also be dangerous because it can become dislodged from the original site and gravitate to the larynx. It is also vital never to *clamp* blindly.

Shock. After the initial examinations have

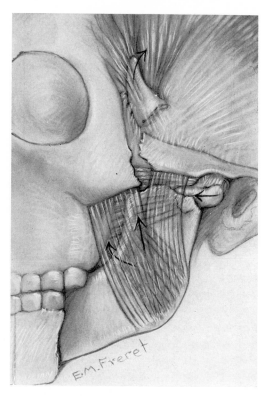

Fig. 28. Wide displacement of fragments due to strong muscular pulls.

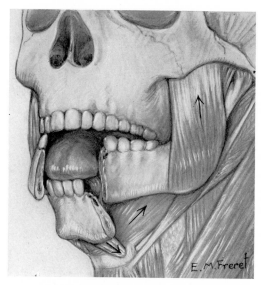

Fig. 29. Displacement of central fragment in bilateral mandibular fracture and resulting increase in distortion from muscular pull. Note pull on tongue.

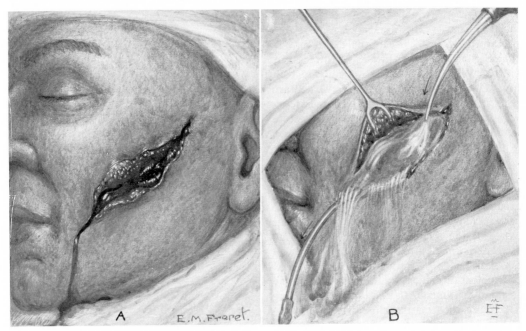

FIG. 30. (A) Typical contused traumatic laceration of cheek. (B) Irrigation of wound depths with copious amounts of water.

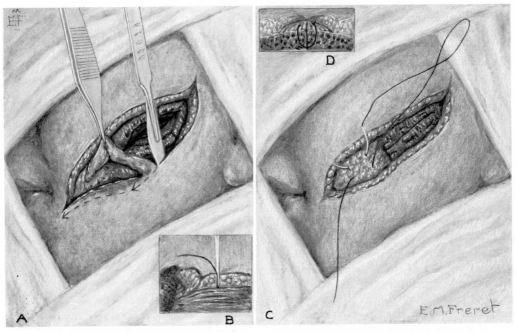

FIG. 31. (A) Débridement of devitalized tissue. (B) Débriding incision at right angles to plane of the skin. (C and D) Suture of deeper layers in anatomic planes.

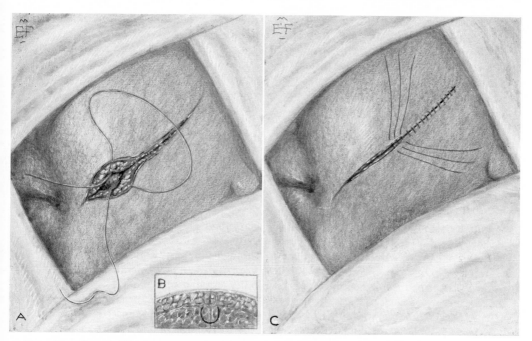

Fig. 32. (A and B) Accurate subcutaneous suture to allow early skin suture removal. (C) Suturing the skin.

been completed, immediately survey the general status of the patient to establish the presence or absence of shock or whether it seems to be impending. Treatment, of course, is standard; if the occasion calls for it, never hesitate to do a "cut down" in order to insert the right sized needle for the administration of whole blood or other fluids. If this is done, insert at least an 18-gauge needle of a polyvinyl cannula in order to have a lumen of adequate size. In treating a patient who is in obvious or impending shock, *beware the use of morphine*, because of its cumulative effect. When its use is unavoidable, it should be administered intravenously.

Treatment. One of the most important steps in treatment is *gross débridement*. It is axiomatic that the ideal time to receive a patient in this condition is immediately following injury, for the more time that elapses before definitive surgery is begun, the greater the possibility of infection and other complications. Thorough *cleansing* with soap and water is the ideal method of preparation for débridement (Fig. 30). All wounds should be thoroughly exposed down to their depths and, of

course, all foreign material removed. Extreme care should be exercised to make sure that no residual *glass particles* remain in a wound. These are frequently overlooked. Where there has been a puncture with a small point of entrance, the wound should be injected with a dye and the entire tract dissected out.

All devitalized and questionable tissue should be excised with a sharp scalpel (Fig. 31). Since the facial bones are fibrinous, when there have been fractures of the bones of the face, attempt to save *all bony particles,* particularly those which are attached to soft tissue, for the remolding of these fragments frequently results in satisfactory healing with re-established contours. If, subsequent to excision of devitalized tissue, closure can be accomplished by direct approximation, this should be completed as quickly as possible. Reposition all tissues in their normal relations if possible. Muscle should be approximated to muscle and the facial planes accurately re-established (Fig. 31 C and D). Avoid closing any wound under too much tension and, if necessary, make lateral incisions for relaxation. The fewer sutures required to gain adequate closure, the better. Use enough buried sutures to approximate deeper soft tissues and eliminate dead space (Fig. 32). Because of the small risk of infection in the head, the neck and the face, it is seldom necessary to insert drains. If there is any question, however, this should be done, removing them within 36 to 48 hours.

In the management of these types of wounds, certain principles are extremely important and cannot be overemphasized:

1. Fixation and immobilization are fundamental. It is recognized that immobilization of the head and the neck is difficult. However, with a little vision and forethought, much can be achieved by the use of Barton bandages. In instances of extensive complications, it may be necessary to apply a bit of ingenuity in devising a plaster skullcap which incorporates wire outriggers made from coat hangers, adhesive tape, Steinman pins and rubber bands.

2. Never attempt to manipulate the nose in the presence of rhinorrhea; consultation with a neurologic surgeon should always be solicited in such instances.

3. Make sure that the patient can swallow. If there is any question about this, suction apparatus should be provided and kept constantly by the bedside.

4. Where possible, avoid complicated external fixation devices designed for holding jaw fractures in alignment by a multiplicity of inserted pins. Treatment in all these cases should always be directed by a surgeon experienced in their management and in the many complications which are common to them.

5. When the patient is unable to close his eyelids, these should be examined carefully, making sure that there is no underlying injury to cornea, sclera or conjunctiva which would contraindicate sealing the lids. Horizontal mattress sutures should then be passed through the upper and the lower lids and tied over rubber tubing to seal the lids together in order to avoid corneal ulcers.

6. If there is extensive posterior nasal bleeding, consider the insertion of a pack in this area (Figs. 33 and 34). In these instances, make certain that good lighting and suction are available.

7. If there is *any question whatever* regarding an airway, do a tracheotomy.

8. Beware of loose or fractured teeth. If

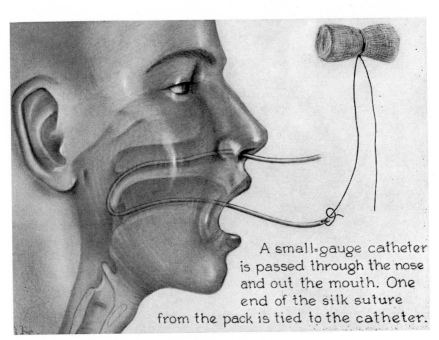

A small-gauge catheter is passed through the nose and out the mouth. One end of the silk suture from the pack is tied to the catheter.

FIG. 33. Packing of posterior nose.

teeth or parts thereof show up missing, make sure, by roentgenographic and other suitable methods, that they have not been aspirated.

9. All teeth in a fracture line must be extracted.

10. Deep lacerations of the tongue should be sutured immediately.

11. Be wary in the use of occlusive dressings when placed over the neck because of the possibility of blocking the airway and also their possible effect on the position of fractures.

12. Blueness in tissue flaps means venous congestion; moderate pressure dressings over these frequently help. Definite blanching, dead whiteness or blackness in a flap means arterial insufficiency, and here viability is always dubious.

13. Use antibiotics routinely.

14. Tetanus antitoxin or a booster injection of toxoid should also be routine.

15. A high calorie, high protein, liquid diet is indicated. If necessary, a gastric tube should be left in place for the maintenance of an adequate intake of this diet.

16. Dietary requirements should be supplemented with intravenous feeding and an adequate vitamin intake.

NEW GROWTHS

GENERAL CONSIDERATIONS

A basic item in any discussion of new growths found in the head and neck region is that, since these tissues are of endodermal,

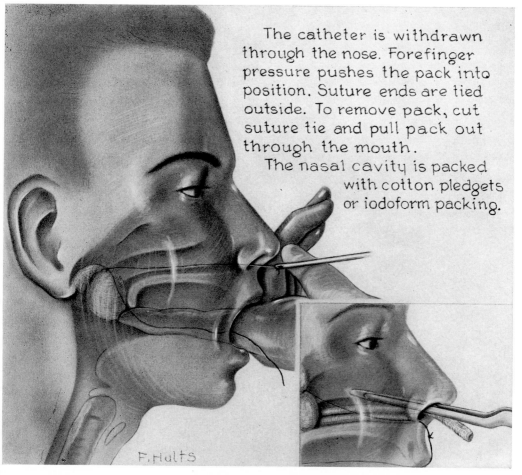

The catheter is withdrawn through the nose. Forefinger pressure pushes the pack into position. Suture ends are tied outside. To remove pack, cut suture tie and pull pack out through the mouth.
The nasal cavity is packed with cotton pledgets or iodoform packing.

F. Hults

FIG. 34. Adjusting pack in position.

mesodermal and ectodermal origins, malignant potential exists in all of them. Ordinarily, however, malignancies that the plastic surgeon sees are readily accessible, and a thorough examination should detect early changes wherever they may be found. Blood and nerve supply around the head and the neck is rich, thus enhancing healing and acting as an excellent protection against infection. However, this is a two-edged sword, since the spread of malignancy may also be enhanced. Examination should always be systematic and should never neglect the nasopharynx, which all too frequently is the primary site of an unsuspected malignancy.

The importance of a biopsy is obvious; any lesion which is worthy of removal is worthy of a biopsy. This should be done at the time of excision by means of a frozen section. The microscope is the final authority in diagnosis and prognosis in malignancy. It is imperative not only that we establish a diagnosis immediately on excision but also that the growth is adequately removed, around the margins as well as in depth. If these conditions are met, the conscientious surgeon will know that he has done all that it is possible to do at that time. We have seen, all too frequently, instances of patients being treated for a considerable length of time without any effort being made to establish a positive diagnosis. Clinical appearance can merely develop a suspicion; the final diagnosis is established only after excision and examination by a competent pathologist.

Surgery vs. Irradiation. If a neoplasm is discrete and amenable to surgical excision, there is, in our estimation, little argument about the advantages of surgical excision over irradiation. The following brief list summarizes our opinion:

1. One-stage complete excision vs. multiple irradiation treatments.

2. Assurance of complete eradication in surgical incision vs. doubt in irradiation therapy.

3. Rapid healing after surgical incision vs. substitution for lesions of radiodermatitis and its sequelae after irradiation therapy.

4. Increased bleeding, if the irradiation is recent.

5. Irradiation before surgery presents the surgeon with scar and fusion of all dissecting planes, if the irradiation is old.

6. Unstable irradiation scars which are potentially malignant.

7. Difficulty, even for experts, in sparing hair, mucous and secretive surfaces, eyes, teeth, etc., from undesirable irradiation.

Irradiation is unquestionably the treatment of choice when (1) the lesion is radiosensitive and a positive cure can be assured; (2) age and general condition of the patient do not warrant surgery; (3) the neoplasm is too far advanced or too widespread to permit surgery; (4) the neoplasm involves vital structures which would have to be eradicated with surgery.

BENIGN NEOPLASMS

Nevi. Nevi are variously classified as raised, pigmented or unpigmented, hairy or warty, epidermal, junctional, intradermal, mixed, blue, linear, etc. Regardless of their type or color, particularly if they are on weight-bearing or frequently traumatized areas, nevi are potentially dangerous, and no one can determine which nevus will turn malignant under constant irritation. Always excise (1) all nevi of toes or feet, in belt or brassière line, in any area subject to irritation during shaving, on the forehead, in the hairline (where irritated by comb), or in areas over the back if they are liable to chronic irritation by weight-bearing; (2) any nevus showing the slightest evidence of growth or breakdown.

Frozen section of any doubtful lesion is essential, since nevus cells may be seen microscopically beyond the pigmented margins. If malignant change is established, radical excision should be done immediately and a skin graft or pedicle shift carried out. Electric or chemical cauterization is to be strongly condemned.

Hyperkeratosis. This condition is premalignant. If these lesions do not disappear but continue to grow under palliative treatment, such as adequate skin cleansing, application of cold cream and avoidance of exposure to the sun, they should be excised. Many of these appear to be perfectly innocent when examined clinically, yet on microscopic section they often show incipient malignancy. Eradication should be carried out with an excision which is several millimeters wide of the visible margin and the specimen checked immediately by a pathologist.

Warts. In general, warts may be electro-desiccated or excised surgically. Plantar warts in particular should be excised surgically rather than irradiated.

Sebaceous Cysts. Surgical excision is the treatment of choice. Excision should include the removal of a small, central ellipse of skin in order to permit complete extirpation without perforating the cyst wall, but excision should *not* be carried out when there is inflammation. Do not forget that sebaceous cysts arise and grow within the epidermis, and malignancy occasionally does develop in such growths.

Dermoids, Branchial Cysts and Thyroglossal Cysts. To avoid recurrence, a dermoid[12] must be completely enucleated, even though this requires excision of a portion of bone. Where there is an associated tract, injection of dye is a great help. Appearance of a new growth in the midline of the nose should be evaluated carefully, and differential diagnosis made between dermal cyst and meningocele. A thyroglossal duct cyst, when properly removed, usually requires excision of a tract which may go through a portion of the hyoid bone and extend upward to the base of the tongue. Complete eradication of the entire tract must be carried out.

Keloids. It is highly important to differentiate between a true keloid and a keloidlike or hypertrophied scar.[7] When such a scar is the result of a burn, one can always be fairly certain that it is hypertrophied and not a true keloid, unless, of course, there is evidence in the *presence of true keloids* not associated with the burn. In the light of present thinking, the preferred treatment is surgical excision within the borders of the keloid until the growth is semiquiescent, followed by complete excision at a later date, taking all precautions to cause minimal trauma. Subsequently, the application of light irradiation may be beneficial.

Hemangioma. As a rule, the *capillary* type of hemangioma can be suitably cared for by injections of sodium morrhuate. Where there is a positive history of growth, treatment should not be delayed. Eradication of these by sclerosing agents is important if they arise in anatomic locations which would entail extensive excision if surgery were attempted. Lesions involving the eyelids, the nose, the lips or the ears are good examples. It must be established in the mind of the patient that injection of a sclerosing agent may leave a residual scar which, if it causes sufficient concern later, may require surgical excision. However, after the tumor has been adequately sclerosed, excision of the scar is a relatively minor procedure.

The *cavernous* type of hemangioma may be either diffuse or discrete. These frequently involve either the upper or the lower extremity. In the upper extremity, the forearm is involved more often; in the lower, involvement is found more often below the knee. Surgery is usually indicated; discrete areas lend themselves readily to adequate surgical excision. On the other hand, the diffuse type may be quite invasive, involving subcutaneous tissue, fascia, tendon, muscle and bone. Occasionally the invasion is so extensive that amputation of the limb may be required. Diagnosis is not always easily made, as typical coloration may not be present. Frequently the area shows a dark blue color and may be associated with a visible and palpable tumefaction (particularly if the lesion is discrete). Another characteristic is *pain*. Pressure over the involved area often elicits a painful reaction. Some cases show sufficient roentgenographic evidence to permit diagnosis by this method; not infrequently, typical *phleboliths* are seen. Surgery is indicated for the diffuse type. Often these may be arrested by a combination of partial excision and strangulation of the exposed portions of the tumor by mattress sutures. This latter procedure aids by destruction and arrest of the tumor growth through the production of excessive scar. We have also used sodium morrhuate injections into exposed tumors.

Lipoma. These are characterized by a rubbery feeling and usually have a rounded, bulbous appearance. Surgical excision is the treatment of choice. When excising a lipoma of considerable size, it is often advisable to use drainage.

Leukoplakia. This condition is definitely premalignant. All areas of leukoplakia should be excised and sent to the pathologist. On the lips or inside the mouth, carefully check dental bridges, ill-fitting dentures, or for jagged teeth. If the patient is a habitual pipe smoker or chews tobacco or dips snuff, these should be prohibited. Any sort of chronic irritation predisposes to the development of this condition. Irradiation or cauterization are contraindicated.

MIXED CELL TUMORS OF THE PAROTID

Surgical excision is the treatment of choice; in excising these tumors, be most careful to remove the entire growth *without rupturing its capsule or spilling its contents.* Be doubly careful of injury to the facial nerve, which should always be saved if at all possible. Recurrence of these mixed cell tumors from residual seeding puts the patient that much closer to the realm of malignancy. Excision of an extremely large tumor of the parotid may cause accidental severing of Stenson's duct. If this occurs, repair immediately and insert within the lining of the duct a small drain or tube which goes into the mouth. *Carcinoma of the salivary glands* may simulate these mixed cell tumors. However, do not be fooled by a large stone in Stenson's duct which may simulate metastasis to the floor of the mouth. Simple removal of the stone will give immediate relief.

MALIGNANT NEOPLASMS

The most conservative treatment for malignancy is radical excision at the earliest possible moment. Palliation is folly; procrastination is conducive to more extensive invasion and, in all too many instances, metastatic spread. *Biopsy* of any growth worthy of excision should be mandatory. A frozen section of the lesion should be made while the patient is on the operating table at the first excision. A wide, sharp dissection into normal tissue is usually best. If there is not adequate tissue to permit this, and one is faced with the possibility of inadequate excision (as in cases where cancer has invaded periosteum or bone), actual *cautery* should be used to destroy and seal the lymphatics and blood vessels and to avoid spread. Bone invasion always dictates thorough cauterization.

Subsequent to excision, the surgeon assumes the obligation of following up these patients by giving them a postoperative survey at least once a month for 2 years, then at least every 6 months for the next 3 years, particularly in cases of *squamous cell carcinoma.* This survey should be followed by annual examinations for the next 5 years. When dealing with squamous cell carcinoma, a surgeon should be alert to the possibility of metastasis and carefully check any regional nodes. *Never curet* a possible malignancy, particularly when the growth is sufficiently isolated or discrete to permit surgical excision. Any *chronic or rodent ulcer* should be suspected as being malignant, and basal or squamous cell carcinoma should always be ruled out in these instances. It is frequently impossible to distinguish between basal cell and squamous cell types without benefit of a biopsy.

Melanoma. Melanomata are notoriously invasive and have a high degree of malignancy with an extremely low proportion of cures. When the diagnosis has been established, wide excision should be carried out. Most authorities recommend complete block dissection of the *regional lymph nodes.* Many suggest *amputation* for melanoma located on an extremity when it is associated with regional metastases. As a prophylactic measure, any *mole* showing change in size, color or shape should be completely dissected and a thorough microscopic study made. To be completely on the safe side, perhaps *all* moles, whether pigmented or not, that are situated in areas subject to constant trauma should be removed.

CONGENITAL ANOMALIES

One of the constant and immediate consequences of congenital anomaly is the severe psychic shock suffered by the parents of the afflicted child; they experience a sense of guilt when they discover that he has been born with a defect. Except in rare instances, inherent transmission of these defects is difficult to establish. However, there is a small group in whom, historically, transmission of some defect can be traced for several generations. When this is true, it is well to caution such persons that their chances of producing a defective child are greater than normal.

Whenever feasible and surgically judicious, congenital defects should be corrected before the child reaches school age. When such children are enrolled in classes with normal children, they are almost certain to become the focus for the natural cruelty and ridicule of their mates and to suffer considerable psychic trauma as a result. Every possible effort should be made by parents, teachers and others to impress upon the child that he is really no different from others, difficult though this often may be.

Harelip and Cleft Palate

The vast majority of parents of children born with this type of defect are eager to have corrective procedures done as soon as possible. Their next concern, as a rule, is the *feeding* problem. In reality, it is rare that these infants present any major feeding difficulty. Occasionally they may have trouble in suckling and have to be fed with a Brecht-type feeder.

Correction of these defects is never an emergency procedure and should be delayed until such time as optimal conditions prevail. As a rule, it is safe to wait until the child is in good health and has reached a weight of $10\frac{1}{2}$ or 11 pounds—at about 3 months of age. Because the deformity of the lip is the more obvious and because of the psychic sequelae, as well as the lesser surgical trauma, this should be closed first. Among other beneficial results of early closure is that the patient more easily retains food in his mouth, which, in turn, enhances his general physical development. Repair of the lip is also paramount in molding the *alveolus* and the *premaxilla*, which invariably show some distortion.

Repair of clefts in the palate should be modified according to the age at which the child can tolerate the necessary surgery. Tissues should be sufficiently well developed to permit the required maneuvers. It is important to begin the repairs before speech patterns are established. As a rule, a child may be 12 months of age or older before subjecting him to operation. A careful survey should be made to rule out *otorrhea, acute respiratory disease* or any other acute condition which would make surgery a hazard. Be sure that the *blood count* is adequate and that *bleeding* and *coagulation times* are within normal limits. *Anesthesia* should be in the hands of a competent anesthetist and preferably should be endotracheal, in order to control aspiration of fluids or blood.

Types of Operation. Lip. Clefts of the lip[11]

vary from a unilateral notch to complete double clefts involving both lips with a protrusion of the premaxilla segment, or any combination of these. Many operations have been proposed, but a complete analysis probably would reduce the selection to (1) the Blair-Mirault (triangular), (2) the Hagerdorn-LeMesurier-Steffensen (quadrangular) flap repair[2] or (3) a variation on one of these. To obtain good lip repair, one should aim for (1) accurate skin, muscle and mucous membrane union; (2) symmetrical nostril floors; (3) symmetrical vermilion borders; (4) slight eversion of lip; and (5) minimal scarring.

Many surgeons feel that bilateral defects should be closed in 2 stages because it is "safer." Where there is any question regarding tension of tissues, the condition of the child or the length of the operation, the procedure should definitely be in 2 stages. With a protruding premaxilla, where the projection is sufficient to make closure of the soft tissues over it difficult, refrain from removing a wedge of the vomer, as has sometimes been suggested. The *vomer represents the growth center of the middle portion of the face; it is imperative to preserve it intact.* Any disturbance may lead to distortion of growth and the so-called dish-face deformity. In bilateral clefts, always bear in mind the growth potential of the small, underdeveloped prolabium.[1] Abnormally long lips are extremely hard to shorten without further increasing the appearance of flatness. Undermine the tissues to relax all flaps adequately, bearing in mind that a tight lip affects growth of the maxilla. Considerable differences of opinion exist as to whether nasal defects associated with clefts of the lip should be corrected at the time of the original repair or deferred to a later date.

Palate. Repair of a cleft palate should aim for a sufficiently long and mobile structure to permit normal speech, proper deglutition and minimal scarring or interference with maxillary, alveolar or dental growth. Frequently, to fulfill all of these criteria is difficult. Reliable data are now available which bring out the fact that extensive clefts should be *repaired in several stages* and in a manner which will obviate the necessity for extensive undermining of palatal tissues to permit approximation of the borders of the defect. Bear in mind that the surgeon's responsibility is to prepare the patient for subsequent *speech training,* for this is the chief ultimate goal in this type of repair. *Prosthodontic* treatment is almost always necessary in these children. Tissue approximation should be free and easy. Where it is necessary to undermine soft tissue to accomplish palatal closure, one should be very careful of the neurovascular bundle which has to be dissected out of the bony canal. The palatopharyngeal musculature should be loosened with extreme caution, and the aponeurosis should be severed on the nasal side. The margins of the cleft should be pared, split and closed with mattress sutures, loosely tied for approximation, since sutures tied on tension frequently cut off the blood supply, thus seriously interfering with healing. *Complete hemostasis* is of the utmost importance. The surgeon should be extremely cautious in the use of *gelfoam* to obtain hemostasis, for this may become loosened and fall into the larynx.

Postoperative Care. LIP. Arm cuffs extending from the wrist to above the elbow on both arms should be applied during the initial healing period. Always insert tongue sutures, leaving them intact until several hours after the child has fully reacted from the anesthetic. Postoperative feeding should be by aseptosyringe, since this causes the least possible damage. Skin sutures should be removed within 48 to 72 hours. The line of closure should be adequately supported by suitable dressings to relieve tension for a minimum of 3 weeks. At all times the suture line should be kept completely clear of blood clots or contaminants. Contaminants may be loosened by moistening and careful use of a toothpick covered with wet cotton.

PALATE. These children also should have cuffs applied from the wrist to well above the elbow. Always have a tongue suture left intact until several hours after the child has fully reacted from the anesthetic. It is well to withhold milk for the first 48 hours to avoid gumming up the suture line; also, no irritating types of food should be given. Good suction and light should be available by the bedside, and no straws or other implements should be offered to the child or inserted past his lips. The child should be put on a high calorie, liquid diet, and after 48 to 72 hours, puréed

foods may be given. If nonabsorbable sutures are used, these should be left in for 2 to 3 weeks.

Complications. Numerous complications may occur following operations for the correction of cleft lip and palate. If considerable oozing is noted inside the mouth, carefully examine the line of incision and particularly inspect the area about the palatine artery. If persistent ooze is found, as a rule it can be brought under control by using small sponges dipped in Adrenalin. If the palatine vessel has been torn within the bony canal, hemostasis may be difficult. One of the simplest methods of bringing it under control is to insert the sharpened end of an applicator stick into the foramen, leaving it for perhaps 36 to 48 hours.

Perforations in palate closures may occur and usually result from tension on the flap where sutures are too tight. Not infrequently trauma from poor nursing care is responsible for perforation. This usually results from hard food or utensils being inserted into the mouth. The insertion of the child's own fingers can be prevented by the application of arm cuffs, as previously suggested.

A child with an unsatisfactory blood picture may show inadequate healing. If the red cell count, hemoglobin or hematocrit are below normal, these should be built up before subjecting the child to surgery. It should be borne in mind that, in some quarters, figures for red cell count, hemoglobin or hematocrit are accepted as normal when they are considerably lower than the adult norm. We have found that children respond much better if these readings approach very closely to the normal for adults.

DEFORMITIES OF THE EAR

These defects are always very noticeable and may produce considerable psychic trauma. Many attempts have been made to fabricate sculptured prosthetic ears to be attached to the skin. However, the attitude of these patients is such that they are prone to reject these and, as a rule, will be unhappy with anything short of a "reasonable facsimile" made from the patient's own living tissues.

These deformities vary considerably, ranging from complete absence of the external ear to various degrees of microtia and cupping and a variety of auricular appendages. Hearing may or may not exist on the affected side. Meatal atresia is common with microtia.

Hearing should always be evaluated by special tests; the presence or absence of an external bony canal and pneumatized mastoid cells should be determined by roentgenogram. Pneumatization of the mastoid cells is highly suggestive that hearing does exist. In the light of current thinking, it is the concensus that if there is roentgenographic evidence of such pneumatization, and at least a rudimentary auditory canal, together with good conductive hearing, and if the deformity is bilateral, it might be worthwhile to attempt surgery. On the other hand, if the deformity is unilateral and normal hearing exists on the opposite side, the risks involved in the operation are not worth the improvement in hearing, which as yet has seldom been increased above 30 decibels. However, this statement cannot be accepted as a final dictum; as research progresses, we hope, through surgery, to be able to create significant improvement in hearing. In any event, we feel that in answer to parents' inevitable questions, we should explain that, where feasible, reconstruction of the ear should be attempted before the child is subjected to the psychic trauma of school contacts. Even when this is not practical, in many instances, parts of the reconstruction may be carried out by the age of 8 to 10 years.

In rebuilding an ear, we must remember the anatomic landmarks; the helical insertion should be in line with the outer canthus of the eye, the lobule insertion at the level of the commissure of the mouth, and the tragus in line with the ala of the nose.

Operation. Reconstruction of marked deformities of the ear[10] is one of the most difficult and extensive—as well as extended—procedures which the plastic surgeon is called upon to make. It is wise to think in terms of a minimum of 3 to 8 stages. Trying to utilize all bits of available tissue is a real challenge to the surgical imagination.

As a rule, the *first stage* involves rotation of the lobule to its normal location and the repositioning of some of the soft tissues. In this procedure an attempt should be made to lay down a foundation of soft tissue that will

permit the surgical reconstruction which is to follow.

The *next stage* consists of the implantation of a sharply contoured cartilage graft, carved to resemble the landmarks of a normal ear. This may be preserved or autogenous cartilage. An incision is made, usually superior and slightly posterior to the gross outline of the ear; through this a pocket is developed by blunt dissection, taking care to avoid bleeding. The graft is then inserted into this pocket, the incision is closed by interrupted sutures, and a pressure dressing is applied.

After the graft has been in place for $2\frac{1}{2}$ to 4 months, it is safe to elevate the newly formed ear, including the cartilage graft, exposing the tissue adherent to its posterior surface. A skin graft may then be applied to the posterior surface of the cartilage graft. If the curved helix is unsatisfactory and the outline fails to imitate a normal ear, a small tube pedicle from the skin of the neck may be attached around the outer margin to round it into a more acceptable contour.

Recently accumulated evidence shows that preserved cartilage is not always entirely satisfactory. Much of this evidence points to the desirability of using the patient's own cartilage, which, of course, entails at least one more major operation. Autogenous cartilage is undoubtedly always preferable, but there is the price to pay of difficulty in procuring it, as well as possible complications. It is perhaps safer to establish, with the consent of the family, a waiting period of at least 6 months between the time of implanting the cartilage and the time of elevating it and applying the skin graft behind it. At the time of the implantation of the cartilage, apply a type of dressing which makes the skin conform to the undulations of the cartilage graft, so that it will adhere and the landmarks show. It is important to develop an accurate technic for applying dressings, for this must be done perfectly; otherwise one runs the risk of applying too little pressure in some areas, allowing accumulation of serum and subsequent complications, or, worse yet, too much pressure over the high points, which will result in necrosis and slough (Fig. 35).

At the time of elevating the cartilage for the reception of a skin graft, by all means avoid exposing the cartilage, and again remember the axiom that *the thinner the cartilage* for the graft, *the better the outlook*. In the hands of a few of those who have attempted it, the technic of Peer in developing cartilaginous outlines out of *diced cartilage* has given satisfactory results. (We must confess that we have never mastered this technic to our own satisfaction.)

In the various stages of reconstruction, be constantly aware of the possibility of injuring the facial nerve, for anatomic landmarks are likely to be grossly distorted in most of these patients. Whenever possible, dissect with the benefit of a nerve-stimulating apparatus. Other complications which may confront the surgeon in this type of reconstruction are (1) resorption of cartilage; (2) hematoma; (3) infection; and (4) necrosis, either from poor circulation or too much pressure.

LOP EAR

This defect is basically an overdevelopment of the entire ear with underdevelopment of the antihelix. It may be associated with a cupping deformity which exaggerates the protruding effect of the cartilaginous support.

Operation. The proposed antihelix is

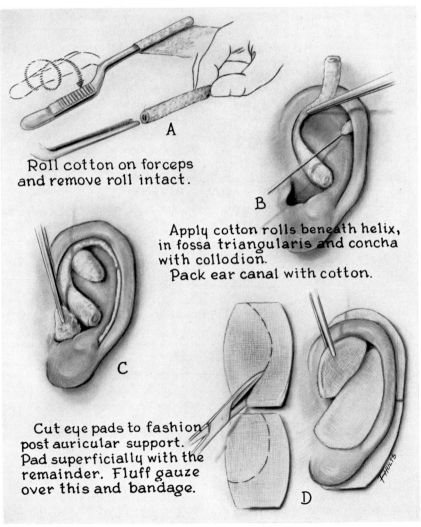

FIG. 35. Manner of dressing the ear. Pressure dressing over this.

marked with through-and-through punctures of needles dipped in methylene blue. Incisions are made in the postauricular skin and the perichondrium is then elevated. The cartilage may then be scored in order to break its spring along the dye-marked, underdeveloped antihelix line. The ear is brought into a backward position and there fixed by appropriate sutures.

Errors and Pitfalls. Local anesthesia is preferable for better dissection and minimal bleeding. Avoid "buttonholing" the skin over the anterior surface of the ear when scoring the cartilage. Place trial stitches of nonabsorbable suture material, without tying, to determine the exact appearance and position of the ear before placing permanent sutures.

Dressings are vitally important following this operation. Without the use of proper dressings over an adequate period of time, the whole procedure may fail (Fig. 11). It is wise to apply a pressure dressing and keep it on for a full month following the operation. The dressing should be designed to avoid twisting of the ear while the patient is sleeping.

Complications. These may include (1) slough from a dressing which has been applied too tightly or from too tight sutures; (2) hematoma; (3) chondritis; (4) infection; (5) palsy of the facial nerve from pressure or direct damage.

PTOSIS OF THE EYELID

Ptosis may be partial or complete, unilateral or bilateral.[5] It may be a congenital deformity, post-traumatic, postparalytic or associated with other disease conditions such as metastatic lesions. In evaluating patients with this condition, make a careful examination to determine (1) the cause; (2) the associated disturbance of all residual motion and whether or not it results from defects of the musculature (the *levator palpebrae* and associated movement in the *frontalis* muscle); (3) the amount of vision which exists (before operation); (4) the age and the general condition of the patient.

Operation. In general, there are 3 types of operation to improve this condition: (1) supportive-sling procedures; (2) attachment of the lid to the superior rectus muscle; and (3) shortening of the levator palpebrae muscles.

In our hands, repair has always been accomplished by means of the fascial-sling operation, since this is more truly a reconstructive procedure. We feel that the other operations cited should be carried out by a qualified ophthalmologist. This applies whether the condition be partial, complete, unilateral or bilateral.

The normal position of the lid is covering the upper iris, the ciliary margin being between the upper edge of the pupil and the upper rim of the iris. In doing the fascial-sling type of correction, be sure to insert the fascia at the proper level above the ciliary margin and to bury it under the frontalis at a point which will be correct in length. The two arms of the fascia should be directed upward from their points of insertion above the ciliary margin of the lid, going deep in the soft tissues to penetrate the muscle beneath the eyebrow at a suitable depth and to emerge above the brow through incisions which are just at its upper level. The fascia should be inserted into the substance of the muscle in order to secure a firm attachment and achieve animation through the pull of the sling to the eyelid below. The tautness of the sling should be sufficient at first to overcorrect the position of the upper lid so that the ciliary margin is above the upper border of the iris. When edema has subsided, downward pull on the lid usually results in a position which is approximately normal.

Following the operation, the eyes should be protected continuously with an antibiotic ointment which is not injurious to the cornea. An eye shield should be worn constantly for several days postoperatively to avoid corneal abrasion.

FACIAL HEMIATROPHY

The cause of this spectacular deformity, which leaves in its wake a distorted, underdeveloped half of the face, has not yet been determined. In planning correction, always remember that the defect is dual. Repair should be aimed not only at counteracting the result of the arrested growth on one side but also at balancing it with the normal growth on the unopposed, opposite side, since otherwise the defect increases as the victim grows. Correction of this defect necessarily entails a certain amount of compromise in each case. It invariably calls for a multiple-stage procedure, consisting of building up contour by means of transplanted homogenous or autogenous material either of one or a combination of types (such as bone, cartilage or dermofat grafts). In using dermofat grafts, always remember that there will be 30 to 50 per cent resorption, and *overcorrect* correspondingly. Extreme care should always be used to avoid infection subsequent to the implantation of tissues. A firm pressure dressing should be applied for at least 4 weeks. Antibiotics should be used in large doses. Try to avoid the formation of abscesses in the face of liquefaction of fat.

PORT-WINE STAINS

There has been considerable discussion about the proper treatment of these unsightly birthmarks. In many places *nothing* is done, because heretofore all approaches entailed a certain amount of compromise. The end-result may well be the substitution of a grotesque deformity for the initial condition. When the lesion is characterized by a moderate degree of coloration, it is questionable whether surgery is indicated; a pigmented cosmetic may be used to advantage instead. Some authors recommend the use of a *split-thickness graft* after excision of the involved area. This is always a compromise, because large grafts of this type almost always contract considerably in healing, and one deformity is merely being substituted for another. *Tattooing* has been recommended in some quarters, but again this usually results in a more marked defect. In many instances *gradual partial excision* of the involved areas has produced good results (Ferris Smith). Blair favors a *full-thickness graft* in order to obtain a better color match and less contraction. Other authors feel that the best treatment is *surgical excision* and filling of the defect with a *pedicle-flap transplant.*

RETROGNATHIA

This condition is a congenital defect[3, 6] which varies in degree, consisting, in mild cases, of a slight recession of the chin, and in extreme instances, of sufficient retrusion to represent a serious hazard to life in the newborn. It is frequently found in association with cleft palate or harelip (q.v.). In the severe form, we frequently see a posterior prolapse of the tongue with marked interference with respiration, particularly when the baby lies on its back. If the situation is not corrected promptly, death may result. The child should be watched constantly and should always be kept on his abdomen. When such urgency exists, we suggest correction by the method of Beverly Douglas, which is, in effect, a surgical adhesion between the inferior surface of the tip of the tongue and its anterior third and the surface of the lower lip. This is frequently a lifesaving measure. If there is still a question of respiratory interference, do a *tracheotomy*. Feeding can be extremely difficult in these infants, making correction still more urgent.

A procedure which can be quite efficacious in overcoming maldevelopment of the lower jaw is to place the baby on a device referred to as a "bottle crutch." This is a mechanism attached to the feeding bottle in such a manner that a metallic bar rests on the upper lip, holding the nipple sufficiently far from the normal sucking position to make the baby reach forward with his lower lip and jaw in his attempt to grasp it. If this is used consistently over a period of time, it is amazing to see what rapid growth of the underdeveloped lower jaw will result.

SYNDACTYLISM

Parents should be cautioned that syndactylism is one deformity that is strongly hereditary. Congenital defects involving the extremities have a greater tendency to pass from one generation to the next than almost any other type of anomaly. For this reason, parents with such defects should be warned to expect abnormality in at least some of their children. The condition may vary from a partial web between 2 fingers to a complete web enveloping several fingers or even an entire hand, as well as partially amputated or completely missing fingers. In some instances the hand will also show an extra digit.

Because of the variety of these defects, each case is an individual problem. Wherever possible, correction should include the use of a portion of each web to fashion a skin-flap cover for as much of the defect as possible. Almost all require additional skin grafts. Where the webs are tight and the use of flaps is limited, a larger graft is indicated. The

neurovascular bundle and the tendinous attachments, as well as the joint capsule, should
not be disturbed. Operation should be deferred
until the child is between 3½ and 5 years of
age, unless the web comes down to the distal
end of 2 fingers of disparate length. In these
instances, growth of the longer finger will be
hindered and modified by the disproportion
with the shorter one; consequently, early
separation between the distal phalanges should
be carried out to allow more normal development. It is axiomatic to avoid a ventral scar,
i.e., to locate the scar on the side of the finger
whenever possible and to try to break up a
linear scar. When embryonic amputation of
the fingers has occurred, length can be added
by tubed pedicles and subsequent bone grafts.
This procedure improves both function and
the cosmetic effect. The tubed pedicles should
be so designed that innervation runs normally
from the stump of the fingers distally in order
to allow for possible later neurotization and
restoration of sensation.

HYPOSPADIAS

Correction of hypospadias has a long historic background, evidenced by approximately
150 authors all of whom claim some degree
of originality in surgical repair. Almost all of
these procedures are based on an initial stage
to correct the *chordee*.

Operation. There are 5 general types of
operations employed to correct this deformity:

1. Free graft of tissue wrapped around a
urethral mold and subsequently buried in the
penile tissues. Our objections to these operations are (a) difficulty in insertion and fixation; (b) difficulty of maintaining uniform
pressure; (c) accumulation of blood clots;
(d) fistulization and possible subsequent contracture of the graft.

2. Stretching or freeing up of the urethra
in an attempt to draw the free portion out to
the glans penis. The major objections to this
procedure are (a) increase of the ventral deformity with growth; (b) limitation of the
operation to those cases involving only penile
hypospadias; (c) tendency to contracture and
stenosis at the distal end of the urethra;
(d) possibility of inadequate blood supply
which may result in necrosis with loss of a
portion of the urethra.

3. Reconstruction of the urethra utilizing
a portion of penile skin for construction of a
urethral tube and penile skin flaps to cover
the neo-urethra. The difficulties in this procedure are (a) subsequent contracture; (b) fistulization; (c) necrosis of both the urethral
tube and the overlying skin flaps; (d) stenosis
of the distal end of the neo-urethra; (e) recurrence of the central curvature seen before
correction of chordee.

4. Reconstruction of the urethra by leaving
a strip of intact skin to epithelize into a complete urethral tube around the catheter, and
covering of this with a flap of penile skin
raised in advance from the side of the penis
and sutured over the strip.

Despite the recent popularity of this procedure, it is difficult to envision how an extremely long, intact, rectangular strip of epithelium, regardless of the adequacy of its
blood supply, can form a circular tube by
simply being covered with skin flaps. This
structure *may* function satisfactorily, but we
feel that a tube developed in this manner is
contrary to all the principles of tissue growth
which we have ever observed. Aside from
every other objection, this operation as a rule
requires diversion of the urinary stream.

5. Reconstruction of a urethra from penile
skin covered by means of scrotal skin flaps.

In our hands, reconstruction in this manner
has given the most consistently satisfactory
results.

EPISPADIAS AND EXTROPHY OF
THE BLADDER

Extrophy of the bladder presents one of
the most difficult problems in reconstructive
surgery of the genito-urinary tract. A patient
with this condition must undergo a long series
of major operations, regardless of the approach used.

Operation. Many surgeons advise ureteros-
tomy for diversion of the urinary stream, after
complete excision of the isolated bladder, and
prior to covering the defect by abdominal
flaps. This is perhaps the *easiest* approach.
A reconstruction which will preserve the bladder and the urethra is a far greater challenge,
yet offers much greater satisfaction to the
surgeon who can accomplish it. In some instances, by gradually dissecting and everting

the margins of the bladder into a fashioned bladder cavity, while, at the same time, shifting lateral flaps of soft tissue and skin from the midline, a reconstructed pouch to cover the exposed bladder can be made satisfactorily. One of the chief difficulties, aside from continuous contamination by urine and the resulting infection, is our inability to exert intracavity pressure in the newly formed bladder to expand its size. This is made the more difficult by absence of any sort of sphincter and the usual spread of the pelvic bones in the pubic regions where a pathologic separation always coexists. Subsequently, of course, one is faced with the problem of the epispadias and the production of some type of sphincter for urinary control; the sphincter is always missing in these cases. Use of the gracilis muscle is sometimes helpful. As a rule, correction of the epispadias may be carried out by simply suturing the margins of the tissue which goes into the formation of the epispadial urethra, but there is usually insufficient skin to bridge the defect with a roof over the built-up tube. However, some type of sphincter for urinary control is imperative.

COSMETIC SURGERY

Any approach to the field of cosmetic surgery must be undertaken first and foremost with a sincere understanding of the patient's problem from his own point of view. The surgeon must recognize that those seeking his help are unwilling or unable to accept and adjust to the reality of their deformities, be they congenital or acquired, real or imagined. Furthermore, it should be remembered that such a patient is deeply concerned and, not infrequently, vaguely resentful of what he considers a great personal misfortune. Therefore, it is obvious that the problem should be studied not only from the physical standpoint but also in terms of personality shortcomings and emotional instability, which, in many instances, may be considerably more crippling than the physical defect. It should also be borne in mind that latent or hidden personality defects are often dramatically brought out into the open after the completion of a cosmetic operation, most particularly if there are complications.

It behooves the cosmetic surgeon then to have a fully adequate background of training and experience not only in the technical aspects of his art but also in evaluation of such cases from an over-all point of view. Anyone who does cosmetic surgery is certainly aware of the medicolegal pitfalls which, in this day and age, are notorious. For this reason, the importance of explaining to the patient in detail exactly how much to expect and the limitations of this type of surgery cannot be overemphasized. It goes without saying that keeping careful and accurate records will pay in saving the surgeon possible untold headaches later on.

RHINOPLASTY

Classification of Deformities. 1. Congenital: hump nose, abnormal width associated with a bulbous or overhanging tip; partial or total absence of nose; cleft or bifid nose; various degrees of atresia of nostrils; defects due to prenatal disease, notably syphilis.

2. Acquired due to trauma: these are increasing at a tremendous rate with the increase in numbers of automobile accidents.

3. Postoperative: e.g., where portions of septal cartilage have been removed resulting in "saddle-back" defects.

4. Postinfectious: frequently the result of lues, septal abscess or other forms of disease causing necrosis of the septal cartilage and resulting in "saddle-back" defects; also from destruction by neoplasia, leprosy and other diseases.

5. Rhinophyma.

Operations. RHINOPLASTY. The standard operative procedure to correct congenital deformities of the nose has not varied to any considerable degree in the past 30 years. Basically, all these operations are directed toward achieving the same end, i.e., the reduction of the nasal hump, the adjustment and reduction of the lateral cartilages, infracturing or narrowing of the nose with or without shortening of the tip by the excision of a small portion of the inferior septal cartilaginous margin, and a reduction of the tip by revision of the alar cartilages.

SEPTAL RECONSTRUCTION OR REVISION. This operation should definitely be differentiated from *submucous resection* as commonly practiced by the otolaryngologist. The septal reconstruction as practiced by the plastic surgeon entails the freeing up of the mucous covering of the septal cartilage over the deviated anterior or posterior septum. In this manner the distorted septal cartilage is exposed, and all deviations from the norm are corrected by scoring or crosshatching the cartilage to replace it into the midline and in correct relation to the vomer. Any distortion of the bony septum is removed by excision of the blocking segment. Subsequently, the septal cartilage is fixed either with a suture or a pack so that it rests in the midline of the nose and re-establishes an adequate airway in each vestibule.

Precautions and Pitfalls. 1. Always plan the desired nasal reconstruction to match the particular face. Sedulously avoid the so-called "standard nose."

2. Prior to operation, the nose should be packed with cocaine and Adrenalin pack to effect adequate shrinking of the membranes and to lessen bleeding. Use local anesthesia whenever possible.

3. Remember that a more depressed bridge is found in children than in adults. Surgery should be delayed, when possible, until adolescence, remembering that the nose grows with the individual.

4. External incisions should always be avoided since they leave disfiguring scars. Intranasal surgery should not raise the incidence of infection.

5. The surgeon should always make minimal scars in the nasal vestibule in order to prevent contracture and should disturb the nasal physiology as little as possible.

6. When a surgeon is confronted with a problem involving a distorted septum in a nose which needs a rhinoplasty, generally he should attempt to do both operations together. Never excise the septum below the inferior border of a nasal bone if it can be avoided. It is the only support for that portion of the nose, and where this precaution is not heeded, a "saddle-back" deformity invariably will follow.

7. Posterior deviations may be resected at the time of a rhinoplasty or an anterior septum replaced in the midline, if no excision is indicated.

8. Do not fail to separate upper lateral cartilages from the septum, since they have a tendency to apply a "guy-wire" pull on the superior septal edge.

9. When removing a nasal hump, always in-fracture or the patient will have a flat, square dorsum.

10. In doing osteotomies of the maxillary bone, beware of injury to the lacrimal duct and the lacrimal sac. Go sufficiently low in making these osteotomies to avoid a shelving appearance externally.

11. Beware extensive or hard chiseling, as the chisel may go into the frontal sinus.

12. Keep in mind that (a) resection of the nasal hump lowers the profile; (b) in-fracturing narrows the nose; (c) excision of lower free ends of the septum shortens the nose and corrects the nasolabial angle; (d) trimming of the upper borders of the alar cartilages and defatting fashions the shape of the nasal tip and reduces bulbousness; (e) excision of the junction of the medial and the lateral crura of the alar cartilages shortens the length of the nasal tip; (f) trimming of the upper lateral cartilages reduces thickness through the sides of the nose above the tip.

13. Packing may or may not be used. If the septum is repositioned, always pack firmly. If there is any sign of bleeding at the end of the operation, always pack.

14. Beware of mucosal perforations in septal work. If one side is perforated, healing may occur; if both sides are perforated in positions which overlie each other, a permanent defect will result. Small perforations may be repaired; large ones cannot be.

15. Splinting is a "must" following rhinoplastic procedures.

16. The patient should wear a splint approximately 2 weeks, but during this period the nose should be scrupulously cleansed at regular intervals.

Reconstruction about the Nose. 1. Loss of nasal substance, if small, may be repaired by local flaps from the cheek or adjacent regions.

2. Always provide an adequate lining for nasal reconstruction when tissue is shifted over a defect involving the entire thickness of the nose. Unless this is done there will be shrinking and distortion.

3. Alar defects may be replaced by a pedi-

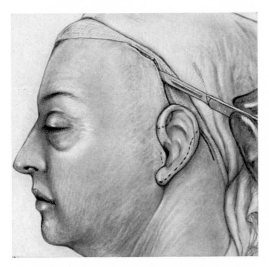

FIG. 36. Incision in the hairline and around the ear to hide all scars.

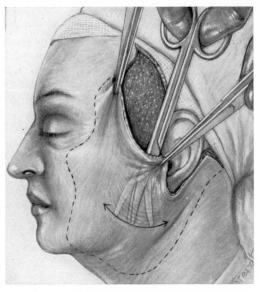

FIG. 37. Undermining. Note extent.

cle from near or far, or from compound grafts from the ears.

4. Major defects must be repaired by tissue brought out from other regions than those adjacent to the nose. In selecting tissue to repair these defects, keep in mind the necessity for accurate color match. Where possible, forehead flaps are preferable. If forehead flaps are not available, one may have to resort to a substitution of tissue from the neck, since this area gives reasonably satisfactory color and texture match. Where this tissue is not available, one may have to fall back on the Italian method of using skin from the inner side of the arm. It should be understood and explained to the patient that there will be some variation in color following such transplantation.

5. "Saddle-back" deformity may be repaired by cartilage or bone grafts. Autogenous grafts are always best. Where glabella and maxillary sinus supports are available, L-shaped cancellous bone from the hip is excellent.

Nasal Fractures. 1. Roentgenograms may or may not be of value. Frequently an adequate diagnosis can be made by observation and palpation.

2. A lateral blow may cause septal displacement and dislocation of the vomer.

3. Frontal blows produce severe septal fracture dislocation with flattening of the nose and telescoping of fragments.

4. Source of bleeding should be located as soon as possible and hemostasis effected immediately. A fractured septum cannot be adequately reduced in the face of active hemorrhage.

5. Cocaine and Adrenalin packs should be applied in the nose if there is troublesome oozing.

6. Always clip the hair from inside the nose before attempting any sort of manipulation or surgery. Otherwise you will find a nasty coagulum at the first dressing.

7. Where possible, reduce the fracture in a manner which causes the least amount of added trauma to the nose. Frequently it is possible to reduce some of these fractures by thumb pressure. In cases where this is not possible, use the Walsham forceps to dislodge impacted fragments. In this event, always look for displacement of the septal cartilage. When found, replace it in its anatomic position by a simultaneous upward lift and lateral shift.

8. After manipulation of a fractured nose, a splint should be applied; postoperative treatment is identical with that of any rhinoplasty.

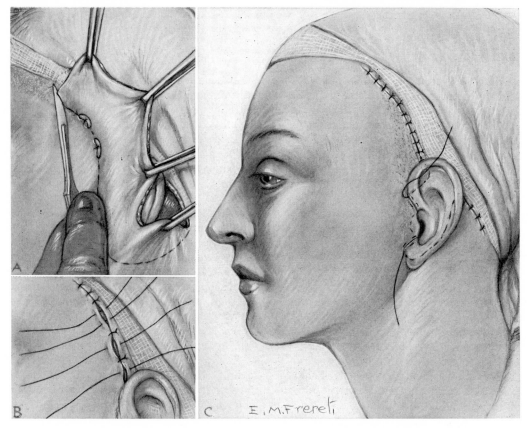

Fig. 38. (A) Excising excess skin. (B) Anchor sutures. (C) Final result.

9. When rhinorrhea is evident, *do not manipulate!*

10. After a displaced septum has been relocated correctly, always insert a pack.

Complications. HEMORRHAGE. 1. When hemorrhage occurs, the first requisites are to procure good light and to institute suction.

2. Insertion of an Adrenalin pack with pressure is usually sufficient to effect hemostasis.

3. In the face of posterior bleeding, it may be necessary to use a bolus pack through the pharynx (Figs. 33 and 34).

4. Beware slow postnasal hemorrhage which is swallowed and does not show up until the patient vomits large clots or goes into shock.

INFECTION. It goes without saying that this should be avoided and all precautions taken to prevent it. Fortunately, with the advent of antibiotics, its incidence is lessened considerably.

STRUCTURAL AND MECHANICAL DIFFICULTIES. 1. There may be loss of the sense of smell and consequently of taste following extensive injuries to the nose.

2. There may be trouble in breathing.

3. Changes in nasal physiology may result from scarring or perforation.

4. The nares may be excessively narrowed.

5. Chiseling too high on the side of the nose may give a shelving appearance over the infracture line.

6. There may be interference with lacrimal function.

DISTANT SEQUELAE. 1. Embolism or atelectasis.

2. Pneumonia or empyema.

3. Psychic disturbance.

WRINKLES

The skin may lose elasticity because of advancing age and the changes incident to it. Loss of elasticity related to rapid loss of weight is also seen. Patients so affected frequently present severe personality problems and, because of them, are extremely hard to please. They should all be warned of the limitations of the corrective procedure and should be cautioned in every instance that the results may not be permanent since their tissues are showing changes inevitable with advancing years.

Operation (Figs. 36, 37 and 38). 1. The principle of repair in these cases is (a) wide undermining and pulling to normal tension after (b) excision of the excess skin with (c) an approximation suture of the defect following the excision.

2. Undermining should be on a subcutaneous plane and should go to the nasolabial fold medially and to the mandible inferiorly in order to achieve maximum correction.

3. Eyelid wrinkles are corrected in much the same way, except that not only should the excess skin be removed but also the herniation of infra-orbital fat (frequently associated with eyelid "bags") should also be corrected. Scrupulously avoid the removal of *too much* skin, as this may result in ectropion.

Errors and Pitfalls. 1. Tension must be judged carefully, otherwise an expressionless mask may result. In appraising this, take into consideration the distention which results from local anesthesia.

2. In correcting wrinkles of the eyelid, be very careful about measurements, otherwise ectropion may follow.

3. Always beware the possibility of damage to the facial nerve. It is frequently advisable to use a nerve stimulator while dissecting.

4. Scars can and should be completely hidden along the line of the ear and in the hairline.

5. Do not perform surgery in the presence of dermatitis or any sort of inflammatory reaction, and beware the hazards of *dyed hair*.

6. During operation seek complete and perfect hemostasis.

7. Subsequent to operation, adequate pressure dressings should be applied to avoid formation of hematomata.

8. Incisions should be supported for several weeks to avoid *scar spread*.

PITTING SCARS OF THE FACE

Abrasion is highly effective in the improvement of old, quiescent acne scars, scars resulting from smallpox and freckles. This procedure should be done in several stages, as excessive abrasion can result in complete skin loss. For this reason it is advisable to explain this to the patient beforehand and to be guided by his desire for subsequent procedures. Care should be taken to determine whether or not a patient is liable to keloid formation; otherwise, a horrible masking defect may follow. We advise the use of hand abrasion for various reasons, the most important being that accuracy is difficult to achieve with the use of machine-driven abrasives. After frank bleeding is encountered, proceed with the utmost caution and level only superficial pits; *do not attempt to remove all pits at one sitting. Never* abrade nevi or cutaneous lesions.

Firm pressure dressings over Merthiolate rayon gauze should be applied and maintained for at least 10 days. This dressing should not be removed mechanically, as it will destroy the regenerating epithelium. The dressing will dry completely after a few days and is easily removed with cold cream. Patients should be warned that they will have a *red skin* for as long as 6 weeks to 3 months.

One should use an abrasive that shows the least amount of shedding. The skin should be thoroughly washed at the completion of the treatment.

Consider modified face lifting after maximum abrasion has been done, as this will place the skin under more normal tension, thus minimizing any remaining pit scars.

MAMMAPLASTY

This procedure is performed for simple hypertrophy or excessive sagging of the breasts. Remember that simple hypertrophy can be acutely uncomfortable for the patient. It can limit activity. It can cause great misery from the pull of brassière straps as well as chafing and irritation beneath the breasts, especially in hot weather. Even psychic disturbance may develop as a result.

A mammaplasty must be planned carefully

and carried out with the utmost care. Circulation is variable in anatomic location and must be appraised individually. The optimum aim is to (1) restore breasts to normal size; (2) give adequate support to the glands; (3) restore normal position of breast on thorax; (4) restore nipples to normal location.

Operation. There are numerous types of breast operations, all having in common (1) careful preoperative markings in both supine and upright positions; (2) dissecting the areola free from surrounding skin and either leaving it attached to the gland or making a free nipple transplant by dissecting it off as a full-thickness graft; (3) incising and wide undermining of skin flaps; (4) excision of redundant breast tissue from quadrants where circulation will be least affected; (5) excision of excess skin; (6) fixation of breast glands for support; (7) fashioning a skin brassière from remaining underlying flaps and suturing.

The operation described by Robert J. Wise for correction of severe hypertrophy of the breast is perhaps the best that has been devised. In our opinion, it offers the most accurate planning and gives the most consistently satisfactory results.

Errors and Pitfalls. 1. The skin must be undermined carefully at the proper planes, otherwise necrosis may follow.

2. Do not interfere with the circulation of the nipple if it is to be left attached during the procedure.

3. Placement of nipples must be symmetrical.

4. If free transplant is used, a better chance of complete "take" is assured if recipient site is not dissected out to full thickness of the skin. In this manner, the nipple is applied to partially denuded skin rather than to fat only.

5. Drainage is frequently valuable.

6. Dress with firm pressure and keep the patient quiet in bed for at least 1 week. In the event of considerable hemorrhage, replace this blood loss to assure adequate healing.

7. Patients should be warned of the probable effects on the results of pregnancy and lactation.

Complications. These are (1) slough resulting from interference with circulation; (2) hematoma—when it develops, always evacuate; (3) liquefaction of fat with drainage; (4) infection and abscess; (5) destruction due to tension, slough, poor healing or a combination of any or all of these.

TRANSPLANTATION OF TISSUE

The science of transplantation has grown tremendously during the past 10 years and has been the subject of much active research. It has been established conclusively that it is extremely hazardous and unjustified to use imbedded ivory, paraffin or other foreign materials of this nature. Where the need for transplanted tissue to build out contours or to correct defects of contour is obvious, always turn to the patient's own living tissue. Foreign implants are practically always rejected by the system, with considerable inflammatory reaction, separations, slough and abundant scarring.

DEFINITIONS

Free Graft. A transplanted portion of tissue which is completely detached from its original site and transferred to another area, depending for its blood supply on the area to which it has been transferred.

Compound Graft. A graft consisting of more than one tissue element, such as skin with cartilage or subcutaneous tissue with bone.

Flap.[9] A segment bearing full-thickness skin with its underlying tissue and carrying its own blood supply, which is attached at a site where it can develop a new blood supply before the original one from its base is severed.

Autograft (autogenous graft). A graft obtained from the body of the same person in which it is being implanted.

Homograft (homogenous graft). A graft obtained from another individual of the same species.

Heterograft (heterogenous graft). A graft obtained from an individual of another species.

Simple Flap. A flap consisting of skin and subcutaneous tissue only.

Compound Flap. A flap containing cartilage or bone in its structure.

Open Flap. A flap with a raw surface uncovered.

Blind Flap. A flap with a raw surface grafted.

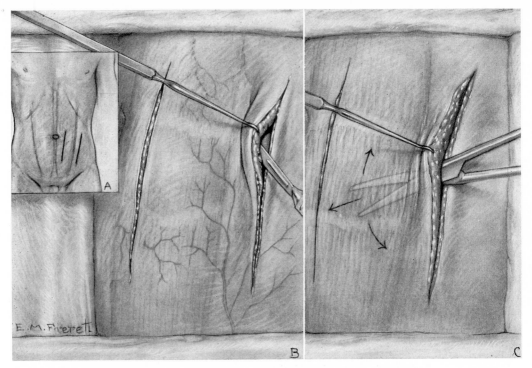

Fig. 39. (A) Selection of site preferably over specific vessels. (B) Incisions. (C) Undermining in subcutaneous plane.

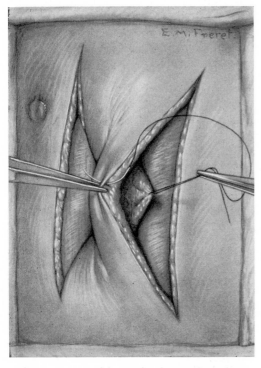

Fig. 40. Anchor stitch inserted to begin tubing.

Tubed Flap. A flap with its edges sutured to each other (Figs. 39 to 43).

SKIN

Skin may be transplanted in any thickness from *epidermis only* to *full thickness*. In general, the thinner the graft, the better the chance of a "take," but the greater the subsequent contracture and the less stable the final result. The converse is also true.

Skin grafting is the most rapid and effective method of converting an enlarged, denuded surface into a closed wound, provided that there is enough circulation to maintain the transplant. Grafting may be a lifesaving procedure; when there is not sufficient autogenous material available, one may have to resort to homografts as a temporary substitute.

Free Grafts. To obtain the graft: (1) pick donor site for best color match; (2) if there is a choice, select a site which will cause the least cosmetic damage (e.g., the lower abdomen or buttock); (3) if a greater amount of graft is cut than is needed to cover the defect, the excess should be placed in a sterile container and stored in a freezer in order to estab-

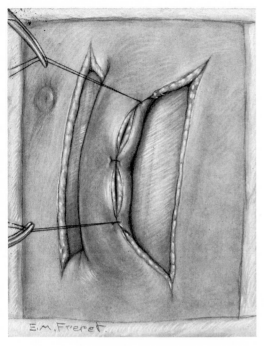

Fig. 41. Anchor stitches in each corner for eversion of tube.

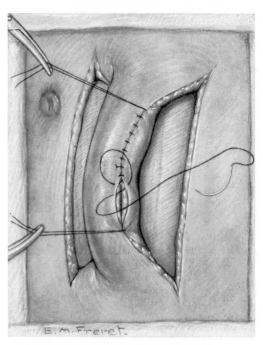

Fig. 42. Suture completed.

lish a "skin bank" for this particular patient in the event that some portion of the graft fails; (4) beware the variable thickness of proposed donor sites in different parts of the body, since age and location affect the thickness of the skin; (5) avoid the use of harsh chemicals in preparing the skin and the donor sites; ether, alcohol and a very dilute solution of iodine are quite adequate; (6) beware the use of detergent or soap on donor sites, since the dermatome glue will not hold on a surface with even a thin film of soap.

CARTILAGE

Cartilage is an ideal supporting material which may be successfully transplanted and which, as a rule, is readily available. It may be used also as an autogenous transplant from a living donor or from a cadaver. It is easily carved or diced. It is fairly rigid and does not change shape (unless absorbed) and may be used either as a supporting pillar in blocks or struts or it may be diced as a filler to build out concave defects. Its commonest uses are

in the reconstruction of the ear, the correction of a "saddle-back" defect of the nose or the correction of depressed defects in the orbital rim.

Precautions and Pitfalls. 1. There is mounting evidence that homogenous preserved (banked) cartilage is very likely to be absorbed. Autogenous cartilage from the patient's ribs is to be preferred when available and is mandatory when preserved implants have been absorbed. Maternal ear cartilage has been tried, but the incidence of curling and absorption indicate that it is not the ideal choice.

2. Make sure that all implants are covered adequately by soft tissue. If cartilage is left exposed, infection usually occurs and is most difficult to control.

3. Observe a cartilage graft for evidence of resorption for 3 to 6 months before continuing with further work.

4. The best preserved cartilage from a cadaver is found in individuals 14 to 40 years of age. Always ascertain that the material is *free from blood- or lymph-borne disease* which might be transmitted.

BONE

Volumes have been written on the use of bone grafts;[8] the reader is referred to the current literature for details.

Bone is the tissue of choice where one rigid support is needed (e.g., in jaw work). Ideally, bone should be replaced by bone, when the patient is young enough to have still intact his bony regenerating and substituting mechanisms. Contact should be made between fresh and grafted bone. Bone grafts may be used only where there is no existing or potential infection. Most schools of thought hold that bone cells are substituted by the host, and only the framework of the graft remains. If periosteum is present, vascularization and solidification occur more readily. However, it is not essential for success of the graft. Probably the best source for bone graft is the ilium,[4] since it is easier to get at and subjects the patient to less hazard than the removal of a graft from a rib or a leg. Bone may be used as a strut support or, as cancellous chips, for filler material.

Precautions and Pitfalls. One must always (1) be sure that the grafts are in contact with living bone; (2) be sure of immobilization and fixation; and (3) avoid infection at all costs.

DERMIS AND FAT

These grafts are used mostly as filler material for soft tissue voids. Sources of supply

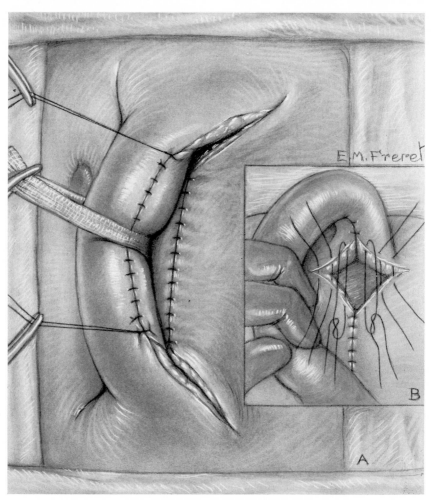

FIG. 43. (A) Donor site closed primarily by undermining and approximation. (B) Manner of closing corners.

are plentiful, the most common being the lower abdomen. Fat is extremely prone to liquefaction and infection; anticipate shrinkage of 30 to 50 per cent in any fat graft and remember the necessity for *overcorrection.*

Precautions and Pitfalls. 1. Beware of infection; strict asepsis is essential. Heavy dosages of antibiotics are routine.

2. If liquefaction occurs, it should be removed promptly with a syringe; avoid, if possible, the insertion of a drain.

3. Firm pressure is important, but excessive pressure may hasten necrosis.

4. Where dermis is implanted, the dermal side should be placed outward to facilitate drainage of possible sebaceous collections.

5. Never make incisions directly over implant sites; always cut away from the defect. Undermine, draw the graft into place with Keith needles, and secure by passing sutures from the graft through the skin and tying over a gauze bolus.

Fascia

The principal use of fascia grafts is to make slings for support in postparalytic corrections. The usual source for this material is the iliotibial band. The advantages of fascia are (1) it is readily available; (2) it affords a tough, living, homogenous tissue which does not resorb or change; (3) it may be used as living ligature on a carrier instrument.

Foreign Substances

There is no room in plastic surgery for *organic* foreign materials such as paraffin, ivory, etc. This has been pointed out previously. Active research for a rigid and pliable substitute for such implant materials is being carried out; among those being tried are:

1. Vitallium. This is a strong, light, inert material which is used extensively in neurosurgical work for replacement of skull defects and in orthopedic work in reconstruction of joints.

2. Acrylic. This is a tough, inert, plastic material frequently used in orthopedic work.

3. Polyvinyl Sponge. This has been employed chiefly as a space filler and is being used experimentally at present. In many instances this material has reacted unfavorably, and there is evidence to support the possibility that it may even play a role in the later production of cancer.

Research is now being carried out on the inert textile materials, such as Nylon, for reconstruction of blood vessels and ureters. These uses are all still in the experimental stage.

REFERENCES

1. Adams, W. M., and Adams, L. H.: The misuse of the prolabium in the repair of bilateral cleft lip, Plast. & Reconstruct. Surg. **12**:225, 1953.
2. Brauer, R.: A consideration of the Le-Mesurier technic of single harelip repair, Plast. & Reconstruct. Surg. **12**:275, 1953.
3. Converse, J. M., and Shapiro, H. H.: Treatment of developmental malformations of the jaws, Plast. & Reconstruct. Surg. **10**:473, 1952.
4. Dingman, R. O.: The use of iliac bone in the repair of facial and cranial defects, Plast. & Reconstruct. Surg. **6**:179, 1950.
5. Figi, F. A.: Plastic surgery of the eyelids, Plast. & Reconstruct. Surg. **5**:403, 1950.
6. Kazanjian, V. H.: Secondary deformities of cleft palate, Plast. & Reconstruct. Surg. **8**:477, 1951.
7. Kitlowski, E. A.: The treatment of keloids and keloidal scars, Plast. & Reconstruct. Surg. **12**:38, 1953.
8. Peer, L. A.: Autogenous bone transplants in humans, Plast. & Reconstruct. Surg. **13**:56, 1954.
9. Smith, F.: Flaps utilized in facial and cervical reconstruction, Plast. & Reconstruct. Surg. **7**:415, 1951.
10. Steffensen, W. H.: Comments on the total reconstruction of the ear, Plast. & Reconstruct. Surg. **10**:186, 1952.
11. ———: Further experience with the rectangular flap operation for cleft lip, Plast. & Reconstruct. Surg. **11**:49, 1953.
12. Webster, J. P., and Crawford, J. R.: Congenital dermoid cysts of the nose, Plast. & Reconstruct. Surg. **9**:235, 1952.

EMANUEL M. SKOLNIK, M.D., and DAVID O. DALE, M.D.

5   The Neck

Those who undertake such major surgery as laryngectomy, neck dissection for removal of potentially fatal new growths or en bloc dissections must be constantly aware of the vital importance of an accurate anatomic knowledge of the field before accepting the responsibility of treatment of any patient for metastatic or other surgical disease involving the neck area. This may seem to be a truism, but, in view of the evidence, it cannot be repeated too often.

The procedures to be discussed here include tracheotomy, laryngectomy and those neck dissections which are concerned primarily with the preservation of life and only secondarily with cosmesis. However, where feasible, technical errors, particularly in areas where disfiguring scars and defects will be so obvious, should be avoided on esthetic grounds.

It is pertinent to review the anatomic reasons for those complications which may occur during and subsequent to surgery of the neck, as well as to suggest safeguards. The indications for tracheotomy, laryngectomy and neck dissections, as well as the technics of these

operations, are well standardized, hence they will not be included in this discussion. For purposes of simplicity and emphasis, sources of damage to related structures will be discussed in detail; these encompass the rich vascular supply, the muscle masses and their function, the nervous elements, miscellaneous structures and scars.

TRACHEOTOMY

When performed in extreme emergency, this lifesaving procedure is primarily concerned with *establishing an airway*, regardless of the ultimate cosmetic effect. The simplest method is to plunge a knife blade into the cricothyroid membrane—the area palpable inferior to the thyroid cartilage ("Adam's apple") in the region of the midline of the neck. This crude technic should be avoided if possible because of the danger of injuring the important complete ring of cricoid cartilage. However, if this approach is most expedient at the moment, a low tracheotomy should be substituted, as soon as the patient's condition permits, to minimize the danger of destruction

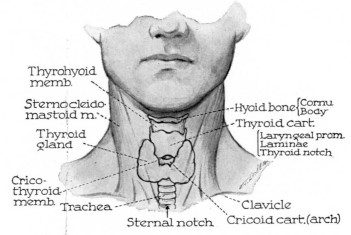

FIG. 44. The bony and cartilaginous framework of the neck (Thorek, P.: Anatomy in Surgery, Philadelphia, Lippincott).

of the cricoid by infection. The only imperative safeguard at this time is to control bleeding from the cricothyroid vessels which run parallel with the superior border of the cricoid cartilage in the cricothyroid membrane.

The conventional tracheotomy is through a midline incision in the center of Jackson's triangle (Fig. 44), an area having as its base the cricoid cartilage, its apex at the suprasternal notch, and as its lateral borders, the sternomastoid muscles. To replace an emergency operation by a tranquil procedure, an airway may be established by inserting an intratracheal tube or a bronchoscope through the obstructed pharynx or larynx. This eliminates the hazard of obstruction during the dissection and is of particular value in infants and children, as well as in adults for whom the tracheotomy is being performed because of a tumor in the neck. The approach of choice is a collar incision, as this is considered by some to leave a less obvious scar. The vertical cut through the skin extends from the inferior border of the thyroid cartilage to the suprasternal notch. Frequently this results in marked contracture of the skin, with resultant difficulty later on. In the male patient, shaving may become a problem. If the contracture is severe, any of several procedures may have to be employed to correct this disfigurement.

With either incision, the dissection is carried downward to the midline through the fascial planes to expose the thyroid isthmus. The only blood vessels of importance here are the anterior jugulars and their communicating veins that may cross the field of surgery (Fig. 45). These should be clamped, ligated and cut before proceeding. The strap muscles of the neck are not involved in this surgery, other than to retract them to gain adequate exposure of the field. If the thyroid isthmus obstructs the view, it is best to clamp it in the midline, cut and then suture the severed ends for hemostasis and to facilitate exposure of the trachea. At this point of the operation, avoid marked lateral dissection in order to safeguard against the development of subcutaneous emphysema or mediastinitis. After a suitable tracheotomy tube has been inserted, the skin incision is sutured loosely, the edges near the tube being left open to permit drainage and to eliminate a complicating subcutaneous emphysema which could prove to be a considerable hazard.

NECK DISSECTION AND LARYNGECTOMY

These two procedures are so closely allied that we may consider the principal complications and safeguards relative to both within this discussion. Damage to muscles represents

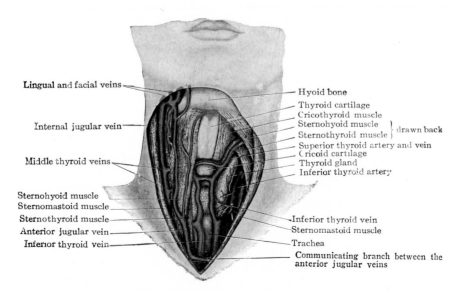

Fig. 45. Diagram showing parts involved in operations on thyroid gland and air passages. (Davis: Applied Anatomy, Philadelphia, Lippincott)

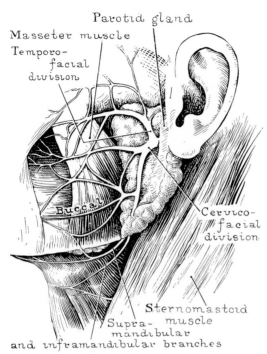

Parotid gland
Masseter muscle
Temporo-
    facial
    division
Buccal
Cervico-
facial
division
Sternomastoid
    muscle
Supra-
    mandibular
and inframandibular branches

FIG. 46. Diagram showing anatomy of facial nerve where it passes through parotid gland; anterior portion of gland removed. (After Sistrunk)

the least incapacitating injury, and in planned operations. such as neck dissection, the sterno-cleidomastoid and omohyoid muscles are, of necessity, sacrificed. In laryngectomy, as a rule the strap muscles are also sacrificed, since this is usually a wide-field procedure. In either case, this loss produces only a very mild deformity which is justified in the light of the gravity of the condition being treated. Loss of the digastric and stylohyoid muscles in neck dissections and removal of the sterno-thyroid and sternohyoid muscles in resections of the larynx or the thyroid afflicted with malignant disease results in nothing worse than loss of tissue bulk with practically no deformity.

The nerves traversing the field of dissection are the most important structures as regards possible postoperative complications. The sensory nerves from the cervical plexus are not significant and must be severed in order to reach the main field of operation. The first

important nerve encountered in either neck dissection or laryngectomy is the mandibular branch of the facial (Fig. 46), which frequently is injured when the upper skin flap is prepared, rather than, as many believe, during dissection of the tail of the parotid gland. Injury to this nerve produces drooping of the corner of the lip and frequently causes difficulty in chewing. Drooling of saliva from that corner of the mouth also causes considerable concern to the patient. This difficulty may be avoided by making the incision at least 3/4 of an inch below the mandible.

Anatomically, the mandibular branch lies in the region of the mandible and crosses the external maxillary vessels just beneath the platysma muscle. This muscle is a valuable landmark in that all the important vessels and nerves lie beneath it, and there is no danger of damage to these vital structures until this muscle is cut.

After preparation of the flap, the neck dissection is started from below. The omohyoid muscle is identified and is significant in that it locates the area of the middle layer of deep cervical fascia and further aids in fascial-plane dissection, helping to avoid injury to the phrenic nerve which is related to the deep layer of cervical fascia (prevertebral).

As the areolar tissues are elevated from the retroclavicular area, the next nerves encountered are those of the brachial plexus. The upper, most lateral cord is the one most often severed in this dissection. However, when one keeps clear of the deep layer of cervical fascia, the brachial plexus does not present a serious threat of complications. During medial dissection, after the posterior triangle has been cleaned out, the sternocleidomastoid muscle is severed at its attachment to the clavicle, and the internal jugular vein is identified. This large vessel is carefully dissected free from the surrounding structures, especially the vagus nerve which runs perpendicularly between the internal jugular vein and the carotid artery and must be preserved. Prior to dividing the internal jugular vein, it is of utmost importance to inspect its undersurface to identify the tenth cranial nerve, to secure its position and to avoid severing it.

The phrenic nerve arises from the anterior ramus of C-4 and receives branches from C-3 and C-5. Therefore, it starts deep to the prevertebral fascia and, as its destination is the diaphragm, it has no occasion to pierce this fascia. Rather, covered by prevertebral fascia, it descends nearly vertically in naked contact with the obliquely placed anterior scalene muscle, crossing it from its posterior to its anterior border. It should not be a source of complication, provided that the upper plane of dissection is superficial to the deep fascia. However, should the fascial plane be distorted, dissection can readily be carried too far and into the scalene muscle, damaging the phrenic and resulting in paralysis of the diaphragm on that side and associated postoperative atelectasis.

As dissection is carried upward, the next nerve to be considered is the spinal accessory or eleventh cranial nerve; this must be considered expendable for adequate exposure of the posterior triangle. This nerve appears from under cover of the digastric between the internal jugular and internal carotid vessels. It crosses the internal jugular vein, which separates it from the transverse process of the atlas, and disappears into the deep surface of the sternocleidomastoid from ½ to 2½ inches below the tip of the mastoid process. Here lymph nodes surround it, and the sternomastoid branch of the occipital artery accompanies it. On making its exit from along the anterior border of the sternomastoid muscle, the accessory nerve can readily be found at this point and be traced upward to the digastric where it meets the twelfth cranial nerve.

The spinal accessory nerve is found to divide the posterior triangle into 2 equal parts as it makes its exit from the posterior border of the sternocleidomastoid muscle and enters the trapezius. Severance of this nerve produces a right-angle neck deformity resulting from paralysis of a part of the trapezius muscle. However, it must be kept in mind that the sternomastoid has been severed and removed during the procedure. Preservation to avoid the shoulder droop secondary to trapezius-muscle denervation is considered justified in this instance. However, bear in mind that the surgical procedure for eradication of disease is far more important in saving the life of the individual than prevention of any deformity that might follow.

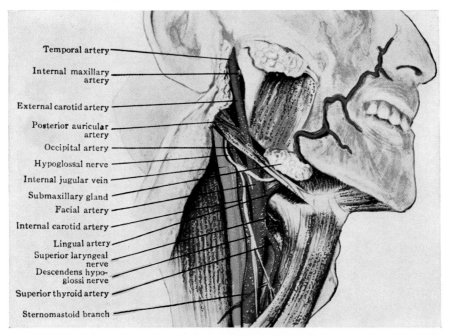

Temporal artery
Internal maxillary artery
External carotid artery
Posterior auricular artery
Occipital artery
Hypoglossal nerve
Internal jugular vein
Submaxillary gland
Facial artery
Internal carotid artery
Lingual artery
Superior laryngeal nerve
Descendens hypoglossi nerve
Superior thyroid artery
Sternomastoid branch

Fig. 47. Carotid arteries and branches. (Davis: Applied Anatomy, Philadelphia, Lippincott)

The ansa hypoglossi nerve which innervates the strap muscles of the neck and is expendable, either in laryngectomy or neck dissection, rises medial to the internal jugular vein and offers an excellent "direction finder" for identification of the main hypoglossal nerve (Fig. 47). In any of these procedures, it is a primary concern that the hypoglossal nerve be identified and preserved. This nerve appears from under cover of the digastric in contact with the accessory nerve or just medial to it. This is the motor nerve of the tongue and, in the adult, is found to curve forward superficial to every artery it meets, viz., the internal carotid, the external carotid and the lingual arteries and, commonly, the superior thyroid and the facial arteries as well. It passes under the cover of the posterior belly of the digastric a second time and so enters the digastric triangle, where it again crosses superficial to the lingual artery. The hypoglossal nerve is most readily found just above the posterior end of the greater cornua of the hyoid bone and thence traced backward.

In connection with the digastric muscle, it is of interest to note that only 3 structures cross it superficially. These are (1) the 2 main tributaries of the common facial vein, (2) the great auricular nerve and (3) the cervical branch of the facial nerve. These are not of great importance, and the posterior belly of the muscle may be exposed freely without risk of doing damage. Passing deep to the posterior belly of the digastric, and thereby placing it in a commanding position, are the 3 great vessels, the last 3 cranial nerves and the sympathetic chain. In fact, all structures in the carotid triangle reach to higher levels deep to the posterior belly of the digastric and stylohyoid muscles.

Other nerves of significance are likely to be found in the field of critical dissection during operation. The first of these is the lingual branch of the fifth cranial nerve, which innervates the anterior two thirds and lateral surface of the tongue; when this nerve is severed, the patient complains postoperatively of lack of sensation in that area.

As the dissection nears its completion in the middle portion of the submandibular triangle, the nerve supply to the submaxillary gland becomes apparent. The lingual nerve may often be short before the main nerve completes its course beneath the mylohyoid muscle. Anatomically, its course is described as a spiral around the submaxillary duct, lying successively above, laterally below and medially above the duct. It is at this point (removal of the submaxillary gland and duct) that the nerve is frequently injured. Careful dissection in the region of the submaxillary duct will result in preservation of the lingual nerve with no impairment of the sensory innervation of the tongue and the floor of the mouth on that side. The other major nervous structure is the cervical sympathetic chain, which only rarely is involved in complications of these surgical procedures. The reason for this is that, anatomically, it lies behind the carotid artery and rarely is damaged except if there is unusual tension in this area. While a Horner's syndrome resulting from its division is not incapacitating, its occurrence is unfortunate and usually unnecessary. However, in most instances where the nerve is damaged due to the stress or pulling, the Horner's syndrome disappears within a few months following the injury.

Preservation of the recurrent laryngeal branch of the vagus nerve is of utmost importance in order to preserve an intact larynx for voice production. However, in laryngectomy, the recurrent laryngeal nerve must be sacrificed.

The vascular structures to be considered are both the arteries and the veins, as well as the lymphatic channels (Fig. 48). The last named are included for one of two reasons; either because obliteration of metastatic malignant disease involves removal of the lymph-bearing channels or because the thoracic duct enters briefly into the field of dissection. The most important artery to be considered is the common carotid. There have been reports of this artery being ligated in error in a hyperextended neck where adequate identification was not carried out, as well as of injury to it during dissection requiring anastomosis or ligation. If ligation of the common carotid is done, the surgeon is in for serious trouble; the patient may die, or hemiplegia may develop, the latter being the more common and presenting itself anywhere from 3 to 5 days following the ligation. If injury to the artery,

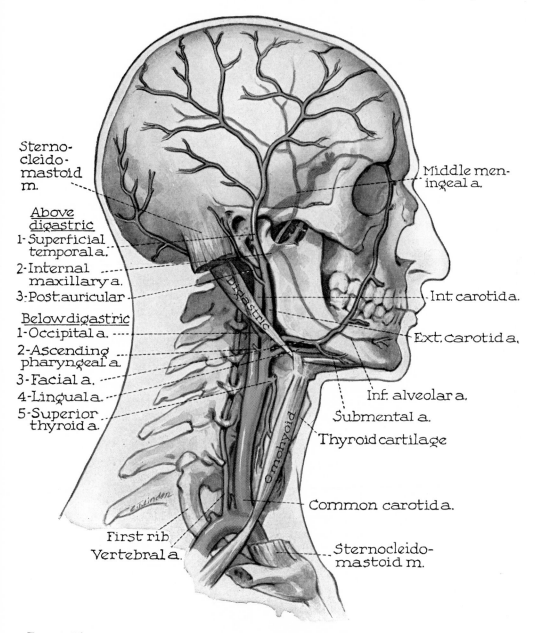

Sterno-
cleido-
mastoid
m.

Above
digastric
1- Superficial
temporal a.
2- Internal
maxillary a.
3- Post. auricular

Below digastric
1- Occipital a.
2- Ascending
pharyngeal a.
3- Facial a.
4- Lingual a.
5- Superior
thyroid a.

First rib
Vertebral a.

Middle men-
ingeal a.

Int. carotid a.

Ext. carotid a.

Inf. alveolar a.
Submental a.
Thyroid cartilage

Common carotid a.

Sternocleido-
mastoid m.

FIG. 48. The carotid arteries. (Thorek, P.: Anatomy in Surgery, Philadelphia, Lippincott)

such as incision with scissors or knife, occurs, it is better to attempt repair of the damage rather than to ligate the vessel.

It has been suggested that vein grafts can be placed in the carotid system when sacrifice of a segment of the vessel is essential to the operation. The internal carotid circulation must always be preserved. There have been reports in the literature of cases in which a segment of the *external* carotid (which can be ligated with impunity) has been anastomosed to the cut end of the *internal* carotid, thus maintaining the blood flow in the more essential structure. Homologous preserved *arteriografts* may be of value in specific instances, but the magnitude of the pressure and the paucity of supporting tissues in this area do not appear to justify utilization of autogenous *venous* grafts.

Occasionally it becomes necessary to sacrifice the internal carotid artery specifically, as in the case of tumors of the ganglion nodosum or glomus jugulare in the neck. Under such circumstances, the prognosis is extremely poor and should be anticipated preoperatively. It has often been difficult to anastomose this area in view of the very short stump of the interior carotid that existed.

In performing a routine laryngectomy, the only vessels of importance that must be ligated are the superior laryngeal artery and vein in the region of the superior horn of the thyroid. Failure to ligate these vessels frequently results in severe hemorrhage or, rarely, if not identified early, in the death of the patient.

Ligation of the transverse scapular and transverse cervical arteries (which are branches of the thyrocervical trunk) occasionally presents complications. These vessels are usually obvious and readily ligated. However, in very aged patients with arteriosclerotic vessels, complete ligation may result in the necessity of tying off the thyrocervical trunk at its origin.

Venous structures may be ligated unilaterally or, for all practical purposes, bilaterally, in the standard neck dissection, without fear of complications. However, in the bilateral ligation of the internal jugular vein, mortality or morbidity may be very high due to the severe cerebral edema that ensues. Because of the significant pressure placed on the ligature adjacent to the innominate vein, particularly that attendant on postoperative coughing or straining, double ligatures should be placed at this proximal position. In all routine dissections, No 1 black silk is best suited for ligating large arteries and, of course, for the internal jugular vein, with double ligatures frequently employed for added security.

Care should also be taken with the external jugular vein in the clavicular area, for here the vessel may be sizable and the potential complications would be fatal. In the course of a radical dissection, no other single vein to be ligated has such potentialities for carrying a fatal air embolism. This complication does not occur with the smaller veins, and the internal jugular has sufficient retrograde flow to flood the field completely should its ligature slip; but the external jugular can produce a fatality with its valve and sucking action.

The major lymphatic structure encountered in the lower portion of the dissection on the left side is the thoracic duct. Injuries to this are not common. However, should the presence of a clear or milky fluid be noted in the lower part of the field, the thoracic duct should be identified and ligated in order to prevent persistent drainage, which has been reported to last over a period of several months.

In laryngectomy, the larynx may be removed without disturbing the hyoid bone, but most operators feel that removal is of advantage, particularly in facilitating closure of the larynx. However, the reason most often given is that this is done to eliminate the pre-epiglottic space completely. This is important, especially in cases in which the lesion involves the ventricles or ventricular bands. As the larynx is lifted upward and forward, the superior cornua of the thyroid cartilage should be dissected free rather than amputated.

Immediately after removing the cornua, the superior laryngeal vessels should be identified and ligated. Ordinarily, they are seen entering the thyrohyoid membrane a little above the edge of the thyroid cartilage and somewhat anterior to the cornua. Closure of the pharynx should be performed carefully in order to avoid development of a fistula. Any tension on the suture line should be avoided.

Miscellaneous tissues that may present a source of complication are relatively few. Such a temporary disturbance in this group is parotid salivary gland fistula, which may result when the lower portion of the parotid gland is resected. The complication usually subsides within a week to 10 days at the most. However, fistulas from the submaxillary gland cannot occur, for, in the radical operation, this gland is entirely removed.

A pneumothorax may be created early in the course of the dissection by tenting the apex of the mediastinal tissues and pulling the pleura up into the field. Fortunately, this too is a rare complication.

In all cases of neck dissection it is of particular importance to follow up the patient, in order to rule out or observe early the presence of cervical metastases.

HAROLD C. VORIS, M.D.

6   The Brain and the Peripheral Nerves

BRAIN AND CRANIAL NERVES

GENERAL CONSIDERATIONS

This section is devoted to a discussion of errors that could be made in the course of operations on the contents of the intracranial cavity and will include procedures carried out on the cranial nerves within the skull. A thorough knowledge of the anatomic relationships of the skull, its covering and its contents is essential to the neurologic surgeon.

Scalp. The scalp differs in structure from the skin elsewhere. The galea (aponeurosis) is a dense fibrous membrane bound to the overlying skin by many fibrous septa. It is continuous in each temporal region with the fascia of the temporal muscle, anteriorly with the frontalis muscle and posteriorly with the occipitalis muscle through which it is attached to the superior nuchal line. It has a rich blood supply from 6 paired arteries, the supraorbital anteriorly, the superficial temporal laterally and the occipital posteriorly. Wounds and surgical incisions of the scalp bleed freely. Ligation of the small vessels is difficult because of the retraction of the cut vessels. However, approximation of the cut edges of galea and skin readily controls bleeding, as the fibrous septa prevent appreciable bleeding into the scalp itself. This approximation is readily accomplished during operation by the use of some type of scalp clip (ordinary Michel skin clips make a satisfactory substitute for the special clips that have been devised by Adson, Raney and others) or by ordinary artery forceps placed on the galea so as to pull it up against the skin. Careful separate approximation of the galea and the scalp at the time of closure is a safeguard against hemorrhage after the sutures are placed. If the galea is not approximated, large hematomas may develop between the scalp and the skull, as the galea is only loosely attached to the pericranium and can readily be dissected and elevated from it by collections of blood, fluid or pus. Thus, subaponeurotic abscesses may become very large and spread diffusely over the entire cranium.

Skull and Dura. The skull is composed principally of membrane bone, the vault entirely so. This bone forms directly from membrane without an intervening cartilage stage. The outer layer of the split membrane becomes the *pericranium*, the inner layer becomes the outer layer of the *dura*. Thus, the cranial dura is always closely applied to the overlying bone and is densely adherent to it at the base, and, in infancy and old age, over the vault of the skull as well. The splitting of the original membrane by the formation of bone can be well seen at the anterior fontanel in the young infant. The fontanel membrane is the only barrier between the subaponeurotic and the subdural spaces. Hence, in a *subdural tap in the infant,* as soon as the needle passes through the fontanel membrane, it enters the subdural space.

Blood Supply. The blood supply of the scalp, the skull and the dura is mainly from the external carotid artery and its branches; the supply to the leptomeninges (pia-arachnoid) and the brain is from the internal carotid and the vertebral arteries. However, the dura receives small branches directly from the vertebral and the internal carotid or from the ophthalmic arteries, the last being branches of the internal carotid. The ophthalmic arteries represent the most profuse connections between the external and the internal carotid systems. They supply the structures of the orbit and the skin of the forehead and anastomose extensively with branches of the external carotid.

The operation of "trapping" aneurysms of the cavernous portion of the internal carotid artery between a ligature in the neck and a clip or ligature on the intracranial portion of the artery has been performed many times. This operation also "traps" the ophthalmic artery, but only rarely has visual impairment followed, because the anastomoses of the ophthalmic artery with branches of the external carotid usually are sufficiently profuse to nourish the retina.

The vessels of the pia-arachnoid and the brain are branches of the internal carotid and the vertebral arteries. The arrangement of their larger branches at the base of the brain into the circle or heptagon of Willis is of great importance in understanding the mechanics of cerebral circulation and in planning the surgical treatment of aneurysms and vascular malformations. According to Padgett,[15] less than half of a large series of specimens had a "normal circle of Willis." In a "normal" circle of Willis, the anterior communicating artery is one half to two thirds the size of the anterior cerebral, which, in turn, is half the size of the internal carotid. The posterior communicating artery is half the size of the posterior cerebral, which, again, is half the size of the basilar. The anterior communicating artery was present and of normal size in at least 90 per cent of Padgett's cases; duplication was the most frequent anomaly. Less than half of the specimens had normal posterior communicating arteries. Abnormalities of the circle of Willis occur nearly twice as often in cases of aneurysm.

The arteries of the brain are not end-arteries, but their collateral circulation is often physiologically inadequate to maintain sufficient nutrition of brain tissue. The two anterior cerebral arteries send branches across the midline to the opposite hemisphere, also anastomosing with branches of the middle cerebral arteries of the same side. A patient usually will survive occlusion of one anterior cerebral artery (distal to the anterior communicating) without significant neurologic deficit. However, loss of both anterior cerebral arteries will produce definite mental and per-

sonality changes. The middle cerebral artery early divides into several branches; loss of one or more of these will cause noticeable motor disturbances. Occlusion of the main trunk artery will be disastrous, resulting in death or profound hemiplegia. Posterior cerebral artery occlusion is followed by *homonymous hemianopsia* because of the inevitable occipital lobe involvement.

Occlusion of the basilar artery will be fatal, as it causes loss of circulation to the brain stem. The vertebral arteries are often unequal in size, and one may even be rudimentary. In such cases, occlusion of the larger vertebral will be fatal, unless the posterior communicating arteries are of sufficient size to carry the load of the basilar circulation. As this is not true in the majority of cases, vertebral or basilar occlusion is a very serious condition.

Cerebrospinal Fluid. A knowledge of the cerebrospinal fluid, its formation, pathways and circulation, is important to the neurologic surgeon. It has been generally considered that the cerebrospinal fluid is formed by a secretion or filtration process from the choroid plexuses of the lateral ventricles. Hassin[10] pointed out that tissue fluids draining through the perivascular spaces into the ventricles and the subarachnoid spaces provide a large source of the cerebrospinal fluid. Probably both mechanisms are important. Certainly an obstruction in the third ventricle, cerebral aqueduct or fourth ventricle will produce an obstructive hydrocephalus with enlargement of the ventricular system anterior to the point of obstruction. This indicates that the cerebrospinal fluid is formed, to a considerable extent, in the lateral ventricles. After draining through the third ventricle, the cerebral aqueduct and the fourth ventricle into the posterior cistern via the foramina of Magendie and Luschka, the fluid appears to diffuse anteriorly through the basilar cisterns and over the convexity of the hemispheres, where the Pacchionian granulations appear to play an important role in its absorption.

Since the brain and the spinal cord have no lymphatics, the cerebrospinal fluid and its pathways are probably analogous to the lymphatic circulation found elsewhere in the body. The fluid itself contains about the same amount (slightly less) of electrolytes as blood plasma. Its protein content is much less than that of blood plasma, indicating the selective mechanism of its production. Its pressure is frequently used as an index of intracranial pressure, although there are certain errors to be avoided in such usage. Lumbar manometric pressure will not necessarily reflect intracranial pressure, particularly if any block or obstruction exists in the pathways. When the volume of cerebrospinal fluid is low, as in certain types of supratentorial tumors with collapse of the ventricles and cerebral subarachnoid spaces, even the ventricular pressure may not truly reflect intracranial pressure.

Factors in Intracranial Pressure. Intracranial pressure depends on a number of factors. Systemic blood pressure, systemic venous pressure, volume of cerebrospinal fluid, volume of other intracranial contents and gravity all play an important role in the production and the maintenance of intracranial pressure, whether normal or increased. The effect of the position of the head on the intracranial pressure indicates that the intracranial cavity cannot be considered as a completely closed box, since if it were, changes in position should have no effect. With an individual in the upright position, the lumbar subarachnoid pressure usually will not equal that at the level of the foramen magnum. Soft tissues over a skull defect are generally depressed when the patient is in the upright position, indicating that, under normal conditions, in the upright position, intracranial pressure is less than atmospheric pressure. This is of great importance in operations on the cranial cavity or the cervical spine with the patient in the upright position, because, under these circumstances, the danger of embolism is very real whenever venous channels are opened.

Under experimental conditions, systolic blood pressure and even systemic venous pressure can often be raised to high levels without significantly affecting intracranial pressure. Yet, the neurologic surgeon is well aware of the augmented swelling of the brain and consequent increase in intracranial pressure which is associated with rises in venous pressure, especially those due to obstruction of venous return from the head. The Queckenstedt test depends on the direct effect of the increase of intracranial venous pressure on intracranial

pressure in general. Finally, the decrease in intracranial pressure brought about by hypotensive anesthesia emphasizes the role that systolic blood pressure plays in maintaining the pressure within the cranium.

The effect of fluid retention on cerebral swelling or edema and of intracranial masses, either neoplasm, abscess or hematoma, on intracranial pressure is obvious. The surgeon must realize that it normally depends on a number of interlocking factors, and that extensive compensatory mechanisms are brought into play when one or more of these factors are disturbed. Significant changes in intracranial pressure occur only when the compensatory mechanisms fail. The mere existence of disturbance in one or more of these mechanisms will not produce a change in intracranial pressure unless the tolerance of the mechanisms is exceeded.

Intracranial Cavity. The intracranial cavity can be divided into areas accessible to the neurologic surgeon. These subdivisions are related partly to the natural contours of the skull and partly to certain dural partitions, the *tentorium* and the *falx cerebri*. The tentorium separates the intracranial cavity into supratentorial and infratentorial regions. The infratentorial is often referred to as the *posterior fossa*. The *cerebellum*, the *medulla* and the *pons* occupy the posterior fossa. The supratentorial cavity contains the *cerebral hemispheres* and the anterior part of the *brain stem*, the *midbrain*, the *thalamus* and the *hypothalamus*. The *supratentorial cavity* is further divided into 2 halves by the falx cerebri. The *cerebral hemispheres* are traditionally divided into 4 lobes or areas, *frontal*, *temporal*, *parietal* and *occipital*.

Cranial Nerves. The cranial nerves are of surgical importance, some more than others. The first pair, the *olfactory nerves,* are in the anterior cranial fossa and are frequently involved in fractures and basofrontal neoplasms. One of these nerves is necessarily sacrificed in *transfrontal craniotomy* in order to permit the elevation of the frontal lobe out of the anterior cranial fossa.

The second pair of intracranial nerves, the *optic nerves,* are of great functional importance, and lesions in the neighborhood of these nerves, the optic chiasm and the optic tracts are often accurately localized by the characteristic changes in the visual fields. The *third, fourth, fifth* and *sixth cranial nerves* course through the middle fossa to gain access to the *orbit* or to leave the skull through the floor of the middle fossa.

The *third cranial nerve* not infrequently is injured by trauma. It is also injured or involved by lesions of the internal carotid artery or neoplasms in the region of the cavernous sinus. The incisural herniations of the *hippocampal gyrus* alongside the brain stem will produce damage to the third cranial nerve, with consequent oculomotor palsy. The *sixth cranial nerve* has the longest course of any cranial nerve and is apt to be involved in markedly increased intracranial pressure. Consequently, lesions of this nerve have little localizing value and generally denote merely an increase in pressure within the cranial cavity. The *fourth cranial nerve* has a rather complicated course but is seldom injured. Its lesions are difficult to recognize and, consequently, it is not of great surgical importance. The *fifth cranial nerve*—like the third, fourth and sixth—arises from the brain stem in the posterior fossa and runs anteriorly into the middle fossa, where its sensory ganglion lies. It almost immediately divides into 3 branches: the *ophthalmic* which passes through the superior orbital fissure to enter the orbit, the *maxillary* which passes through the foramen rotundum into the pterygoid fossa and the *mandibular* which passes through the foramen ovale into the infratemporal fossa. The *trigeminal nerve* may be involved in neoplasms or aneurysm of the middle fossa, but its greatest surgical importance is in operative treatment of *trigeminal neuralgia*. The remainder of the cranial nerves, the seventh, eighth, ninth, tenth, eleventh and twelfth, are all found in the posterior fossa.

SURGICAL CONDITIONS

Surgery in Head Injuries. Injuries to the head constitute an important part of intracranial surgery. The number of craniocerebral injuries in this country has risen steadily in the past 3 decades, running parallel with the steady rise in all types of bodily trauma with which damage to the brain is frequently associated. While injuries to the scalp and the skull cannot be completely disregarded, it is the cerebral damage which is of greatest importance. Injuries to scalp and skull are generally significant only as they may provide an avenue for the entrance of infection. However, in *depressed skull fracture,* fragments of bone may contribute to injury or compression of the brain.

Indications for surgery in head injuries can be stated concisely. First, compound wounds of the head, whether involving scalp alone, scalp and skull, or involving the brain as well, all offer indications for surgical treatment. *Extradural and subdural hematoma,* as well as traumatic subcortical hematoma, constitute the other early indications for surgical intervention. Cerebral injury per se, without hematoma, is not, in the opinion of the writer, an indication for surgical intervention. However, drainage of cerebrospinal fluid from the nose and the rare *traumatic aerocele* are also indications for early surgical interference. In the author's experience, drainage of cerebrospinal fluid from the ear has never been persistent and, consequently, has never required surgical intervention. On the other hand, drainage of cerebrospinal fluid from the nose may be persistent. It is a grave error to allow it to persist for more than a few days; after that, operation, with closure of the torn dura, should be done. This is a major neurosurgical procedure that should be carried out only when adequate facilities are available. Traumatic aerocele should be observed carefully with frequent roentgenograms. If the air continues to accumulate or persists, it indicates that the opening is still present and surgical treatment is indicated.

Late indications for surgery in head injuries include chronic subdural hematoma and certain cases of post-traumatic epilepsy. The recognition of extradural and subdural hematomas is of the greatest importance since, if unrecognized, these conditions are usually fatal; but if they are recognized and surgically removed in time, good results are obtained.

Extradural hematomas are a rare but important complication of head injury. According to Munro,[13] they occur in only 3 per cent of all head injuries. Kearns[11] found extradural hematoma to be the cause of death in

93, or 18 per cent, of 510 cases of fatal head injury. They are rare in children and the aged and are most common in young adults. This is apparently due to the greater adherence of the dura to the skull in infancy and in old age, since an extradural hematoma must necessarily dissect the dura from the skull as it forms. Acute subdural hematomas are usually associated with severe brain injury, either contusion or laceration, and are usually fatal. However, recovery of patients who were operated on for acute subdural hematoma has been reported by a number of authors. We owe to Wilfred Trotter[20] the recognition that chronic subdural hematomas are usually of traumatic origin and that the source of the hemorrhage is generally a rupture of a cerebral vein as it crosses the subarachnoid and the subdural spaces to enter the dural lacunae. Usually it is a superior cerebral vein that is torn, but the inferior veins that enter the sphenoparietal sinus and also those that enter the lateral sinus from the posterior inferior surface of the temporal lobe and the anomalous cerebral veins which may enter the dura from the convexity of the hemisphere all may at times be sources of hemorrhage.

Subdural hydroma has recently received a great amount of attention as a complication of meningitis, especially in children. However, it is often of traumatic origin. Munro[13] considers it as representing a subdural hematoma which has become greatly diluted by osmosis and consequently appears as xanthochromic fluid. The protein content of such fluid is often very high, but, surprisingly, the fluids do not coagulate when removed. In one case, the fluid removed at operation contained 2,000 mg. per 100 cc. of total protein but still did not coagulate on standing. DaCosta and Adson[3] considered subdural hydroma to be a separate clinical entity, and they reported a case in which a tear of the arachnoid was demonstrated at operation. This tear apparently had allowed cerebrospinal fluid to enter the subdural space but had acted as a valve to prevent its return to the subarachnoid space. It is likely that both mechanisms are responsible for post-traumatic chronic subdural hydromas. Adequate proof of a subdural hydroma should consist of a demonstration of a tear in the arachnoid, the presence of neomembranes

or xanthrochromic spinal fluid with a high total protein content, significantly higher than that of the cerebrospinal fluid.

CHANCES OF ERROR. It is often difficult to recognize extradural and acute subdural hematomas, although in so-called typical cases it may be easy. In many instances, it is hard if not impossible to differentiate acute subdural from extradural hemorrhage, and the two conditions should be considered together from a clinical standpoint. The earlier the onset of symptoms, the more extradural bleeding should suggest itself because of the usual arterial origin of the extradural bleeding. When there is no severe associated brain injury, a classic "lucid interval" will be present, and there will be an uncomplicated development of localizing signs. The typical patient who has suffered a head injury will undergo a brief period of unconsciousness, from which he apparently recovers. However, during the next few hours, or perhaps within the next day or two, he will become progressively drowsy and stuporous, then sink into coma, with perhaps a prelude of restlessness, confusion or delirium. As he becomes comatose, one pupil dilates and a *contralateral hemiparesis* or *hemiplegia* develops. Localized contralateral convulsive seizures may occur. Roentgenograms of the skull on the side of the dilated pupil may show a linear fracture crossing the groove of the middle meningeal hemorrhage. (Such a patient almost always has such a middle meningeal hemorrhage.)

Many cases of extradural bleeding and most cases of acute subdural hemorrhage are complicated by associated brain injury, the patients being stuporous or comatose from the onset, with localizing neurologic signs that are due to the brain injury. A few patients show a gradual onset of symptoms over several days to a week. In these cases, the first arterial hemorrhage has been small and probably stopped spontaneously, but the initial separation of dura from bone has ruptured emissary veins, which continue to bleed. Progressive dissection or separation of the dura from the bone occurs, with progressive rupture of more emissary veins. The hemorrhage from these emissary veins probably also ceases spontaneously but continues from freshly torn vessels. Thus the clot slowly grows. The clinical signs in such cases consist of progressive drowsiness, stupor and slowly developing neurologic manifestations. These cases simulate clinically subacute or chronic subdural hematoma and cannot be differentiated from these preoperatively.

The suspicion of extradural or subdural hematoma must be entertained when there is alteration in the state of consciousness, restlessness or outright delirium in previously quiet and rational patients. The progressive development of drowsiness, stupor and coma or the deepening of pre-existing stupor or coma are very significant. Dilation of the homolateral pupil is a dependable localizing sign, especially if it develops while the patient is under observation. *Convulsions,* particularly if localized to one extremity or one side of the body, are of great diagnostic value, as are unilateral weakness or paralysis of the extremities. These signs are usually contralateral to the lesion, but occasionally, with large hematomas, the contralateral peduncle is pressed against the incisurea of the tentorium so that the hemiparesis and pyramidal-tract signs are homolateral to the hematoma. Slow pulse rate and elevated blood pressure are also of significance. In chronic subdural hematoma, papilledema occurs, and the spinal fluid is xanthochromic in three fourths or more of the cases. The separation of subdural hematomas into acute and chronic types may be questioned from the pathologic and the etiologic standpoint, but it is justified clinically.

Acute subdural hematomas are large collections of liquid or clotted blood without the neomembranes which are nearly always associated with severe brain injury; they carry a high operative mortality. On the other hand, chronic subdural hematomas are originally small and generally associated with mild brain injury; the hematoma may be organized, have neomembranes and show a low operative mortality.

Surgery of Intracranial Tumors. Intracranial tumors are classified as *intracerebral* or *extracerebral* and as *primary* or *metastatic*. The second group includes both extracerebral and intracerebral growths, although the majority are intracerebral. In certain cases the meninges are involved in so-called meningeal sarcomatosis or carcinomatosis. The most common source of metastatic intracranial tumors is primary tumor of the lung, though a primary carcinoma of the gastro-intestinal tract, the kidney, the thyroid or the breast may metastasize to the intracranial cavity. In most cases of intracranial metastasis from other than lung tumors, the route is via the lung, while at the same time there may be metastases to the lung. However, direct metastasis to the brain from other parts of the body may occur without involvement of the pulmonary circulation. A *persistent foramen ovale* accounts for some of these cases; another avenue permitting tumor cells to reach the brain without passing through pulmonary circulation is the profuse anastomosis of the vertebral veins, with veins to the head and the neck on the one hand and to the trunk and the abdomen on the other. These anastomotic channels have been well demonstrated by Batson.[2]

Surgery of Hydrocephalus. An infant with an enlarged head may have a subdural hematoma and should always have a bilateral subdural tap through the anterior fontanel as a safeguard. If this procedure does not reveal a subdural hematoma, then the ventricles may be tapped, again through the anterior fontanel. If they are enlarged, a dye test may be carried out to determine if the hydrocephalus is communicating or obstructive. Five cc. of 0.8 per cent indigo carmine may be injected into one ventricle. The dye will appear immediately in the fluid from the other ventricle. If it does not, the foramen of Monro is obstructed. The dye can be recovered promptly by spinal puncture, unless there is an obstruction between the lateral ventricles and the lumbar subarachnoid space.

At a second stage, ventriculography may be performed. This may reveal the location of obstruction, especially if it is a tumor, and will give information on the severity of the hydrocephalus. If there is less than 2 cm. of space between the ventricle and the skull, cerebral destruction is so severe that the child is not likely to develop normally. In such cases, operative intervention is an error.

There are a number of operative procedures which are of value in the treatment of hydrocephalus. Where hydrocephalus is obstructive, a shunt from the ventricles into the cerebral

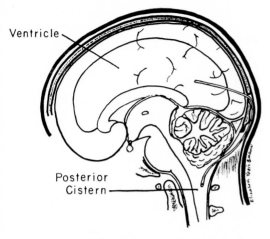

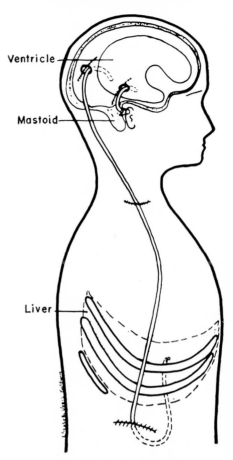

FIG. 49. Diagram of sagittal view of head and intracranial cavity illustrating ventriculocisternal shunt (Torkildsen procedure). Note catheter extending from posterior horn of lateral ventricle to posterior cistern.

subarachnoid spaces generally is indicated. The so-called Torkildsen procedure or ventriculocisternal shunt (Fig. 49) is well-known and is most satisfactory when the posterior cistern is normal. This operation consists of leading a rubber or plastic catheter from the posterior horn of the lateral ventricle beneath the scalp and the occipital muscles, or beneath the skull and the occipital muscles, into the posterior cistern. When this procedure is not applicable, *third ventriculostomy* can be carried out. Third ventriculostomy requires a dilated third ventricle and intact basilar subarachnoid cisterns. In the infant, it is best to follow the route originally advocated by Dandy,[7] with elevation of the temporal lobe out of the middle fossa and puncture of the lateral wall of the floor of the third ventricle. When the third ventricle is dilated, the lateral aspect of the floor is readily accessible in the triangle formed by the third nerve below, the anterior carotid artery anteriorly and the elevated tip of the temporal lobe above. This triangle will be crossed by the posterior communicating artery which, if large, should be preserved. In the adult, third ventriculostomy is performed most easily through the anterior route advocated by Stookey and Scarff.[19] Transfrontal craniotomy is done first; the

FIG. 50. Diagram illustrating ventriculo-antral shunt (Nosik) and ventriculoperitoneal shunt.

frontal lobe is elevated, and the thinned-out lamina terminalis is punctured above the optic chiasm. In properly selected patients, third ventriculostomy is a very satisfactory procedure for obstructive hydrocephalus.

When the cerebrospinal fluid spaces are obliterated, or absorptive mechanisms are inadequate, shunting of the cerebrospinal fluid to another body cavity becomes necessary. Various shunts have been proposed but given up for one reason or another, and, at the present time, there is still no method in widespread use which gives general satisfaction. One proposed by Nosik[14] drains the cerebrospinal fluid into the mastoid antrum (Fig. 50). A small rubber or plastic tube is led from the temporal horn of the ventricle into the mastoid antrum, which is readily exposed even in the

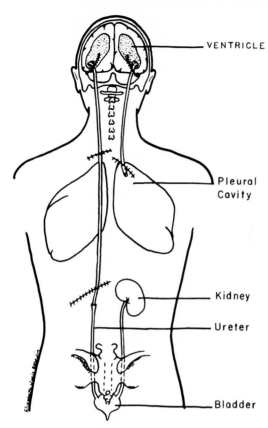

VENTRICLE

Pleural Cavity

Kidney

Ureter

Bladder

FIG. 51. Diagram illustrating ventriculopleural and ventriculo-ureteral shunts.

infant. The fluid drains through the middle ear and the eustachian tube into the nasopharynx. This has the advantage of maintaining fluid and electrolyte balance, as these are reabsorbed from the gastro-intestinal tract. It has the grave disadvantage of providing an avenue for intracranial infection from the nasopharynx, and most of the reported cases have succumbed eventually to meningitis. It must be considered as an undesirable procedure with possible limited temporary advantage in certain cases. Theoretically, shunts of the ventricle to the pleural or peritoneal cavities (Fig. 51) are advantageous since there is no disturbance of fluid and electrolyte balance, as the ventricular fluid is reabsorbed from both of these cavities.

The difficulty lies in keeping the drainage apparatus open, and in the majority of reported cases frequent revision of the shunt has been necessary. Sacrifice of a kidney and drainage of either the spinal subarachnoid space or the ventricle through a rubber or plastic catheter into the ureter was revived by Matson.[12]

The problem of maintaining fluid and electrolyte balance is often difficult, especially in infants after dismissal from the hospital. As the child grows, revision of the shunt, with introduction of a longer tube, may be necessary. Apparently retrograde infection from the bladder has not been a problem, but sacrifice of the kidney remains a significant objection.

Recently Pudenz[17] and his associates have revived the idea of establishing a communication between the cerebrospinal fluid pathways and the vascular system. This is the most physiologic method of treating hydrocephalus, as it returns the cerebrospinal fluid directly to the venous system. These investigators establish a shunt between the lateral ventricle and the right auricle. A silicone rubber tube is passed from the ventricle into the common facial vein and internal jugular vein and hence into the right auricle. A silicone slit-and-core valve is molded into the tip of the cardiac end of the tube. This valve is constructed to open when the pressure in the tube exceeds 30 mm. of water. The valve must be so located that it floats in the pool of blood in the auricle. A valve that remains in the lumen of a vein will be enveloped by the vessel wall and cease to function in a short time.

At present, none of the shunts described can be depended on to function indefinitely, and revision may often be necessary. However, it is known that in many cases of hydrocephalus a spontaneous arrest occurs, with the development of a balance between production and absorption of cerebrospinal fluid. Consequently, any procedure is justifiable which may prevent progressive cerebral damage or death until spontaneous adjustment can occur.

Intracranial Aneurysms. The surgical treatment of intracranial aneurysms consists of (1) simple ligation of the internal carotid artery; (2) trapping of an aneurysm by intracranial clips on either side or, in cases of aneurysm of the internal carotid, especially the cavernous and infraclinoid portions, by a ligature in the neck and a clip on the intracranial portion of the carotid; (3) placing a clip on the neck of the aneurysm; (4) surgical extirpation of the aneurysm; and (5) packing muscle about the aneurysm or within its cavity.

The choice of form of treatment depends on the location of the aneurysm and whether it is pedunculated, sessile or fusiform. The ideal operative treatment is its extirpation or occlusion of its neck without interference of circulation through the vessel of origin. However, many aneurysms are sessile, some are fusiform, and, even when pedunculated, the neck is often fragile and easily torn. The arachnoid adhesions with which it is surrounded frequently make its exposure and mobilization difficult and may result in its being torn during the procedure. Consequently, a direct attack on an aneurysm is generally dangerous and may lead to disaster. With the use of hypotensive anesthesia the danger of uncontrollable hemorrhage is lessened. If hypothermia is combined with hypotensive anesthesia it becomes feasible to occlude temporarily both anterior cerebral arteries or the middle cerebral artery for periods up to 15 minutes without permanent damage to cortical neurons. Such temporary occlusion can be effected by means of removable clips such as those devised by Olivecrona and Schwartz. Extirpation of an aneurysm or at least packing its cavity with muscle is thus often feasible. Both simple ligation of the internal carotid artery in the neck or trapping the aneurysm, with occlusion of the vessel of origin, remain the safest methods of surgical treatment in most cases. These procedures require the presence of an adequate collateral circulation through the circle of Willis so that the vessel of origin can be sacrificed without producing serious neurologic deficit.

Bilateral carotid angiography is an essential preliminary to surgical attack on most aneurysms. Bilateral intracranial aneurysm is not infrequent, and it is embarrassing to operate successfully on an intracranial aneurysm only to have the patient succumb later to hemorrhage from another, previously unrecognized. If possible, competency of the circle of Willis should be demonstrated by angiography. The value of the Matas test, or preliminary digital compression of the carotid vessels, has been stressed by some authors and

minimized by others. Ligature of the common carotid artery instead of the internal has been advised by a number of writers. Carotid pressure studies carried out by Bakay and Sweet[1] suggest that in the majority of cases ligation of the common carotid is just as dangerous as that of the internal. Dandy[8] occluded the internal carotid artery as a preliminary procedure. If the patient showed no untoward symptoms after 10 minutes of preliminary compression, he then ligated it. If the patient indicated an inability to tolerate initial complete ligation, partial ligation was carried out, and 1 to 6 weeks later, complete ligation was performed. His report of 4 deaths in a series of 105 ligations of the internal carotid artery has been bettered only by Poppen's[16] series of 101 carotid ligations with 3 deaths.

The arterial clamp devised by Selverstone permits gradual occlusion of the internal carotid artery over a period of several days and is a valuable method of dealing with patients who require occlusion of the internal carotid artery but whose preoperative tests indicate inability to tolerate initial complete ligation. Carotid pressure studies carried out at the time of exposure of the internal carotid artery are a valuable safeguard and are likely to prove to be the best method of determining whether or not the patient would tolerate immediate occlusion. Bakay and Sweet[1] have shown that if there is a drop of more than 70 per cent in the carotid pressure distad to occlusion, the patient probably will not tolerate complete ligation.

Delayed (over 6 to 8 hours) onset of contralateral hemiparesis and hemiplegia after the internal carotid artery is ligated may be due to a propagating thrombus or embolism from the site of the ligature, or from the aneurysm itself, or it may represent peripheral spasm with cerebral thrombosis in the presence of lowered intravascular pressure in the cerebral vessels on the ligated side. In the former situation, removal of the ligature is of no avail; in the latter, improvement of the patient's condition may well follow removal, and a number of such cases have been reported.

Spontaneous Subarachnoid Hemorrhage. The following plan is advised for the management of the patient with spontaneous subarachnoid hemorrhage who has survived the first few hours after the initial hemorrhage or leak. If his condition stabilizes without further bleeding being evident, he may be observed for 5 or 7 days, when, if the spinal fluid no longer contains fresh red blood cells, *angiography* may be performed. On the other hand, if there is evidence of further or repeated bleeding, angiography should be carried out as an emergency procedure and surgical treatment instituted.

Ligation of the internal carotid artery (Fig. 52) is generally the only procedure to be attempted in the acute cases. Mortality is greatest during the first week after subarachnoid hemorrhage. An aneurysm in the cavernous portion of the internal carotid artery should be treated by ligation—either

initial or fractional—of that vessel. After ligation of the internal carotid artery has been accomplished in the neck, at the same or at a later sitting, the intracranial cavity may be opened by a transfrontal craniotomy and the aneurysm may be trapped by a clip distal to the aneurysm but proximal to the bifurcation of the artery. Pedunculated aneurysms of the intracranial portion of the internal carotid artery above the cavernous sinus or its branches may be excised in selected cases, or may be treated by trapping or by cervical carotid ligation alone. Sessile or fusiform aneurysms in the internal carotid artery between the cavernous sinus and its termination must be treated by trapping or by cervical carotid ligation alone. Aneurysms of the

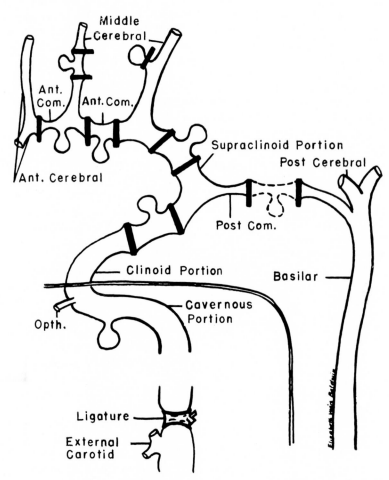

FIG. 52. Diagram of carotid circulation, illustrating the surgical treatment of various aneurysms.

branches of the middle cerebral artery must be attacked directly. There is considerable risk of permanent neurologic sequelae.

Ligation or trapping of an aneurysm of the anterior cerebral artery between its origin and the anterior communicating artery is always feasible if the filling of the opposite anterior artery can be demonstrated by contralateral carotid angiography. Aneurysms of the anterior cerebral artery distal to the anterior communicating artery can usually be operated on directly with satisfactory results. Aneurysms in the anterior communicating artery itself are very difficult to treat surgically. The artery is so small that there is seldom room to trap the aneurysm and leave the anterior cerebral arteries intact. Sacrifice of one anterior cerebral artery can be tolerated, but sacrifice of both anterior cerebral arteries usually will result in serious mental and personality defects. Aneurysms of the vertebral or basilar arteries are seldom accessible to surgical treatment. Fortunately, only about 25 per cent of intracranial aneurysms occur on the basilar artery or its branches.

Direct attack on an intracranial aneurysm is not feasible if (1) it is located at the bifurcation of a major vessel; (2) it is on the anterior communicating artery; (3) there is more than one aneurysm; and (4) the aneurysm is too large to permit exposure of its origin. However, in the last named case, with the use of hypotensive anesthesia, the aneurysm may be opened and packed with muscle or gelatin sponge.

The surgical removal of angiomatous malformations of the brain is being attempted more often. It is now realized that these lesions are frequently the cause of intractable and progressively severe seizures and that they may cause death from subarachnoid hemorrhage. It is important to determine, as well as possible, both their arterial supply and their venous drainage by cerebral angiography, preferably serial. In the surgical attack, every effort must be made initially to control the arterial supply. Once that has been accomplished, the venous drainage may be dealt with at leisure. Since the lesions to a considerable extent *replace* instead of *displace* brain tissue, increased intracranial pressure is not usually a problem, and, unless they are deep-

seated, requiring extensive incisions into the brain substance, they can often be removed without injury or destruction of valuable cerebral tissue. The introduction of hypotensive anesthesia and most recently of hypothermia have made surgical attack on the more formidable of these lesions much more feasible.

A patient who has evidence of *spontaneous subcortical hematoma* should be operated on as soon as his general condition permits accurate localization of the lesion and surgical attack upon it. Most of these lesions are located in the temporoparieto-occipital area. If the patient's condition permits determination of the visual fields, the presence of a homonymous hemianopsia will indicate its location. A posterior parietal burr-hole or a trephine opening permits adequate exploration of the brain with a blunt needle which will localize the hematoma in most cases. Then it can be removed by aspiration, but if removal seems to be incomplete, or if the patient does not improve on repeated aspiration, then osteoplastic craniotomy should be carried out, with removal of the hematoma through a transcortical incision or by uncapping it. In many cases these collections of old blood intermixed with fluid are of large size, often 30 to 60 cc. Usually there is no difficulty with further bleeding after the removal of the hematoma, but the open surgical exposure of a lesion has the advantage of permitting adequate hemostasis within the cavity after evacuation of the hematoma. Rehabilitation measures should be instituted as soon as possible.

DIAGNOSTIC PROCEDURES

History Taking. The foundation of an accurate neurosurgical diagnosis is a well-organized record of a patient's symptoms and complaints. While such a record should be concise, it must be sufficiently detailed and is best written in narrative form, with careful attention to chronologic sequence. Experience and practice in history taking and particularly in interpreting a patient's statements are essential. It is important for the examiner to be certain that the patient understands his questions and that he, in turn, understands the statements made by the patient. For example, dizziness often means one thing to the examiner and another to the patient; unless it is established what the patient means by dizziness, a gross misinterpretation of the patient's symptoms will result. The history should not be confined to neurologic symptoms, as often signs referable to involvement of the nervous system are the first evidence of systemic disease.

Examination. Many patients come to the neurologic surgeon after having received a thorough general examination and diagnostic study. However, it is an error to omit a routine general examination if it has not been carried out recently by a competent examiner. Evidence of malignancy of the prostate may be found on rectal examination and thus provide the explanation for a patient's paraplegia. Clinical or x-ray examination of the chest may disclose a primary carcinoma of the lung which has metastasized to the brain, causing symptoms of intracranial involvement. Examination of the nasopharynx may reveal the source of a tumor at the base of the skull with multiple cranial nerve palsies.

A clinical neurologic examination should not be merely a routine examination of the cranial nerves and the motor and sensory systems but should also include special diagnostic procedures such as perimetric fields, examination of the vestibular apparatus of the auditory sense and the determination of olfactory acuity. The competent diagnostician will be able to carry out these procedures himself. Others may find it necessary, or at least more convenient, to call in the services of specialists from allied fields, particularly the ophthalmologist and the otolaryngologist. In any case, a complete neurologic examination should always precede the employment of complicated, often uncomfortable, and sometimes actually dangerous special diagnostic procedures.

Electroencephalography can hardly be considered to be a routine clinical procedure. It is not available in many localities. It is generally expensive and often fails to be of any diagnostic value. It has been particularly disappointing insofar as the recognition and the localization of intracranial tumors are concerned. However, it is of value in patients with convulsive seizures and in some cases of head injury. Unfortunately, few neurologists and fewer neurologic surgeons are competent themselves to interpret an electroencephalographic record. Consequently, the services of a trained and expert electroencephalographer are essential in the use of this procedure.

Radioisotope studies, like electroencephalography, are not uncomfortable or dangerous to the patient. Unfortunately, like electroencephalography, in the hands of many observers, these studies have proved to be inaccurate in attempts to recognize and diagnose brain tumors. The average of accuracy for both of these procedures is, in most reports, no more than 60 to 70 per cent. When one considers that mere lateralization of a cerebral tumor is, from a surgical standpoint, often wholly satisfactory, it is apparent that these procedures leave much to be desired.

Angiography has become an important diagnostic procedure. It is uncomfortable and at times carries significant danger. The ideal contrast medium has not yet been found, and the materials in general use have a specific effect on the blood-brain barrier and the vascular endothelium. Consequently, circulatory complications (generally vasospasm and thrombosis) often occur. Angiography has the further disadvantage of requiring injections into at least 3 arteries (both carotids and one vertebral) in order to survey the intracranial circulation completely. Recently, technics have been described which eventually may provide us with a complete cerebral angiogram after 1 or 2 injections. This will represent a great advance. Arterial puncture requires considerable skill on the part of the angiographer, and errors are frequent. The open methods do not demand so much skill, but they do not safeguard against the disadvantage of surgical incision and exposure of the arteries, with occasional loss of the vessel.

Though angiography is not entirely dependable for recognition of intracranial tumors, when such tumors have a specific vascular pattern, angiography will locate them accurately and also give considerable information regarding their probable nature. Avascular lesions can be known only by the displacement of major blood vessels. Lesions in the posterior part of the cerebral hemisphere often do not significantly displace major blood vessels and, consequently, may not be recognized. Experience with vertebral angiography has not yet supplied sufficient data to make it an entirely accurate diagnostic procedure for tumors of the posterior fossa. Angiography has its greatest value in aneurysms and angiomatous malformations. In these conditions the other diagnostic procedures cannot be substituted. At the present time, angiography carries a moderate amount of risk (at least in the elderly patient), entails considerable technical difficulty and requires special roentgenographic equipment.

The injection of air into the intracranial cavity, as first recommended by Dandy in 1918,[4] is the most dependable procedure for the diagnosis and the localization of intracranial neoplasms. The route of injection depends on the individual case. In most clinics, the spinal route[5] (encephalography) is considered to be dangerous and inadvisable where there is papilledema or definitely suspected intracranial neoplasm. The spinal route is more uncomfortable to the patient. However, the advantages are that shaving of the head, incisions into the scalp and openings into the skull are not required. Ventriculography is less upsetting to the patient and safer in cases of increased intracranial pressure. In infants, where the fontanel is not yet closed, ventriculography is technically easier than encephalography and is usually preferred, especially since it carries less risk to the infant. Diagnostic air studies carry little risk in the absence of increased intracranial pressure, except in debilitated patients. These studies are very accurate in the recognition and the localization of intracranial tumors, provided that the tumor has reached a size that produces distortion or malformation of the ventricular system. Midline tumors of the brain stem which fail to block or distort the ventricular system will not be recognized in air studies, nor will small neoplasms which have not produced significant ventricular distortion. Technical skill in giving spinal air injections is very important, and considerable experience in the interpretation of the roentgenograms is necessary before satisfactory accuracy can be expected.

Preoperative Care

The preoperative care of the neurosurgical patient differs only in detail from that of the general surgical patient. The principles involved, as well as the errors that can be made, are the same. Patients with intracranial lesions frequently have headaches, which generally can be controlled by Empirin and codeine or by codeine alone. Morphine should never be used in cases of increased intracranial pressure because of the danger of depressing the respiratory center. *Vomiting* may be present in patients with intracranial lesions and should be controlled if possible. The straining connected with vomiting is dangerous and may lead to the quick death of the patient through the mechanism of suddenly produced foraminal or incisural herniation. The temporary limitation of oral intake and the use of intravenous fluids usually suffice to control vomiting. Chlorpromazine is of great value in reducing the tendency to vomit. *Constipation* may be present, and straining at stool should be avoided if possible. There is considerable disagreement as to whether the use of enemas or laxatives contributes more to straining at stool. It is the writer's opinion that cathartics, particularly saline cathartics, are less dangerous than enemas.

Unconscious, debilitated and paraplegic patients must have special attention paid to the care of their *skin*. It is essential to nurse them meticulously and turn them frequently. The alternating-pressure air mattress has been of great value in preventing the development of trophic ulceration. *Feeding* unconscious or semiconscious patients presents a special problem. In the hospital, intravenous or subcutaneous fluid injections are a ready means of controlling fluid intake. However, nutrition cannot be maintained adequately by intravenous feedings. A nasal tube passed into the stomach generally should be installed where parenteral feedings prove to be necessary for longer than 2 or 3 days. If a patient vomits persistently, the stomach tube cannot be used satisfactorily, but it does permit the administration of oral medication so that many injections may be done away with. *Tracheotomy* may be lifesaving in a severely injured patient. It is the safest and most satisfactory way to handle the unconscious patient who is having difficulty with his airway.

General Safeguards

Anesthesia. It is very important to select the proper anesthetic agent for intracranial surgery. The older neurosurgeons, recognizing the dangers of ether, especially of its *improper* administration, often used local anesthesia. Cushing, in particular, did the majority of his work under local anesthesia. The improvement of rectal and intravenous anesthetic agents, particularly *Avertin* and *Pentothal Sodium,* has led to their widespread use. *Ether* still remains a satisfactory anesthetic for intracranial surgery, but many anesthetists fear its employment in the neurosurgical operating room where some type of electrosurgical unit is generally in use. However, ether by the endotracheal technic is safe because of the extensive draping and consequent shielding of the operative field that is commonly used in neurosurgical cases. At the present time it is popular to employ different anesthetic agents, counteracting their side-effects with the administration of various auxiliary drugs. At times the administration of an anesthetic takes on the aspects of a controlled pharmacologic experiment rather than a sound and well-balanced clinical procedure. However, anesthesiologists must be given credit for bringing to the neurosurgical operating room technics which are proving to be of tremendous value.

Hypotensive Agents. The development of safe hypotensive agents has made it possible for the neurologic surgeon to remove large vascular tumors and to operate safely on aneurysms and on large vascular malformations. It has been known for a long time that cooling of tissue markedly reduces its metabolism and that not only a limb or an organ but the entire body can be subjected to marked reduction in blood supply under conditions of artificial cooling without permanent tissue damage. The elaborate equipment required to establish either local or general hypothermia was impractical for operating-room use until it was possible to produce hypothermia by chemical means. Now this technic can be readily carried out in the operating room and is almost a matter of routine in some clinics. This makes it possible to interrupt temporarily the blood supply to various portions of the brain, or even to the entire intracranial cavity without the permanent serious consequences that otherwise would follow. For this reason, some previously inoperable lesions, especially aneurysms and vascular malformations, can now be attacked successfully. The

use of either or both of these technics requires highly skilled and educated anesthesiologists, as well as the aid of adequately trained and experienced operating-room personnel.

Choice of Procedure in View of Anesthetic. It is important to remember that a complicated procedure is not always the best, and that the difficulties or risks of anesthesia should never be greater than those of the operative procedure itself. Consequently, complicated technics should be reserved for difficult and complicated operations, and routine procedures should be performed under an anesthetic which has been tested and proved to be simple and safe. Many diagnostic procedures, particularly encephalography and ventriculography, usually should be carried out under local anesthesia. The use of general instead of local anesthesia for cerebral angiography is still questionable. However, the technical difficulties of arterial puncture and the necessity for immobilization of the head while roentgenograms are being taken often make general anesthesia desirable. Although some insist that the procedure is safer under general anesthesia, there is still some doubt, since the addition of general anesthesia to a minor operation appreciably increases the risk. At the present time, in anesthetic circles it is popular to minimize the risk of anesthesia in skilled hands. However, some degree of risk will always remain, no matter how well safeguarded.

Error of Excessive Use of Isotonic Fluid. Neurosurgical thinking regarding fluid and blood balance during operations has changed in the past 25 years. The availability of intravenous fluids and of whole blood has made it possible to replenish the blood loss completely during an intracranial operation, and this should be the aim of the surgeon. The administration of large quantities of isotonic fluids during an intracranial operation is inadvisable because of the possible production of cerebral edema. Some anesthesiologists are unaware of this and have to be cautioned not to administer an excessive quantity of such fluids.

Technics and Instruments. The basic principles of intracranial surgery do not differ from those of surgery in general, but their details do. Opening the skull demands special technics. The control of hemorrhage from intracranial structures has required the development of special procedures and implements. Power-driven instruments are popular for opening the skull, and various types of cranial burs and saws powered by electric motors have been developed. It is the writer's opinion that little time is gained in craniotomies by using power-driven instruments; a good hand instrument, carefully used, remains the tool of choice.

The development of special technics for control of bleeding from fragile, thin-walled intracranial vessels supported by soft, easily injured cerebral tissue has been very important in intracranial surgery. The methods of opening the intracranial cavity are old. Asepsis was then and is now a necessary prerequisite if the entrance to the intracranial cavity is to be accomplished without danger of infection. Cushing first brought suction, together with refined methods of handling cerebral tissue, to the field of intracranial surgery. Retraction was carried out gently over moist cotton. Capillary oozing was controlled by suction on moist cotton. Hemorrhage to larger vessels could not be thus controlled; therefore, Cushing invented the special hemostatic silver clip. These clips could be applied to thin-walled vessels and left in situ rather than using the cumbersome method of clamping and ligating.

However, silver clips cannot be easily applied to small vessels, and the control of oozing points still necessitated time-consuming suction over moist cotton. The adaption of the Bovie electrosurgical unit to neurologic surgery made it possible to produce hemostasis rapidly in the operative field. It was learned by experience that the electrocoagulating current did more damage to tissue than was grossly apparent at the time of application and was not safe to use about the brain stem and the spinal cord. The development of 2-point or bi-polar electrocoagulation by Greenwood[9] has increased the safety of this method of controlling hemorrhage. Since the current passes only between the 2 tips of the coagulating forceps, vessels can be safely coagulated on the surface of the brain or the spinal cord. Tissue destruction is minimal and is confined to the vessel being coagulated.

The control of oozing points or venous hemorrhage by human fibrin sponge and thrombin came into use during World War II. The expense and the scarcity of human fibrin sponge made the development of other types of special coagulating agents imperative. Now gelatin sponge and oxidized cellulose gauze can be applied to bleeding points and oozing surfaces or can be used for packing tumor cavities and left to absorb. The search still goes on for a satisfactory substitute for dura mater and an agent which can be introduced between raw surfaces to prevent adhesions from forming. At the present, gelatin film appears to be the best, readily obtainable agent, although it leaves much to be desired, especially from the standpoint of prevention of adhesion. Human fibrin film is preferable to gelatin film, but it is expensive and scarce.

POSTOPERATIVE CARE

Fluid and Electrolyte Balance. Recently, the thinking about fluid and electrolyte balance in the neurosurgical patient after operation has changed materially. It is no longer considered to be advisable to dehydrate the postoperative brain-tumor patient. However, these patients must not be given excessive amounts of sodium chloride, and, if possible, the retention of fluids by cerebral tissue must be prevented. The neurosurgical patient should receive a minimum of 2,000 cc. of fluid in 24 hours, administered orally if possible. If necessary, fluids may be given parenterally, but not more than 9 Gm. of sodium chloride should be given in 24 hours unless there is specific loss of sodium chloride, as in occasional persistent vomiting, diarrhea or spinal-fluid fistula. This amount may be secured by the use of 2.5 per cent glucose in 0.4 per cent sodium chloride solution or the limitation of normal saline solution to 1,000 cc. in 24 hours. Diuresis may be advisable, and the good results that follow the administration of hypertonic glucose or sucrose solution may be due to their diuretic effects. Cathartics and enemas are the oldest methods of reducing increased intracranial pressure. The combination of 2 ounces of magnesium sulfate, 11 ounces of magnesium citrate or 3 or 4 ounces of phospho-soda is a valuable method of bringing about fluid elimination. In unconscious or stuporous patients, magnesium sulfate enemas may be used in the same way. A 50 per cent magnesium sulfate solution may even be given by Murphy drip.

Sedation. Neurosurgical patients are often restless and at times delirious. In some cases, the pain following craniotomy may be controlled satisfactorily by codeine. A grain of codeine can be given to most neurosurgical patients every 4 hours if necessary. Codeine does not control restlessness well, and some type of sedation is often necessary. Barbiturates may be used, but paraldehyde remains one of the best agents for the control of restlessness; its margin of safety is high. It may be administered by the oral or the rectal route or even parenterally, and it is excreted rapidly. This is important since prolonged sedation may lead to failure to recognize signs of compression due to the formation of a postoperative hematoma. Chloropromazine or reserpine often help to quiet the restless patient. These drugs are also of value in preventing hyperthermia, a common complication after intracranial operations. They also seem to potentiate other sedatives and anodynes.

Hyperthermia. This may be a serious postoperative complication, and its control is essential. The usual methods of alcohol sponging and placing ice bags about the patient will control the milder forms. In more severe cases, large doses (10 to 20 gr.) of amidopyrine may be given orally or rectally, and in intractable cases, cold enemas, even of ice water, may be necessary. Where available nursing care permits, packing the patient in ice or wrapping him in cold, wet sheets is also advisable.

Position of Patient. Most patients may be sitting up in bed or even in a chair within a day or two after craniotomy or even suboccipital craniectomy. Intracranial pressure and the tendency to serious oozing are less in the upright position; consequently, moderate elevation of the head after operation is desirable. However, in the unconscious patient, the lateral horizontal position maintains a better airway and should be maintained until he is fully conscious.

POSTOPERATIVE COMPLICATIONS

Long and complicated intracranial operations increase the danger of wound contamination because of the numerous personnel and the complex equipment needed in the operating room. Careful asepsis and meticulous technic are the mainstays in prevention of postoperative infection, but after long and intricate operations, the prophylactic use of antibiotics is desirable. A distressing complication of intracranial surgery is *postoperative venous or arterial thrombosis*. This is more apt to happen in elderly arteriosclerotic patients, but it may occur in patients of any age. It is easy to make an error in distinguishing between venous and arterial thrombosis. The prognosis is better in the venous form, as permanent tissue damage is less likely to occur, and collateral venous circulation is established more readily. The use of anticoagulant therapy may appear to be indicated, but surgeons usually hesitate to use it because of the increased danger of postoperative hemorrhage. The differentiation between postoperative vascular thrombosis and cerebral compression from postoperative hematoma is not easy to make, and errors are frequent. A patient may be progressively stuporous and have localizing neurologic signs, such as Jacksonian convulsions or progressive hemiparesis or hemiplegia, in either condition. Where consciousness is retained, and progressive impairment of neurologic function takes place, vascular thrombosis is likely, but when the patient is continuously more stuporous and comatose, postoperative hematoma is a strong possibility. Unless the surgeon is certain that there is no postoperative hematoma, he should reopen the wound without delay. Prompt evacuation of a postoperative hematoma and control of the source of the hemorrhage may mean the difference between survival and death or between complete neurologic recovery and permanent disability.

Postoperative psychosis is apparently metabolic or psychogenic in origin. It follows neurosurgical operations as well as others. The treatment consists of adequate sedation, with a high fluid, caloric and vitamin intake. The principles of treatment of toxic delirium are the same, whether it occurs in an alcoholic, a general surgical or a neurosurgical patient.

SPECIFIC INTRACRANIAL OPERATIVE PROCEDURES

Trephination. The oldest type of intracranial operative procedure is the *bur-hole*, or *trephination*. Today, this has very limited application and is used only as a primary procedure for the diagnostic injection of air and for the drainage of chronic subdural hematomas. When employed in diagnostic injection of air, it is generally placed in each parieto-occipital region, so as to permit so-called posterior ventriculography. The posterior horns or body of the ventricles are then entered with a cannula.

A satisfactory location for the bur-hole for posterior ventriculography is 7 cm. above the external occipital protuberance and 4 cm. from the midline. It may be placed in the frontal region, at the hairline for frontal ventriculography, and should then be not over 2 cm. from the midline, since the anterior horns of the lateral ventricles are much closer to the midline than are the posterior horns. For drainage of a chronic subdural hematoma, the bur-hole is best placed in the postero-parietal region, above the insertion of the temporal muscle. If the patient is in the supine position, with the head of the table elevated, such bur-holes will not only disclose the majority of subdural hematomas but also will permit of their drainage by gravity.

Since defects of the size of the ordinary cranial bur are insignificant from a cosmetic standpoint, usually no attempt is made to repair them. However, when exploring for a possible chronic subdural hematoma, there is need for a slightly larger opening to permit adequate manipulation of a catheter to wash out the hematoma. In view of possible liability cases, it may be undesirable to leave any defect in the skull. Therefore, it is better to use a 1-inch trephine and remove a button of bone, which is later wired back in place, than to make a bur-hole and enlarge it with rongeurs. In cases of suspected subdural hematoma, it is sometimes necessary to make more than one bur-hole in order to uncover the clot, since the subdural hematoma may be far anterior over the tip of the frontal lobe or low in the temporal region over the temporal lobe. A subdural hematoma may occur in the posterior fossa and require an occipital bur-hole to reveal its presence and permit of its evacuation. Multiple exploratory bur-holes ("woodpecker surgery") are not often indicated. If a suspected subdural hematoma is not found by routine posteroparietal bur-holes, it is better to proceed with ventriculography or angiography.

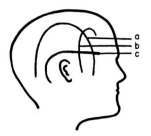

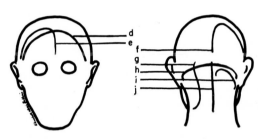

Fig. 53. Diagram illustrating various incisions for intracranial operations. (a) Lateral osteoplastic craniotomy. (b) Hockey stick incision for anterior subtemporal decompression. (c) Penfield incision for subtemporal decompression. (d) Souttar incision for bilateral frontal craniotomy. (e) Naffziger incision for transfrontal craniotomy. (f) Sachs incision for occipital craniotomy. (g) Adson incision for unilateral suboccipital decompression. (h) Cushing crossbar incision for bilateral suboccipital decompression. (i) Dandy incision for unilateral suboccipital decompression. (j) Midline incision for suboccipital decompression.

Craniectomy. Decompressions or craniectomies are generally subtemporal or suboccipital (Fig. 53). Harvey Cushing popularized the so-called "crossbow incision" for exploration of the posterior fossa. This gave a wide approach to the posterior fossa and permitted exploration of both cerebellopontine angles and cerebellar hemispheres. Today, lesions in the posterior fossa can be localized more accurately. The use of the upright position has facilitated operations in this region, and removal of the lateral pole of the cerebellar hemisphere exposes the cerebellopontine angle better than retraction of the hemisphere. This has led to the use of unilateral incisions for exploration of either cerebellopontine angle and midline incisions for exploration of the fourth ventricle. These straight muscle-splitting incisions are rapidly and easily made and closed, and they heal more rapidly than the extensive "crossbow incision" or its modifications.

In the upright position, intracranial pressure is less, bleeding, especially venous, is decreased, and the procedure can be carried out more rapidly. However, the upright position has 2 dangers. The first is *postural hypotension,* which is best guarded against by wrapping the lower extremities with an elastic bandage and applying a good abdominal binder. Hypotensive anesthesia cannot be used with the patient in the upright position. The second danger is *embolism.* It is essential to occlude all veins carefully as soon as they are exposed or severed and to wax the edges of bone carefully in order to prevent the entrance of air into the diploic spaces. With these safeguards, air embolism should not occur. The risks of the upright position are more than offset by its advantages.

Subtemporal decompression remains a satisfactory method of exposing temporal-lobe lesions. It can be carried out in 3 ways. The routine *hockey-stick or question-mark scalp incision* with a muscle-splitting incision of the temporal muscle is generally used for anterior subtemporal decompression. Bone is then removed over the posterior part of the frontal lobe and the anterior part of the temporal lobe. If a patient is placed with the head hanging, this approach permits the adequate exposure of the sphenoid ridge, the posterior communicating artery, the anterior choroidal artery and the lateral aspect of the brain stem. A modification of this procedure, with the patient in the upright position, is used for the extradural temporal approach to the gasserian ganglion and its sensory root.

When adequate exposure of the middle and posterior parts of the temporal lobe is desired, *subtemporal craniectomy* may be carried out through a so-called English type of subtemporal decompression, with the scalp and the temporal muscle reflected as a musculocutaneous flap through a horseshoe-shaped scalp incision. Penfield modified this by reflecting the musculocutaneous flap anteriorly, using a scalp incision that begins over the mastoid process and extends upward and then forward along the line of insertion of the temporal muscle. When using a musculocutaneous flap, do not make the error of removing bone above the line of insertion of the temporal muscle. When the wound is closed, the temporal muscle is anchored by silk or wire sutures to the bone edge, using punch or drill holes at 1-cm. intervals. This gives a firm and adequate closure and prevents the development of unsightly temporal bulging. The Penfield subtemporal decompression method has proved to be very satisfactory for giving access to lesions of the posterior part of the temporal lobe. It will adequately expose any lesion of the posterior part of the temporal lobe which is causing a *homonymous field defect.* It is the procedure of choice for such lesions.

Routine subtemporal decompression is a palliative measure for increased intracranial pressure. It is seldom used today except occasionally in the treatment of deep-seated brain tumors. Some surgeons prefer to employ subtemporal decompression and irradiation in the treatment of tumors of the thalamus and the third ventricle, and it is of value in cases of so-called pseudotumor (serious arachnoiditis) with persistent papilledema. However, the latter condition can often be treated satisfactorily with a low sodium diet and limitation of fluids.

Craniotomy. *Krause's osteoplastic craniotomy* has been variously modified by many surgeons. The most notable modifications are Naffziger's for transfrontal craniotomy and Sachs's for occipital craniotomy. Both of these permit more adequate exposure of the frontal or the occipital lobes and avoid badly placed scalp incisions which heal poorly or produce cosmetic deformity. *Naffziger's transfrontal craniotomy* may be used for lesions of the anterior part of the frontal lobes, the floor of the anterior fossa, the optic chiasm, for pituitary tumors and for aneurysms of the carotid, the anterior cerebral or the anterior communicating arteries. In order to permit adequate retraction of the frontal lobe, it is a safeguard to carry out spinal drainage during this operative procedure, unless it is certain that the ventricles can be tapped sufficiently to decrease intracranial pressure. Hypotensive anesthesia will also generally permit the adequate retraction of the frontal lobe without undue damage to it. The patient should be in the supine position and the head rest slightly lowered so as to tilt the head backward, using gravity to aid in retraction of the frontal lobe. In transfrontal craniotomy, it is important to place the bone flap as low as possible on the forehead. However, the anterior margin of the bone flap should not enter the frontal sinus; with a large frontal sinus it may be necessary to sacrifice some ease of exposure in order to avoid entering the frontal sinus. *Sachs's approach to the occipital region* is preferable to the routine lateral craniotomy, though this remains the best approach for parietal lesions and routine explorations of the cerebral hemisphere. Parasagittal lesions, particularly meningiomas, often need to be approached on either side of the midline, so the coronal or Souttar incision, with either bilateral bone flaps or a single large free bone flap, is the best procedure.

The original Krause method of reflecting together the skin, the temporal muscle and the bone in osteoplastic craniotomy best preserves the blood supply of the bone. However, the preservation of the blood supply of the bone flap often makes it difficult to control bleeding from the undersurface of the bone. Consequently, many surgeons partially free the bone flap from the temporal muscle. The logical extension of this is to reflect the scalp and the temporal muscle separately, removing the bone as a so-called free bone flap, replacing it at the end of the operative procedure. Unfortunately, hematomas then sometimes form between the scalp and the bone and, unless promptly recognized and evacuated, lead to eventual breakdown of the wound and chronic infection. Then the devitalized bone flap falls a ready prey to chronic infection, becoming a sequestrum which must be removed. Hypotensive anesthesia and even the use of hypothermia are valuable safeguards in the removal of a large vascular tumor. Adequate replacement of blood and wide exposure of the tumor, together with patience and skill on the part of the surgeon, are all essential. Multiple-stage procedures are not used as frequently as formerly, but in debilitated patients or in young children they are still often desirable.

Surgery for Intracranial Aneurysms. *The surgical treatment of intracranial aneurysms should be undertaken only after careful evaluation of the aneurysm and the collateral circulation by preoperative angiography.* Operation on an aneurysm should usually be carried out under hypotensive anesthesia. Danger of rupture is thus lessened, and, if it does occur, it is usually possible to control the bleeding sufficiently to permit occlusion of the artery or clipping the neck of the aneurysm. The addition of hypothermia makes it possible to occlude the major cerebral vessels, even both carotid and vertebral arteries simultaneously, for several (up to 12 to 15) minutes. This may permit the resection of otherwise inoperable lesions or inaccessible aneurysms.

Surgery for Trigeminal Neuralgia. The surgical treatment of trigeminal neuralgia is still an important field in intracranial surgery. The new procedure of so-called decompression of the gasserian ganglion and its sensory root (Taarnoj operation) may not stand the test of time, so it is possible that sectioning the sensory root of the trigeminal nerve will remain the only method of guaranteeing these patients permanent relief. Sensory-root section can be carried out through a unilateral suboccipital craniectomy or by a subtemporal approach. While a few men, especially those trained by the late Walter Dandy,[6] choose the suboccipital route, the majority of neurologic surgeons prefer the temporal approach. Most use the extradural approach to the ganglion, although, as suggested by Wilkins, some make use of the intradural route. The temporal approach is best carried out with the patient in the upright position, through a small, anteriorly located subtemporal decompression, usually made through a short muscle-splitting incision. Control of bleeding, from the middle meningeal artery is an essential safeguard when using the extradural approach. This may be done in various ways, but it is easiest to coagulate the vessel at the foramen spinosum. Then, if desired for additional protection, the foramen spinosum can be plugged with bone wax or with a small wooden plug such as a matchstick. Some surgeons advise an attempt to preserve the greater superficial petrosal nerve, feeling that it tends to lessen the danger of trophic lesions of the cornea. However, unless care is taken to avoid traction on the dura along the petrosal ridge, tardy or delayed facial palsy will occur in a certain proportion of cases. Therefore, it is best to section the dural fibers carefully along the petrosal ridge, even at the risk of sacrificing the greater superficial petrosal nerve or of opening the superior petrosal sinus. The control of venous oozing about the gasserian ganglion and along the petrous ridge has been greatly facilitated by wedging small pieces of gelatin sponge between the dura and the bone. These may be left in place permanently. It is necessary occasionally to section the superior or medial third of the sensory root in order to control pain in the ophthalmic division of the nerve. It is advisable at times to section this root prophylactically in elderly or debilitated patients in order to obviate the necessity of reoperation on these patients if they should later develop pain in the ophthalmic division. If this is done, *special care of the cornea* after operation is essential. This can be accomplished satisfactorily during the first few days after operation by placing a suture in the upper eyelid and taping it down to the cheek. This keeps the cornea covered by the upper lid except when the nurse may elevate the lid in order to irrigate the eye. This suture is removed after 2 or 3 days, and some type of protective shield or goggle is used for permanent protection of the cornea.

Surgery for Intracranial Infection. The treatment of intracranial infection has changed greatly in the last 15 years. Neurologic surgeons have learned that intracranial abscess is much less common because of the use of antibiotics for treatment of infections of the ear and the sinuses and as a prophylactic measure after head injuries, especially those with compound wounds, otorrhea or rhinorrhea. The actual treatment of brain abscess is also greatly facilitated. Instead of marsupialization and exterior drainage of an abscess, with the gradual obliteration of its cavity over a period of days and weeks, total resection of the abscess and its capsule is often the procedure of choice. Total resection is safer and

easier, if an abscess is well localized and encapsulated. However, radical removal of an area of suppurative encephalitis is better than allowing a patient to succumb because of inability to localize the infection.

Surgery for Brain Abscess. The surgical treatment of brain abscess is now often carried out through craniotomies instead of being confined to limited operative exposures through bur-holes or trephine openings. The ideal treatment of brain abscess is to remove all grossly infected and devitalized brain tissues and leave a clean cavity which can be washed out repeatedly, postoperatively, by means of a drainage tube, instilling penicillin or other antibiotic solution. Such a cavity will heal with a minimum of scar tissue. With this method, post-traumatic epilepsy should be much less frequent than with the old method of marsupialization and external drainage, which always resulted in a dense fibrous scar extending from scalp and dura down into the brain.

Surgery for Skull Fractures. With the use of antibiotics, it is no longer necessary to divide compound, depressed skull fractures into those cases in which the condition of the patient will permit surgical treatment within the first few hours after injury and those in whom, because of initial shock and collapse, it is necessary to postpone surgical treatment. These cases can be safely operated on when the condition of the patient permits. However, the longer the delay the more thorough and radical must be the *débridement,* not only of scalp, temporal muscle and skull, but also of brain tissue. In the delayed cases, it is an essential safeguard to remove all contused and devitalized brain tissue so as to leave a clean cavity, lined by relatively normal brain substance. Repair of the dura is imperative, and, if necessary, a graft of either temporal fascia or fascia from some other part of the body should be used. Primary repair of the bone defect is seldom advisable, especially in contaminated wounds, and should be postponed until a later date. Primary repair of the scalp is important and should be accomplished by using whatever plastic procedures are necessary. If complete repair of the scalp defect is not possible, it is even more essential to obtain tnitial repair of the dura. Then, later, satisfactory skin-grafting procedures can be carried out on the granulating dura.

Surgery for Skull Defects. The repair of skull defects often appears to be more important to the patient than to the surgeon. In the past, neurologic surgeons have tended to be neglectful of skull defects since they were so conscious of their therapeutic value. Laymen frequently are so concerned about the presence of skull defects that their repair may become necessary for psychological reasons, if not for cosmetic or protective values. It is impossible for many patients with skull defects to earn their livelihood because they are refused employment. So, for one reason or another, most skull defects of more than 1 or 2 cm. in diameter eventually need to be repaired.

METHODS OF REPAIR. The neurologic surgeon has a variety of metallic and plastic materials at his disposal for such repairs. Tantalum is the most satisfactory of the various metals which have been used in the past. It is ductile and malleable and can be fashioned and shaped at the operating table to fit the defect. It is difficult to use it for repair of the orbital ridge as, unless it is very carefully conformed so as to avoid pressure on the overlying scalp, the scalp eventually becomes eroded over it, causing a breakdown. It requires time and patience to form tantalum to large or complicated defects satisfactorily. Until recently, the use of plastics required a prolonged or 2-stage procedure. However, Spence[18] has introduced a plastic which can be polymerized at the operating table and molded to the shape of the skull defect. The plastics are not radiopaque, so they do not interfere with later roentgenographic examination of the skull, especially in air or angiographic studies. However, autogenous grafts of bone and cartilage remain the safest method of repair of skull defects, since they never set up reactions necessitating removal of the graft. It requires additional operative procedures to obtain autogenous grafts, and the cosmetic result is often not as satisfactory as with the alloplastic material. Nevertheless, they continue to be preferred by conservative surgeons.

When alloplastic materials are used, exercise due caution to avoid errors. They should never be introduced into freshly contaminated wounds; such wounds must be healed for at least 3—and preferably 6—months before an attempt at cranioplasty is made. When there has been chronic infection or drainage, a minimum period of 6 months should be required before the operation is undertaken. Great care must be used to prevent pressure by the plate on the overlying scalp, and the scalp wounds must never be closed under tension. If fluid accumulates between scalp and skull, it must be removed by repeated aspiration with aseptic technic until it no longer occurs. Otherwise, the wound will break down and a draining sinus will develop, eventually necessitating removal of the plate. Polythene plates are poorly tolerated in patients with a dural defect with exposed brain or open ventricle. Tantalum plates may be better borne in such cases, but autogenous grafts are better still. If possible, repair of the dural defect should precede cranioplasty.

Surgery for Meningoceles. So-called *spurious meningoceles* are seen occasionally (usually in children) as a result of trauma. These are accumulations of cerebrospinal fluid between scalp and skull, usually found at suture lines where the dura is most adherent to the skull. They are the result of the simultaneous tearing of the dura with the skull fracture. This is most apt to happen in young children when the dura is adherent to the skull, especially at the suture line. These collections of fluid beneath the scalp differ from hematomas in that they are diffuse and lack evidence of infiltration or induration at their border. They may become very large and may increase in size over a period of several days. If there is a doubt about their nature, it can be resolved by diagnostic aspiration under aseptic conditions, though it is better not to aspirate, since they can easily be infected. It is an error to aspirate in the hope that they will not recur, because they will recur rapidly until the dural tear has healed. Once this takes place, the fluid will be absorbed and the swelling disappear.

In rare instances, it has been necessary to carry out an operative procedure. In 2 patients who were operated on by the writer, a small protrusion of arachnoid was found incarcer-

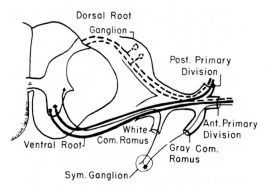

FIG. 54. Diagram of motor, sensory and sympathetic components of a spinal nerve.

ated in the fracture, preventing its healing and permitting the continued escape of cerebrospinal fluid.

This complication of combined skull and dural injury with persistent drainage of cerebrospinal fluid is frequent in fractures of the floor of the anterior cranial fossa and results in persistent rhinorrhea. Operative intervention is likely to be necessary in these patients. The prophylactic use of antibiotics lessens the risk of meningitis in persistent rhinorrhea, but it is an error to delay surgical intervention too long in these cases. When traumatic cerebrospinal rhinorrhea persists longer than 10 to 14 days, operative intervention should be undertaken, including careful repair of the dural defect. There have been reports of operative intervention in traumatic otorrhea, but in the author's experience, this condition has always subsided spontaneously within 10 to 14 days.

WORDS OF CAUTION

The neurologic surgeon must be prepared to study and evaluate his patient carefully before operation. He must expect to carry out not only routine but also special diagnostic procedures and to survey patients from both the general and the neurosurgical standpoints before subjecting them to an operative procedure. The careful selection of the anesthetist, as well as the anesthetic agent to be used, and the training of competent operating-room personnel and assistants are the responsibility of the surgeon himself. Unless he can provide the necessary adjuncts to the opera-

tion and the care of his patient, he should not attempt to do elective neurosurgical procedures. After the operation, the surgeon must be prepared to follow up the patient carefully and to see him personally at frequent intervals until the immediate postoperative convalescence is over and the wound is healed.

PERIPHERAL NERVES

GENERAL REMARKS

The only way to safeguard against errors in the surgical treatment of the peripheral nerves is to acquire a thorough knowledge of their histology, together with technical skill of the highest order, to be obtained only by long years of experience.

Peripheral-nerve injuries are of frequent occurrence, especially in industry. It is essential to diagnose and treat these injuries properly in order to avoid prolonged or permanent damage. While they are seldom, if ever, dangerous to life, these injuries may induce serious and lasting disability and so impose a great burden upon both the individual and the society that must support or recompense him for his disability.

The trunk of a peripheral nerve contains fibers of 3 categories: motor, sensory and sympathetic (Fig. 54). The *motor fibers* arise from the anterior horn cells of a given spinal segment and enter the converging filaments of an anterior root to reach a *mixed spinal nerve*. Here they divide into 2 groups; one group enters the *posterior primary ramus* of the nerve and proceeds distally to reach the lateral muscular branch of that ramus, while the other takes its course through the *anterior primary ramus* to be distributed at various intervals to those muscles that the nerve supplies. The *sensory components* of a peripheral nerve arise from nerve endings in a variety of somatic structures, cutaneous and subcutaneous tissue, tendons, joint tissue, periosteum and skeletal muscles. They have their cell bodies in the posterior root ganglion. The peripheral fibers join the motor fibers in the mixed spinal nerve. The central processes enter the spinal cord and then follow various routes in accordance with the type of sensibility which they transmit.

The *sympathetic pathway* between the

spinal cord and the periphery consists of 2 groups of neurons, preganglionic and postganglionic. The *preganglionic fibers* originate in cells in the intermediolateral cell column of the gray matter of the first thoracic to the second lumbar segments. They pass through the anterior spinal roots and the mixed spinal nerves to the *anterior primary ramus*. They then split off from the proximal part of this ramus to form the *white ramus communicans,* which extends to various sympathetic ganglia where a connection with the postganglionic neuron is made. The *postganglionic fibers* make up the *emergent gray ramus communicans.* On reaching the anterior primary ramus, the postganglionic fibers split into 2 groups, one passing in the posterior primary ramus and the other pursuing its course through the branches of the anterior primary ramus. These latter fibers innervate blood vessels, sweat glands and the erector muscles of the hair.

The *peripheral nerves to the limbs* all undergo considerable rearrangement in the brachial and lumbosacral plexuses before forming the main nerve trunks to the extremities. These plexuses and their peripheral nerves are all subdivisions of the anterior primary rami of the spinal nerves. The ultimate distribution of nerve fibers to muscles is contingent not only on their rearrangement in the limb plexuses but also on regrouping at more distal points. Thus, throughout the course of a peripheral nerve, there are intraneural plexuses in which descending fibers are regrouped in bundles or funiculae before leaving the nerve trunk, either as an independent or a collateral (anastomatic) branch. An *individual funiculus or nerve clump* is formed at a varying distance proximal to its emergence from the nerve. On the average, for a distance of a few centimeters, the funiculus is independent of other fibers in the nerve, but, on occasion, the funiculus is much longer, as in the funiculi in the musculocutaneous nerve to the coracobrachialis and in the ulnar nerve to the flexor carpi ulnaris.

Diagnostic Aids. The regularity of the emergence of individual nerve branches constitutes an important aid in the localization of the level of a nerve injury. For example, a lesion which paralyzes the brachioradialis muscle but not the triceps obviously lies in

the *radial nerve,* between the origin of the branch to the brachioradialis muscle and the branches to the triceps muscle. On the other hand, a lesion below the origin of the branches to the brachioradialis muscle and the primary extensors of the wrist may still paralyze the extensors of the thumb and the index finger, as in the dorsal interosseous branch of the radial nerve at the level of the head of the radius.

Nerve Regeneration. When there is anatomic interruption of a medullated nerve fiber, the axon degenerates peripherally to the point of injury, and the sheath of Schwann, together with the myelin sheath, gradually break up and disappear. This disappearance of the myelin sheath and degeneration of the nerve fiber is known as Wallerian degeneration. Degeneration of nerve fibers begins a few days after injury to the nerve, and within 10 days regenerating nerve fibers may be found in the connecting tissue, between the central and the distal ends of the nerves, if these have been approximated accurately. *Regeneration of the myelin sheath* takes place less rapidly than that of the nerve fiber. In some cases, return of volitional muscle control may occur before myelinization is complete. Under favorable conditions, the rate of regeneration is about 1 mm. a day. The length of time before clinical evidence of regeneration of an injured nerve appears depends on a number of factors, of which the *level of the injury* is perhaps the basic one. The mechanics of nerve repair, the condition of the nerve ends, of the wound and of the nerve bed, as well as the interval between the receipt of the injury and the time of suture, are also important factors. If the nerve ends are not in continuity, the downgoing axons from the proximal end of the nerve meet obstruction in the shape of scar tissue and are forced to turn back on themselves, so that they form a *bulbous enlargement of the proximal stump* (neuroma). This enlargement is usually very sensitive and may even be intensely painful if in an area subject to pressure. The pain is usually referred to the original distribution of the nerve, so paresthesias in that distribution will be produced by pressure or stimulation of the neuroma.

Causalgia. When a nerve is injured, but without complete interruption of its fibers, a syndrome known as causalgia may develop. These patients have pain in the distribution of the sensory fibers of the affected nerve and often show marked hyperesthesia of the skin in the course of its distribution. This pain, at times, may be so severe that the patient will take every precaution, such as wrapping the limb with cold, moist cloths, to prevent irritation or stimulation of the affected cutaneous surface. Autonomic changes, such as excessive perspiration and increased warmth of the affected part, may be noted. *Atrophy of the subcutaneous tissues* causes thinning of the skin of the affected areas, so that, for example, the fingers or the toes will become thin and tapering. The median nerve in the upper extremity and the tibial nerve in the lower, containing a large number of sympathetic fibers, are those most frequently involved.

At times the painful area is larger than that usually attributable to the nerve in question. The obvious vasomotor disturbances, the influence of emotion on the patient's pain and the usual relief of the symptoms by sympathetic block indicate that the sympathetic component of the irritated peripheral nerve is responsible for the symptoms. Surgical measures directed to the point of the injury often are sufficient to relieve the symptoms. The nerve may be freed from scar tissue and transplanted to a bed free from scar. Hersage, with longitudinal incisions in the nerve, may be carried out to relieve the constriction of scar tissue within the substance of nerve. In other patients, some type of temporary or permanent sympathetic block is necessary. Sympathetic denervation of an extremity *should not* be carried out without a previous demonstration that procaine block of the sympathetic supply to the limb can temporarily alleviate the patient's discomfort. In some cases, several procaine sympathetic blocks alone will relieve causalgia permanently.

Diagnosis

History Taking. The study of a patient with peripheral nerve injury must include a careful history. Particular attention should be paid to the location and the age of the injury, whether it was a *closed injury* or an *open wound* and whether it was *sharply incised* or *contused*. The possibility of spontaneous recovery from a closed nerve injury must always be kept in

mind. On the other hand, when it is obvious that a nerve is interrupted anatomically, exploration and nerve suture as soon as possible are indicated. It is important to find out whether *weakness* or *paralysis* with sensory disturbance appeared gradually or were immediately present after the injury. In the first situation, the lesion is likely to be scar tissue involving the nerve secondarily or compression of the nerve by callus. If paralysis was present from the onset, the nerve is interrupted anatomically or has suffered severe damage.

Examination. The examination of the patient must include careful inspection and palpation of the region of injury to determine the extent of scar tissue and the possible presence of callus or neuroma. Palpation of a nerve trunk may determine the exact level of the injury and whether anatomic continuity is sustained. If aneurysm is suspected, adjacent structures, especially large vessels, must be examined carefully. In penetrating wounds of the extremities, due to projectiles or incision, the site of nerve injury usually can be told accurately by the situation of the scar of entrance and of exit (if present). Careful analysis of the motor function of the limb is essential. It must be kept in mind that gross movements of the limb are often of little diagnostic value, since they can still be accomplished when there is total paralysis of one or more of the limb's nerves. However, in the case of all major nerves to a limb, movements of certain muscles or muscle groups innervated by the nerve in question cannot be well imitated or simulated by other muscle groups. Among such movements are extension of the wrist, as well as the distal phalanges of the fingers and the thumb, in lesions of the radial nerve; abduction of the fifth finger in the plane of the palm in injuries of the ulnar nerve; flexion of the distal phalanges of the thumb and the index finger in median-nerve injury and dorsal flexion of the foot and the ankle in injuries of the peroneal portion of the sciatic nerve.

In like manner, although there is a considerable degree of overlap and variation in the sensory distribution of the limb nerves, there are always isolated areas innervated by the nerve in question. The *tip of the little finger is supplied exclusively by the ulnar nerve and will always be anesthetic when that nerve is injured.* The tip of the index finger is supplied exclusively by the median nerve, and in radial-nerve injury there is usually a zone of analgesia on the dorsum of the hand, between the first and second metacarpals. Observation of reflexes is important, but their status is subject to certain qualifications, chief of which is the lack of response of a portion of a muscle group when nerve interruption is *partial.*

Thus, the *triceps reflex* may be present if the long head of the triceps muscle has been spared. The *Achilles reflex* may be active when the only muscle of the calf that is capable of contraction is the soleus. Alteration of sweating is an important indication, since if a peripheral nerve is severed or otherwise interrupted, sweating no longer takes place in its field of distribution. *Sweating tests* may be carried out by the use of indicators, such as starch-iodine or sodium chinizarin 2.6 disulfonate, or the electrical resistance of the skin may be studied with suitable electrical apparatus (dermometer).

Trophic disorders are especially apt to occur when pain is present, as in causalgia. The hands and the feet are sites of predilection. The delicate indentations of the skin become more shallow, and the skin grows inelastic and smooth and, in time, becomes translucent, shiny, glossy and mottled. Fibrosis of subcutaneous tissue may occur, and trophic ulcers may develop when a region of sensory loss is subjected to pressure, trauma or excessive cold or heat. Such trophic ulcers are most likely to appear in the fingers in median or ulnar nerve palsies and in the toes, the sole or the heel of the foot in tibial nerve injuries. Shrinkage of subcutaneous tissue may take place; finger tips are most subject to this and may show a considerable degree of tapering. Fingernails become brittle, ridged or curved, and pallor of the skin or cyanosis, or a combination of the two, may exist. There may be coldness of the part with the pallor or increased warmth with hyperemia. *Edema* is probably due to disturbances in the lymphatic circulation coincident with lack of use. It usually extends beyond the field of disturbed sensation.

Tingling or formication provoked by percussion, or by general pressure to the distal part of an injured nerve trunk, is known as the *sign of Tinel.* The sensation is experienced in the distribution of the nerve and not at the spot stimulated. When Tinel's sign is sought, to indicate nerve regeneration, percussion should start distally and continue proximally along the course of the nerve. It must consist of single taps by one finger only. The significance of Tinel's sign is disputed and it is not always a dependable indication of nerve regeneration. However, it may serve a useful purpose until return of motor power or sensation becomes evident.

Electric examination of affected muscles is of considerable value in diagnosis and also in observing the progress of regeneration. *Chronaxia* has considerable advantage over testing with faradic and galvanic current because degeneration and regeneration may be determined much earlier than with the faradic and galvanic current. *Electromyography* is the most valuable test of all, largely because it uses fine insulated needles that make possible a record of electrical activity of individual muscles or, at best, a few individual muscle fibers. Thus, it may be possible to obtain definite evidence of degeneration or regeneration in isolated muscle groups long before such evidence is available by other methods. The drawback of electromyography is the extensive and complicated equipment required.

OPERATIVE PROCEDURES

The indications for operative intervention may be stated as follows: (1) the presence or suspected presence of anatomic severance of a nerve; (2) the progressive development of motor or sensory disturbance in an injured nerve; (3) the failure of return of function in a nerve that has been injured but is presumed to be in anatomic continuity.

There is considerable disagreement as to whether primary nerve suture should be carried out at the time of the primary repair of a compound wound of the extremities. It was the experience in both World Wars that, under combat conditions, primary nerve suture was not justified at the time of initial *débridement* and repair of a compound wound. At primary repair, the nerves, if possible, should be identified and their ends tagged, but nerve suture should be reserved for more optimum circumstances, to be carried out after the primary wound has been well healed for several weeks. Many authorities believe that this is also true in civilian practice.

It has been pointed out that, theoretically, nerve regeneration into the distal segment of a nerve will be more rapid after Wallerian degeneration has taken place; therefore, it has been concluded that primary nerve suture at the time of injury is undesirable. However, under favorable circumstances, where wounds are not grossly contaminated, primary nerve suture at the time of the initial repair is the procedure of choice. Some of the best results in peripheral-nerve surgery have been obtained under such conditions. Yet, where a wound is grossly contaminated or where extensive mobilization of the nerve trunks is necessary to effect suture, primary suture should not be carried out until several weeks after the wound is well healed. If, after injury to an extremity, signs of nerve involvement gradually develop, exploration of the nerve in question is indicated and should be carried out as soon as the signs of its involvement are apparent. The most difficult decisions arise in cases of closed nerve injury, such as injuries to the facial nerve in basal skull fracture or damage to the brachial plexus. Where the continuity of the trunk presumably has not been interrupted, but recovery does not soon take place, it may not be desirable to wait for spontaneous regeneration, since that might mean 18 to 24 months, if the injury is proximally located. In such cases, if there is any possibility that the nerve lesion can be improved, either by suture or relief of constriction by scar tissue, operation should be carried out, especially if there is any significant degree of disability.

Proper exposure is very important. It is frequently necessary to mobilize nerves for a considerable distance in order to accomplish end-to-end apposition after removal of scars and neuromas. Therefore, it is important to approach nerves through fascial planes rather than by penetration through muscle substance. If a muscle is penetrated, it should be done by splitting in the direction of its fibers. Where it is necessary to divide a muscle, it should be severed at its point of fascial attachment so that it may be repaired easily. Skin incisions that are perpendicular to flexion creases must be avoided since a traction scar probably would result. Not only the skin but also fascial layers and subcutaneous tissues are involved in the production of flexion scars. Proper placement of incisions for exposure of peripheral nerves will avoid much deformity.

Identification of the ends of a nerve that are imbedded in an extensive soft-tissue scar is often extremely difficult. It is necessary to identify the nerve at a point where normal anatomic relationships are present both above and below the scar and then trace the proximal segment of the nerve downward and the distal segment of the nerve upward into the scar. Often the two ends will be found separated by scar tissue over a distance of a centimeter or more. Where anatomic interruption of nerve fibers is complete, stimulation of the proximal portion of the nerve will not result in any motor activity below the level of the injury. In the conscious patient, such stimulation will, of course, produce paresthesias in the distal distribution of the nerve. Where degeneration of axons has taken place, stimulation of the distal segment of the nerve will induce no response. Where Wallerian degeneration has *not* taken place, stimulation of the distal segment of the nerve will produce contraction of the muscles which it supplies, but in the conscious patient, no sensory phenomena can be elicited.

Many peripheral-nerve operations can be carried out satisfactorily on conscious patients, provided that local anesthesia is adequate. However, peripheral-nerve procedures are often prolonged and at times require positioning of the limbs in uncomfortable postures. Consequently, many patients will insist on general anesthesia, particularly for secondary procedures.

After a nerve has been mobilized, if it is found to be interrupted, the ends that are involved in scar tissue must be resected, otherwise satisfactory regeneration cannot be expected. However, before the neuroma and the scar are actually resected, an estimate should be made as to whether, after mobilization and possible rerouting of the nerve trunk, the ends can be brought into apposition. Otherwise, it will be better to suture the neuromas with the limb in flexion; then, after the suture line is healed, nerve stretching may be carried out. Re-exploration with resection of the neuromas and end-to-end apposition of the nerve trunks may then follow. When a nerve is in continuity, but is thickened and offers increased resistance to palpation of the involved area, it is known as a *neuroma in continuity*. If function is severely impaired, resection of the neuroma and resuture of the nerve may be the best procedure, but, in most cases, the problem is the relief of pain, as satisfactory function of the nerve is present.

The procedure of hersage is an attempt to relieve the constriction of nerve fibers due to scar tissue. It consists of longitudinal incisions in the sheath of the nerve at different points on its periphery. In the case of a sizable nerve, such as the ulnar or the median at the elbow, 5 or 6 or even 8 of these incisions may be carried out. They should be carried down through the sheath of the nerve and discontinued as the normal funicular structure of the nerve becomes apparent. If they are made carefully, using a sharp knife, and are exactly parallel with each other, few, if any, functioning nerve fibers will be severed.

After extensive mobilization of the central and peripheral ends of a nerve trunk, it may still be necessary to reroute it in order to accomplish satisfactory suture. Transference of the ulnar nerve to the anterior aspect of the elbow is the best example of such a rerouting procedure, as flexion of the elbow will reduce a previous gap in the ulnar nerve by 5 to 7 cm. Transposition of a nerve, or rerouting, has definite limitations, since usually it cannot be done without sacrificing some of the nerve's branches. Attempts to do it without such sacrificing of branches that interfere with the transposition will reduce the distance gained by the transposition. When a nerve passes anterior to a joint, its flexion is of great value in reducing a gap. For example, flexion of the wrist and the fingers will reduce a gap in the median nerve above the wrist as much as 4 cm. Rotating the head to the side of the lesion will reduce a gap in the radial nerve of 2 cm., while elevation and adduction in the arm will reduce a gap of 8 cm. Flexion of the elbow will reduce gaps in the median and radial nerves of 5 to 6 cm., and in the ulnar nerve, similar reductions may be added to the effect of transposition. Flexion of the knee can be used to reduce a gap of 10 cm. in the sciatic nerve.

The use of peripheral nerve grafts should be considered when gaps cannot be overcome by mobilization, transposition, positioning of the limb or by 2-stage stretching of the nerve. In the experimental animal, heterogenous grafts have been used with considerable satisfaction, but the few reported successes in humans have been with autogenous grafts. Only a few nerves can be sacrificed for autogenous grafts. These are the superficial branch of the radial, the medial cutaneous nerve of the forearm, the external saphenous nerve on the dorsal aspect of the leg and the internal saphenous nerve of the thigh. Preserved nerve grafts from cadavers have not been satisfactory up to this time. However, the possibility of using frozen segments of nerve as homografts must be considered, since such homografts could be removed at autopsy and quick frozen for later use in bridging defects in large nerves.

In autografting, the cutaneous nerve to be used is exposed and the segments of desired length are then cut on either a moist tongue depressor or moist gauze, whence they are transferred to the point of suture. If sutures are passed through the ends of the cut grafts before they are sectioned, their handling is greatly facilitated. After transfer to the recipient site they are sutured to the sheaths of the nerve ends so as to approximate the ends of the graft to the funiculi. Shifting of the grafts must be avoided, and, as far as possible, the grafts should be sutured to funiculi of similar size at each end of the nerve. It has been suggested that after a few weeks the wound should be re-explored and section and resuture carried out at the distal end of the graft in order to prevent scar tissue from interfering with the growth of the regenerating fibers through the grafts into the distal segment of the nerve. The actual technic of nerve suture is the final step in any nerve repair and is very important. Resection of neuromas and scar tissue in the ends of the nerve is done piecemeal so as to avoid the needless sacrifice of normal nerve tissue. The resection starts from the lesion and proceeds in both directions, cutting clean right-angle sections with a sharp knife or razor at intervals of 3 to 5 mm. until the funiculi appear to be normal. In larger nerves there is often troublesome bleeding from the end of the central artery, and if this does not respond to pressure with moist cotton, it will be necessary to hold a small piece of muscle or of gelatin sponge firmly against the nerve for several minutes. This will control the bleeding. The nerve ends must be approximated so that their previous anatomic alignment is restored as nearly as possible. The nerve sheath is then drawn together with fine silk, and tantalum or wire sutures are passed through the periphery of the ends. These sutures are placed 1 to 2 mm. apart and include only the sheath of the nerve. It may be necessary to transfix the two ends of the nerve with heavier silk or wire suture to permit sufficient traction to bring the ends of the nerve into apposition while the multiple fine sutures in the sheath are tied. For this, fine silk or tantalum wire sutures (5.0 to 7.0) again are used. The so-called "plasma-clot method" of nerve suture was developed by Torlov and his associates. This requires special apparatus, and there is a chance of error in the possibility of separation of the nerve ends after the suture is accomplished.

POSTOPERATIVE CARE

Protective splinting is often necessary after peripheral nerve repair when the limb has been placed in flexion to overcome a gap in the nerve. In such cases the splinting must be maintained for 3 to 4 weeks, or until it is certain that firm union has taken place at the point of suture. Then the splint may be removed and the nerve stretched by gradual extension of the limb.

As soon as that has been accomplished, or, in other cases, as soon as the wound has healed, physiotherapy should begin. This may consist at first of gentle massage and later of active and passive movements of the limb, together with galvanic stimulation of the paralyzed muscles. The aim of physiotherapy is to maintain the tone and the contractility of the paralyzed muscles and to prevent contractures or deformity of the limb because of the presence of the paralysis. In severely paralyzed limbs, during intervals between physiotherapy treatments and manipulations, some type of protective splinting may be necessary to prevent contracture. Such protective splinting should be in the neutral position of the limb in order to prevent stretching of the paralyzed muscles.

CRANIAL NERVES

Injuries to the cranial nerves must be included in any discussion of peripheral-nerve injury. The cranial nerves most frequently injured are the facial, the spinal accessory, the hypoglossal and the recurrent laryngeal branch of the vagus. Peripheral injury to the facial nerve should be treated by exposure of the branches of the nerve and primary suture. The surgeon frequently is called upon to treat cases of spontaneous paralysis of the facial nerve (so-called Bell's palsy) or injury of the facial nerve due to basal skull fracture.

Facial nerve paralysis is sometimes produced by the surgeon when completely removing tumors of the cerebellopontine angle, especially acoustic neuromas. Here the surgeon may use a so-called nerve-crossing or anastomosis operation, in which the function of one nerve is sacrificed in order to obtain regeneration in another, more important one. In the case of the facial nerve, the spinal accessory, the hypoglossal or the glossopharyngeal nerves are available for repair. While, from physiologic and embryologic standpoints, the glossopharyngeal nerve should be the most satisfactory, from a technical standpoint, it is the most undesirable because it is so small and inaccessible. Consequently, most surgeons use the hypoglossal or the spinal accessory nerve.

Incisions for the exposure of the facial nerve at its emergence from the stylomastoid foramen and the hypoglossal or the spinal accessory nerves in the neck should not parallel the anterior border of the sternocleidomastoid muscle (as recommended in some quarters) but rather should parallel the angle of the jaw. Such an incision causes much less cosmetic deformity. If the hypoglossal nerve is sacrificed, deviation of the tongue on protrusion, with atrophy of its homolateral half, will result. This, it seems to the author, is preferable to the weakness and atrophy of the shoulder muscles produced by spinal accessory paralysis. The latter is undesirable in women for cosmetic reasons and in active men from the standpoint of shoulder function.

After hypoglossofacial anastomosis, *physiotherapy to the facial muscles* is essential to prevent atrophy and loss of muscle tone. After evidence of regeneration appears, a long training period for the patient is necessary to overcome the tendency toward association of movements of the face with those of the tongue and also to establish satisfactory voluntary contraction and emotional control of the facial muscles. In the case of the facial nerve, perfect results cannot be expected from nerve crossing because of the difficulty of getting symmetrical movements of the face on emotional expression. The patient will obtain functional results in direct proportion to his voluntary efforts.

Words of Caution

Primary nerve suture must not be attempted in contaminated or infected wounds. Delay in operation and especially in suture should not exceed a year after the injury. Attempts at nerve grafting should be reserved for those cases where transposition of nerves, positioning of the limbs and 2-stage stretching do not reduce gaps effectively. Nerve crossing or anastomosis has a very limited application, generally used only in injury to the facial nerve proximal to the stylomastoid foramen.

Nerve suture must be accurately performed with very fine suture material. The sutures are passed only through the perineurium, and the nerve ends must be approximated without tension. Physiotherapy is of great importance both before and after surgery. *The treatment of peripheral nerve injuries should not be undertaken unless adequate facilities for physiotherapy are available.*

REFERENCES

1. Bakay, L., and Sweet, M. H.: Cervical and intracranial intra-arterial pressures with and without vascular occlusion, Surg., Gynec. & Obst. **95**:67, 1952.
2. Batson, O. V.: The function of the vertebral veins and their role in the spread of metastasis, Ann. Surg. **112**:138, 1940.
3. daCosta, D. G., and Adson, A. W.: Subdural hydroma, Arch. Surg. **43**:559, 1941.
4. Dandy, W. E.: Ventriculography following the injection of air into the cerebral ventricles, Ann. Surg. **68**:5, 1918.
5. ———: Roentgenography of the brain after the injection of air into the spinal canal, Ann. Surg. **70**:397, 1919.
6. ———: Section of the sensory root of the trigeminal nerve at the pons, Bull. Johns Hopkins Hosp. **36**:105, 1925.
7. ———: Hydrocephalus *in* Lewis, D. (ed.): Practice of Surgery, vol. 12, Hagerstown, Md., Prior, 1932.
8. ———: Intracranial Arterial Aneurysms, Ithaca, Comstock, 1944.
9. Greenwood, J.: Two point or interpolar coagulation; review after a 12-year period with notes on addition of a sucker tip, J. Neurosurg. **12**:196, 1955.
10. Hassin, G. B.: Cerebrospinal fluid; its origin, nature and function, J. Neuropath. & Exper. Neurol. **7**:172, 1948.
11. Kearns, J. J.: Difficult diagnostic problems resulting from trauma, Indust. Med. **9**:25, 1940.
12. Matson, D. D.: Ventriculo-ureterostomy, J. Neurosurg. **8**:398, 1951.
13. Munro, D.: Craniocerebral Injuries, New York, Oxford, 1938.
14. Nosik, W. A.: Ventriculomastoidostomy; technique and observations, J. Neurosurg. **7**:236, 1950.
15. Padgett, D. H.: The circle of Willis *in* Dandy, W. E.: Intracranial Arterial Aneurysms, p. 67, Ithaca, Comstock, 1944.
16. Poppen, J. L.: Specific treatment of intracranial aneurysms; experiences with 143 surgically treated patients, J. Neurosurg. **8**:75, 1951.
17. Pudenz, R. H., Russell, F. E., Hurd, A. H., and Sheldon, C. H.: Ventriculo-auriculostomy; a technique for shunting cerebrospinal fluid into the right auricle, J. Neurosurg. **14**:171, 1957.
18. Spence, W. T.: Form-fitting plastic cranioplasty, J. Neurosurg. **11**:219, 1954.
19. Stookey, B., and Scarff, J.: Occlusion of the aqueduct of Sylvius by neoplastic and non-neoplastic processes with a rational surgical treatment for relief of the resultant obstructive hydrocephalus, Bull. Neurol. Inst. New York **5**:348, 1936.
20. Trotter, W.: Subdural hemorrhage of traumatic origin and its relation to pachymeningitis hemorrhagica interna, Brit. J. Surg. **2**:271, 1914.

JAMES W. WATTS, M.D., AND JOSÉ H. MATEOS, M.D.

7 The Spine and the Spinal Cord

In this chapter no attempt is made to cover all phases of surgery of the spine. Emphasis is placed on the safeguards and the errors in performing surgery of the spine and the spinal cord. Important but well-standardized methods may be omitted entirely, while some minor point in diagnosis or management may be discussed at length.

LITERATURE ON SPINAL CORD SURGERY

By the end of World War I, two important monographs on the spinal cord had been published in America. The first was Charles A. Elsburg's *Diseases of the Spinal Cord and Its Membranes* and the second was *Surgery of the Spine and Spinal Cord* by Charles H. Frazier. Tumors of the spinal cord were rarely reported. Little was done about congenital anomalies. Fractures of the spine with cord compression were operated on, but with disappointing results. Postoperative care of paraplegics with decubitus ulcers and genitourinary infections was heartbreaking. Spinal operations had such a reputation that even patients with *curable* conditions, such as benign tumors, were reluctant to submit to surgery and often postponed treatment until too late.

At that period, major emphasis was on surgery of brain tumor, head injuries, brain abscess, tic douloureux and the like. It was quite natural that neurosurgeons should have been looked upon as "brain" surgeons.

Then, three events occurred which resulted in a change of surgical attitude and emphasis. The first of these was the establishment of the protruded intervertebral disk as the chief cause of low back pain and sciatic pain. The second was the discovery of antibiotics and the third was the acceptance and the development of *physical medicine* as a method of therapy and rehabilitation.

Although there had been isolated reports earlier, it was only in 1934 that a paper appeared which shifted the focus of neurosurgeons' attention from the brain to the spine. This was a report by Mixter and Barr which established protruded intervertebral disk as the cause of low back pain and sciatic pain. At the present time, more disk operations are performed than any other surgical intervention in the average neurosurgical clinic. The mortality is low, complications are rare, and results are reasonably good. As a consequence, the fear that used to be associated with spinal operations has largely disappeared. Patients will now submit to these procedures, believing that even if surgery does not cure, at least too great a risk is not involved. This has led to reinvestigation and study of conditions which had long been given up as hopeless.

Urinary infection, one of the chief causes of death among neurosurgical patients, can now be controlled by antibiotics. Pulmonary atelectasis develops less frequently into terminal bronchopneumonia.

During World War II, the large number of young men with severe injuries of the spinal cord presented an obligation and a challenge to our Army and Navy. During the Pacific campaign, the Navy established a program of rehabilitation under the direction of Dr. Henry H. Kessler, who, soon after World War I, had inaugurated the first state rehabilitation program in New Jersey. Under the leadership of Dr. Howard Rusk, an active program of rehabilitation, based on the earlier work of Dr. Kessler and Dr. George Deaver of New York and Dr. Donald Munro of Boston, was undertaken by the Army. Many new technics enabling paralyzed veterans to

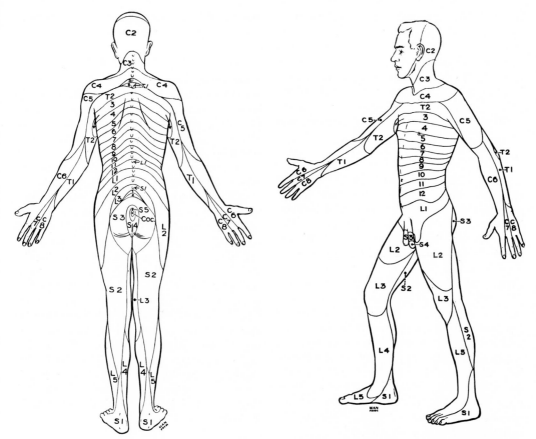

FIG. 55. (*Left*) The dermatomes from the posterior view. (*Right*) A side view of the dermatomes. (After Haymaker and Woodhall: Peripheral Nerve Injuries, Philadelphia, Saunders)

become self-sufficient and ambulatory were discovered. Widespread utilization of these methods and experience in the management of other types of injury so impressed the medical profession that it accepted physiotherapy, occupational therapy and other rehabilitation services and established physical medicine and rehabilitation as an approved specialty.

Before considering the safeguards and the errors associated with specific conditions such as congenital anomalies, protruded intervertebral disk and tumors and injuries of the spinal cord, we shall discuss several topics which have a general application (Fig. 55).

GENERAL CONSIDERATIONS

Position During Surgery

The *prone position* is used for most patients in performing lumbar and thoracic laminectomy. In lumbar laminectomy, the spine is flexed by breaking the table, with the apex of the break in the midlumbar or lower lumbar region. *Flexion of the spine* separates the laminae and allows the surgeon to perform an interlaminar operation in many cases of protruded intervertebral disk. *Hyperextension* must be avoided, as it brings the laminae closer together.

A few surgeons prefer the *lateral position*.

Operations on the cervical vertebrae may be performed in either the prone or the upright position. The neck is flexed and the chin brought down toward the chest. A head rest is required. Most disk operations are done in the upright position. When there is a combined cervical laminectomy and suboccipital craniectomy, the upright position is to be preferred. Venous bleeding is reduced, and when bleeding does occur, it runs out of the wound instead of pooling. Air embolism and subdural hematoma have been reported but are rare, and the risks of these complications must be balanced against the advantages of full exposure. Hyperextension must be avoided. Children and debilitated patients are operated on in the prone position.

ANESTHESIA

Endotracheal anesthesia is used in all spinal operations when a general anesthetic is employed. Induction is with Pentothal Sodium. Nitrous oxide and oxygen are given by inhalation. The anesthetist has control of the airway in both prone and upright positions. Care must be taken to ensure free pulmonary exchange. Maintenance of blood pressure has not been a serious problem. We recall only one instance when it was necessary to shift the patient from the upright to the horizontal position because of a fall in blood pressure.

Some surgeons employ spinal anesthesia, but we agree with Williams[12] that it should be reserved for those circumstances where other forms of anesthetic agents are, for one reason or another, inexpedient. While complications are rare, they may be serious.

Choice of local anesthesia is infrequent, though it is still used by a few neurosurgeons who have perfected a technic using local combined with procaine block. These surgeons constitute a small minority.

PROGNOSIS

Misunderstanding can be avoided by explaining to the patient and his relatives what the operation may be expected to accomplish. If the results fall far short of what the patient had anticipated, disappointment and dissatisfaction are sure to occur.

SPINAL FLUID EXAMINATION

To avoid errors when spinal puncture is performed, careful manometric studies should be carried out to determine whether *subarachnoid block* is present. The protein content of the fluid should be checked, since it is elevated when there is a block. It must be kept in mind that increased spinal fluid protein can be due also to other causes, such as inflammation or degeneration. However, elevation of the spinal fluid protein is always indicative of organic disease of the nervous system.

ROENTGENOGRAPHY

In getting roentgenograms, an error which sometimes occurs is failure to include the diseased or damaged area of the spine on the plates. To safeguard against this, the surgeon should state specifically the level and the views which he requires.

In addition to anteroposterior and lateral views, *special* exposures are often helpful. In a case of cervical spine injury, it is necessary to have films taken with the mouth open in order to determine if there is a fracture of the odontoid process. Oblique views of the cervical spine are necessary in order to visualize the intervertebral foramina. Lateral views of the seventh cervical and the first thoracic vertebrae are difficult to secure because of the numerous overlying structures. By pulling the shoulder down, or slanting the tube, one may get a more satisfactory picture. As an additional safeguard, when examining the lumbar vertebrae, the oblique position is necessary in order to visualize the articulating facets. Evidence of sclerosis at the articulations may be an indication of instability.

MYELOGRAPHY

Myelography is an important diagnostic aid in determining the presence of protruded intervertebral disk, spinal cord tumor and other causes of spinal cord compression. *Pantopaque* is the contrast medium most generally used. Safeguards and errors in connection with myelography will be considered in more detail later in this chapter.

MANAGEMENT OF THE BLADDER

Before the days of antibiotics, there were strong differences of opinion about the management of the "cord bladder." Catheterization usually led to cystitis and pyelitis in patients with spinal cord injuries. Attempts were made to establish an "automatic" bladder by compressing it. The bladder was allowed to become distended, finally catheterization was performed, and it was usually necessary to carry out a suprapubic cystotomy.

At the present time, catheterization is performed promptly, an indwelling catheter inserted and tidal drainage, as recommended by Munro, employed. In addition to this, the patient is put on regular doses of a drug such as Gantrisin. We use 0.5 Gm., 4 times daily.

CONGENITAL ANOMALIES

Spina Bifida Occulta

One should be aware that congenital disorders may give rise to complications or progressive loss of neurologic function as growth proceeds.

Spina bifida occulta is often discovered when a routine roentgenogram of the lumbosacral spine is taken. If it is causing no symptoms, it requires no treatment. We believe that Matson's[5a] closing remarks, following his paper on *Surgical Treatment of Congenital Spinal Disorders,* present concisely the best view of this problem:

I like to think that the way to approach lesions associated with spina bifida occulta is radical investigation combined with very conservative surgical treatment. There certainly is little or nothing to be gained by manipulation of the cord itself, or the cauda equina, whether the lesion is a dermoid cyst or one of the so-called lipomas (I like to avoid this term because I think we may get to think of them as discrete tumors, which they are not). These fatty masses may extend everywhere from the skin right on down into the substance of the cauda equina, and one may injure the neural tissue any time after the skin incision is made if he is not aware of the simple fact that the overlying fascia, muscle, bone and meninges may all be defective.

Insofar as one can remove any structures that are compressing or distorting the cord or the cauda equina, divide fibrous bands, remove intraspinal meningoceles, excise discrete masses of fat, and remove dermoid cysts, surgical intervention is extremely worth while, but even then it must be carried out very carefully. Beyond that, I think it is meddlesome to feel that one must explore every patient simply because neurologic signs are present.

The treatment of meningoceles and meningomyeloceles associated with spina bifida is an individual problem in which each case must be considered on its own merits. The neurosurgeon often sees infants on the day of birth. If there is leakage of the cerebrospinal fluid from the sac, the defect must be closed promptly in order to avoid infection. If the skin of the meningocele is healthy, we recommend waiting 3 to 6 months to allow time to determine whether hydrocephalus will develop.

The simple meningoceles without nerve involvement constitute a minority.

If the infant has meningomyelocele, associated with paraplegia, loss of bowel and bladder function and hydrocephalus, little can be accomplished by operation. In any event, a careful neurologic examination is essential to determine the degree of paralysis, and before any surgical treatment is undertaken, the prognosis should be carefully explained to the parents and to the patient's physician.

Dermoid and teratomatous lesions of the spinal canal should be approached conservatively, with emphasis on the contents of cysts, removal of the solid tumor and cyst wall which is freely mobilized, with no attempt at sharp dissection from neural tissue itself.

PROTRUDED INTERVERTEBRAL DISK

The symptoms of nerve root pressure due to protruded intervertebral disk have become so well known that a patient often comes to the office or clinic complaining of a "slipped" or "ruptured disk." He may have a friend who was operated on, with complete relief of pain. Therefore, he sees no reason to postpone operation, as he is confident that he has the same condition and will have the same result. Yet another patient consults the surgeon reluctantly because he knows of someone who had a disk operation with disappointing results. Naturally, an individual's ideas are colored by the one case that he knows.

The greatest error the surgeon can make is to feel that he can cure every pain in the neck or the low back by a disk operation. The most important safeguard is the taking of a careful history.

Many factors influence the results of disk surgery—the condition of the back before the disk injury, the type of work the patient does, the personality of the patient and the compensation and liability considerations.

Disk surgery is primarily for relief of nerve root pressure. If the symptoms are mainly nerve root manifestations and the nerve is not badly injured, the results of operation should be good.

LUMBAR DISK

Disk protrusion can occur at any level, but approximately 90 per cent are found at the lumbosacral level, or between the fourth and fifth lumbar vertebrae, where they cause low back pain and sciatic pain. A few patients give a history of severe back strain, with immediate development of low back pain radiating down the back of the thigh into the lower leg and the foot. On examination, they reveal local back tenderness, hypalgesia on the lateral part of the foot and the leg, absence of ankle jerk and limitation of straight leg raising. In a case like this, the diagnosis is obvious and the relation of the symptoms to the accident definite. Most patients have a history of several episodes of low back pain, which may have kept them in bed from a few days to a week, with the symptoms clearing up in a couple of weeks. Then, after some minor accident, back pain recurs and, this time, is associated with extension of pain into the leg. In some, the back pain improves when the leg pain develops. Neurologic examination confirms the diagnosis of nerve root compression due to protruded disk.

Limitation of straight leg raising on the ipsilateral side is, perhaps, the most common finding in nerve root pressure at L^4-L^5 and L^5-S^1. If there is no limitation of straight leg raising, doubt is cast on the diagnosis. An exception may occur when the protrusion or rupture is in the midline.

Roentgenograms of the lumbosacral spine are of little diagnostic value in making a diagnosis of protruded disk, but they are essential to exclude spondylolisthesis, malignant neoplasm, hypertrophic arthritis, etc. Loss of the normal lumbar lordotic curve is usually present in ruptured and protruded disk. The disk space may be narrowed, but a minor degree of narrowing is not significant.

FUSION

When is fusion of the spine indicated? When leg pain is the major complaint and back pain the minor one, a simple disk operation is performed. In our clinic, relatively few fusions are done at the time of a primary disk operation. Exceptions to this are patients with a history of chronic low back pain and instability, with roentgenographic evidence supporting this. Fusions are carried out in patients who continue to have back pain after a simple disk operation and in those who develop a recurrent disk protrusion.

Pantopaque myelography is used routinely in every patient before disk operation by some members of our department; others use it only in selected cases. It is employed when the symptoms are sufficient to require operation in order to verify the diagnosis and establish the level of the protruded disk. We find it to be correct in 90 to 95 per cent of our cases.

A "needle defect" may simulate a protruded disk. As a precaution to avoid this error, the needle is inserted at a space above or below the suspected disk. A well-defined filling defect on the side of the pain at the suspected level is diagnostic of protruded disk. Absence of filling of the nerve sleeve at the suspected level on the side of the pain, with normal filling on the opposite side, is consistent with a diagnosis of protruded disk. An hourglass defect may be produced by a midline protruded disk but sometimes may result from an artefact. A normal myelogram with a narrow spinal canal does not exclude a laterally placed disk as a cause of nerve root compression.

Air myelography has had no value in our hands. Studies with air myelography, employing a 1,000,000-volt machine, now in progress at the Walter Reed General Hospital in Washington, D. C., may revive the use of air as a contrast medium. When myelography fails, discography will demonstrate the lesion in certain ruptured disks. It is of special value when there is absence of protrusion into the spinal canal.

CERVICAL DISK

Cervical disks which require operation occur most often between C-5 and C-6 or C-6 and C-7. A posterolateral protrusion between C-5 and C-6 characteristically causes pain in the neck with extension to the thumb, numbness of the thumb and weakness of the biceps muscle with diminished biceps reflex. A disk compressing the nerve root between C-6 and C-7 usually produces pain and numbness in the index finger and often in the thumb and the ring finger, with associated numbness, weakness of the triceps muscle and diminished triceps reflex. Cervical arthritis and the anterior scalene or thoracic outlet syndrome must always be considered in differential diagnosis. Compression by a disk usually affects the thumb and the index finger. Compression by the anterior scalene affects chiefly the little and the ring fingers, and the symptoms and signs are less well-defined, less limited to a single nerve root distribution. Hypertrophic cervical arthritis may give rise to pain and stiffness of the neck with extension to the arm and the hand. The pain is less well-defined than with protruded disk, and the oblique roentgenograms will show encroachment on numerous neural foramina.

Myelography has been found to be a valuable and reliable diagnostic procedure which is used regularly. As a safeguard, bed rest and traction should be employed before resorting to operation for cervical disk.

The upright position, with endotracheal anesthesia, is usually employed for operation. When the disk protrusion is cartilaginous, nucleus tissue is removed, as in the lumbar region. When one finds a "hard disk," i.e., a disk covered with bone or a bony spur, the nerve root is decompressed by removing the posterior part of the foramen, which may be sufficient.

Midline protrusion or rupture of a cervical disk often impinges on the spinal cord without producing pain in the arms. Prompt action is then necessary to prevent paralysis. Even by myelography there is a chance of error when trying to differentiate between disk and tumor. Laminectomy of the vertebra above and below the protrusion is necessary. If the bulge into the spinal canal is bony or cannot be removed, decompression is accomplished by cutting the dentate ligaments.

In the *Yearbook of Neurology, Psychiatry and Neurosurgery* for 1955, attention is called again to the necessity of excluding compression of the cervical cord in patients with atypical multiple sclerosis, amyotrophic lateral sclerosis and other degenerative conditions of the cervical cord.

While rare, as compared with lumbar and cervical disk protrusion, protrusions of thoracic intervertebral disks are beginning to attract attention. Reports indicate that they may simulate cardiac, pulmonary or abdominal disease, as well as intercostal neuritis. Special precautions must be taken during myelography. Slow movement of the column of oil in both oblique positions with from 9 to 18 cc. of Pantopaque is advocated by Abbott and Retter.

Causes of Failure

There are a number of causes of failure in the disk operations. There may be a recurrence at the same level, or a second disk may be protruded, or it may rupture at a later date. Greenwood has found that disk tissue may work its way well up under the lamina of the vertebra or into a neural foramen. If we are confident that a protruded disk is present, and if it is not discovered through an interlaminar exposure, we do not hesitate to perform a hemilaminectomy to obtain adequate exposure. Loose nucleus pulposus has been found under the lamina in several instances.

SPINAL CORD INJURY

When injury to the spine occurs, without damage to the cord, it is primarily an orthopedic problem. Mild injury to the cord may cause only transient weakness, while more severe damage results in permanent paralysis.

Concussion

Spinal cord concussion implies physiologic interruption of function but without any anatomic change, such as a contusion, a laceration or a compression. Concussion is often difficult to differentiate from *contusion* of the spinal cord, because contusion may occur with or without fracture of the spine. When injury to the cervical cord is associated with head injury, the presence of blood in the cerebrospinal fluid cannot be considered as evidence of laceration of the cord.

Contusion

Contusion may occur as a result of hyperflexion or hyperextension. When dislocation or compression fracture can be demonstrated by roentgenogram, contusion is much more probable. Compression of the cord can be produced by dislocation of the vertebrae, fragments of bone in the case of fractures and

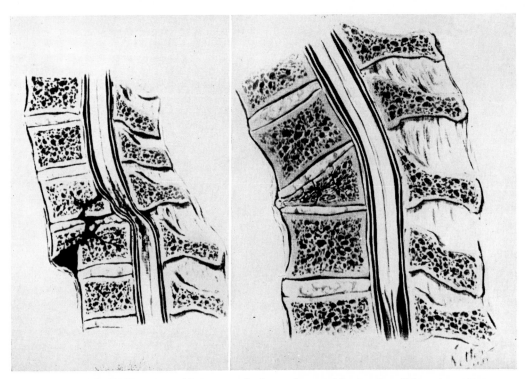

FIG. 56. (*Left*) Fracture of lower cervical vertebrae with anterior dislocation of upper segment and injury to cord. (*Right*) Compression fracture of twelfth thoracic vertebrae with wedge-shaped deformity of vertebral body. (Netter, F. H.: The Ciba Collection of Medical Illustrations)

occasionally by a ruptured intervertebral disk (Fig. 56).

Tarlov[9] and his associates have demonstrated experimentally that complete recovery can take place if the compression is relieved in adequate time when the symptoms are due more to mechanical pressure than to anoxia. Unfortunately, as Tarlov points out, surgery cannot always be performed as promptly in man as in the experimental animal.

Two excellent studies have been made recently. One, by Wannamaker,[10] is based on early treatment of 300 consecutive cases of patients with spinal cord injuries in the Tokyo Army Hospital. The other is a survey of the neurologic results of 858 spinal cord injuries by Comarr and Kaufman,[3] who state that, "While most authors agree in general upon proper methods of treating the complications of paraplegia, one apparently unsolved question still remains: When is laminectomy indicated?" And after a study of their statistics, the question remains unanswered.

We are inclined to agree with Naffziger and Boldrey, who state that, "In general the more experienced the surgeon, the fewer the cases that will be judged suitable for operation." We are also in accord with Crutchfield,[4] who believes that, "When properly applied, skeletal traction is the safest, most effective and simplest method of treating patients with acute injuries to the cervical spine. Furthermore, when used to its full advantage, it leaves few, if any, indications for laminectomy, spinal fusion or plaster supports."

Laminectomy is obviously demanded when there is evidence of compression of the cord. It may also be indicated when the symptoms point to nerve root compression at or near the site of the fracture.

IMMEDIATE TREATMENT

In connection with safeguards and errors in the management of injury to the spine, more important than operative technics is the first aid and handling immediately after entering the hospital. Ambulance personnel should be properly instructed. A patient with suspected injury to the spine should not be allowed to sit up, nor should he flex his head. He should be moved by 2 or 3 individuals who can keep him in the neutral position. A rigid support or stretcher is necessary. If a kyphos is present, hyperextension during transportation is advised. If the fracture was produced by hyperextension, slight flexion is recommended. If the conditions under which the injury was produced are unknown, the patient should be transported in the supine position with the body straight.

Special precautions should be taken in making roentgenograms when fracture to the cervical spine is suspected. It is advisable for the patient to be accompanied by the resident, who can control movements of the head and the neck. Manual traction or halter traction may be indicated. The special views required are discussed in an earlier part of this chapter.

If the patient is a quadriplegic, it is helpful, on admission to the hospital, to place him on a Stryker frame or a Foster bed. Roentgenograms can be taken with the patient on these special frames, and in the Foster bed, the Crutchfield tongs may be applied without transferring to an operating table. By using the double litter turning method, decubitus ulcers usually can be prevented. Tidal drainage should be instituted promptly. Abdominal distention can be cared for by means of the Wangensteen suction apparatus and the rectal tube.

With rehabilitation in mind, physical therapy should be initiated within a few days to a week, or as soon as the patient's condition permits.

SPINAL CORD TUMOR

Metastasis to the Spine without Cord Involvement

Metastasis to the spine may be from carcinoma of the breast, the lung, the prostate or the kidney. In consultation, we have seen a patient who had been discharged from the Army with a neuropsychiatric disability. He was obviously psychoneurotic, with somatic complaints ranging from his head to his heels, including pain in the back. A neurologic examination was negative, as were roentgeno-grams of the spine. Yet his nervous symptoms became so unbearable that he voluntarily sought admission to a mental hospital, where neurologic examination and roentgenograms of the spine again were negative. About 3 months after our examination, he wrote a highly critical letter—declining to pay his bill—stating that more recent roentgenograms had shown that he had cancer of the spine. It is easy to understand this patient's feelings, but it illustrates that destructive changes in the spine may not be revealed by roentgenograms for several months after the onset of pain. In doubtful cases, it is necessary to follow the patient and repeat the roentgenograms.

Hemangioma

Hemangioma of the vertebrae is uncommon but important. A vertebra may suddenly collapse at the site of the lesion, as in one patient who, while walking about the room, suddenly fell to the floor and said that he felt as if he had broken his back. Roentgenograms showed the characteristic appearance of coarse trabeculations of the vertebral body and partial collapse of the vertebra.

Multiple Myeloma

Multiple myeloma may also result in collapse of the vertebrae, but there is usually sufficient other evidence of myeloma to lead to the correct diagnosis.

Epidural Space Tumors

Carcinoma often metastasizes to the epidural space, invades the epidural fat and forms a sleeve around the spinal cord which cuts off the venous circulation and gives rise to myelitis by compression and ischemia of the spinal cord. In some patients, this is slowly progressive, and one has time to evaluate the conditions. In others, it proceeds very rapidly, as in a 68-year-old man who was well until one Saturday night when he developed retention of urine. Sunday morning, his right leg was paralyzed. By noon, his left leg was also paralyzed, and by the time he was admitted to the hospital in midafternoon, he was partially paralyzed in both arms. A myelogram and laminectomy were performed the same evening, and he gradually improved sufficiently to be able to walk with the aid of aluminum Loftstrand canes.

In addition to carcinoma, lymphosarcoma or Hodgkin's disease may also invade the epidural space. At times in the past, when a patient began to develop evidence of cord compression, we tried x-ray therapy and resorted to laminectomy only when the paralysis became advanced, but the results were disappointing. At the present time, it is our policy to perform a laminectomy promptly when signs of cord compression develop and follow later with x-ray therapy.

INTRADURAL EXTRAMEDULLARY TUMORS

The management of meningiomas and neurofibromas is well standardized. If the symptoms are not too far advanced, the results of operation are excellent. In operating for a dumbbell neurofibroma, a laminectomy should be done first and the intraspinal part removed. Since neurofibromas are sometimes multiple, the possibility of a second intraspinal tumor must be borne in mind. If the patient does not follow the course which one anticipates, the myelogram should be repeated in order to establish the diagnosis.

TUMORS OF THE FORAMEN MAGNUM

Tumors of the foramen magnum are particularly difficult to recognize since there is no typical syndrome for an accurate clinical diagnosis. Love, Thelen and Dodge[8] emphasize the need for a high index of suspicion in patients complaining of cervical and suboccipital pain, peculiar peripheral paresthesias, weakness of the upper extremities and difficulty in walking. Some patients give evidence of increased intracranial pressure on funduscopic examination and by x-ray study; in others, the diagnosis can be made by myelography. "Platybasia" and the Arnold-Chiari malformation may also give symptoms referable to the region of the foramen magnum and, to avoid error, must be considered in patients with an atypical multiple sclerosis and amyotrophic lateral sclerosis.

INTRAMEDULLARY TUMORS

Ependymomas and astrocytomas are the most common tumors of this group. Syringomyelia is sometimes associated with spinal cord tumor and may be indistinguishable from it.

The absence of a sensory level, and the inability of children to describe their symptoms in detail, may cause one to miss spinal cord tumor, which can masquerade under a diagnosis of poliomyelitis or Guillain-Barré syndrome. When disturbance of bladder function is the chief symptom in a child, it may in error be looked upon as a behavior problem.

Widening of the spinal canal and thinning of the pedicles is definite evidence of an expanding intraspinal lesion. Spinal puncture gives evidence of subarachnoid block and elevation of the protein content of the fluid. A lumbar myelogram will demonstrate the lower level of the block. However, this may be misleading, as the main part of the tumor may lie higher in the canal, and the block may be due to accompanying edema caused by the tumor. If the tumor is not visualized when the dura is opened, a catheter should be passed up and down the intradural space to determine the location of the mass.

RELIEF OF INTRACTABLE PAIN

When the cause of pain cannot be cured, and the pain is unbearable, it becomes necessary to destroy the nerve pathways which conduct the pain.

SUBARACHNOID ALCOHOL

Subarachnoid alcohol is of limited value. Its chief usefulness is in patients with terminal carcinoma accompanied by pain in the lower extremities and the perineum, who have only a few weeks to live. It may also be used to control pain and reduce spasticity in paraplegia due to injury and other causes.

POSTERIOR RHIZOTOMY

Rhizotomy of spinal sensory roots is performed to relieve pain which is well localized. Its value is limited because of the wide overlap of the sensory fields, and the neurosurgeon is often disappointed to find that following operation the patient has pain somewhat above or a little below the anesthetic area.

ANTEROLATERAL CHORDOTOMY

The most effective way of relieving pain in the lower part of the body is by anterolateral chordotomy. This consists of sectioning of the spinothalamic pathways. Bilateral section is usually required in carcinoma patients. The incision into the cord is made at a different level on the two sides to avoid interfering with circulation. Bilateral chordotomy often interferes with bladder control.

PREFRONTAL LOBOTOMY

When anxiety and drug addiction are present, in addition to pain, prefrontal lobotomy, transorbital or bimedial, is sometimes used to control suffering.

REHABILITATION

In many patients, relief of pain by simple removal of a protruded intervertebral disk brings about complete rehabilitation and enables a prompt return to regular employment. If nerve damage occurred before the disk was removed, corrective exercises may be required.

Removal of a meningocele where there is no nerve root involvement may restore an infant to normal. When a meningomyelocele with paraplegia is present, repair of the meningocele is only the beginning of treatment. The child requires orthopedic maneuvers to correct the foot deformity and often will also need braces and perhaps tendon transplants. Bladder dysfunction requires medical and sometimes surgical attention from a urologist.

The paraplegic war veteran and the injured industrial worker have presented a challenge to the medical profession. In the past, attention was focused on the paralyzed lower extremities. Now, the "physiatrist" gives his attention to the arms and other parts of the body which have retained good function. The enthusiasm and optimism of these physicians are contagious. Munro has stated that anyone with a good pair of shoulders can learn to ambulate.

Rehabilitation is not completed when the laminectomy incision is healed; neither is it complete when the patient has learned to ambulate. Occupational therapy is necessary to keep joints mobile and muscles functioning, but one additional step is required. If the individual cannot return to his old job, he has to undergo a period of *vocational* training so that he can secure employment in some other type of work and resume his place in the community. While a team which includes physicians and social agencies is necessary to accomplish these results, the surgeon must be aware of all the possibilities.

OCCUPATIONAL SAFEGUARDS

Many handicapped individuals have proved to be excellent, efficient workers. However, the viewpoint of the employer must not be overlooked; the compensation aspects should be reviewed so that the employer will not be required to take too great an additional risk. The "second injury" clause is receiving study in some communities and may bring about an improvement in this situation.

REFERENCES

1. Bancroft, W. F., and Pilcher, C.: Surgical Treatment of the Nervous System, Philadelphia, Lippincott, 1946.
2. Bradford, F. K., and Spurling, R. G.: The Intervertebral Disc, ed. 2, Springfield, Ill., Thomas, 1947.
3. Comarr, A. E., and Kaufman, A. A.: A survey of the neurological results of 858 spinal cord injuries, J. Neurosurg. **13**:95, 1956.
4. Crutchfield, W. G.: Evaluation of skeletal traction in treatment of cervical spine injuries, J. Internat. Coll. Surgeons **22**:63, 1954.
5. Haymaker, W.: The Nervous System *in* Karsner, H. T.: Human Pathology, ed. 8, pp. 823-906, Philadelphia, Lippincott, 1955.
6. Ingraham, F. D., and Matson, D.: Neurosurgery in Infancy and Childhood, pp. 5-81 and 345-368, Springfield, Ill., Thomas, 1955.
7. Kahn, E., and Bassett, R. C.: Correlative Neurosurgery, pp. 238-243, 327-348 and 363-388, Springfield, Ill., Thomas, 1955.
8. Love, J. G., Thelen, E. P., and Dodge, H. W.: Tumors of the foramen magnum, J. Internat. Coll. Surgeons **22**:1, 1954.
8a. Matson, D. D.: Surgical treatment of congenital spinal disorders (Abstr. and Disc.), J. Internat. Coll. Surgeons **22**:59, 1954.
9. Tarlov, I. M. *et al.*: Spinal cord compression studies. Part I, A.M.A. Arch. Neurol. & Psychiat. **70**:813, 1953; Part II, *Ibid.*, **71**: 271, 1954; Part III, *Ibid.*, **71**:588, 1954; Part IV, *Ibid.*, **72**:43, 1954.
10. Wannamaker, G. T.: Spinal cord injuries, J. Neurosurg. **11**:517, 1954.
11. White, J. C., and Sweet, W. H.: Pain: Its Mechanisms and Neurosurgical Controls, p. 210, Springfield, Ill., Thomas, 1955.
12. Williams, J. W.: Focal spinal arachnoiditis complicating anesthesia, J. Internat. Coll. Surgeons **22**:18, 1954.

FRANCIS L. LEDERER, M.D., and FREDERIC J. POLLOCK, M.D.

8 The Ear, the Nose and the Pharynx

THE EAR

DESCRIPTIVE ANATOMY

The ear is divided into 3 portions. The *external ear* consists of the *auricle* and the *external auditory canal*. The *middle ear* is made up of pneumatic spaces separated from the external auditory canal by the *tympanic*

membrane (eardrum). The middle ear is connected to the *nasopharynx* by a bony and cartilaginous passage, the *eustachian tube*. The mastoid air cells, which fill the mastoid portion of the temporal bone, are continuous with the middle ear. The middle ear contains 3 tiny ossicles: (1) the *malleus*, one process of which is imbedded in the tympanic mem-

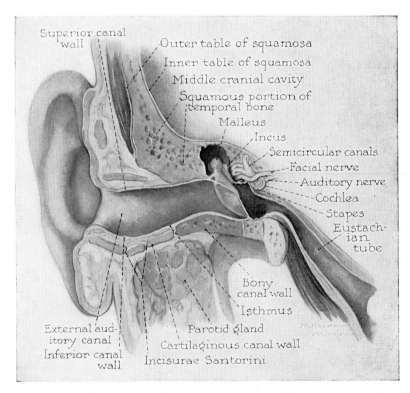

FIG. 57. Sagittal section through external and middle ear. The inclination of the tympanic membrane and the relation of the malleus, incus and stapes are indicated. The squamous portion of the temporal bone is seen to be the roof of the external auditory canal, thereby placing the latter directly below the middle cranial fossa. (Lederer, F. L.: Diseases of the Ear, Nose and Throat, Philadelphia, Davis)

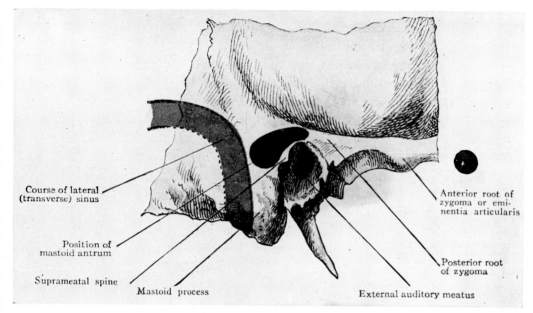

Course of lateral
(transverse) sinus

Position of
mastoid antrum

Suprameatal spine

Mastoid process

Anterior root of
zygoma or emi-
nentia articularis

Posterior root
of zygoma

External auditory meatus

FIG. 58. Lateral view of the temporal bone, showing relations of the lateral or transverse
sinus and mastoid antrum. (Davis: Applied Anatomy, Philadelphia, Lippincott)

brane, (2) the *incus,* and (3) the *stapes,* the
footplate of which is in contact with the inner
ear through the *oval window* (Fig. 57). There
are vital structures which are located in close
proximity to the middle ear and the mastoid
process. The *dura* of the middle and the posterior fossa is separated from the middle ear
and the mastoid cells by a thin layer of bone,
the *tegmen.* The *lateral dural sinus,* which
continues into the neck to form the internal
jugular vein, is in close apposition to the
mastoid cells (Fig. 58). The *facial nerve* has
an intimate relationship to the middle ear.
The *inner ear* consists of 2 portions: (1) the
labyrinth, including the semicircular canals,
which controls equilibrium and (2) the
cochlea which contains the *organ of Corti,* the
end-organ of hearing. The labyrinth communicates with the *subarachnoid space.*

SURGERY OF THE EXTERNAL EAR

Foreign Bodies. The most common foreign
body of the external canal is *cerumen* (ear-
wax). If this secretion is present in a large
quantity, it will cause diminution of hearing.
It is an error to attempt to remove cerumen
with a probe, a hook or a curet because it can
damage the skin lining the external auditory

canal, with resulting external otitis. The tympanic membrane may also be injured, causing
an acute otitis media. The best method of
removing cerumen is to use a metal ear syringe
filled with lukewarm water, aiming the stream
along the posterosuperior canal wall. The
water reaches the tympanic membrane and
pushes the cerumen from behind (Fig. 59),
forcing it out. It is important to determine
whether the patient has a history of a perforated drum or a chronic discharging ear. In
such instances, syringing should be carried
out with warm alcohol, 95 per cent, or the
cerumen may be *carefully* removed along the
antero-inferior portion of the canal under
direct vision.

Other foreign bodies that may be present
in the exterior canal include insects and
organic or inorganic material. Insects should
first be rendered inactive by the instillation of
alcohol, then washed out. Organic material,
such as beans or seeds, should not be flushed
out with water, as they are hygroscopic and
will swell, making removal much more
difficult. In place of water, 95 per cent
alcohol should be used, or the object may
be *cautiously* removed with a curet. With any
foreign body, care must be taken not to force

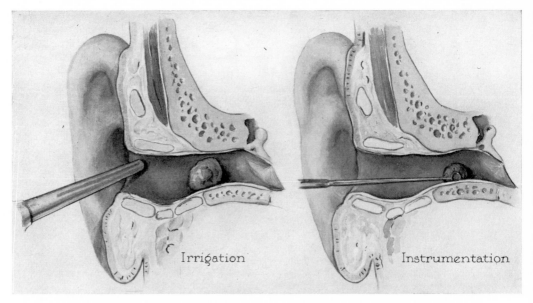

Irrigation   Instrumentation

FIG. 59. Methods of removing foreign bodies from the external auditory canal. (Lederer,
F. L.: Diseases of the Ear, Nose and Throat, Philadelphia, Davis)

it beyond the isthmus or narrowing of the canal or through the tympanic membrane. In children, general anesthesia is desirable in order to be able to control the patient and safeguard against more serious damage. Rarely, in the case of pebbles and the like, a postauricular incision is necessary to remove a foreign body.

Traumatic rupture of the tympanic membrane may result from a sharp, concussive-like blow on the ear or from basal skull fracture. Bleeding usually stops spontaneously. The recommended treatment is a "hands off" policy. *Frequent examinations or wiping are to be avoided*. The clot is left undisturbed; no syringing is to be carried out and no ear-drops are to be used. Parenteral antibiotics are in order. A piece of sterile cotton should be placed in the meatus and the ear bandaged, if necessary, to ensure cleanliness. After a period of 2 weeks, the canal may be gently cleansed of its dried blood. Tuning fork tests and audiometric evaluation are essential in determining auditory function.

Paracentesis of the Tympanic Membrane. Paracentesis of the tympanic membrane is a procedure that is indicated for the evacuation of fluid or pus from the middle ear; in acute

suppurative otitis media, when the drum is bulging, or where drainage through a small existing perforation is inadequate, *incision of the drum* is frequently necessary (Fig. 60). Acute otitis media is usually treated with antibiotics, which halt the progress of infection and leave a sterile fluid which partially or completely fills the middle ear cavity. Hearing then becomes impaired. The drum is not inflamed but has a yellowish color, and a fluid level may be observed. The fluid may be removed by aspiration with a No. 20 gauge, blunt-end needle, using mild suction, or an incision of the drum followed by inflation of the eustachian tube.

In children, paracentesis or aspiration of the tympanic membrane is best done under general anesthesia with Vinethene or the like, as it permits ample time to make a proper incision or to direct the needle without too much emotional trauma. At home, a small child may be securely mummified in a sheet and told that it will hurt momentarily. In adults, local application of a solution made up of equal parts (1 cc.) of cocaine, phenol and menthol may be employed but can be dispensed with if the initial pain is described to the patient. Paracentesis requires utmost

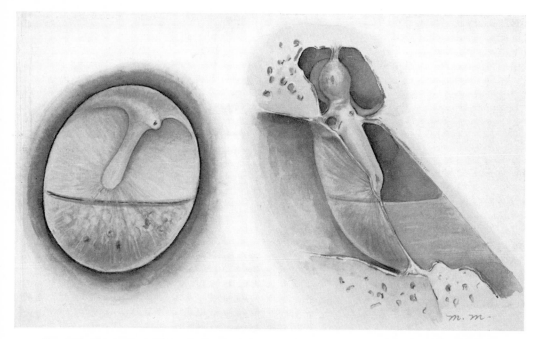

Fig. 60. Exudative otitis media may produce a picture of a fluid in the middle ear. There is a line of demarcation (niveau). If the eustachian tube is inflated, bubbles will be observed behind the tympanic membrane. The middle ear may be completely filled with fluid. (Lederer, F. L.: Diseases of the Ear, Nose and Throat, Philadelphia, Davis)

aseptic precautions, the incision being made in the postero-inferior quadrant (Fig. 61). Care should be taken to avoid making the incision in the canal wall or dislocating the stapes. The mesial wall of the middle ear is occupied by the base of the *cochlea* (promontorium) which is about 3 mm. from the tympanic membrane.

Acute Otitis Media and Mastoiditis. As the middle ear and the mastoid process form a connected series of pneumatic spaces lined by mucous membrane, an inflammation of the mastoid cells is present in all cases of suppurative otitis media. This inflammation may terminate in 1 of 4 ways: (1) complete resolution of the inflammatory process; (2) development of a chronic suppuration; (3) sterilization of the fluid, with the development of a subacute secretory otitis media; or (4) progression of the suppuration and breakdown of the bony walls of the mastoid cells to produce a surgical mastoiditis.

The employment of chemotherapy and anti-

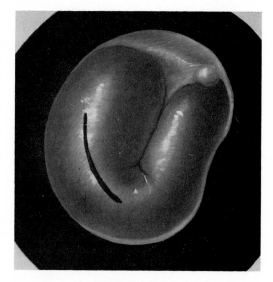

Fig. 61. Incision of tympanic membrane is preferably carried out in the posterior inferior quadrant. (Lederer, F. L.: Diseases of the Ear, Nose and Throat, Philadelphia, Davis)

biotics has reduced the frequency of acute surgical mastoiditis, but the classic signs and symptoms of the condition may be so masked by the use of these drugs that greater caution must be taken to avoid error in the close clinical observation of these cases. The following are significant of developing mastoiditis:

1. Recurrent episodes of pain during an acute otitis media.

2. Fever present after the third week of acute otitis media.

3. Sudden cessation of discharge in acute otitis media when accompanied by an exacerbation of pain and/or fever.

4. Increase in amount of discharge and development of a pulsating character to the secretion.

5. Mastoid tenderness persisting after the third week or appearing at that time.

6. Retroauricular swelling of an edematous or fluctuant character occurring over the mastoid process.

7. Roentgen-ray evidence of thickening of the mucosa and of a breakdown or absorption of the bony walls (trabeculae) of the mastoid cells.

It is important to emphasize the fact that with the employment of antibiotics, many of the above signs may be lacking. X-ray study should be done in cases of otitis media in which discharge persists for several weeks, even in the absence of swelling, pain, tenderness and/or fever.

TREATMENT OF ACUTE MASTOIDITIS. The treatment may be either medical or surgical. In the event of an impending or presenting intracranial complication, surgery is imperative. Decision as to whether a mastoidectomy is necessary depends on comprehension of the underlying pathologic conditions, the symptoms, the otologic signs and the exercise of surgical judgment.

Incision (either endaural or postauricular) should be done carefully, as dehiscence or destruction of the bony cortex of the mastoid may lay underlying structures open to damage. In the use of mallet and gouge, to prevent injury, the direction should be away from the dura and the lateral sinus. Present-day mastoid surgery favors the employment of the electric bur. The course of the facial nerve, as it runs deep to the posterior part of the external canal, must be kept in mind. Unless a phlebitis is suspected, the lateral sinus should not be exposed. It is considerably thinner than the dura and is easily damaged. Exposure of the dura or the lateral sinus does not ordinarily lead to complications unless these structures are traumatized. In the event that either is exposed, the bony covering should be removed over a larger area than was first planned in order to prevent the sealing off of possible infection.

If the lateral sinus is opened accidentally, there will be a profuse welling up of venous blood. A pack over the tear in the sinus wall will stop the flow. It will be necessary to expose the sinus by carefully removing the bony covering in each direction. A small rolled pack is placed between the bone and the sinus wall at each end so as to compress the sinus completely. Packing directly into the lumen of the sinus must be avoided. These packs are to be left in place for about 1 week. Removal is best carried out in the operating room under aseptic conditions, for if bleeding occurs on their removal, repacking may be necessary.

COMPLICATIONS OF OTITIS MEDIA AND MASTOIDITIS

Infection of the middle ear and the mastoid cells is potentially dangerous because of the proximity to vital intracranial structures. It is the involvement of these areas that causes so much concern. The spread of infection may be contiguous or the result of a vascular thrombophlebitis.

Meningitis. The *meninges* are separated from the *middle ear* and the *mastoid antrum* by only a thin bony *tegmen* or roof. The *labyrinth* has such a close connection with the meninges that a purulent labyrinthitis easily leads to a meningeal infection. When a patient with meningitis is first seen, it is important to determine whether there has been any history of previous ear infection. The ears must be inspected carefully to ascertain whether an otitis media is the cause of the more serious infection. Spinal puncture is an important aid in making the diagnosis. Smear and culture should be done in order to determine the offending organism and to institute proper and adequate chemotherapy.

The prognosis in meningitis has improved greatly since the advent of antibiotics and chemotherapy. However, the eradication and the evacuation of the primary focus of infection in the mastoid must still be accomplished in order to bring about a cure. If the meningitis is otitic in origin, a simple or (in the event of chronic suppuration) a radical mastoidectomy must be done, with exposure of the dura, in order to eradicate the disease which has produced the meningitis.

Extradural Abscess. This is an infection which has traversed the tegmen (roof of the mastoid), resulting in collection of pus between the bone and the dura. Headache is the predominant symptom. Characteristically, this headache is of a deep, boring type, most often worse at night. If extradural abscess is suspected, mastoidectomy should be carried out, widely exposing the dura of the middle and the posterior fossae. When purulent material is encountered, the dura should be exposed in all directions until normal covering is found. Usually this suffices to effect a cure. However, the patient should be watched carefully for possible evidence of beginning invasion of the subarachnoid space or of the brain tissue proper, as this may lead to an extension of the infectious process.

Brain Abscess. Extension of infection into

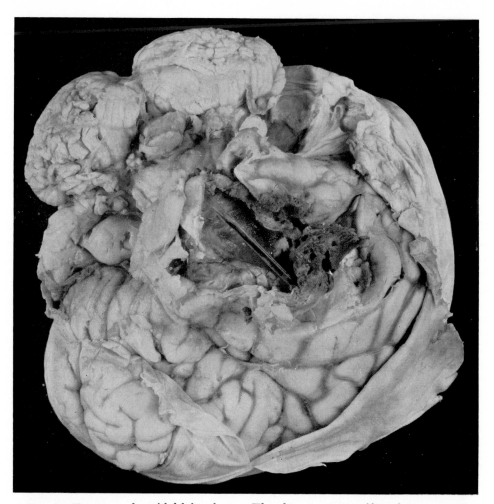

FIG. 62. Temporosphenoidal lobe abscess. The abscess was manifested 20 years after a chronic ear ceased to discharge. This abscess ruptured spontaneously into the zygomatic region. (Lederer, F. L.: Diseases of the Ear, Nose and Throat, Philadelphia, Davis)

the nearby brain tissue may take place in an acute or chronic otitis media or in mastoiditis. The spread may be into the temporosphenoidal lobe or into the cerebellum. This may occur along the course of blood vessels or by direct extension. In the temporosphenoidal lobe, signs of increased intracranial pressure, headache, lethargy and bradycardia point toward involvement (Fig. 62). Neurologic examination, spinal fluid study and determination of ocular fields and fundus changes aid in the diagnosis. As always, skill and sound surgical judgment are important factors in successful management. The abscess should be given time to wall off and then be drained through the mastoid cavity. In this manner the disease of the mastoid is eradicated simultaneously. Extension into the posterior fossa gives rise to a cerebellar abscess, the signs and symptoms of which consist of increased intracranial pressure, headache, in-co-ordination, nystagmus and bradycardia. Neurologic study and determination of spinal fluid changes aid in the diagnosis. The prognosis has always been poor, but, of late, treatment by antibiotics and establishment of surgical drainage have increased the recovery rate.

Lateral Sinus Phlebitis and Thrombosis. Inflammation of the wall of the lateral sinus is usually a result of direct extension of infection from the mastoid process. If the inflammation traverses the bone and causes a *collection of pus* to develop between the sinus wall and the bone, a *perisinus abscess* is produced. When the wall of the sinus is infected, a *mural thrombosis* often forms, and if the process continues, an *obturating thrombus* will develop.

Chills and fever are the most characteristic signs of lateral sinus involvement. The "swinging" or "iceberg" type of temperature curve, with fluctuations between 99° and 106°, is characteristic. True chills are experienced, during which time the blood cultures often will be found to be positive. Metastatic abscesses may occur. When the diagnosis is made promptly and surgical treatment instituted at once, the prognosis is good. Treatment consists of elimination of the infective focus and drainage of the affected venous sinus. Mastoidectomy should be carried out and the bone over the lateral sinus removed.

A needle may be introduced into the lumen at an acute angle in order to prevent perforation of the opposite sinus wall. If there is no bleeding, it indicates that the sinus has been obliterated by a thrombus. The sinus should be exposed in either direction until a section of normal wall is encountered. Packs are then placed at either end, between the sinus wall and the bone. The sinus is opened longitudinally, and the clot is removed. An attempt must be made to secure free bleeding from either end. The packs are left in place for 5 to 7 days. Ligation of the internal jugular vein in the neck has been advocated to prevent emboli from entering the general circulation, but this procedure is not always necessary if the clinical progress is smooth.

Labyrinthitis. Secondary inflammation of the inner ear may complicate the course of a suppurative otitis media. Invasion of the labyrinth is manifested by vertigo, nystagmus, loss of hearing, nausea and/or vomiting. Spread of the infection from the labyrinth may cause a meningitis or a cerebellar abscess. When the disease remains localized, mastoidectomy for removal of the offending focus may be sufficient. If a diffuse purulent labyrinthitis is present, a radical mastoidectomy with destruction and drainage of the labyrinth may be necessary if it is apparent that there is a threat of spread to the meninges, regardless of whether the ear is functioning or nonfunctioning.

Facial Paralysis. This may be a result of inflammatory disease of the middle ear. The nerve may be affected by toxins, by direct extension of the infection with disease of the surrounding bone or by trauma during the course of surgery of the ear. If the paralysis occurs early in an acute otitis media, the treatment may consist only of watchful waiting, as the paralysis frequently disappears spontaneously (Fig. 63). If direct extension of the infectious process causes facial paralysis, along with other signs of mastoiditis during the course of acute or chronic middle ear disease, surgery on the mastoid with the uncapping of the nerve is recommended. If the nerve is injured in the course of surgery, revision and exposure of the site of the injury, in combination with one of the indicated and accepted methods of repair, are advocated.

Chronic Otitis Media and Mastoiditis. In chronic suppurative otitis media, the patient has a continuing or intermittent aural discharge. This may be scanty or profuse, but it is foul-smelling and is accompanied by a conductive form of hearing loss to a lesser or greater degree. These symptoms in themselves are not serious, but the importance of chronic otitis media lies in the fact that it can cause all of the intracranial complications, such as meningitis, extradural or brain abscess, lateral sinus thrombosis, labyrinthitis or facial paralysis, that have been described previously. Treatment must be directed at relieving the patient of the dangers associated with the disease and at producing, if possible, a dry ear with adequate hearing.

Unfortunately, chemotherapy and antibiotics are of very little value in the treatment of chronic otitis media. In the course of this disease, especially in attic or in marginal perforations, the formation of *cholesteatoma* is characteristic. These consist of masses of desquamated epithelium and cholesterin crystals. Such masses tend to enlarge, causing destruction of the bone by pressure necrosis, eventually leading to the exposure of vital structures and intracranial complications. Water has a deleterious or exacerbating effect on a chronic otitis media, so that water or watery solutions are to be avoided in bathing or in treatment. *Polyps* originate in the middle ear and project into the external canal. They may

be removed under aseptic precautions by means of a small snare. Never tear or pull polyps away by force, as they may be attached to important structures of the inner ear, and pathways for infection to the dura might thus be opened.

The surgical treatment of a chronic otitis media is indicated to prevent such complications as have been discussed. Symptoms of impending catastrophe, such as headache, nausea and vomiting, facial paralysis or vertigo, lead to the consideration of surgery. By the technic of radical mastoidectomy, with either the electric drill or the gouge, the middle ear, the mastoid antrum and the remaining mastoid cells are transformed into one large cavity, freely communicating with the external auditory meatus. The cholesteatomatous material and granulation tissue are removed and the resulting cavity lined by a skin flap from the membranous canal.

Safeguards in Radical Mastoidectomy

Radical mastoidectomy may be carried out by the postauricular or endaural approach. *The position of the dura is to be borne in mind at all times.* Uncovering the dura, in itself, does not result in complications, but care must be exercised *not to injure or tear it.* The facial nerve in its course through the middle ear may be injured inadvertently. It is well to avoid the area of the nerve and not to attempt to remove granulations from it, as the

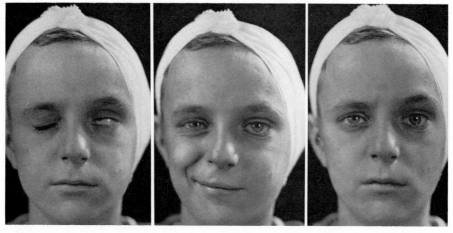

FIG. 63. Facial nerve paralysis (peripheral) occurring during an acute suppurative otitis media. Recovery was uneventful following a simple mastoidectomy. (Lederer, F. L.: Diseases of the Ear, Nose and Throat, Philadelphia, Davis)

nerve itself may have been exposed by the disease process. The horizontal semicircular canal can usually be seen. Here, too, in order to avoid injury, granulations over a fistula should not be disturbed. In the posterior part of the cavity, the lateral sinus may be exposed by the disease or through surgical removal of bone.

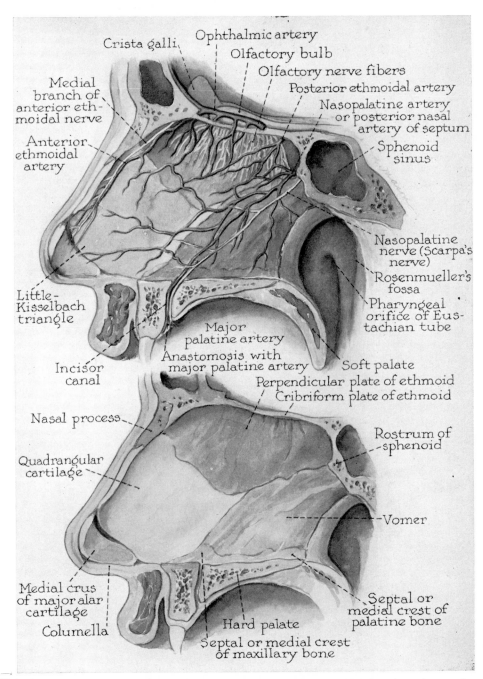

FIG. 64. Nasal septum, showing its structural arrangement, blood and nerve supply. (Lederer, F. L.: Diseases of the Ear, Nose and Throat, Philadelphia, Davis)

THE NOSE

DESCRIPTIVE ANATOMY

The external nose consists of a bony and cartilaginous pyramid covered with skin. The lower portion curves outward on each side, forming the *nasal alae*. These constitute the lateral part of the openings, the *nostrils*. In the midline, between the *nares*, is the *columella*, made up of cartilage covered by skin. The entrances to the nasal cavity through the nostrils are known as the *nasal vestibules*. Here the skin makes a transition to the nasal mucous membrane. The skin of the vestibule contains numerous hairs (vibrissae).

The nasal cavity is divided into 2 parts by the mesially placed *nasal septum*. This is supported by 4 bones, the *perpendicular plate* of the *ethmoid*, the *vomer*, the *nasal crest of the maxilla*, the *nasal crest of the palatine bones* and the quadrangular cartilage. Both sides are lined by mucous membrane (Fig. 64). The periosteum and the perichondrium of the underlying structures form the submucosa of the mucous membrane and cannot be separated from it. The lateral wall of the nasal cavity is convoluted by 3 or 4 nasal turbinates (Fig. 65). Beneath each turbinate is a passage leading to a meatus. The mucous membrane of the inferior turbinate, the warming and moistening component, contains numerous cavernous spaces filled with blood. The roof of the nasal cavity is very narrow, and a portion of the ethmoid bone, the *cribriform plate*, separates the nasal cavity from the anterior cranial fossa.

The *paranasal sinuses* are bony spaces in the skull lined by mucous membrane which is continuous with the mucosa of the nasal cavity. The *frontal sinuses*, located in the frontal bone, may be absent bilaterally or unilaterally and may vary greatly in size and contour. The opening into the nose is by way of the *nasofrontal duct* which leads into the middle meatus. The *maxillary sinus* is located within the maxillary bone. It also has a natural opening into the middle meatus. The *sphenoid sinus* lies in the body of the sphenoid bone and opens into the posterior-superior portion of the nasal cavity. The *ethmoid sinuses* consist of a series of air cells or spaces within the ethmoid bone. Each cell group has its own

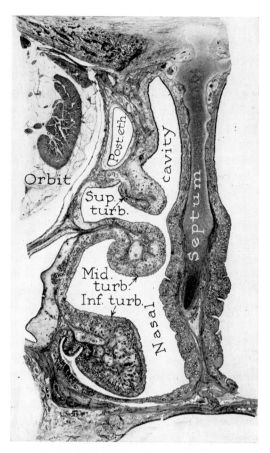

FIG. 65. Lateral wall of nose and septum (6-week-old infant). The inferior turbinate is almost in contact with the flat floor of the nose. Note that the perichondrium of the cartilaginous septum is reflected below; at this point, then, perichondrium is opposed to periostium (vomer). (Lederer, F. L.: Diseases of the Ear, Nose and Throat, Philadelphia, Davis)

opening, the anterior group leading into the middle meatus and the posterior group into the superior meatus.

SURGERY OF THE NOSE

Furuncle of the Nasal Vestibule. This type of inflammation is frequently due to infection originating in the hair follicles. Pain is severe, and redness and swelling of the nose occur in proportion to the degree of involvement. Treatment is conservative, with dry or moist heat combined with chemotherapy or antibi-

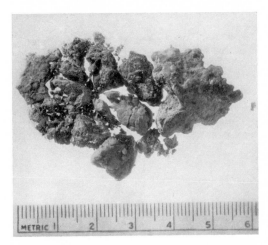

FIG. 66. Rhinolith removed from one side of the nose which it had practically occluded. (Lederer, F. L.: Diseases of the Ear, Nose and Throat, Philadelphia, Davis)

otics. Manipulation or incision of a nasal furuncle may lead to serious complications, particularly *venous thrombosis* by way of the angular vein. This may reach the dural sinuses and lead to a cavernous sinus involvement. It is a serious error to pull out vibrissae, and all manipulation in the infected area should be scrupulously avoided.

Fracture of the Nasal Bone. This is a fairly common type of injury. The diagnosis depends on the history of the trauma, a noticeable external deformity and a feeling of crepitus on gentle manipulation. X-ray studies may be helpful. Reduction of the fracture can usually be carried out readily but is best done within the first 10 days after injury. Under anesthesia—local in adults, general in children—the nose is manipulated by employing an elevator in the nasal cavity and thumb pressure from the outside. A depressed fracture cannot be forced back into place until the fragment has been elevated from within the nasal cavity.

Septal Abscess. This is a complication of nasal trauma, most often seen in children following a hematoma of the nasal septum. The common error is to *overlook* such an abscess. The history is one of nasal injury which is usually followed by bilateral obstruction of the nose. Examination shows the septum to be ballooned out into each nostril. Aspiration will reveal purulent material. The treatment is wide incision along the mucocutaneous junction on one side of the septum, suction and the insertion of a suitable drain.

CAUTION. Because the infection may destroy the cartilaginous support of the external nose, the patient should be apprised of the fact that a depression of the bridge occasionally may follow a septal abscess.

Foreign Bodies. These are usually introduced into the nose by children or psychotics, or they may result from overlooked cotton or gauze. The most constant symptom is a *unilateral nasal discharge,* usually of a purulent character. When a patient presents himself with a history of a persistent nasal discharge from one nostril, a foreign body must be suspected. Opaque foreign bodies will be evident by roentgenogram. Removal under good illumination and visualization is essential. General anesthesia is required in children. The nasal mucosa should be packed with a shrinking agent, such as epinephrine or ephedrine, to ensure maximum visability. The object may be grasped by a nasal forceps, or a blunt hook may be inserted behind it. Care must be exercised not to push it into the nasopharynx, whence it might be aspirated into the lungs. Also, take care not to injure the nasal membrane, bringing on unnecessary bleeding. At times, calcareous deposits may form around a foreign body to develop into a rhinolith (Fig. 66). These and other sharp foreign bodies must be removed with studied gentleness.

Deviations of the Nasal Septum. If surgical correction of irregularity of the nasal septum is contemplated, it must be ascertained first that there is no other cause of obstruction. The presence of nasal polyps or a neoplasm, choanal atresia, hypertrophic and allergic rhinitis first must be ruled out. Surgical treatment of septal deviations consists of elevation of the mucoperichondrial and the mucoperiosteal layers from the cartilage and the bone on one side (Fig. 67). A vertical incision is then made through the cartilage (but not the mucoperiosteum on the opposite side), and the opposite mucosal lining membrane is elevated. First, the cartilage and then the bone are removed by means of cutting forceps. Gentleness is the established technic to avoid the error of tearing the mucosa and producing a perforation or bringing about a fracture which might extend into the *cribriform plate*. Packing of the nose should be firm and carefully placed to remain in situ for 24 hours, to obliterate any space between the mucosal flaps in order to prevent formation of a hematoma.

Enlargement of the Turbinate. Surgery of the turbinates is rarely necessary unless they are diseased. If these structures are hypertrophic, there is usually an underlying cause which must be found and corrected. The *inferior turbinate* is covered by a mucous membrane very rich in cavernous spaces, so that any cutting operation on this tissue is accompanied by danger of hemorrhage and its removal leads to a disagreeable atrophic state. If treatment is given with a view to reducing the size of the turbinates, submucous electrocoagulation or streaking with a caustic agent (chromic acid, trichloracetic acid, silver nitrate) or the injection of sclerosing solutions are the methods of choice. The use of shrinking agents, such as nose sprays or drops, over a period of time will cause marked swelling (rebound reaction) of the soft tissues of the nasal cavity. Cessation of the use of these agents often will allow the mucosa to return to normal.

Sinusitis. Unless there is an overwhelming infection, evidence of retention or signs of osteomyelitic involvement of the bone, acute sinusitis should be treated conservatively, without resort to surgery. In an *acute frontal sinusitis*, where there is pus under pressure which does not drain spontaneously through the nasofrontal duct, an external trephination into the floor of the frontal sinus may be necessary. However, in the subacute stage, intranasal shrinkage and irrigation through the nasofrontal duct are usually possible.

In *chronic sinusitis*, treatment is carried out surgically to allow elimination of pus from the sinus cavity and to remove the infected hypertrophic lining. In the case of the maxillary sinus, irrigation may be carried out in 1 of 2 ways: (1) by use of a cannula which is inserted through the natural ostium located in the middle meatus, or (2) by means of a puncture of the thin bony wall beneath the inferior turbinate with a straight needle or a curved trocar. Dangers of antrum irrigation include hemorrhage, air embolism and emphysema of the soft tissue of the cheek or the orbit, which is occasionally followed by infection.

In chronic sinusitis which does not respond to local treatment, external surgery may become necessary. In maxillary sinus disease, a sublabial approach combined with an intranasal window is carried out. Incision is made at the gingival-buccal border, the periosteum is elevated, and the sinus is entered through the thin bone of the canine fossa. The purulent material and hypertrophic mucosa are removed. An opening is made through the in-

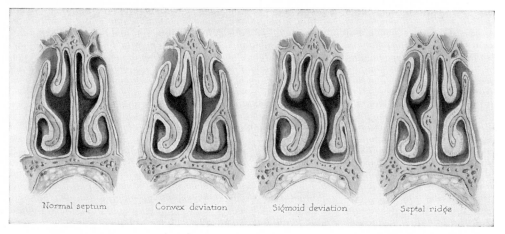

Normal septum   Convex deviation   Sigmoid deviation   Septal ridge

Fig. 67. Nasal septum in its midline position, mild convex deviation, sigmoid deviation and septal ridge. (Lederer, F. L.: Diseases of the Ear, Nose and Throat, Philadelphia, Davis)

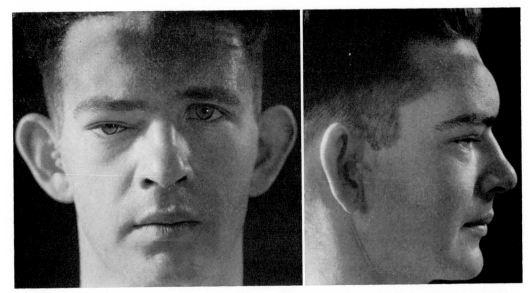

FIG. 68. Large mucocele of right frontal sinus. (Lederer, F. L.: Diseases of the Ear, Nose and Throat, Philadelphia, Davis)

ferior meatus to allow drainage from the sinus. There is some danger of osteomyelitis developing after maxillary sinus surgery. Tissues must be handled carefully and the periosteum preserved. There may be a dehiscence found in the posterior wall of the sinus, so care should be exercised in removing the lining membrane.

In chronic frontal and ethmoid disease, external surgery occasionally may become necessary. When the opening of the frontal sinus or of an ethmoid cell is obstructed permanently, the secretion is retained in the sinus, thereby causing erosion of the bony walls and an external swelling (mucocele).

The diagnosis of a *mucocele* is aided by roentgenographic study (Fig. 68). Differential diagnosis from an osteoma or other neoplasia must be made. Treatment is surgical by an external approach, the incision being made through the eyebrow, curving downward midway between the inner canthus of the eye and the bridge of the nose. In reflecting the periosteum of the floor of the frontal sinus, the pulley of the superior oblique muscle must be preserved and reflected with the periosteum. Entrance into the sinus is made through the floor. The lining membrane of the mucocele may or may not be removed, but this

should be done if possible, because an abscess may lurk behind it. Bony sequestra are removed. The posterior wall may have been eroded and the dura exposed, so *great care*

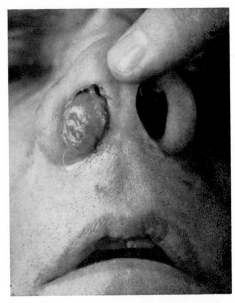

FIG. 69. Nasal polyp in the anterior naris. (Lederer, F. L.: Diseases of the Ear, Nose and Throat, Philadelphia, Davis)

must be taken in this area. The opening into the nose must be re-established; a tube can be inserted from the sinus into the nose and sutured to the closed external skin overlying the sinus. This tube is kept in position for sufficient time to allow epithelialization of the tract (6 weeks). Diplopia, osteomyelitis, meningitis and frontal lobe abscess are among the possible complications which may be encountered.

Nasal Polyps. These may develop singly or in groups in the course of a chronic maxillary or ethmoid sinusitis in the presence of infection and/or allergy (Fig. 69). They are usually pedunculated, smooth, gray or pink translucent masses which originate from the nasal or the sinus mucous membrane. Nasal obstruction is the predominant symptom. Surgical intervention is usually required. This is best carried out by a cold snare, under topical anesthesia. The polyp should be cut cleanly and never removed by grasping and tugging, as the mucosa to which it is attached may be

covering a dehiscence in the ethmoid roof which would offer a direct opening to the meninges. It is important that all polyps be carefully subjected to microscopic examination, since a neoplasm may be similar in its gross appearance.

Osteomyelitis. Osteomyelitic involvement of the frontal bone or maxilla may follow as a complication of sinusitis (Fig. 70). This may occur as a fulminating infection or as a chronic or latent inflammatory process involving the soft tissues of the bone. In the rapid type of destruction, high fever, intense frontal pain, headache, prostration and edema spreading beyond the borders of the sinus are observed. X-ray study does not always reveal the total extent of the involvement. Removal of the diseased bone and a surrounding portion of healthy osseous tissue is frequently necessary. Adequate antimicrobial therapy is essential but is not in itself curative. Meningitis, epidural infection and brain abscess may result from this type of infection. In the fulmi-

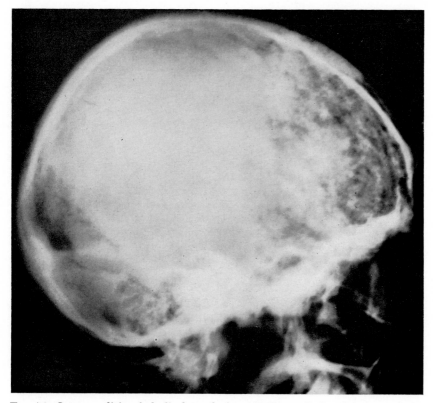

FIG. 70. Osteomyelitis of skull; lateral view. (Lederer, F. L.: Diseases of the Ear, Nose and Throat, Philadelphia, Davis)

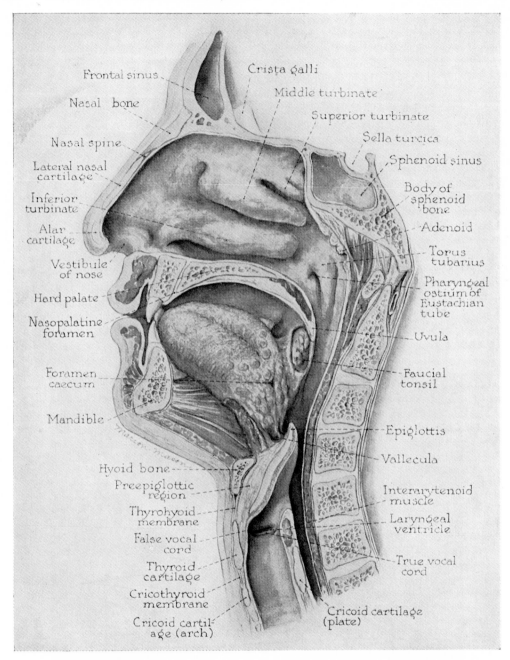

Frontal sinus

Crista galli

Middle turbinate

Nasal bone

Superior turbinate

Nasal spine

Sella turcica

Lateral nasal cartilage

Sphenoid sinus

Inferior turbinate

Body of sphenoid bone

Alar cartilage

Adenoid

Vestibule of nose

Torus tubarius

Hard palate

Pharyngeal ostium of Eustachian tube

Nasopalatine foramen

Uvula

Foramen caecum

Faucial tonsil

Mandible

Epiglottis

Hyoid bone

Vallecula

Preepiglottic region

Interarytenoid muscle

Thyrohyoid membrane

Laryngeal ventricle

False vocal cord

True vocal cord

Thyroid cartilage

Cricothyroid membrane

Cricoid cartilage (plate)

Cricoid cartilage (arch)

FIG. 71. Sagittal section through the head, showing the nasal cavity, pharynx, tongue and larynx. (Lederer, F. L.: Diseases of the Ear, Nose and Throat, Philadelphia, Davis)

nating form of infection, it is important to remove bone as widely as possible inasmuch as the infection continues to spread with too conservative removal. In the chronic type of osteomyelitis, removal of sequestra and clearing up of the infected bone margins are vital.

Patients with these conditions should be carefully and continuously observed, since the infection frequently remains latent, only to flare up again at a later time.

Tumors. Neoplasia of the nose and the sinuses may be either benign or malignant.

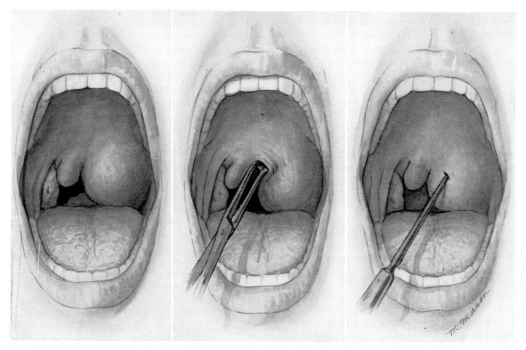

Fig. 72. Peritonsillar abscess involving the left side, illustrating the evacuation through the supratonsillar fossa with a curved forceps and opening through the anterior pillar with a bistoury knife. (Lederer, F. L.: Diseases of the Ear, Nose and Throat, Philadelphia, Davis)

Papilloma, osteoma and dermoid cysts may be observed, the latter as a midline tumor on the nasal dorsum. Carcinoma, sarcoma and melanoma also occur, but with less frequency. The maxillary sinus and the ethmoid labyrinth are the commonest sites for malignancy. Any hyperplastic tissue in the nose, especially if there has been a history of bleeding, should be suspected of being malignant, and a biopsy should be performed routinely. Surgical excision, to be adequate, should be carried out widely by means of an incision externally along the nose and through the lip (Ferguson-Weber incision). If the orbital plate is involved, exenteration of the orbital contents is advisable in order to increase the possibility of a cure. Resection of the superior maxilla with removal of the palate is usually necessary to eradicate the disease and ensure adequate inspection. Postoperative radiation may be employed, either in the form of radium packs directly into the created cavity or by external irradiation.

THE PHARYNX

Descriptive Anatomy

For anatomic consideration, the pharynx is divided into 3 portions: (1) the *epipharynx*, (2) the *mesopharynx* and (3) the *hypopharynx*. Actually, it is one continuous muscular tube with no divisions of the lining mucous membrane (Fig. 71). The epipharynx (nasopharynx) opens forward into the nasal cavities, through the choana, and joins the mesopharynx (oropharynx) at the level of the palate. The eustachian tubes lead from the middle ear to an opening on each lateral aspect of the nasopharynx. The roof of the nasopharynx contains lymphoid tissue (adenoid) which is thrown up into folds. The oropharynx extends from the level of the palate to the base of the tongue and communicates anteriorly with the oral cavity. As the posterior edge of the palate curves downward toward the base of the tongue, it divides into 2 muscular bands, the anterior and the posterior pillars. Embedded in the space between the pillars is the *palatine tonsil*. This lymphoid structure is covered on its free surface by stratified squamous epithelium and has a fibrouslike capsule by which it is attached to the lateral pharyngeal wall. The blood supply of the tonsil is from the *external carotid artery* by way of the *ascending palatine artery* and branches of the *internal* and the *external maxillary arteries*. The hypopharynx (laryngopharynx) is the lowest portion of the pharynx, extending from the base of the tongue to the opening of the esophagus. This muscular tube divides around the larynx, the divided portions being known as the *pyriform sinuses*.

Disease of the Nasopharynx

The nasopharynx may be the seat of an acute infection, such as an *acute adenoiditis*. This usually occurs in association with an *acute tonsillitis. Cysts and tumors* are frequent in the nasopharynx. Anaplastic types of *malignant tumors,* such as transitional cell carcinoma, lympho-epithelioma and reticulum cell sarcoma, are encountered not infrequently in this area. The original lesion may be quite small, so that the first signs or symptoms noted will be mild conductive hearing loss, nasal blockage and masses in the neck which are malignant metastases to the cervical lymph nodes. The common error in diseases of the nasopharynx is an error of omission, this region frequently being overlooked in the examination of patients. By means of a nasopharyngeal mirror, an electric nasopharyngoscope or a suitably constructed speculum, the nasopharynx may be inspected adequately.

Acute Tonsillitis. This is the commonest manifestation of an acute pharyngeal infection. When the patient complains of a severe sore throat, has a high fever and shows redness and swelling of the tonsils with exudative material in the crypts, the diagnosis is assured. The treatment of acute tonsillitis is medical. It is an error to perform tonsillectomy during the acute phase as there is danger of spreading the infection, with a resulting phlegmon of the pharynx and involvement of the deep structures of the neck. It is best to wait for 3 to 6 weeks after an acute tonsillitis has subsided before attempting surgery.

Peritonsillar Abscess. An acute infection of the tonsils may spread to the loose peritonsillar tissue, producing a peritonsillitis or a peritonsillar abscess ("Quinsy sore throat"). Dysphagia becomes so severe that the patient cannot swallow his own saliva, so that "drooling" is characteristic. The voice will have a nasal twang, and marked trismus will be present. The palate on the affected side will be swollen and tender, and there may be some degree of fluctuation present. The tonsillar swelling toward the midline pushes the uvula to the opposite side.

Early treatment should be conservative, by means of warm irrigations and antimicrobials, but later the abscess must be incised. Topical anesthesia (Pontocaine or cocaine) used at the site of incision will relieve the pain caused by the procedure (Fig. 72). General anesthesia is best avoided, as there is great danger of aspiration of pus. A cataract knife with adhesive tape wrapped around it so as to expose no more than about $3/8$ of an inch of the blade or a long-handled knife with a bistoury-type blade can be used. The incision is spread with a long, curved forceps. Incision is best done with the patient in a sitting position so that the purulent material may readily be expectorated. The most serious danger is that of hemorrhage.

Tonsillectomy and Adenoidectomy

These 2 procedures will be considered together, although either one frequently is performed alone. The detailed indications for these surgical procedures need not be discussed here. When an absolute indication exists, the operation may be performed by those with special skill and experience on patients of any age. If operation is not urgent, it is preferably not done until after the age of 5. However, age need not be the final determining factor. Operation should be postponed in the presence of acute infection, contagious disease or pulmonary disorder or where the risk of operation exceeds the risk of the disease. A history of severe bleeding after small cuts or of bruising readily should cause the surgeon to suspect a bleeding tendency.

In children, general anesthesia is required. The preparation of the patient (both emotional and laboratorywise) is very important. The clotting time should be determined and the urine examined. The child should be told in advance that he is going to have tonsillectomy and adenoidectomy; it should never be carried out as a "surprise attack." The heart and the lungs should be re-examined on the day of the intervention, and even a slight rise in temperature considered as contraindicative for surgery. It is important that the child have nothing by mouth after retiring the night before the surgical intervention (if the procedure is to be carried out in the morning). Premedication should include atropine, in order to lessen the amount of secretion. Ether is still the anesthetic of choice for children. Rectal Pentothal Sodium, administered by a trained anesthetist in the child's room prior to transporting him to the operating theater, serves to allay the emotional trauma of induction of the anesthetic. Laryngeal intubation aids in maintaining an adequate airway and in preventing the aspiration of blood during surgery. The teeth should be inspected and loose ones removed in order to prevent

their later dislocation and aspiration into the tracheobronchial tree.

Removal of the tonsils can be carried out by dissection and cold snare or by means of enucleation with a Sluder or a Beck tonsillatome. In the dissection technic, it is important initially to locate the cleavage line between the tonsillar capsule and its bed (Fig. 73). The posterior pillar must be preserved by careful dissection. The arch of the palate and the uvula should not be traumatized, as scarring in this region will alter the normal anatomic relations of the parts. Bleeding from the tonsillar bed is abundant at the time of the enucleation, but much of it can be controlled by careful application of gauze sponges. The bleeding vessels should be grasped individually in a hemostat, and a ligature or a suture applied. It should be remembered that the vessels run from the superior to the inferior portion of the tonsil bed, so the hemostat should be applied across the area. Care in suturing all bleeding vessels will result in a dry cavity

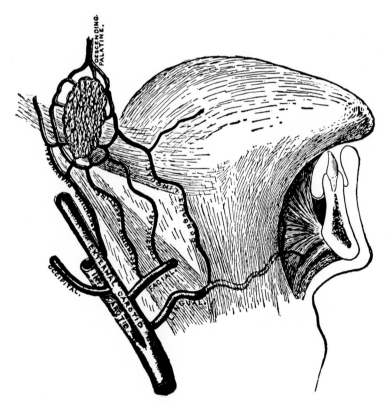

FIG. 73. Diagram illustrating blood supply of faucial tonsil. (Davis: Applied Anatomy, Philadelphia, Lippincott)

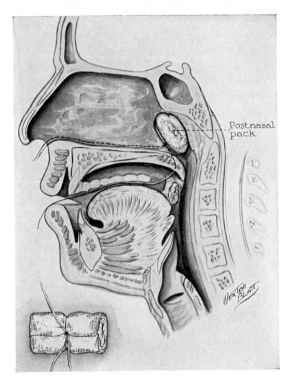

Postnasal pack

Fig. 74. Posterior nasal pack. This type of pack is extremely useful in emergencies and frequently has to be resorted to for the control of postnasal hemorrhages. (Lederer, F. L.: Diseases of the Ear, Nose and Throat, Philadelphia, Davis)

and fewer of the harrowing experiences with secondary hemorrhage.

Adenoidectomy is, at best, a "blind" operation, accomplished with the La Force adenotome, followed by the use of an adenoid curet. After the large mass of adenoid tissue has been removed, the nasopharynx can be directly inspected with the aid of the Love or a similar type of palate retractor, and the remaining lymphoid tissue may then be removed with a punch under direct vision. Bleeding from the epipharynx may be profuse but usually can be controlled by pressure of a gauze pad or a hemostat. Suturing is practically impossible in the adenoid region. If the bleeding cannot be controlled, it may be necessary to insert a postnasal tampon (Fig. 74), allowing it to remain in place for 24 hours. No child should be returned to his room without making sure that all bleeding has stopped. Each cavity should be reinspected to be certain that all are dry before allowing the child to come out of the anesthesia. Additional precaution is observed by continuing to watch the patient in a properly equipped recovery room.

Postoperative hemorrhage may be primary (within 12 hours) or secondary (usually from the fourth to the seventh day). When the child expectorates bright red material and has blood coming from his nose, it is well to check on its source. It must be borne in mind that blood may be swallowed continuously, so that the first symptom may be the emesis of a large quantity of dark material. A constant check on the pulse is essential to safeguard against this possibility.

General anesthesia should never be given in the presence of postoperative hemorrhage. A portion of clot may become dislodged, be aspirated and cause a laryngeal, tracheal or bronchial obstruction. *Intravenous anesthesia is never to be employed.* The clot should be removed and the area inspected. If the bleeding is arterial, the vessel should be ligated by careful suture technic. If it is a general venous ooze, gentle pressure with a gauze sponge should be exerted. Tannic acid-Adrenalin mixture applied to the surface may control the bleeding, though sometimes only temporarily. A postnasal tampon may be necessary for the control of adenoid hemorrhage.

TUMORS OF THE PHARYNX

These may be benign or malignant. The most common type of *benign lesion* is the single, small, pedunculated *papilloma,* which usually occurs on the palate, in the tonsillar area or on the pharyngeal wall. At times papillomas are multiple or can become so. These tumors can be removed by dissection aided by electrocoagulation of the base. Malignant growths include *carcinomas* and *sarcomas.* Lymphosarcoma of the tonsil will not ulcerate but will cause an enlargement of the entire structure. When one tonsil is observed to be larger than the other, a neoplasm must be suspected. Tumors of the pharynx are best considered with the discussion of laryngeal lesions. In all tumors of the pharynx, especially those which have a tendency to enlarge or to ulcerate, a threat to the airway and hemorrhage are the important emergencies. Therefore, tracheotomy and/or ligation of the external carotid artery come in for consideration.

ARNOLD S. JACKSON, M.D.

9   The Thyroid

ANATOMY

The thyroid is a ductless gland composed of two lateral lobes connected by an isthmus and often a pyramidal lobe extending upward from the latter (Fig. 75). The gland varies in weight but approximates 30 Gm. and is situated on either side and in front of the trachea at about the level of the second to the fourth tracheal cartilages. The thyroid is reddish brown in color and varies in size and weight, depending on age, sex, place of residence and general health of the person.

The upper portion of each lateral lobe is designated as the upper pole and the lower portion as the lower pole. The thyroid and the cricoid cartilages, the esophagus, the trachea, the inferior laryngeal nerve, the inferior constrictor of the pharynx and the posterior part of the cricothyroid muscle are situated on the inner side of each lobe. Posterior to each lobe lies the carotid sheath, containing the common carotid artery, the jugular vein and the vagus nerve. The prevertebral fascia and muscles, the parathyroids and the inferior thyroid artery are also behind the gland. The sternohyoid, the sternothyroid and the omohyoid muscles lie on the anterolateral surface of the gland. The sternocleidomastoid muscles just cover the lateral border. A loose fibromuscular capsule surrounds the gland. The thyroid isthmus is absent in about 10 to 15 per cent of cases.

BLOOD SUPPLY

The thyroid is one of the most vascular organs in the body and is supplied by 3 vessels—the superior, the inferior and the thyroidea ima arteries. The superior thyroid artery is a branch of the external carotid. As it enters the upper pole of the gland, it divides into the anterior and posterior branches and gives off a small branch to the suspensory ligament. The first part of the subclavian artery

gives rise to the inferior thyroid artery, which divides into 2 or more branches at varying distances from the gland. The thyroidea ima artery arises from the arch of the aorta or from the innominate artery and passes upward over the anterior surface of the trachea and terminates in the isthmus; this vessel is not always present. The superior and inferior arteries form a rich anastomosis in the gland.

VEINS

The distribution of the veins in the thyroid is not consistent. The superior thyroid vein usually terminates at the junction of the thyroid, lingual and facial veins. The middle vein empties into the internal jugular vein. The inferior thyroid veins end in the left innominate vein. The imae veins empty into the innominate vein of both sides. Thyroid veins are valveless, so the danger of air embolism is always present. In performing a thyroidectomy, great care must be taken to avoid injury to the veins. Tearing of the middle vein may lead to serious hemorrhage. In the removal of an intrathoracic goiter there is always the danger of venous bleeding.

NERVES

The vagus nerve supplies the thyroid gland with two important nerves—the superior and the inferior recurrent laryngeal nerves. Injury to the former is relatively unimportant, but bilateral injury to the latter may result in death and, at best, aphonia.

The superior laryngeal nerve arises from the inferior ganglion, passes downward and medially and crosses behind the internal carotid artery, dividing into the internal and the external laryngeal nerves. The latter accompanies the superior thyroid artery, but in a deeper plane, and supplies the cricothyroid and the inferior constrictor muscles. As pointed out, care must be exercised to clamp only the artery and the vein when ligating these vessels lest this nerve be injured.

Because the recurrent (inferior) laryngeal nerve may vary greatly in its location, the surgeon must be prepared to find the same anatomic variations as in performing surgery of the biliary tract. These nerves may penetrate and transverse the gland or remain in the tracheo-esophageal groove.

In safeguarding this nerve, Dr. Philip Thorek points out that in performing a thyroidectomy when the gland is dislocated forward and medially, the nerve usually hugs the side of the trachea. It is then located not in the tracheo-esophageal groove but on the posterolateral aspect of the trachea. It always passes posterior to the joint that exists be-

tween the inferior cornu of the thyroid and the cricoid. This cartilaginous prominence formed by the joint is a valuable guide to the nerve. On the right side the nerve crosses the first part of the subclavian artery, turns upward and medially behind that artery and the common carotid and travels in the groove between the esophagus and the trachea. It ascends in this groove to the lobe of the thyroid gland and crosses or is crossed by the inferior thyroid artery. On reaching the lower border of the inferior constrictor muscle, it passes deeply to it so as to gain access to the muscles of the larynx. It supplies the muscles that act on the vocal folds and also sensory branches to the mucous membranes of the larynx below the folds. On the left side the

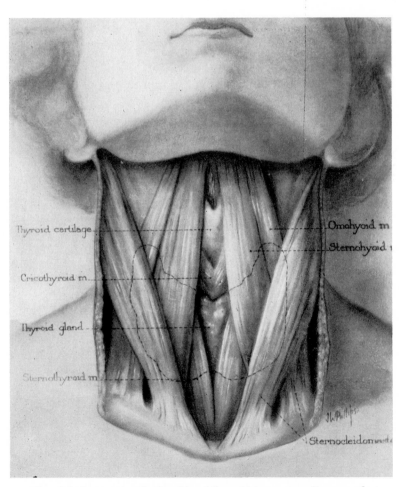

Fig. 75. Anatomic relationship of thyroid to surrounding muscles. (Jackson, A.: Goiter and Other Diseases of the Thyroid Gland, New York, Hoeber)

nerve turns around the arch of the aorta and ascends in the tracheo-esophageal groove.

The importance of the surgeon being familiar with the exact location of these nerves is stressed since their injury results in one of the most distressing complications in surgery.

The thyroid is supplied by an extensive lymphatic system. More important is its nerve supply. The vagus and the sympathetic (median and inferior cervical) ganglions and the superior laryngeal supply it. The inferior laryngeal nerve, although in close contact with the gland, does not supply it.

THE PARATHYROID GLANDS

These are usually four in number and are situated on the posterior surface of the thyroid gland. The upper pair usually are embedded in the gland substance, while the lower pair are in intimate contact with the branches of the inferior thyroid artery and the recurrent laryngeal nerve.

ERRORS AND SAFEGUARDS

In no place in the body is it more important for the surgeon to have a complete understanding of the anatomy than in the field of thyroid surgery. He should have a clear conception of the location and the relationship to the surrounding structures, of the vascular supply, of the superior and the recurrent laryngeal nerves and of the parathyroid glands. Failure to so inform himself may result in serious if not fatal complications, such as immediate or delayed hemorrhage, paralysis of the vocal cords, air embolism and tetany.

Although the special dangers which the surgeon encounters when dissecting the blood vessels and the recurrent laryngeal nerves will be considered in detail later, when discussing operative complications, it is important now to point out the following significant sources of error when performing a thyroidectomy.

The location of the superior thyroid artery varies a great deal, and so does its caliber, so that even the experienced surgeon may be confused at times. It is important to remember that the superior laryngeal nerve is located in close proximity to the artery (usually a little higher), and if a hemostat is applied too high, the nerve may be clamped, resulting in temporary dysphagia and voice impairment. As the vessel is under considerable tension, it

is well to apply 2 hemostats above and 1 below before dividing, in case 1 clamp slips or is defective.

If the inferior thyroid artery is to be ligated separately—a method employed by some surgeons—it is especially important that its location be well understood. In his text, *Anatomy in Surgery,* Dr. Philip Thorek gives the best description of its anatomic relationship that we have seen.

Although the superior vessel enters the superior pole, the inferior thyroid does *not* enter at the inferior pole of the gland. It travels upward along the medial border of the scalenus anterior muscle as far as the level of the sixth cervical vertebra and turns medially behind the vagus nerve and the common carotid artery; it passes in front of the vertebral vessels and, continuing downward, reaches the posterior border of the gland to which it is finally distributed. To do this it makes a hairpin turn, the summit of which varies considerably as to its level. It also supplies the larynx, the pharynx, the trachea, the esophagus and the surrounding muscles. As the artery reaches the thyroid it is crossed either in front or behind by the recurrent laryngeal nerve. A large branch of the vessel ascends along the posterior border of the gland to anastomose with a descending branch from the superior thyroid artery.

Unless the exact relationship of this artery to the nerve is realized, the latter may be injured by either a hemostat or a ligature when ligating the vessel. Ligation of the inferior thyroid artery separately does ensure better hemostasis. It is also important to avoid the parathyroids.

The thyroidea ima varies considerably in size and, unless ligated, may occasionally prove to be annoying in performing a thyroidectomy or a low tracheotomy.

Even though all the major vessels are ligated, the blood supply to the thyroid is adequate because of a rich collateral blood system.

PATHOLOGIC CONDITIONS OF THE THYROID GLAND

Congenital Anomalies

The thyroid gland may be deficient in size (hypoplasia), absent (aplasia) or the isthmus or a lobe may be lacking. The pyramidal lobe is absent in two thirds of all the cases coming to operation but, when present, may extend to the hyoid bone. Failure to remove this lobe may result in its increasing in size and, if toxic, causing a recurrence of symptoms with disfigurement. Accessory thyroid glands may occur at the base of the tongue or be attached to the trachea or the larynx and, if not removed, may cause persistent symptoms following thyroidectomy. Aberrant thyroid tissue is also found in the abdomen, as in teratomas of the ovary.

THYROIDITIS

Either acute or chronic inflammation of the thyroid gland may occur.

Acute Thyroiditis. This condition may and probably often does follow a virus infection, rhinitis, laryngitis, tonsillitis or sinusitis. It may also follow a systemic disease such as typhoid, or it may occur as the result of trauma. The gland becomes swollen and tender, and one or both lobes may be involved. The patient may complain of pains in the neck or behind the ear or of vague generalized aches and pains, together with fever and malaise.

TREATMENT. Antibiotics, antithyroid drugs, cortisone and x-ray therapy have all been tried with varying success. None of these has proved to be satisfactory in the experience of the author, who advocates thyroidectomy in any case of persistent symptoms.

In those rare instances in which the condition has progressed to the purulent stage, surgery with incision and removal of involved tissue and drainage is definitely indicated.

Chronic Thyroiditis. This may be manifest by 2 forms: (1) struma lymphomatosa and (2) Riedel's struma.

STRUMA LYMPHOMATOSA (HASHIMOTO'S DISEASE). This condition of unknown etiology is usually seen in middle-aged women and is characterized by a uniformly enlarged firm gland, nonadherent to the surrounding structures. The gland is avascular and, on section, appears grayish yellow in color. The thyroid

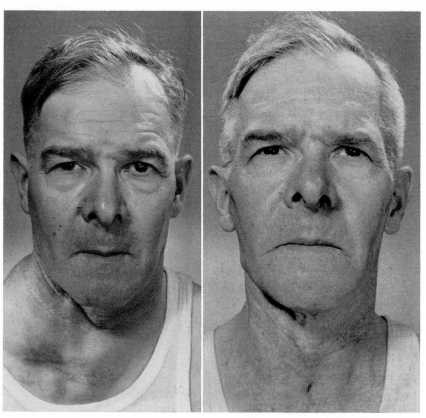

FIG. 76. (*Left*) Case of Hürthle cell carcinoma. (*Right*) Same patient after thyroidectomy.

may be tender, and the patient may complain of pain and an enlargement in the neck with some discomfort on swallowing or breathing. The treatment of choice is subtotal thyroidectomy. The author prefers a conservative operation performed with the electrosurgical loop, in which each lobe is hollowed out within its capsule.

RIEDEL'S STRUMA. This entity is also known as iron struma and is relatively uncommon. The thyroid gland becomes a dense, hard mass that may tightly constrict the trachea, causing severe cyanosis and dyspnea. In contrast with Hashimoto's disease, the inflammatory process in this condition extends to the surrounding structures, tending to obliterate anatomic landmarks. Often only pathologic diagnosis differentiates it from malignancy. It occurs in both sexes and most frequently in middle life. While it may be only necessary to divide the isthmus to afford relief, the author prefers thyroidectomy performed by the electrosurgical knife. Extreme care must be used to avoid injury to the adjacent structures. It may be necessary to use postoperative thyroid therapy.

MALIGNANT LESIONS

Great difference of opinion exists concerning the classification of malignant tumors of the thyroid gland. Among the less complex and more easily understood of such classifications is one used at the Mayo Clinic as follows:
1. Papillary adenocarcinoma
2. Carcinoma in adenoma
3. Diffuse adenocarcinoma
4. Epithelioma
5. Sarcoma

A nodular goiter, particularly in a child or in a male adult, should be regarded with suspicion until proved to be benign. If this appears as a "clinically solitary nodule," the chances are much greater that it is malignant, the incidence running as high as 40 per cent in the male (Fig. 76). The author is among those who advise the removal of all thyroid tumors unless there is some special contraindication, such as senility, advanced cardiovascular disease or some other malady.

Papillary Adenocarcinoma. The term lateral or aberrant thyroid gland was discarded some years ago after Pemberton, Black, Eberts, Clay and others showed that this conception was incorrect. Instead of malignant lesions arising in so-called fetal rests, it is now recognized that these lesions are actually metastases from the thyroid malignancy to the adjacent lymph glands. This condition comprises about one third of all malignant lesions of the thyroid, is seen most often in children and young adults and is of a relatively low-grade malignancy. When recognized early, it may be only necessary to do a total lobectomy of the involved side, together with a removal of all the glands, a subtotal resection of the opposite lobe and a follow-up with deep x-ray therapy. Though there is no uniformity of opinion concerning the treatment of this lesion under this plan, the author has seen a long period of survival in a group of cases.

Adenocarcinoma in an Adenoma. Why some adenomas never undergo malignant change and why others do so only after 40 or 50 years of existence remains a mystery. There are those who feel that the malignancy arises not from the adenoma (Crile) but from the gland itself, but this view is not supported generally. On the basis of our present knowledge, it seems logical to advise prophylactic subtotal thyroidectomy for nodular adenomatous goiters. These tumors invade the capsule only in the late stages, but they metastasize early by way of the blood stream and may not be recognized by the clinician or the surgeon but only by the pathologist. Such recognition may be too late. In a series of 774 cases of cancer seen at the Mayo Clinic, Pemberton found 38.1 per cent of the cases to be in this group. The pathologic picture may vary widely and prove to be confusing, so that even the most eminent pathologists may not concur in their opinion. There are instances in which it is most difficult to establish clearly the criteria of malignancy.

Diffuse Adenocarcinoma. This is a highly malignant condition which may arise from either the gland or an adenoma. When the condition can be established clinically, there is little or no hope for the patient, because it is highly malignant, grows rapidly and metastasizes by way of either the lymph or the blood stream. About one third of the malignant lesions of the thyroid belong in this group, and, since they are often inoperable when first seen, the prognosis is poor.

Squamous Epithelioma. This condition is extremely rare, occurring in only about 1 per cent of all malignancies of the thyroid. As a consequence, it is not an important clinical entity.

Sarcoma. This is also rare, although the author has observed 3 instances in approximately 100 malignant thyroid lesions. Diagnosis is established by pathologic study; neither radical surgery nor x-ray therapy is of much avail.

Summary. In brief, it may be said that the treatment of malignancy of the thyroid resolves itself into the question of early recognition, early eradication and prophylactic thyroidectomy for adenomatous goiters. The role to be played by radioactive iodine is yet to be determined. Unfortunately, I^{131} so far has

seemed to destroy part but not all of the growth, but at Memorial Hospital in New York City, as well as elsewhere, its use gives promise of prolonging life and of detecting metastatic lesions that, in turn, may be made amenable to treatment.

Safeguard your patient who has an adenomatous goiter by advising its early removal. Do not make the mistake of considering a case of Riedel's struma to be an inoperable malignancy.

MISCELLANEOUS LESIONS OF THE THYROID GLAND

Certain other extremely rare diseases of the thyroid gland have been reported, none of which have any special significance in a discussion of surgical problems. Among these reported conditions are tuberculosis, the various fungoid diseases and lues.

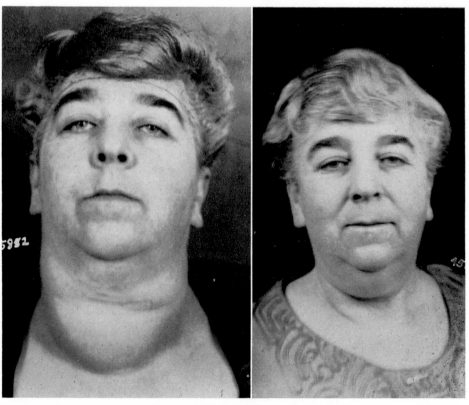

FIG. 77. (*Left*) Case of multiple nontoxic nodular goiter. (*Right*) Same patient after thyroidectomy. (Jackson, A.: Am. J. Surg. 2:228)

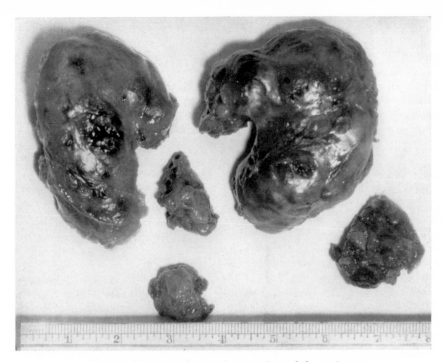

FIG. 78. Gross specimen of nontoxic nodular goiter.

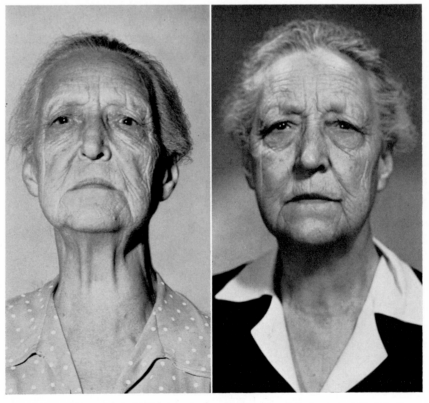

FIG. 79. (*Left*) Toxic diffuse goiter without exophthalmos. (*Right*) Same patient 3 months after thyroidectomy.

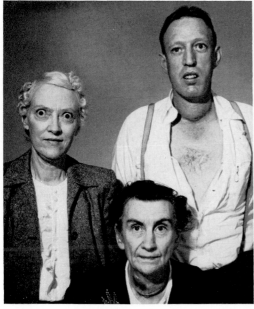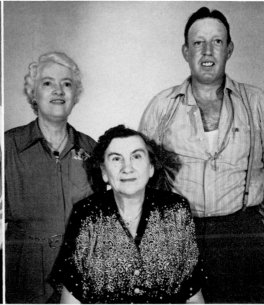

FIG. 80. (*Left*) Three cases of toxic diffuse goiter treated unsuccessfully with I[131]. (*Right*) Same patients 3 months after surgery. (Jonas, K. (ed.): Babcock's Principles and Practice of Surgery, Philadelphia, Lea and Febiger)

GOITER

By far the most important surgical problem of the thyroid gland concerns goiter, a classification of which is suggested as follows:

NONTOXIC:

1. Colloid, simple diffuse
2. Adenomatous, nodular (Figs. 77 and 78)

TOXIC:

1. Adenomatous, toxic nodular, with hyperthyroidism
2. Exophthalmic (Graves' and Basedow's disease), toxic diffuse (Figs. 79, 80 and 81)

Simple Diffuse Colloid Goiter. These are not a surgical problem. They commonly occur in children at puberty and may be prevented by the weekly administration of small amounts of iodine. In adults, large colloid goiters usually are associated with adenomas and should be removed.

Nontoxic Nodular Adenomatous Goiter. These may be seen at any age in both sexes, but in a ratio of 5 females to 1 male. They generally arise in the neglected colloid goiters of youth. They may remain comparatively dormant throughout life or they may become:

1. Enlarged outwardly 71%
2. Substernal 25%

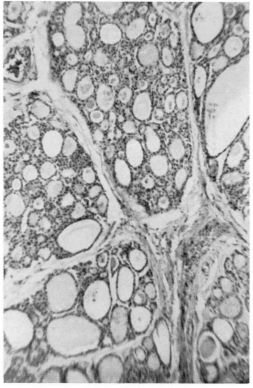

FIG. 81. Photomicrograph of thyroid of patient treated unsuccessfully with I[131]. (Jackson: Missouri Med. 50:777)

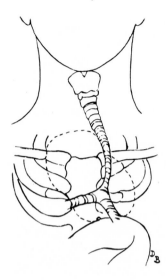

Fig. 82. Compression of trachea by intrathoracic goiter.

Large multiple adenomatous goiters that enlarge outwardly seldom cause symptoms but are disfiguring and, therefore, should be removed.

Toxic Nodular Adenomatous Goiter. These probably are seen more often in the area of the Great Lakes than in any other section of the world. This is in contrast with Europe, particularly Switzerland and Austria, where nodular goiters are endemic but seldom toxic. By middle age, nearly one half of these nodular goiter patients (Fig. 83) seen in the middle western states show some evidence of hyperthyroidism. As has been demonstrated by Dr. Collier and the author, a considerable rise in blood pressure may be observed before an elevation of the basal metabolic rate occurs. Unfortunately, these cases are often treated for years for hypertension and cardio-

3. Intrathoracic (major portion within the chest) 4%
4. Toxic (at 60 years) 50%
5. Malignant—
    clinical solitary ....20% F, 40% M
    multiple .... 4 to 10%

Small nodular goiters are prone to become toxic and malignant. Large goiters of this type seldom become toxic but are apt to become substernal and occasionally intrathoracic. Small nontoxic adenomatous goiters seldom cause symptoms but should be removed to prevent possible future complications.

Intrathoracic Adenomatous Goiter. These are not often toxic but they may cause dyspnea by tracheal compression (Fig. 82) and, though rarely, dysphagia by pressure on the esophagus. Large dilated veins on the neck and the chest may suggest this condition. Roentgenograms, both anteroposterior and lateral, may show the goiter even when it is not seen or palpated on swallowing. Examination of the vocal cords may show some paralysis resulting from traction by the goiter on the recurrent laryngeal nerve. Rarely, edema of the extremities is seen from injected venous circulation. Inspiratory stridor and "brassy" cough may be indicative. Delayed surgical relief endangers the patient and increases the risk of surgery. Such patients have been treated for many years under the mistaken diagnosis of asthma.

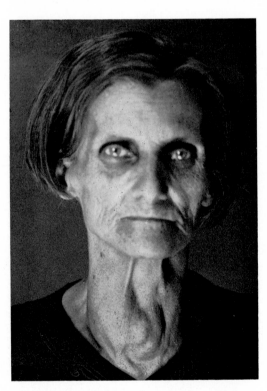

Fig. 83. Advanced case of multiple toxic nodular goiter. (Jackson, A.: Kansas M. Soc. J., June, 1939)

vascular disease before the source of the trouble is recognized.

Cardiac changes manifest by the electrocardiogram are a common sequel, and digitalis is of little avail in the treatment of the resulting auricular fibrillation. Before treating a patient for cardiovascular disease, make sure that a small adenoma of the thyroid is not responsible.

Patients suffering from this condition give a history of gradual loss of weight and strength. Unlike Graves's disease, gastrointestinal disturbances are not seen, nor do exophthalmos, thrills or bruits occur. There is not the ravenous appetite with weight loss. Tremor does occur and also palpitation and nervousness. However, the latter is not the extreme emotional type bordering on delirium, as seen in Graves's disease. The blood pressure is rather typical, with an elevation of both the systolic and diastolic pressures. The basal metabolic rate is elevated but rarely exceeds + 60 per cent. Protein-bound iodine studies may be helpful. Do not confuse the two forms of hyperthyroidism. They are as different as measles and scarlet fever.

Exophthalmic Goiter. On the other hand, exophthalmic goiter occurs more often in young people (the average age is 33), although it is seen in ages from 3 to 80 years (Fig. 84). The duration of symptoms is much shorter— weeks, in contrast with months. The disease may follow a long severe strain, such as the care of a sick relative, or may result from overwork, prolonged anxiety, shock, fear or infection; but the etiology remains unknown, as does the cause of the exophthalmos. The disease progresses in a series of waves, and at their crest a crisis occurs, with fever, vomiting, diarrhea and possibly delirium. A tremendous loss of weight may occur during this period. Fortunately, owing to better understanding and earlier recognition of the disease, crises have become as rare as typhoid fever and, even if they do occur, may be speedily controlled with Lugol's solution. An early symptom is an excessive and even ravenous appetite accompanied by weight

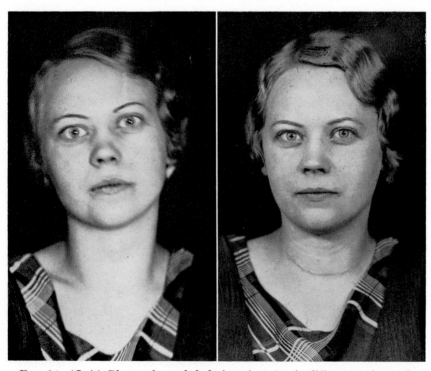

Fig. 84. (*Left*) Photo of exophthalmic goiter (toxic diffuse) patient taken before operation, showing exophthalmos and symmetrical enlargement of the gland. (*Right*) Postoperative photo of the same patient. (Jackson, A.: Am. J. Clin. Med. **50**:70)

loss, such as is seen in only one other dis-ease—diabetes. A marked intolerance to heat, excessive perspiration, weakness on climbing stairs, tremor, palpitation and dyspnea are other early complaints. There is inability to relax, indicated by "purposeful movements without any purpose" (Plummer), such as constantly tossing around in bed until the elbows and the knees become chafed and red. The telltale stare and exophthalmos, from which the disease derives its name, may be absent or slight within the first 3 months of the onset of the disease.

The signs are often pathognomonic. Most characteristic is the blood pressure. Early in the disease the systolic may be normal or ele-vated only slightly, but the diastolic is de-creased, often dropping to 70, 60 or 50 mm. Hg. and occasionally heard all the way to zero. Only aortic insufficiency must be differ-entiated.

So, too, the quadriceps test of weakness may prove to be typical if the patient is asked to step up on the examining table. The basal metabolic rate is markedly elevated and may be between 40 and 80 per cent. Likewise, protein-bound studies may be of diagnostic aid. A basal metabolic rate below 30 per cent should seldom be considered to be diagnostic of the disease, provided that the patient has received no previous medication. In such a case, with the diagnosis still in doubt, all medication should be stopped for 3 weeks and the test then repeated.

One cannot stress too much the great value of a careful clinical history and a physical examination in arriving at a diagnosis of these cases. These two factors and experience are of more value than laboratory aids. Yet, an accurate basal metabolic test made by a reliable technician on a good machine is of great value not only in clarifying the diag-nosis but also in gauging the degree of im-provement before and after surgery. Seldom should one rely on a single test. Even under ideal conditions, the metabolic rate in a nor-mal person can be elevated falsely merely by his being nervous and breathing rapidly.

DIFFERENTIAL DIAGNOSIS

Like syphilis, hyperthyroidism may simu-late many other diseases, particularly those affecting the nervous, cardiovascular or gastro-intestinal systems. Even the most experienced thyroidologists may be confused by these per-plexing cases, so it is well to remember the words of the old master, Dr. Charles H. Mayo, who used to say, "Exophthalmic goiter is never an emergency operation." Also, it is well to remember that the highest achievement of the surgeon is the art of correct diagnosis, and this is of prime importance in the field of thyroid surgery.

CHOICE OF OPERATION OR PROCEDURE

Having correctly established the diagnosis by a careful history taking and a physical examination, with the help of the laboratory aids, one is confronted with the problem of the correct operation or procedure.

The introduction of Lugol's solution by Plummer in 1922 eliminated the necessity of the ligation operation of the superior thyroid artery, a most popular procedure in its day. In 1927, the author published a series of 100 primary thyroidectomies for exophthalmic goiter and never has had occasion to use a ligation operation since 1925, although reports of this procedure appeared in the literature until 1943, when Astwood and co-workers dis-covered thiouracil.

The latter, as well as the more valuable propylthiouracil, Tapazole and other antithy-roid drugs, eliminated the necessity of the 2-stage lobectomy operation in advanced cases of toxic nodular goiter.

If surgery is to be used, primary thyroid-ectomy is now the universally accepted method of procedure for the treatment of both toxic nodular and exophthalmic goiter.

In the latter disease, a difference of opinion exists. Time and a study of a large series of cases alone will determine the most effective method of therapy. A decade has elapsed since radioactive iodine was first used in the treat-ment of Graves' disease, yet the relative merits of I^{131} and surgery are still moot. Pro-ponents of the iodine therapy maintain that the same results can be obtained with less expense, with little or no risk and with fewer complications. It is true that the risk appears to be small, that the danger of the development of malignancy or sterility seems to be remote, that paralysis of the nerve, hemorrhage and tetany do not occur. Yet the author has seen several patients in whom the disease had not been controlled even by competent authorities after prolonged treatment and in whom hyperthyroidism persisted, cardiovascular complications were becoming evident, and exophthalmos was progressing and probably had become permanent. Most of the leading thyroid clinics, where both methods are available, give preference to surgery, except in a few complicated cases involving senility or other diseases or conditions.

GENERAL PREOPERATIVE PRECAUTIONS

No patient should be subjected to thyroid surgery until his case has been carefully studied from every angle and every possible risk eliminated. This study should include a carefully taken history, a physical examination and the use of all laboratory aids considered to be pertinent.

IODINE

For example, a patient suffering from exophthalmic goiter, to all outward appearances, may be ready for thyroidectomy. The weight may be close to normal and the basal metabolic rate below 50 per cent. Yet the all-important point in the history may have been overlooked, namely, that he has been on iodine for weeks or months and has become iodine-resistant, so that after surgery there is little response to iodine and a fatal crisis may ensue. Such a case was reported by the author before the 1927 meeting of the American Association for the Study of Goiter. Yet, even today, occasionally we see patients who have been kept on iodine for long periods of time prior to surgery. *No patient should receive iodine longer than 3 weeks before primary thyroidectomy is to be performed.* In the case just mentioned, a young woman with exophthalmic goiter had been given iodine for 6 months, and she appeared to be in excellent condition for operation, no one having had reported the danger of a patient becoming "iodine-fast." Within 48 hours after operation, a fatal crisis developed.

A patient with toxic nodular goiter who has been prepared for weeks or months with propylthiouracil should not be subjected to thyroidectomy without a resting period of 10 days in which iodine is substituted for the antithyroid drug, the purpose being to reduce vascularity and diminish the great tendency to bleeding, which may be troublesome to even the most experienced surgeon.

OBESITY

This is rarely a serious problem in thyroid surgery, most hyperthyroid patients being underweight. It may be desirable to delay surgery a few weeks until the patient has regained some of the lost weight. An intake of 4,000 or more calories a day may be required to accomplish this.

Occasionally large nontoxic nodular goiters that may be substernal or intrathoracic are seen in obese persons. In such cases it may be desirable to place the patient on a low caloric diet for several weeks or months and reduce weight so as to facilitate surgery and reduce the risk.

CONDITION OF HEART

The condition of the heart is of prime importance in thyroid surgery, and the services of a competent cardiologist are desirable in evaluating the risk of operation as well as in properly preparing the patient for surgery. The electrocardiogram may indicate the need for further preparation.

The author feels that the use of stimulants such as nicotine and caffeine is definitely a factor in preventing the successful treatment of hyperthyroidism, and their use must be forbidden. In this connection, recent studies with the ballistocardiogram appear to indicate definite coronary disease in smokers when no such changes may be seen in the electrocardiogram.

CONDITION OF NERVOUS SYSTEM

The nervous system must be evaluated carefully in hyperthyroidism. If the patient has confidence in his surgeon and in the results of surgery, fear is dissipated and the danger of postoperative reaction is greatly diminished. The patient must be psychologically ready before surgery is attempted. The author has never made any attempt to conceal the time when thyroidectomy is to be performed and prefers to have the patient willing and anxious for surgery.

The role of the entire *house staff* is important in preparing hyperthyroid patients for operation. They can convey much confidence by their reassurance, by letting patients converse with other thyroid patients successfully operated on and by being kind and attentive.

PREPARATION OF THE PATIENT FOR OPERATION

The preoperative preparation depends on (1) type of goiter, (2) condition of the patient, (3) choice of anesthesia and (4) the physician and the surgeon. Today, with the use of iodine and antithyroid drugs, most patients can safely be prepared for thyroidectomy at home.

Since 1928, the following plan has been followed successfully by the author, with variations only in the treatment of toxic nodular goiter.

Type of Goiter

Nontoxic Adenomatous Goiter. Preoperative medication is administered as follows: Nembutal, gr. 1½, the night before and the morning of surgery; scopolamine, by hypodermic, 1 hour before surgery, gr. $\frac{1}{150}$ in persons under 50, gr. $\frac{1}{200}$ in persons over 50; Pantopon, gr. ⅙, by hypodermic, 1 hour before surgery.

Prior to giving the hypodermics, Vaseline cotton is placed in the ears, the eyes are covered, and head towels are applied. Relatives are requested to leave, the room is darkened and kept quiet, and the patient is asked to try to sleep. In the operating room, if the patient is still wakeful, another hypodermic of Pantopon, gr. ⅙, may be given (rarely needed in older persons).

Toxic Adenomatous Goiter. Each patient must be judged individually, and only the experience of the surgeon and the internist will determine the length of time required for preparation and the type of treatment. If one must err—and no one can judge all cases correctly—it is better to err on the safe side and give too long a period of preparation. The late Dr. Frank Lahey preferred to continue preoperative treatment with the antithyroid drugs in these cases until the basal metabolic

rate approximated normal. With due respect for the brilliant record achieved by this eminent surgeon, the author feels that surgery in these cases may often be performed safely with a shorter period of preparation, especially since the basal metabolic rate is not an accurate index of the ability of these patients to undergo surgery safely.

In the milder early cases, no preparation other than that given in the nontoxic cases may be required. Others may need weeks and even months of preparation with the antithyroid drugs. If propylthiouracil is used, the average dosage given by the author is 50 mg. 4 times a day, or a total of 200 mg. This may be increased to 300 or 400 mg., but rarely is a larger amount deemed necessary. If Tapazole is selected, an average dose of 5 mg. given 4 to 6 times a day is used.

Antithyroid drugs are stopped 10 days prior to surgery, and 5 drops of Lugol's solution, 3 times a day, are given instead to diminish bleeding. If decompensation or auricular fibrillation is present, the patient may be digitalized, although the antithyroid drugs will usually prove to be more effective.

The remainder of the preoperative preparation is the same as for the nontoxic adenomatous goiter cases.

Exophthalmic Goiter. All but the most advanced cases can be prepared by giving 10 drops of iodine 3 times a day for from 10 to 14 days prior to surgery. Every effort should be made to have the patient gain weight. He may be prepared at home, provided that he refrains from work. Occasionally, a mild sedative, such as phenobarbital, grs. ¼ or ½, may be required for rest, but it should be remembered that such cases are rather sensitive to the drug and it should be stopped at the first sign of an itching skin eruption.

Patients with advanced disease, in whom the condition has continued for a long period of time, cardiovascular changes have occurred and toxicity is severe, may require preparation for several weeks with an antithyroid drug before iodine therapy.

The only difference in the immediate preoperative preparation and that used for toxic adenomas is that these patients are given 4 doses of 10 drops of Lugol's solution the morning of operation.

In considering special safeguards in the preoperative preparation, the surgeon should be sure that the patient has utmost confidence in him. Elimination of fear is an important factor in performing surgery on toxic goiter patients, and unless the patient's psychology is right, the operation had best be postponed. The nursing and the house staff can assist materially in building up the patient's confidence.

If the operation is to be performed under local or nerve block anesthesia, it is most important that the preoperative medication be administered in exact timing with the surgery. If this is delayed too long, the beneficial effect of the sedation is worn off.

Likewise, it is important that quiet be maintained in both the patient's room and the operating room, as loud talking and noise disturbs the patient and keeps him restless and apprehensive.

If a general anesthetic is given, the anesthetist should be competent and experienced in the use of anesthesia in thyroid surgery. He must be prepared to meet any of the several complications that may develop. Oxygen should be available at all times. Also, a tracheotomy set should be at hand. When operating in the presence of hyperthyroidism, it is well to remember that the patient needs plenty of air.

ANESTHESIA

The type of anesthesia used depends on the preference of the surgeon and the facilities at his disposal. Some use cyclopropane, others use Pentothal Sodium, nitrous oxide and ether, local infiltration or deep and superficial nerve block. The last named has been used with excellent results by the author for the past 28 years. It has many advantages over local infiltration and general anesthesia and is simple to administer. The advantages may be summarized as follows:

1. Anatomic landmarks are not obliterated as with local infiltration.

2. The patient is under the control of the surgeon and not of the anesthetist as in general anesthesia.

3. If the operation is prolonged, the patient leaves the table in much better condition.

4. The problem of postoperative mucus is lessened.

5. There is no postoperative emesis, so the patient is able to take medication immediately by mouth.

6. The patient's cough reflex is retained, so that any overlooked vessel may be detected.

7. There is less shock and postoperative discomfort reaction.

Technic. For superficial cervical nerve block anesthesia, the following technic is used by the author:

Procaine, 1½ per cent, without Adrenalin is preferred. With the smallest needle, a wheal of 2 cc. of procaine is made just above the clavicle at its midportion. The patient's head is then turned to the opposite side, and a 5-inch needle is inserted into the wheal. Ten cc. of procaine is injected as the needle is advanced just beneath the skin and in the direction of the tip of the mastoid. This blocks off the cervical sympathetics coming over the top of the sternocleidomastoid muscle. As the needle is withdrawn, another 10 cc. is injected, making a total of 20 cc. It is most important that the needle be kept constantly in motion as the injection is made; otherwise some procaine might be injected into a vein and a reaction develop. If this does occur, the patient may experience a mild convulsive seizure which can be controlled with oxygen. The use of a barbiturate preoperatively is good protection against this eventuality.

Before making the midline incision through the fascia, a few drops of procaine should be injected. Again, before clamping the superior thyroid arteries, a few drops should be injected adjacent to the vessels to block the sympathetic nerve. The gland itself may also be injected to distend the capsule in small goiters and make them easier to manipulate. Before skin closure, a subcutaneous injection is made along the entire length of both skin flaps. In a secondary operation, the area of the original incision should be injected.

Author's Technic. If certain signs develop during the course of either a local or general anesthetic, it may be necessary or advisable to terminate the operation and complete it at a second stage. Such indications rarely occur today with the properly prepared patient. In hyperthyroidism an elevation of the pulse rate above 130 or a marked increase in the pulse pressure with extreme restlessness may be such an indication, or an increased oxygen consumption should be taken as an indication to stop.

If a general anesthetic is used, an endotracheal tube should be employed to maintain an adequate airway, using the carbon dioxide absorption technic.

Pentothal Sodium is used quite generally today for induction purposes, but it carries a certain risk in prolonged anesthesia. Laryngeal spasm and respiratory embarrassment may be guarded against by spraying the throat with 10 per cent cocaine before administering Pentothal Sodium.

Avertin carries a similar hazard and is apt to have a prolonged effect following operation.

Nitrous oxide and ethylene likewise have the objection that if given in sufficient amount to produce satisfactory anesthesia, the patient is apt to develop anoxia.

Cyclopropane is an excellent anesthetic but is highly explosive and is said to cause cardiac irregularities in certain conditions, particularly hyperthyroidism.

The surgeon must be prepared at all times to co-operate with the anesthetist in the prevention and the treatment of anoxia. In malignant thyroids or in the delivery of large intrathoracic goiters, the trachea may be either damaged or compressed in such a way as to seriously impair breathing. Too forcible traction on attempting to deliver a large nodular goiter may so compress the trachea as to cause respiratory failure. Collapse of the trachea necessitating immediate tracheotomy may be required unless an endotracheal tube is in situ.

Excessive mucus may be annoying, causing the patient to cough and choke, especially when the trachea has been distorted for many years. If preoperative medication with depressant drugs has been used, respiration may be further embarrassed with general anesthesia, and constant aspiration must be maintained.

More serious but unusual complications of anesthesia are carotid sinus syndrome and convulsions. The former is the result of stimulation of a hypersensitive carotid sinus and may result from lateral traction on the carotid artery. A marked slowing of the pulse followed by a severe drop in blood pressure and often reduction of the respiratory rate occur. Immediate removal of the causative factor, together with artificial respiration and lowering of the patient's head to prevent cerebral hypoxemia, is indicated. The area of the bifurcation of the carotid sinus should be injected with 5 to 10 cc. of 1 per cent procaine.

Convulsions may result from injecting procaine into the vein when a barbiturate has not been given preoperatively. If it occurs from any other cause, the intravenous injection of a barbiturate is indicated.

It is most important that the surgeon and the anesthetist co-operate at all times to be sure that the patient does not pass into a state of anoxia. Should an emergency occur during operation, such as a sudden hemorrhage or a tracheal compression, co-operation of the surgeon and the anesthetist will carry the patient safely through the crisis.

POSITION OF PATIENT ON OPERATING TABLE; DRAPING; SCREENING; INSTRUMENTS

The position of the patient on the operating table can add to or detract from the ease of the operation. The patient should be high enough on the table so that the head drops well back, bringing the anterior surface of the neck into a convex position. The author has developed a special table that greatly facilitates the operation and also a "windshield" screen that gives the surgeon a maximum field in which to work and the patient a maximum amount of air space and comfort. Smothering the patient with sheets and towels is annoying to both patient and surgeon. Every effort should be made to give him all possible comfort, particularly if nerve block anesthesia is to be used.

Likewise, the *proper instruments* will facilitate the operation. The old Ochsner straight clamps and the large curved Kellys have no place in a thyroidectomy. Instead, the surgeon should have available 18 small straight and as many small curved hemostats; 4 claw retractors; 2 curved goiter retractors; 2 tissue forceps; a large and a small removable-blade scalpel; a self-retaining spreading retractor;* 2 diamond jaw needle holders; 2 Mastin muscle clamps; a pair of suture and a pair of dissecting scissors and skin clips (Fig. 85).

Sutures are a matter of individual prefer-

* The author's retractor is made by the V. Mueller Co., Chicago, Ill.

ence; some surgeons favor silk, others use cotton or catgut. The author has always used 00 and 000 chromic gut with wedged-on needles (atraumatic).

The matter of *closure* is also one of individual choice. The author prefers 000 plain subcutaneous interrupted sutures with metal skin clips, half of which are removed the day after operation and the remainder the next day. If silk sutures are used, they should be removed not later than the third day, as they tend to leave permanently disfiguring stitch marks.

A combined needle holder and scissors has many advantages. The first assistant can use this to tie knots and to cut sutures, thus saving the time that it would take the second assistant, cutting with the regular scissors, to react.

Since 1928, the *electrosurgical knife* has been used routinely by the author in performing thyroidectomy. This has many advantages and some disadvantages in comparison with the scalpel. First, one must know his machine, as some are far more satisfactory than others. One could do serious harm by "cooking" the nerves or damaging the trachea with too

powerful a unit or too great coagulation. Its use is not as satisfactory in large cystic adenomatous goiters. It is not used to coagulate any large or important vessels, such as the superior and inferior thyroid arteries, the vessels on the outside of the gland or the lateral veins. It is a great timesaver when used to coagulate the vessels on the skin flaps, on the surface of the gland and within the capsule. It eliminates much foreign material from the field and lessens serum. With the loop cautery, it is possible to do an intracapsular resection of the gland without endangering the vital structures and at the same time remove or destroy a maximum amount of hyperplastic tissue far more effectively than with a scalpel.

TECHNIC OF THYROIDECTOMY

INCISION

A 4-inch piece of catgut clamped at each end by a hemostat is used to mark the proposed incision. This should be placed parallel with a natural crease in the neck, slightly curved at either end. Naturally, it should be shorter for small goiters but should always be of sufficient length so as to facilitate the op-

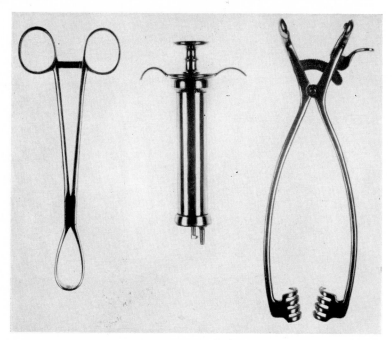

FIG. 85. The author's instruments. (*Left*) Grasping clamp. (*Center*) All-metal syringe. (*Right*) Self-retaining retractor. (Jackson, A.: Surg., Gynec. & Obst. 46:547)

eration. In making the incision, the scalpel at all times should be carried at right angles to the skin so as to prevent postoperative overlapping of a skin flap. The incision should be placed about 1½ inches above the clavicles. If placed too low, it will appear years later across the chest and be disfiguring.

The skin flap is now dissected upward, as the second assistant strongly retracts the flap with claw retractors. No muscle should be removed, for, if one is cut, frequent bleeding occurs.

The upper flap should always be reflected sufficiently high, or else later exposure of the superior poles will be handicapped.

A claw retractor is next placed in the middle of the upper flap and another in the same position in the lower; the latter is dissected for ½ inch in depth the length of the incision.

DRAPING

A *split goiter towel* is then draped over the operative field, and a self-retaining retractor is placed. Too many surgeons handicap themselves with an inadequate incision and exposure of the operative field. Moist wet towels are placed on either side of the neck to prevent drainage to the back.

EXPOSURE

Two straight hemostats are placed on either side of the midline and elevated by the second assistant. A few drops of procaine are injected into the pretracheal fascia and a midline incision made through this tissue. At this point a pair of dissecting scissors should be inserted into this incision and the veins on either side separated. These veins are usually joined just above the sternum and again at the upper end

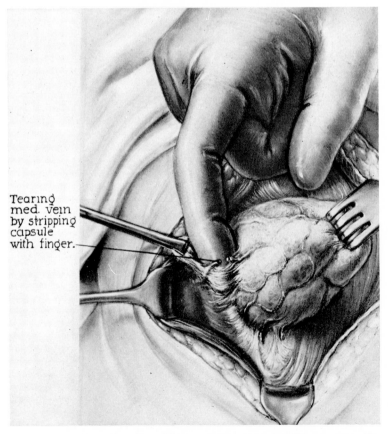

Tearing med. vein by stripping capsule with finger.

FIG. 86. Avoid tearing the median vein by stripping the capsule with the finger.

of the incision, and care must be used to avoid cutting them, as well as those on either side.

The *sternohyoid and the sternothyroid* muscles are next freed from the gland by sharp dissection and retracted or, in the case of a large goiter, divided by use of the Mastin noncrushing muscle clamps. In dividing the muscles, one should be careful not to cut the surface of the gland or the vessels at either end. When large veins are to be cut, it may be safer to ligate them first by suture in order to guard against possible air embolism. The lower muscle clamps are fastened down by towel hooks, and the upper ones are crossed and retracted on the side being resected. One should never hesitate to divide the muscles in order to obtain better exposure. Complications are often the result of inadequate exposure.

The goiter is now gently elevated by traction with a claw retractor, and sharp dissection of the capsule is begun. The superior thyroid artery and vein are exposed, the pole injected, doubly clamped, divided and ligated. Such dissection lessens the tendency of tearing the middle vein. Do not include muscle fibers in the ligation, since retraction of these fibers may loosen the ligature. To guard against sudden retraction of the artery, the upper hemostat is left in situ until the vessel is sutured securely by one or more ligatures of 00 chromic gut. These hemostats should clamp only the vessels and not damage the superior branch of the recurrent laryngeal nerve. The goiter is then rotated upward, thus exposing the lateral veins which may be divided and ligated separately or with the gland. Care must be exercised to avoid tearing these veins either by finger or blunt dissection, in which case annoying and even serious bleeding may result (Fig. 86).

HEMOSTASIS

Hemostats may now be placed on the remaining vessels along the sides of the gland. At all times the relationship of the recurrent laryngeal nerve and the parathyroid glands must be recognized, and the clamps should be placed well above these vital structures (Fig. 87). *Think twice and act slowly before placing a clamp on the lower pole,* the most dangerous area. One should always be able to see gland tissue below the clamp. This may prove to be

friable and vascular, and in a later attempt to control bleeding, the nerve may be injured. For this reason some surgeons prefer first to isolate and ligate the inferior thyroid artery after exposing the nerve. The author feels that, by and large, this technic does not decrease the incidence of nerve injury.

RESECTION

The selected lobe is resected with either the scalpel or the surgical knife. The author prefers the latter, using the loop cautery, especially in cases of exophthalmic goiter. The hyperplastic tissue may be shelled out easily with an intracapsular dissection, as an egg is removed from its shell. Important vessels are sutured, and smaller ones within the capsule are coagulated or ligated.

The amount of tissue removed depends on the type of goiter. In the nodular type, every effort should be made to remove or destroy all adenomas and cysts, although it may not always be possible to do so without endangering

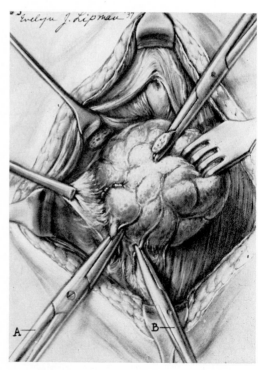

FIG. 87. Avoid placing hemostats too low, thus endangering (A) the parathyroid and (B) the recurrent laryngeal nerve.

the vital structures. In toxic diffuse goiter, all hyperplastic tissue that can be removed safely should be resected.

There is far less chance of the adenomatous goiter recurring than of the toxic diffuse type, especially if it is a toxic adenomatous goiter occurring in an elderly person. A rough estimate would be to leave one third of a normal-sized lobe in a nodular goiter and one fourth of a normal-sized lobe in a toxic diffuse goiter.

In considering the amount of tissue to remove, remember that some tissue undergoes resorption after operation. Few surgeons favor the so-called radical total thyroidectomy except in the case of malignancy.

Next, the edges of the capsule are approximated by interrupted sutures, using an atraumatic needle (Fig. 88). One treats the remaining lobes in the same manner, being sure to search for a pyramidal lobe.

The patient is asked to *cough* several times. If any vessels have been overlooked or not ligated securely, they may be detected and

secured. The operative field must be absolutely dry before closure. Sometimes this is very difficult, and it may be necessary to resort to the use of Gelfoam or even small muscle flaps.

DRAINAGE

If a *drain* is to be used, a soft, split rubber tube not over 1/4 inch in diameter is inserted in the midline. Where excessive drainage is anticipated, a drain may also be inserted at either end of the incision. Drains are not left in situ over 48 hours.

CLOSURE

The pretracheal muscles are approximated by interrupted sutures. This is important in order to prevent a postoperative tracheal adhesion and consequent disfiguring scar when swallowing. The fascia is united by a continuous stitch. Subcutaneous sutures are placed to improve the scar, and skin clips or interrupted dermal sutures close the incision.

A firm pressure bandage is applied, using

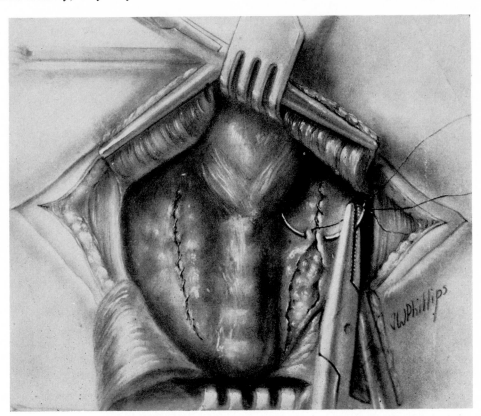

FIG. 88. Suturing the capsule. (Jackson, A.: Goiter and Other Diseases of the Thyroid Gland, New York, Hoeber)

fluffs, mechanic's waste and goiter pads or a towel. One half of the clips are removed in 24 hours, the remainder in 48 hours. The end-result should be a fine, hairline scar.

There are many ways of performing a thyroidectomy, European surgeons in particular using a technic that differs from that of American surgeons. However, an important point to remember is that great speed is no longer an essential requisite, especially when nerve block anesthesia is used. Still, needless delay in bad-risk cases may prove to be a vital factor. Rather than speed, the avoidance of injury to the laryngeal nerves and the parathyroid glands and the removal of sufficient hyperplastic tissue to effect a cure in toxic diffuse goiter cases are the important objectives.

The surgeon should always remember that it is the end-result, the long-time cure, that should be striven for.

The author feels that the method he has developed gives the maximum fulfillment of these objectives. There is less danger of injuring the important structures when an intracapsular resection is performed, and the incidence of recurrence is materially decreased in toxic diffuse goiter by the use of the electrosurgical knife.

POSTOPERATIVE CARE

NONTOXIC ADENOMATOUS GOITER

These cases require little or no postoperative care. Sedation is rarely used. For mucus, steam inhalation without benzoin is effective. The patient should be encouraged to inhale the steam deep into the bronchial tubes and then requested to cough and raise the mucus. In the case of large goiters where a drain has been used, there may be considerable drainage, requiring a change of dressings some hours after surgery in order to spare the patient the discomfort of a soggy dressing. As a rule, patients are more comfortable with the head of the bed elevated.

The *dressing* should be applied so as to give a neat appearance and yet exert firm compression in order to prevent accumulation of serum in a dead space. The author prefers mechanic's waste or sponges beneath a goiter pad to the use of flats. The dressing should be held in place by 1-inch adhesive crisscrossed in front and back with a minimum touching the skin.

Early ambulation is important to prevent complications such as embolisms and atelectasis. Patients are encouraged to be out of bed the day of operation and to drink liquids freely.

TOXIC ADENOMATOUS GOITER

Since neither Lugol's solution nor antithyroid drugs are effective postoperatively, they are not used. As these patients are in the older-age group, sedatives are contraindicated. Most of them have been sufficiently sedated before operation so that they will be drowsy during the day.

EXOPHTHALMIC GOITER

The postoperative care of these patients is most important. The author has not seen a postoperative crisis in the past 15 years and believes that none should occur if the patient is properly treated.

Lugol's solution is the crux of the matter. For the average case, 4 doses of 10 drops each are given the first hour following surgery. During the next 24 hours, 10 to 15 more doses of 10 drops each are given when the patient is awake. It should be used in a small amount of liquid, usually a few ounces; a large volume may cause the patient to vomit.

If *emesis* occurs, the patient should be given Lugol's solution, a drop to a teaspoonful of ice chips or water. If he fails to retain that, 50 drops may be given in a pint of tap water by rectum, or it may be given subcutaneously. On no occasion has it been necessary to give sodium iodide intravenously. If all the above methods fail, the fluid may be given by a Levine tube attached to a metal container at the head of the bed.

Psychology is most important in the aftercare, and patients must be impressed with two things. They must take the Lugol's solution and keep it down, and they must keep calm and be quiet and relaxed. Relatives should be asked to stay out of the room, which should be quiet and dark.

In severe cases these factors are especially important, and in these patients as much as 20 doses of Lugol's solution may be given during the first 24 hours. During the second 24 hours, a dose of 10 drops may be given at hourly intervals if the patient is awake. On the third day the dosage may be cut to 3 drops a day and continued during the remainder of the hospital stay and as long as indicated. All patients are encouraged to be out of bed on the day of operation.

In this field of surgery it is very important for the surgeon to supervise the postoperative care. Patients have been known to leave the operating room in apparently excellent condition, only to go into a state of severe anoxia within the hour from hemorrhage or collapse of the trachea from other causes.

Hyperthyroid patients who appear to be well controlled at the completion of the operation may go into a state of severe thyrotoxicosis before the end of the day if they are not retaining their iodine.

While it should be the duty of a competent house staff to recognize these complications early, it is the major concern of the surgeon, if possible, to anticipate and prevent such possible disasters. The author endeavors to see all thyroid cases within an hour or two after surgery and again at the end of the day. If a toxic diffuse goiter patient is not retaining his or her iodine, steps must be taken at once to remedy the situation.

POSTOPERATIVE COMPLICATIONS AND SEQUELAE

The most important complications and sequelae in thyroid surgery may be summarized as follows:

IMMEDIATE COMPLICATIONS:
1. Hemorrhage
2. Injury to recurrent laryngeal nerve
3. Tracheal collapse
4. Air embolism

DELAYED COMPLICATIONS:
1. Hemorrhage
2. Hematoma
3. Tetany
4. Infection
5. Serum
6. Crises
7. Hypothyroidism
8. Hyperthyroidism
9. Exophthalmos
10. Tracheitis

IMMEDIATE COMPLICATIONS

Hemorrhage. Several causes, such as injury to the internal jugular vein, tearing of the median or lateral veins, tearing of the mediastinal veins, as in removal of an intrathoracic goiter, and injury to the superior and inferior thyroid arteries, may result in hemorrhage. Occasionally, bleeding from a large goiter itself may prove to be annoying and even serious if one or several vessels are injured at the same time. If sudden flooding of the field of operation with blood occurs, compress the respective lobe by compressing and displacing it medially, sponge the field dry and secure the bleeding vessel.

It is in operating for *recurrent* goiters that the jugular vein is most often injured, for it may be drawn up into the normal field of operation by scar tissue and be so adherent to the latter as to be overlooked.

The *lateral veins,* branches of the internal jugular, are the most frequent cause of hemorrhage in a thyroidectomy. Most often the hemorrhage results from too forcible elevation of the goiter or from attempting to lift it by stripping the capsule with finger dissection. To avoid this, the superior thyroid vessels of the lobe that is to be resected should first be clamped, divided and ligated. This permits the gland to be rotated on its axis because of severing the upper pole, and, in turn, this brings the lateral veins into view as the goiter is gradually rotated and elevated by either a claw retractor or an elevating clamp. Then the capsule should be carefully dissected from the gland with the scalpel, care being taken not to cut the veins, which may leave the gland at right angles. Alternating the handle of the knife and the blade, one can carefully dissect, clamp and ligate the vessels. It is not always necessary to take this step; frequently they may be clamped with the gland and later sutured separately.

Tearing of mediastinal veins has been the cause of fatalities in the performance of thyroidectomies. It is a difficult place to control bleeding, and prevention is preferable to treatment. Again, it usually results from too forcible and hurried elevation of the goiter from the thoracic cavity. One would do well to heed the words of Dr. Charles H. Mayo: "An old fox always cleans up his tracks as he goes."

Proceed from the upper pole downward, resecting the gland as it is delivered and completing the ligating and suturing as the goiter is slowly delivered. On one occasion the author was able to stop a vein bleeding deep in the mediastinum by locating it with a light (such as is manufactured by Cameron), picking it up with a long tissue forceps and coagulating it with the electrocautery. It was far too deep and inaccessible to ligate without resorting to thoracic surgery.

If 2 hemostats are placed above and 1 below before dividing the superior thyroid vessels, these should not retract and bleed from use of a defective clamp. The author does not ligate the inferior thyroid arteries but prefers to clamp the lower pole. However, the former is a method used by many surgeons, and one should use special care to avoid injury of the nerve and the parathyroid glands.

Injury to Recurrent Laryngeal Nerve. This is the most serious complication in a thyroidectomy, and every effort should be made to avoid this catastrophe. The Lahey group has preferred to expose this nerve first in order to minimize the danger of injuring it. In general, this is a good principle to follow in surgery, and yet even these excellent surgeons honestly report a definite percentage of nerve injuries. The author has not adopted this method, except on occasion when doing a radical operation for malignancy, but prefers to do an intracapsular operation which appears to have definite advantages.

If the nerve is to be exposed, the inferior thyroid artery must first be located behind the common carotid artery. This is done by retracting the common carotid and the internal jugular vein laterally; the vessel will be found in the tissue between these large vessels and the trachea and the esophagus. In most instances the inferior thyroid artery will appear at about the level of the midportion of the thyroid gland. It can also have various other locations, like the cystic artery.

In most instances the recurrent laryngeal nerve will pass beneath the inferior thyroid artery, but often it will pass over and above the artery. Thus, the nerve can be located according to its relation to the artery, and, if it passes above, it is in much greater danger of injury because, as the thyroid is elevated from its bed, the artery is also elevated and, along with it, the nerve. The field must be dry and the light sufficient in order to locate the nerve (Lahey).

If such an injury occurs, it may be recognized by an inspiratory stridor or dyspnea, and it may still be possible to correct the condition by removing a causative ligature or suture.

Tracheal Collapse. This is a rare complication, and yet the author has seen 5 cases, 2 of which occurred at the operating table. On one occasion, after the removal of a smaller right lobe, the trachea, which had been compressed for many years, suddenly buckled under the pressure of a huge left lobe. With regard for a point just emphasized, this intrathoracic lobe was quickly delivered, with relief of the compression. However, at the same time, the lateral vein was torn, though, fortunately, it was easily located and ligated.

Air Embolism. Another rare but usually fatal complication, which is a most dramatic tragedy, is air embolism. The author's case occurred 30 years ago after the operation was completed and the dressing applied. The patient was about to leave the operating room when she had a violent spell of nervous coughing. Suddenly, she became cyanotic, and at the same time a hissing sound occurred, as if air was escaping from a bicycle tire. In 10 seconds the patient was dead. Autopsy performed immediately showed that a ligature applied to a vein in the sternothyroid muscle had been loosened by the coughing and air had been aspirated. A fairly large number of cases of this sequel to neck surgery have been reported in the literature, and one should constantly be on the alert to prevent such a disaster.

DELAYED COMPLICATIONS

Hemorrhage. Following thyroidectomy, hemorrhage may occur a few minutes, a few hours or a few days after the patient leaves the operating room. The author has seen patients hemorrhage at all of these stages, and this probably has been the misfortune of most thyroid surgeons. Prompt recognition of and attention to hemorrhage is imperative, and all assistants, nurses and house staff members should be trained to recognize it. Do not procrastinate. The patient is often restless, the neck becomes convex instead of concave, and dyspnea and cyanosis follow. A few minutes lost may result in the loss of the patient.

Oxygen should always be available at once to patients who have undergone thyroidectomy. Elevating the head and bending it forward may give temporary relief.

If time permits, the patient should be returned to surgery at once, and, again, if time permits, a sterile "prep" should be done. However, the author has been forced to operate not only in the patient's room but in the elevator as well. In most instances, removal of the skin clips and the subcutaneous and muscle midline sutures will relieve the pressure on the trachea and allow the patient to breathe normally. Hemorrhage in itself is seldom a serious factor and usually can be controlled by pressure of flats. In most cases it results from some small vein in the capsule which was not secured. The next step is to shell out the clots carefully with moist warm gauze and the gloved finger, and with adequate light to seek the source of the bleeding. *Even more care of the vital structures must be exercised than at the original operation.* When bleeding has developed slowly after a day or two, finding the source is not a simple procedure.

Hemorrhage, either primary or delayed, is controlled by gently elevating the gland with the index finger and at the same time compressing it against the trachea. In thyroid surgery one should never permit himself or his assistant to grasp hurriedly for a bleeding vessel lest he damage the nerve or the parathyroids.

Hematoma. If a small oozing vessel is overlooked, especially beneath the skin flap, an annoying and disfiguring hematoma may result. A loosely applied dressing the first day or two after operation helps to further this sequela. While performing the operation, blunt forcible reflection of the skin flaps may lead to extensive ecchymosis of the tissues. Usually the clots may be easily expressed and recurrence prevented by a firmly applied dressing. Warm moist dressings after the third day will clear up the ecchymosis, but it may be well to apply Vaseline strips first to prevent possible blistering of the skin.

Tetany. This is an infrequent but serious complication resulting from injury to or removal of the parathyroid glands. If the patient complains of muscular stiffness followed by a sensation of numbness or tingling of the extremities or around the mouth, tetany should be suspected. Circumoral pallor may occur. Tapping the facial nerve may elicit a positive Chvostek's sign. Trousseau's sign of muscle spasm of the hand and the arm may be produced by applying a blood pressure cuff and raising the pressure. Carpopedal spasm of the hands and the feet and convulsions may follow.

Tetany may be controlled instantly by the intravenous injection of 10 cc. of a 10 per cent calcium chloride or calcium gluconate solution. In addition, large doses of calcium should be given orally. Chronic tetany is treated by vitamin D in doses of 50,000 to 300,000 units daily. A vitamin-A derivative, AT 10, may be used but only with great care and frequent checking of the blood calcium levels which may rise to dangerous heights.

Postoperative tetany must be controlled by these methods, since no permanently successful transplants of parathyroid glands have been performed.

Infection. Despite all precautions, infection occasionally may occur following thyroidectomy and may be persistent and resistant. Serum pockets are precursor factors and, when present, should be probed to prevent the development of infection. If infection occurs, the wound should be probed and irrigated every 3 hours with alternate solutions of saline, peroxide and sulfathiazole powder. Antibiotics may be of value.

Serum. A frequent complication of thyroidectomy is serum, especially following the removal of large adenomatous goiters and, in particular, those which are substernal or intrathoracic. These cases are usually drained for 24 to 48 hours, since serum is to be expected. Some surgeons feel that the use of silk decreases the amount of serum. It probably does, but when infection develops, there may be trouble for months. For this reason, the author feels that the use of the electrosurgical knife lessens the amount of serum by decreasing the amount of suture material. As previously mentioned, a firmly applied dressing, using mechanic's waste to obliterate the dead space, is the best safeguard.

Crises. These are seldom seen any more following thyroidectomy and will not occur if the patient has been properly prepared with Lugol's solution for exophthalmic goiters and with antithyroid drugs for toxic adenomatous goiters. A true crisis occurs only in the exophthalmic type and can be prevented and controlled with Lugol's solution unless the patient is iodine-fast.

Postoperative Hypothyroidism. This is not a serious sequela and can be readily controlled with desiccated thyroid therapy. All patients who have undergone thyroidectomy should have a basal metabolic rate determination a few days following surgery and again in 3 months.

Postoperative Hyperthyroidism. Hyperthyroid patients may require repeated basal metabolism tests until the metabolic level has become normal. No fixed rule can be set for the length of time needed or the dosage of Lugol's solution required in cases of exophthalmic goiter.

Exophthalmos. When persistent or progressing, exophthalmos may be due to either hypothyroidism or hyperthyroidism. The latter may mean that the operation was incomplete, that Lugol's solution was discontinued too soon or that the patient has overdone. When this occurs with hypothyroidism, a rare complication, it may be checked and corrected by thyroid therapy.

Tracheitis. The most frequent sequela of thyroiditis is tracheitis. It is best treated by the deep inhalation of plain steam.

The correction of errors made by other surgeons is not a relatively simple matter. If a bilateral paralysis of the recurrent laryngeal nerves has occurred, an immediate tracheotomy may be indicated to save life if the dyspnea is progressing. From there a different problem is presented, but there is a growing tendency to favor the relatively simple procedure of arytenoidectomy over the King operation.

Where thyroidectomy has failed to effect a cure in toxic diffuse goiter, and Lugol's solution and antithyroid drugs have likewise failed, the surgeon has resorted to either reoperation or I^{131}. A secondary operation complicated by much scar tissue is far more difficult than the original operation and calls for that much more care of the important vessels and nerves. The jugular vein in particular is apt to be drawn up into the operative field by scar tissue and so more easily traumatized.

Before attempting a secondary operation, it is most important to have a competent laryngologist ascertain the status of the recurrent laryngeal nerves. The chest should be x-rayed (anteroposterior and lateral views) to determine the condition of the trachea and the presence of possible overlooked intrathoracic masses.

SUMMARY

Thyroid surgery is a highly specialized branch of general surgery and should not be attempted by the occasional operator. Thyroidectomy is an operation requiring an experienced operative team as well as a competent anesthetist capable of caring for any possible emergency.

Before surgery is considered, the diagnosis must be determined accurately and proper preoperative therapy administered or a fatal postoperative crisis may occur, regardless of how perfect the surgical technic.

The basal metabolic rate can lead the inexperienced surgeon into pitfalls and errors. Not infrequently the rate can be falsely elevated by rapid breathing when hyperthyroidism is not present, and resection of a normal gland might be performed with resultant myxedema.

On the other hand, a relatively low basal metabolic rate in an advanced case of toxic nodular goiter is of relatively little significance. Such patients are often poor surgical risks, regardless of the rate, unless properly prepared by antithyroid drugs.

Remember, too, that a patient with toxic diffuse goiter who is iodine-fast is a dangerous surgical risk and may go into a fatal postoperative crisis unless first given a resting period with an antithyroid drug.

It is well to remember that the small nodular goiter is relatively more dangerous than the large one. It is more apt to be toxic and also more apt to be malignant.

A clinically solitary adenoma is much more likely to be malignant than the multiple type, especially if occurring in the male, and therefore should be removed as soon as possible.

The so-called lateral aberrant thyroids are actually malignant metastases from the adjacent lobe and, as such, should be removed and a total lobectomy performed at the site of the primary lesion.

A biopsy should be obtained even in advanced malignancies. While most malignant thyroids are radioresistant, some show remarkable improvement under therapy.

The most important errors made in thyroid surgery may be summarized as follows: (1) injury to the laryngeal nerves and the parathyroid glands (to be avoided by adequate knowledge of the anatomy and careful hemostasis, with adequate exposure and careful dissection); (2) inadequate removal of tissue in toxic diffuse goiter; (3) overlooking of substernal or intrathoracic nodular masses; and (4) inadequate or improper preoperative and postoperative care.

By following the methods herein outlined, the author feels that all of these errors may be prevented, provided that the surgeon is adequately prepared.

MAX CUTLER, M.D.

10 The Breast

Since my subject is not surgery of the breast, but rather the *errors* which are prone to occur in the performance of such surgery and the *safeguards* which have been devised to avoid them, discussion of other aspects of mammary affections, such as "chronic mastitis," will be omitted.

CYSTIC DISEASE OF THE BREAST

Valpeau (1838), Sir Astley Cooper (1845) and Sir Benjamin Brodie (1846) were the first to describe "benign cystic disease" of the breasts. In 1883, Reclus gave this condition the name of *maladie kystique des mamelles* and stressed the frequency and multiplicity of the cysts and their generalized distribution. The term *Reclus' disease* has been used to designate this state.

For some unexplained reason, the epithelium of the mammary ducts and acini may undergo a process of active hyperplasia of a specific type. The newly formed epithelial cells which result from hyperplasia die and desquamate. This special type of epithelial change has been named *desquamative hyperplasia,* in contrast with another type of epithelial change which has been called *epithelial neoplasia,* or true tumor formation (Cheatle). The desquamative type of epithelial hyperplasia results in the formation of *cysts*; the neoplastic type results in the formation of papilloma and carcinoma.

As a result of this peculiar active epithelial hyperplasia, one or both breasts become the seat of cysts which vary in size from microscopic dimensions to cysts measuring 6 to 8 cm. in diameter and occupying a large part of the mammary gland. It should be borne in mind that the breast may be the early seat of extensive multiple cysts which may be detected only by microscopic examination.

Two *complications* arise as a result of cyst formation: stagnation and tumor formation.

Microscopic evidence indicates that when cancer develops in a cystic area it first passes through the *benign* papillomatous stage. The neoplastic change, as a rule, affects the small cysts rather than the larger ones. The question of the relationship between cystic disease of the breast and carcinoma is obviously a very important one. Unfortunately, the problem is highly controversial. The present author believes that a certain proportion of mammary carcinomas can be traced directly to cystic disease.

ERROR IN MANAGING SINGLE CYST

A common error in the treatment of an apparently single cyst is failure to make a sufficiently wide excision of the mammary tissue which contains it and failure to exercise every precaution against dissemination. As a safeguard, the operator should always be prepared to proceed with the radical operation in the event that the lesion proves to be malignant. After the specimen is removed it should be subjected immediately to careful inspection and palpation, and any suspicious portions should be studied by means of frozen sections under the microscope. If no cancer is discovered the wound may be sutured. In the event that cancer is found in the cyst wall or elsewhere in the tissue, treatment for carcinoma should be instituted at once.

ERRORS IN MANAGING MULTIPLE CYSTS

When the breast is filled with multiple cysts it sometimes becomes necessary to perform a simple mastectomy, leaving intact the pectoral fascia, the muscles and the axillary glands. Efforts to conserve part of the breast frequently make it necessary to perform further operations for the removal of other cysts. The removed mammary tissue must be carefully examined for suspicious areas, including microscopic study of frozen sections as an additional safeguard. In the absence of indications of cancer, the wound is closed. A still further safeguard is study of paraffin sections of the breast to confirm the negative diagnosis.

Never make the mistake of disregarding *a localized nodularity*. It can be a sign of great gravity. As a rule, it is far more serious than one or more solitary cysts, for a localized nodularity usually represents a group of small cysts in which the epithelium may have passed into the more menacing precancerous or even cancerous stage.

BILATERAL MULTIPLE CYSTS

A difficult problem presents itself when one or both breasts of a young woman contain multiple cysts. The question then arises: To what extent is a surgeon justified in performing unilateral or even bilateral mastectomy?

In Favor of a Conservative Procedure. Cysts large enough to be palpable clinically are—with rare exceptions—benign acinous cysts. The chances of carcinoma are no greater than in a breast where no cysts are palpable clinically.

In Favor of Surgical Interference. Near a large cyst there are likely to be small cysts, visible only under the microscope, which may be either *precancerous* or already the site of microscopic cancer.

Unfortunately, we have no means of determining these facts clinically. Moreover, as there is no way we can predict the future course of epithelial cells in the precancerous state, the final decision must be reached individually in every instance. A strong family history of cancer of the breast influences the author in favor of mastectomy *in older patients*. In the absence of such a positive history, the patient's own attitude should be considered. One patient may refuse to take the smallest chance of carcinoma and insist on removal of the breast; another may prefer to take a calculated risk; still another will refuse mammectomy under any circumstances. Fortunately, the condition is uncommon in very young women. Until we have further knowledge which will permit us to interpret the conditions that we find, we must continue to evaluate each case on its own merits and in the light of our present limited understanding of the problem. *In the absence of proved cancer, mastectomy should be avoided in younger women.*

ERRORS AND SAFEGUARDS

With respect to errors and safeguards in cystic disease of the breast, the following is suggested. A common error is to *enucleate* a cyst. The fallacy of this procedure is that the large, clinically palpable cyst, which is the most innocuous, is removed and the smaller cysts, which are by far the more dangerous, are left. To avoid this pitfall one should attempt to include enough surrounding breast tissue to extirpate any microscopic cysts which otherwise might remain as a threat of later development of cancer. In occasional cystic breasts the disease is limited to 1 or 2 ducts and their branches and actually may be eradicated by adequate excision. Unfortunately, in the majority of cases the disease will be found to be more widespread.

Here the surgeon will be faced with a difficult decision. He has 3 choices: (1) to be content with the limited excision and look upon the operative procedure as an adequate substitute for biopsy and exploration; (2) to extend the surgical procedure centimeter by centimeter in an effort to *get around the lesion*; and (3) to perform a simple mastectomy, assuming that the patient's permission for removal of the breast is forthcoming.

Psychological Aspects. It is a matter of delicate judgment to decide which of these 3 courses the surgeon should choose, always keeping in mind that the loss of the breast in a young woman is usually a far more serious matter than is generally realized. The small chances of cancer existing or developing later must be balanced against the emotional trauma in any given case. If the surgeon has taken time to explore the psychological side of the question adequately, such evaluation should not be too difficult.

How to avoid more than a reasonable "calculated risk" and at the same time to save a young woman from a distressing mutilation requires good judgment and delicate tact—the exercise of the true Art of Medicine!

SURGERY OF MAMMARY PAPILLOMATA

Benign papillomas are soft yellowish tumors which vary in size and consistency. They may be so small and delicate that their discovery is difficult, requiring very careful dissection of the duct, or they may grow into large round solid tumors which develop into *duct carcinoma*. Frequently, hemorrhage into the duct obliterates all signs of the tumors, so they will not be discovered until the tissue is examined microscopically. Studies of whole sections of breasts have disclosed that papillomas exist in many instances where there had not been any previous suspicion of their presence. These studies have also demonstrated that papillomas are more often multiple than was hitherto supposed. Papillomas are sometimes solitary, originating in a duct in the nipple, in the ampulla or in one of its main-duct branches. Multiple papillomata commonly affect only one breast, though they may be bilateral (Fig. 89). The number of such tumors is sometimes very great; the entire duct system of the breast may be riddled with these lesions. Again, papilloma may be entirely limited to a single duct and its branches.

DIAGNOSIS

Serous or serohemorrhagic discharge from the nipple is the classic clinical sign of duct papilloma. This discharge is spontaneous and intermittent. However, two facts must be borne in mind. Papillomata may exist without causing a discharge from the nipple, and serohemorrhagic exudate may result from other causes, i.e., trauma or duct carcinoma. In most instances a hemorrhagic discharge from the nipple is due to a single duct papilloma or, more commonly, to multiple duct papillomata. The discharge of blood may cease spontaneously for several months or years and then reappear. Gentle pressure over the areola may help to locate the source of bleeding. Transillumination generally permits localization and helps to determine the extent and the distribution of the lesions, unless they are microscopic (Fig. 90). We have observed many breasts in which transillumination demonstrated papilloma, without ever having detected any discharge from the nipple. The chance of error is evident. So, as a safeguard, both breasts should always be transilluminated. In the examples cited, it is probable that these were dormant papillomata which had not yet developed this sign. Opacities may

sometimes be found in the absence of all clinical signs. Pain may occur in the presence of multiple lesions, but a single papilloma is rarely painful.

Bloody discharge from the nipple may occur in the absence of a palpable tumor. In recent

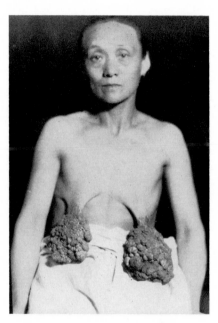

Fig. 89. Bilateral papilloma of nipples. (Cheatle and Cutler: Tumours of the Breast, London, Arnold)

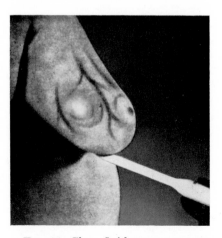

Fig. 90. Clear fluid cyst as seen on transillumination. (Cheatle and Cutler: Tumours of the Breast, London, Arnold)

years, patients have come under clinical observation very soon after such a discharge developed, and when they were first examined, a palpable tumor was rarely discovered. When a tumor is found it may be either a papilloma or a carcinoma of the duct. Unless a carcinoma is sufficiently developed to give unmistakable clinical signs, the differential diagnosis can be established only after removal of the lesion and its gross and microscopic examination.

Prognosis

The prognosis of papilloma of the breast is essentially similar to that of papilloma in other organs, such as the urinary bladder or the colon. Some remain benign for many years, growing to large proportions; others undergo malignant transformation in their early stages. There is increasing evidence that so much time may be required for the supervention of carcinoma upon the papillomatous state that the patient does not live long enough to permit this event to occur. Since there is no clinical method of determining whether or not the malignant transformation has already taken place, nor to predict its time of appearance, *all papillomata of the breast must be regarded as being potentially malignant.*

Treatment

The only safe treatment of a breast papilloma is to regard the whole mammary gland with suspicion regarding its present and future condition. If a tumor is large and occupies the main portion of the breast, simple mastectomy is often indicated. When the tumor is small and its nature is in doubt, it should be excised and examined at operation, both grossly and microscopically (frozen section). If carcinoma is discovered, appropriate treatment must be instituted at once.

On the other hand, if both gross and microscopic study of the excised portion of the breast give no positive evidence of carcinoma, the surgeon must evaluate the indications for a simple mastectomy. No general rule can be set down; each case must be judged on its own merits. In making this decision, the following factors must be considered: (1) whether or not other members of the patient's family have

suffered from breast cancer; (2) the patient's age; (3) the possibility of there being other papillomata in the breast, as indicated by the extent of the disease in the excised specimen, as well as the presence or absence of cysts or papillomata in the lines of incision; and (4) the microscopic appearance of the epithelial cells as regards their degree of anaplasia. Thus the decision is a matter of clinical judgment and so must be highly individualized.

TREATMENT OF CANCER OF THE BREAST

Since surgery continues to occupy a prominent place in the treatment of mammary cancer, the first decision to be made will relate to the question of operability. Generally accepted contraindications are: (1) fixation of the mass to the ribs or the sternum; (2) involvement of the supraclavicular lymph nodes; (3) fixation of axillary lymph nodes; (4) signs of acute fulminating type of disease; (5) carcinoma *en cuirasse*; (6) distant metastasis; and (7) constitutional contraindications to surgery.

In the present state of our knowledge, we recommend and practice the radical surgical operation for presumably operable mammary cancer. In many circumstances we combine irradiation therapy with the surgical operation, and under exceptional conditions we *substitute* irradiation for surgical removal.

Exploratory Operation and Biopsy

As women consult their physicians earlier, the proportion of clinically doubtful tumors increases, and the indications for *exploratory operation* grow more frequent in proportion. Since many localized nodularities are benign, the radical procedure in clinically doubtful lesions must be preceded by exploration and biopsy. Naturally, the proportion of clinically doubtful cases varies to some degree with the experience of the examiner. The chief danger lies in not being sufficiently gentle in handling the tissues, thereby favoring dissemination.

Technic of Exploratory Operation. In planning the skin incision, the lesion should occupy the center of the tissue area to be removed. Do not make the error of regarding the *cosmetic effect* as of greater importance than *the patient's safety.*

In a local procedure the incision should be elliptic with the lesion in its center, extending from the areola to the periphery of the breast. A second, curved incision is then made along the periphery. Thereafter, radial incisions are made through the breast tissues down to the pectoralis fascia, permitting the specimen to be removed en bloc. The specimen is then examined by gross inspection and microscopic study of the frozen sections. In most instances an experienced surgical pathologist is able to establish the diagnosis from gross inspection of the lesion alone. Carcinoma has a characteristic hardness and "grates" on incision, the cut surface is flat or concave, the edges are ill-defined, puckering the surrounding tissues, the cut surface is opaque, characteristically "chalky" points and streaks are usually visible, and the margin is abrupt and hard. No other growth simulates this consistency. A

frozen section should always be made as a safeguard in confirming the diagnosis made from the gross specimen. *If doubt still remains, microscopic evidence should be awaited before removing the breast.*

Interpretation of Frozen Sections. Serious errors may be made if the surgeon does not keep constantly in mind the fact that *the specimen of tissue selected for study may not represent the main lesion.* In many instances the examination of the frozen section at once establishes the diagnosis. In another group, the microscopic features are such as to create considerable doubt. Under these circumstances, the surgeon must accept the full responsibility for the procedure adopted. Unless all other evidence overwhelmingly favors the diagnosis of cancer, the only safe course to adopt is to withhold the radical procedure until there is opportunity to study prepared paraffin sections carefully.

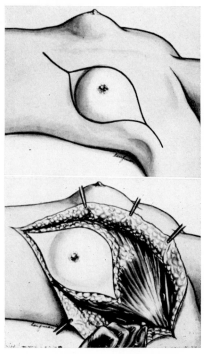

Fig. 91. (*Top*) Skin incision for radical mastectomy. (*Bottom*) Insertion of pectoralis major exposed and ready to be severed.

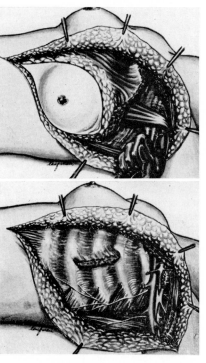

Fig. 92. (*Top*) Pectoralis minor exposed and ready to be severed. (*Bottom*) Operative site after radical mastectomy. Note preservation of long thoracic and subcapsular nerves.

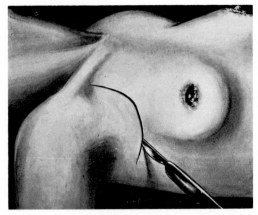

FIG. 93. Transverse curved axillary incision, Greenough technic. Incision extends from midpoint of clavicle to posterior axillary fold. (Taylor and Daland: Surg., Gynec. & Obst. 65:807)

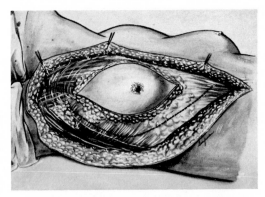

FIG. 95. Wide undermining of flaps in all directions. Dotted line indicates lateral extent of incision into fascia, Greenough technic. (Taylor and Daland: Surg., Gynec. & Obst. 65:807)

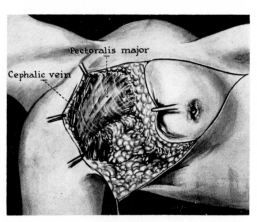

FIG. 94. Exposure of insertion of pectoralis major muscle and axilla, Greenough technic. (Taylor and Daland: Surg., Gynec. & Obst. 65:807)

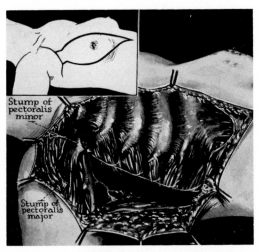

FIG. 96. Both pectoral muscles divided; muscles, fascia and axillary contents removed. (*Inset*) Outline of Greenough skin incision. (Taylor and Daland: Surg., Gynec. & Obst. 65:807)

TECHNIC OF RADICAL OPERATION

The incision should be made so that the tumor occupies the center of the operative field, regardless of where it may be located. The amount of skin which must be removed is an important consideration. Experience clearly indicates the necessity of wide removal of skin. The dominating and guiding principle must be the safety of the patient, not the difficulty of closing the incision. This conception is well illustrated by Halsted's suggestion that the closure of the operative wound be left to the assistant. Undoubtedly this is an excellent safeguard against the temptation to restrict this portion of the operative procedure.

The elliptic skin incision is extended downward far enough to permit removal of the fat and the fascia in the costoxiphoid angle. It is extended upward along the inner and upper aspects of the arm along the convex edge of the pectoralis major muscle, but only far enough down the arm to permit a separation of the sternal fibers of the pectoralis major from the bicipital groove (Fig. 91). This incision must be placed high enough to avoid the axilla, with the error of producing a cicatrix in that region.

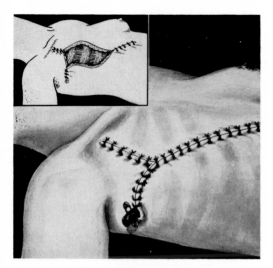

FIG. 97. Complete closure of Greenough incision. (*Inset*) Greenough incision partly closed. (Taylor and Daland:
Surg., Gynec. & Obst. 65:807)

Undercutting the flaps is the next step. The
skin flaps should be as thin as compatible
with their safety, while the undermining must
be carried out widely in all directions so as to
mobilize the flaps for subsequent closure. The
upper flap should be undercut beyond the
midline, the lower flap beyond the outer border of the axilla. The sternal portion of the
pectoralis major muscle is divided at its insertion in the bicipital groove, its upper border
parallel with the clavicle. By gently placing
the fingers under the muscle, it is raised and
its sternal attachments cut. This procedure
exposes the ribs and the pectoralis minor
muscle (Fig. 92). Fat and fascia are dissected
away from the upper portion of the rectus
abdominus and the serratus magnus muscles.
The parts are wrapped in warm towels and
the surgeon's attention directed to the axilla.

In order to gain adequate exposure of the
axilla, the pectoralis minor is excised completely, the axillary contents being removed
gently and completely in a downward and outward direction. The subscapular nerve and the
long thoracic nerve (nerve of Bell) are saved.
The incision is closed either by primary suture
completely, or is only partly closed, the remainder of the wound being grafted by the
Thiersch method, according to indications. A
drain is placed in the axilla through a stab
wound.

ERRORS AND SAFEGUARDS WHEN USING THE GREENOUGH INCISION

Taylor and Daland* have described the
Greenough technic of radical mastectomy as
follows (Figs. 93, 94 and 95).

The incision about the breast has the shape of
an arrowhead. The transverse axillary incision
begins at the lower border of the clavicle near
its midpoint, courses downward and outward,
crosses the free border of the pectoralis major,
and continues to the latissimus border at the level
of the lower end of the scapula. The pectoralis
major muscle is exposed by raising the axillary
skin flap. The cephalic vein is identified but
spared. The remainder of the dissection of the
breast muscles and axillary contents is performed
as in the Halsted operation, the skin incision being
made as seen in Fig. 96. The wound is sutured
and drained as indicated in Fig. 97.

An important error in doing radical mas-
tectomies is *inadequate skin removal,* which
leads to local recurrences. Judgment as to the
amount of skin to be removed is based on
the extent of the lesion, but equally important,
if not more so, is *adequate removal of the subcutaneous fat.* This means making the skin
flaps as thin as possible without causing
necrosis, while extending the dissection widely
in all directions, as indicated in the figure.

Avoid the error of placing the upper part
of the incision too low. It must be high enough
on the chest wall to avoid the scar crossing the
axilla and bending the arm. As in all surgical
procedures, *the gentle handling of tissues is
of paramount importance.* Early motion of the
arm must be encouraged to ensure prompt
normal function. Careful hemostasis is especially important to facilitate healing of the
extensive incision. If these principles are followed, the incidence of postoperative edema
will be reduced to a minimum. In the author's
experience, the small group of those patients
who have developed more than a slight edema
of the arm have been unusually obese women.
It should be borne in mind that, more often
than is generally recognized, this complication
represents uncontrolled disease located along
the axillary vein and the lymphatics rather
than a complication of the surgical procedure.

* Taylor, Grantley W., and Daland, Ernest M.:
The Greenough technic of radical mastectomy, Surg.,
Gynec. & Obst. 65:807-811, 1937.

EDWARD L. COMPERE, M.D.

11 Orthopedic Surgery

The orthopedic and fracture surgeon has been blamed more frequently than any other for bad or unsatisfactory end-results of treatment. The orthopedic surgeon is engaged in the prevention of or the correction of deformities or defects of the spine and the extremities which have resulted or may result from injury or disease. If the end-result of treatment shows persisting deformity, or the patient is just as disabled as he was before the treatment was undertaken, the surgeon is likely to be held responsible. For this reason, the orthopedic surgeon or any physician dealing with the conditions resulting from trauma to the spine and the extremities must be exceptionally alert to avoid errors in the treatment of his patient. Any error may result in deformity or a crippling defect. He must take every safeguard which will protect his patients against any injury that can be attributed to the treatment itself.

GENERAL PRINCIPLES OF BONE AND JOINT SURGERY

Successful surgery on the spine or the extremities frequently requires a long period of postoperative rehabilitation. Oftentimes the surgical procedure itself is but a small part of the total treatment, and several factors must be evaluated when contemplating most orthopedic operations. The age of the patient, his occupation, his mental and economic status, his physical condition and life expectancy all may significantly influence the choice of operation. Extensive long-term reconstructive surgery of an extremity might be properly indicated for one individual, whereas in another patient with a similar local problem but under greatly altered circumstances, amputation would be the wiser choice. Proper application of the factors operating in each case calls for vision and foresight. The overall problem must be constantly reviewed, for errors in surgical judgment often result from

failure to consider the patient "as a whole" before taking up the local definitive problem.

SKELETAL IMMOBILIZATION

Similarly, the *psychological and physiologic* aspects of skeletal immobilization must be kept in mind. It is a common practice to require immobilization of a part of an extremity, an entire extremity or of the body and one or more extremities following, or in conjunction with, orthopedic procedures. The need for diversion, occupational therapy and physiotherapy is very great under such circumstances. Not only do many disturbances in physiology and metabolism result from prolonged immobilization or repeated surgical procedures, but also the patient's emotional stability may be severely tested. The success or failure of some orthopedic operations, as well as other nonsurgical treatment, may be determined in part by the mental adjustments of the patient. When prolonged or extensive immobilization is anticipated, due regard must be given, both preoperatively and postoperatively, to the patient's emotional make-up, his physical status and his usual occupation.

GOALS OF ORTHOPEDIC SURGERY

Most orthopedic procedures are designed to relieve pain, improve function, prevent deformity and occasionally to provide cosmetic improvement. At all times one must bear in mind the goal to be achieved and weigh it properly in each case. To provide cosmetic improvement at the expense of function, to produce a greater range of joint motion with a resultant painful or unstable joint or to jeopardize union of a fracture in a long bone in an attempt to prevent stiffness of adjacent joints are errors to avoid.

SURGICAL APPROACH

For any operation on the extremities, a thorough knowledge of surgical approaches is essential. Many times the task of gaining adequate exposure is the largest and most technical part of the operation. *Errors in approach may prolong surgery,* make it technically very difficult or require unnecessary incisions. In planning the surgical approach, the surgeon should have a well-conceived purpose in mind, and he must give due regard not only to the immediate problem but should also anticipate possible or probable subsequent operations on the same extremity. The proper placing of skin incisions requires consideration not only of the desired approach, with a thorough understanding of the procedure intended, but also the evaluation of the blood supply of the extremity, the vitality of the skin and the presence of pre-existing scars. "Exploratory incisions" are rarely used except for the purpose of opening major joints. It is a mistake to employ multiple or parallel incisions in a small area. *If subsequent procedures are performed in the same or a closely adjacent location, the scar of the earlier procedure should be used for the approach with the incision placed accurately in the old scar, or when the skin relaxation is adequate the old scar should be excised.*

In dealing with the young, growing skeleton of children, the problems differ from those encountered in adults. Generally speaking, a more conservative approach must be cultivated, particularly in the treatment of fractures. Children possess greater powers of repair, the bones heal more rapidly, and physiologic remodeling of the injured bones is usual in the growing skeleton. The potential growth of the various bones must be considered at different age groups. On the other hand, these same factors may work against the surgeon. Some affections of the skeleton may become worse with growth if not treated, making it necessary to adopt a more radical approach. Congenital deformities frequently tend to become more severe and more difficult to correct if allowed to persist untreated. Also, *surgical or other trauma to the epiphyseal cartilages may result in premature epiphyseal closure* which, if asymmetric, may produce unsightly deformities.

Knowledge of Physiology of Bone

A fundamental knowledge of the physiology of bone, its mechanism of healing and its re-

sponsiveness to noxious and other stimuli should be a part of the armamentarium of any surgeon handling orthopedic conditions. These factors must guide the surgeon in making his decision and help him to recognize the dangers and pitfalls of surgical procedures which are either too radical or too conservative.

Precautions

A surgeon should not proceed to perform an open bone operation immediately after he has finished operating on another patient who has an infection. He should also avoid having assistants who have acute colds or suffer from chronic coughs.

Nurses should be trained to *handle all of the instruments and equipment with sterile forceps.* The circulating nurse should be discouraged from using a forceps which is in common use, although such forceps is kept immersed in a bottle with antiseptic solution. Such forceps, when used on other cases, should first be autoclaved before use in a bone operation.

Assistants should be taught *how to sponge* by holding the sponges with forceps and discarding the sponges after each one has been used once.

The proper draping of the patient is considered very important by many orthopedic surgeons; double layers of drapes are safest.

Lost Sponges. The orthopedic surgeon should always request a sponge count before and after operating on the spine, the hip, the shaft of the femur or the shoulder. When the operative wound is large, deep and vascular, only large lap sponges with attached tape and metal ring should be used. Smaller sponges should contain an x-ray-opaque marker. If the sponge count shows a sponge to be missing, a roentgenogram of the operative field should be taken before starting to close the wound. If a sponge marker is shown on the film, the sponge must be located before closing. Damages have been collected from many surgeons because a sponge was left in the wound.

DANGERS AND SAFEGUARDS OF IMMOBILIZATION AND FUNDA- MENTALS OF ITS USE

Immobilization of a part may be secured by traction, external fixation or internal fixation. Each has inherent dangers and pitfalls and each has its proper indication. Each requires knowledge and care if it is to be used safely and successfully. Most disconcerting complications of well-executed orthopedic surgical procedures can arise from errors in the use of immobilization. Any surgeon employing these methods should have a sound knowledge of the potential hazards.

TRACTION

Traction on an extremity may be exerted by means of the skin (skin traction) or through metal fixation to a bone (skeletal traction). Usually skin traction is employed in cases where a small amount of weight is to be employed over a short period of time, and skeletal traction is used when a greater weight is contemplated over a prolonged period of time. In choosing the type of traction, it is necessary to anticipate how much weight will be required and for how long. It is a mistake to apply skin traction as the definitive treatment of a fracture of the femoral shaft in an adult; likewise, it is not wise to utilize skeletal traction for the short period of traction usually employed in the preoperative and postoperative treatment of fractures which are subject to internal fixation.

Skin Traction. Though skin traction may be applied in several different ways, the particular method employed is not so important as are the principles of its use. *When using any form of skin traction, daily critical observation is necessary to prevent complications.* If adequate supervision cannot be had, skin traction should not be utilized. The circulation of the toes, the integrity of the peripheral nerves and the skin over the various bony prominences should be inspected carefully. It is well to unwrap the circular bandages at periodic intervals to examine the underlying skin and then to reapply the circular dressings smoothly and effectively.

In the application of skin traction, the bony prominences (specifically the malleoli, the heel and the dorsum of the foot) should be protected carefully by several layers of sheet wadding or its equivalent. Although the traction adhesive straps must never be placed directly over the head of the fibula, this bony prominence and the peroneal nerve behind it must be protected by padding. The possibility of pressure necrosis of the skin and peroneal nerve palsy are very real and may be produced by a tight elastic circular bandage as well as by traction straps. *The danger of peroneal nerve paralysis* is particularly great when a sling is used under the knee, as with Russell's traction. Under no circumstances should the sling exert pressure back of the fibular head. The sling should be well-padded and should be employed only when frequent, experienced supervision can be exercised.

The *"don'ts"* of skin traction include, besides those described above, the following. *Do not* extend the traction above or proximal to the area treated. Traction applied above the fracture dissipates that applied below it. *Do not* employ skin traction on extremities having manifest evidence of peripheral vascular disease. *Do not* apply skin traction over blisters, abrasions or areas of dermatitis. *Do not* utilize skin traction when the weight required exceeds 20 pounds or when marked overriding of fragments exists. *Do not* use Bryant's overhead skin traction in children more than 4 years of age or in fat, heavy infants more than 18 months old. Circulatory embarrassment to the point of ischemic necrosis and gangrene of the leg have resulted when this warning was ignored.

Skeletal Traction. Skeletal traction utilizes pins, wires, screws or tongs which are inserted through or into a bone (Fig. 98). Obviously, the insertion of these devices must be done under strict asepsis, using a surgically sterile field and instruments. Though desirable, it is not necessary that these procedures be done in the operating room if they can be performed more expeditiously at the bedside. All of the precautions of open surgery must be observed so as to prevent contamination, infection and possible osteomyelitis. The "no-touch" technic is advisable. Skeletal-traction devices must not be employed in any location where doubt exists concerning the cleanliness of the local skin. Small infected areas may be sealed off with collodion prior to surgical cleansing of the area, but active adjacent bone infection with surface drainage obviously contraindicates the *local* use of skeletal traction. When a prolonged period of traction is anticipated, *threaded* Kirschner wires or Steinmann pins should be used. These have less tendency to loosen or migrate, and the likelihood of pintrack infection is lessened. Since there is a direct communication between the bone and the exterior, a sterile dressing should be placed over the projecting internal fixation, and it must be kept scrupulously clean.

The skeletal fixation should have a firm purchase on the bone. In long bones the transfixation must engage both cortices to eliminate the possibility of migration or tearing out of the pin or wire, with resultant injury to soft tissues. When skeletal traction is applied to the skull, only the outer cortex should be pierced. Because of pressure absorption of bone, daily tightening of the tong fixation is necessary. Care must be exercised not to pierce the inner table of the skull. To do this could result in penetration of the superior longitudinal venous sinus, with intracranial hemorrhage or perforation of the meninges and danger of meningitis.

In those cases where moderate to heavy traction is required, countertraction must be employed. For the lower extremity a Thomas

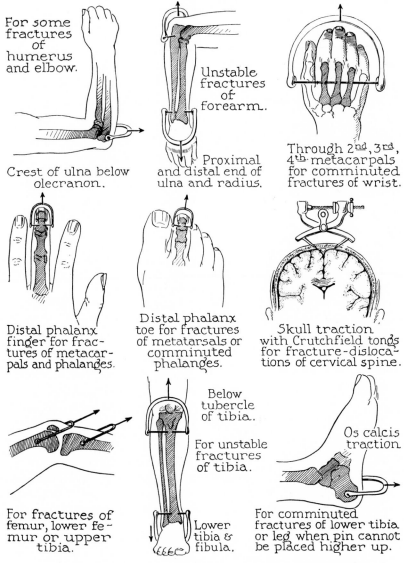

For some fractures of humerus and elbow.

Crest of ulna below olecranon.

Unstable fractures of forearm.

Proximal and distal end of ulna and radius.

Through 2ⁿᵈ, 3ʳᵈ, 4ᵗʰ metacarpals for comminuted fractures of wrist.

Distal phalanx finger for fractures of metacarpals and phalanges.

Distal phalanx toe for fractures of metatarsals or comminuted phalanges.

Skull traction with Crutchfield tongs for fracture-dislocations of cervical spine.

For fractures of femur, lower femur or upper tibia.

Below tubercle of tibia.

For unstable fractures of tibia.

Lower tibia & fibula.

Os calcis traction.

For comminuted fractures of lower tibia or leg when pin cannot be placed higher up.

FIG. 98. Skeletal traction. (Compere and Banks: Pictorial Handbook of Fracture Treatment, Chicago, Year Book Pub.)

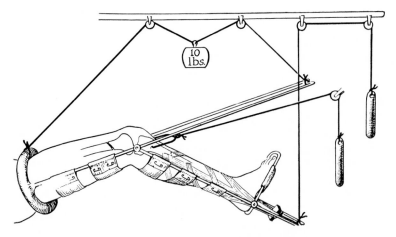

Fig. 99. Balanced traction in a Thomas splint. The Pierson attachment permits motion of the knee while the fracture is healing. (Compere and Banks: Pictorial Handbook of Fracture Treatment, Chicago, Year Book Pub.)

splint is commonly used, and the counter-traction rope is attached to the ring (Fig. 99). This may result in pressure from the ring against the ischium, the pubis or the greater trochanter. To prevent injury to the overlying soft tissues, the patient must be examined frequently and the pressure areas protected.

In some special cases, a form of traction can be employed which incorporates the principles of both skeletal-pin fixation and plaster-of-Paris external immobilization. This is called the "well-leg traction." In this procedure, skeletal traction on the affected leg is exerted against the opposite normal extremity. The inherent dangers of both skeletal traction and external plaster-of-Paris fixation are manifest in these cases. The articular surface of the knee of the well leg can be damaged by the prolonged compression of the joint surfaces against each other.

EXTERNAL FIXATION

This is achieved principally by means of plaster-of-Paris casts, but in its broad sense it includes adhesive strapping. Improperly applied plaster casts can do great injury to tissues compressed by them. When applied over a fresh injury or postoperatively, a constrictive cast can so interfere with circulation in an extremity that Volkmann's contracture or gangrene will result. There is no substitute for common sense and wisdom in exercising the principles of plaster-of-Paris technics. Plaster casts and splints serve a variety of purposes, and individualization is necessary in each case. Unpadded skintight casts serve no

useful purpose. The dangers which attend their use far exceed any theoretical advantage which they possess. A cast applied to immobilize a fresh injury of an extremity should be padded carefully. All bony prominences must be adequately protected, preferably with multiple layers of sheet wadding. The plaster bandage should be rolled smoothly around the extremity and molded carefully about the padded bone prominences. The poorly padded cast or the cast which is permitted to set with creases or indentations in it may produce pressure necroses over the head of the fibula, the ankle malleoli, the back of the heel, the olecranon or any other bony prominence. Cast pressure may produce ulnar or external peroneal nerve paralysis.

Pressure Necroses. Tight bandages or improperly applied plaster casts may produce localized necrosis of tissue or gangrene of a portion of an extremity. These complications can be avoided by the experienced and careful surgeon. The danger zones which require special padding when applying plaster casts are demonstrated in Figure 100. The best padding consists of 10 to 12 layers of sheet wadding. Felt is not as soft, and some felt is so hard that it causes rather than prevents pressure sores. Most sponge rubber is too soft and does not protect bony prominences adequately.

Extensive bone and soft-tissue surgery will be followed by extensive swelling of the adjacent soft tissues. A tight cast with minimal padding should not be applied in these cases. If the toes or the finger tips are swollen or blue, the leg or arm cast must be split from end to end and the cast spread open suffi-

FIG. 100. Areas which should be carefully protected by felt, rubber or cotton pads before incorporating them in a plaster cast. (Compere and Banks: Pictorial Handbook of Fracture Treatment, Chicago, Year Book Pub.)

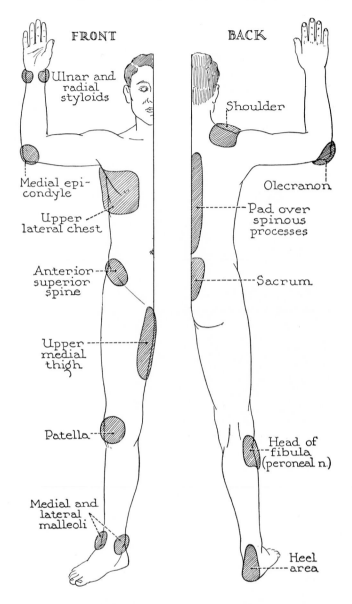

FRONT   BACK

Ulnar and radial styloids

Shoulder

Medial epicondyle

Olecranon

Upper lateral chest

Pad over spinous processes

Anterior superior spine

Sacrum

Upper medial thigh

Patella

Head of fibula (peroneal n.)

Medial and lateral malleoli

Heel area

ciently to relieve all constriction and undue compression. The split in the cast should not be made directly over any operative incision. It should be carried through bandages or sheet wadding to expose the skin and must assure that no constricting strands are left to exert a tourniquet effect.

A patient's complaint of pain within a plaster cast must always be carefully evaluated. Sharply localized burning pain usually indicates excessive pressure with impending skin necrosis and calls for immediate attention. It is negligence to ignore any complaint

of pain which cannot be explained readily, or to mask the pain with narcotics. The cast should be split or removed, as the individual case dictates. A well-reduced fracture or a skillfully executed operation on an extremity can be negated and a disastrous result obtained from soft-tissue necrosis due to cast pressure.

The danger of Volkmann's ischemic contracture must always be uppermost in the mind of the surgeon who is handling injuries about the elbow. Any elbow fracture carries the threat of circulatory embarrassment due

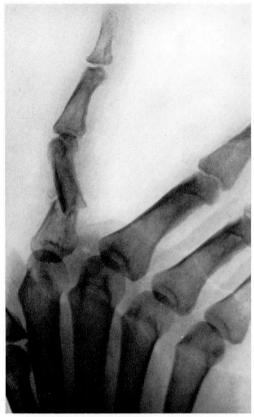

FIG. 101. Malunited fracture of proximal phalanx 3 weeks after injury. A tongue-depressor splint was used. As a result of maintaining the metacarpal-phalangeal joint and the interphalangeal joints in complete extension, these joints are stiff. Fingers should be splinted in moderate flexion. This would have permitted correction of the angulation, and malunion of the fracture and the loss of joint motion would have been avoided. (Compere and Banks: Pictorial Handbook of Fracture Treatment, Chicago, Year Book Pub.)

to swelling, compression of the antecubital vessels by bone fragments, arterial spasm or a combination of these complications. When excessive swelling about the elbow exists or is anticipated, a plaster cast or a splint is dangerous. It is wiser and safer to employ skin or skeletal traction as the definitive or preliminary treatment pending subsidence of the swelling. The cardinal signs of circulatory

embarrassment and impending ischemic necrosis in any extremity are pain, pallor, cyanosis and coldness of the distal parts. When these signs present themselves, the cast must be removed immediately. It is far better to lose reduction of a fracture while preserving a viable extremity than to risk permanent loss of function due to ischemic necrosis.

Walking casts should be snug, and a longitudinal as well as a transverse metatarsal arch should be molded on the bottom of the cast. The rubber heel should be centrally placed and must not be tilted so as to throw a torque on the foot or the ankle upon weight bearing. If an arm cast extends onto the hand, the metacarpals must be molded carefully in the palm to preserve their natural arch and to facilitate grasp. *Under no circumstances should an arm cast extend beyond the metacarpal-phalangeal joint of the hand.* If immobilized for several weeks, the resulting stiffness of the metacarpal-phalangeal joints may become a formidable problem in rehabilitation (Fig. 101). Following the application of any arm cast, the patient must be taught how to *exercise actively all joints which are not immobilized, particularly the fingers and the shoulder.* If the patient does not open and close the hand actively and repeatedly, with all of his strength, crippling stiffness may occur. The development of the signs and symptoms of reflex neurovascular disturbances, such as the "shoulder-hand" syndrome, will not occur if the physician impresses the patient sufficiently and the patient actively exercises the fingers and the shoulder each day while the arm cast is worn.

INTERNAL FIXATION

The recent refinements of metallurgy, as well as improved surgical technics, have made internal fixation of bones a preferred method of treating certain fractures. Certain dangers must be recognized, and errors in the use of internal fixation can result in tragedy. In the hands of inexperienced or inadequately trained surgeons, the hazards of internal fixation far outweigh the advantages. Internal fixation is best accomplished by *slotted plates* or *intramedullary rods*. These permit physiologic compression between the fracture surfaces which promotes rapid healing. The nail or plate must

FIG. 102. Fractures of the ulna near the elbow with dislocation of the head of the radius. Not infrequently the fracture of the ulna is treated, while the dislocation of the head of the radius is not recognized. (Compere and Banks: Pictorial Handbook of Fracture Treatment, Chicago, Year Book Pub.)

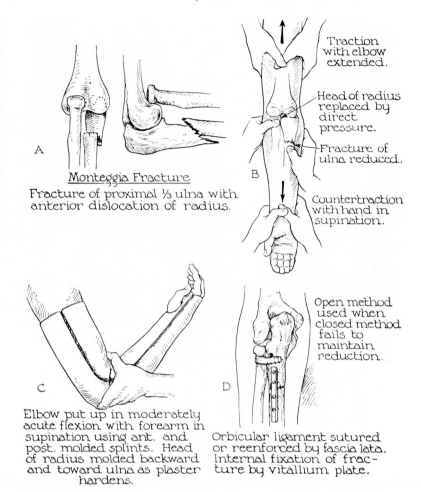

Traction with elbow extended.

Head of radius replaced by direct pressure.

Fracture of ulna reduced.

Countertraction with hand in supination.

A

Monteggia Fracture
Fracture of proximal ⅓ ulna with anterior dislocation of radius.

B

C

Elbow put up in moderately acute flexion with forearm in supination using ant. and post. molded splints. Head of radius molded backward and toward ulna as plaster hardens.

D

Open method used when closed method fails to maintain reduction.

Orbicular ligament sutured or reenforced by fascia lata. Internal fixation of fracture by vitallium plate.

be long enough to afford adequate immobilization. If the fractured bone is the femur, the plate should be attached to each fragment with not less than 4 screws. Each screw should penetrate and firmly engage both the lateral and the medial cortex of the femur. *Never should less than 2 screws be used to attach a metal plate to each fragment of a fractured bone, however small the bone may be* (Fig. 102). *Circular wires or bands* should be used rarely. They afford poor fixation and may cause pressure necrosis and bone absorption. The most common cause of *nonunion of fractures* is distraction of the fragments. If too much traction is used and the ends of the fracture fragments are kept apart, delayed union or nonunion will result. If the older type of metal plate with round holes which rigidly immobilize is applied, without firm

contact between the fracture fragments, nonunion is likely to result (Fig. 103).

When a surgeon opens a fracture to reduce it accurately and apply internal fixation he should always take advantage of the golden opportunity afforded him of placing some type of bone graft across the fracture lines. This may be small osteoperiosteal grafts from the fracture fragments or large tibial grafts (Figs. 104 and 105).

AMPUTATIONS AND DISARTICULATIONS

In the young and robust, the surgeon should not be in a hurry to amputate, no matter how ominous the appearance of the case. It is surprising how rapidly such patients recuperate from extensive injuries, and how limbs which, at the time of injury, seemed to be beyond

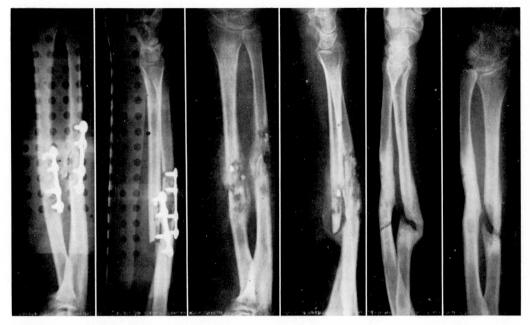

FIG. 103. Simple fracture of both bones of the forearm, complicated by osteomyelitis following attempts at open reduction. (Compere, E. L.: S. Clin. North America 25:58)

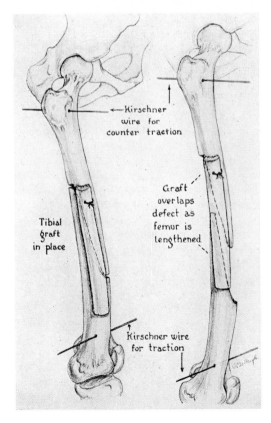

all hope of restoration can regain their complete function and usefulness. Strict asepsis, coupled with the use of oral and local administration of sulfathiazole, and patience in these cases often bring about better results than the most brilliant surgery.

Adams has referred to this point in connection with crushed or compound fractures of the fingers. Since the blood and nerve supply in this region is abundant, restorative repair is the rule, unless there is gangrene.

FIG. 104. A technic which will hasten union and restoration of strength following an oblique osteotomy on any long bone which is to be lengthened by traction after osteotomy is shown in this illustration. A long autogenous tibial bone graft is fastened in place by a heavy catgut suture. The attachment is to one fragment of the long bone so that as lengthening is obtained by means of traction, the tibial graft continues to maintain contact with both osteotomy fragments and subsequently becomes firmly united to both. Similar bone grafts are ideal in treating old ununited fractures. (Compere, E. L.: J. Bone & Joint Surg. 18:692)

FIG. 105. The surgeon who is faced with the problem of trying to promote the healing of old ununited fractures, especially if he is dealing with a congenital pseudarthrosis of the tibia and the fibula, must use long massive bone grafts which will bridge across the sclerotic, almost totally avascular ends of the fracture fragments and make adequate contact with more nearly normal bone proximal and distal to the fracture site. Adherence to this rule will prevent many failures and much heartache. (Compere, E. L.: Bone & Joint Surg. 18:513)

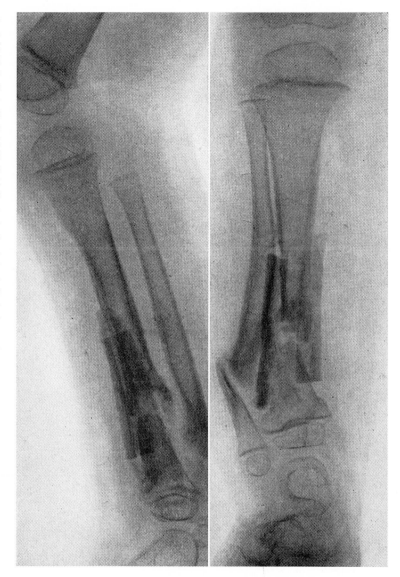

HEMOSTASIS

Before beginning an amputation, the surgeon should make sure that hemostasis is satisfactory and likely to remain so during the entire operation. The tourniquet should be released before the flaps are sutured; otherwise, there may be hemorrhage from some vessel that was not properly secured, with a resulting hematoma. Always leave some avenue of escape for serum.

The danger of later postoperative hemorrhages is always greater when an operation has been carried out in an artificially produced bloodless field.

SEVERED NERVES

All nerves that are severed during an amputation should be pulled out for an inch or more from the wound surface and the ends cut off. This will prevent involvement of the nerve stump in the scar. Experience acquired during and since World War II has shown that better results are obtained if the *nerve* is *not* injected with alcohol.

BLOOD SUPPLY

A good blood supply of a soft tissue flap is a *sine qua non* to success in an amputation stump. If arteriosclerosis is present in the limb

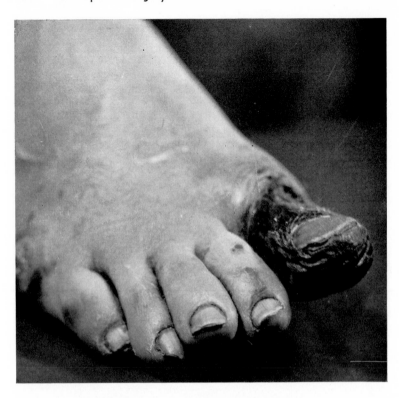

Fig. 106. Arteriosclerotic gangrene of toe. Never use moisture in treating such conditions.

to be amputated, be especially cautious (Fig. 106). Amputation should be done high enough to ensure an adequate blood supply.

Cooling of Saws

Saws used in dividing bones must be cooled while in use. If allowed to become heated, local necrosis of the bone may result, with possible infection or sequestration. Cooling is best accomplished by playing a small stream of normal salt solution onto the saw as it is being used.

Bursae

Never incise bursae; always excise them. As long as the lining of the bursal sac remains, just so long will suppuration continue if infection is present. Before excising a bursa, make sure that it does not communicate with a joint.

Sepsis

In amputations the utmost care is necessary to avoid infection, or the result may be disastrous.

The Stump

Any disarticulation or amputation which leaves a painful stump or one that cannot be adapted to a prosthetic apparatus must be considered a technical failure. The important thing after recovery from an amputation, as far as the patient is concerned, is a good serviceable stump.

The points to be considered in connection with a good stump are three: (1) the shape of the stump shall present sufficient surface to fit the prosthesis snugly; (2) the stump shall be painless and have a good blood supply; (3) the flaps should be sufficiently large to cover the end of the bone well.

Flaps

Avoid stretching and tension of flaps. An inexperienced surgeon may shape the amputation flaps too short and not allow for retraction. There is marked retraction of muscle and skin, especially in the neighborhood of joints such as the knee, following an amputation. Nature sometimes accomplishes rather neat amputations (Fig. 107).

Scars

Scars must be so situated that they are out of the way of pressure when the stump is placed in a prosthesis. The patient will have

Fig. 107. Spontaneous amputation of foot following gangrene resulting from frostbite.

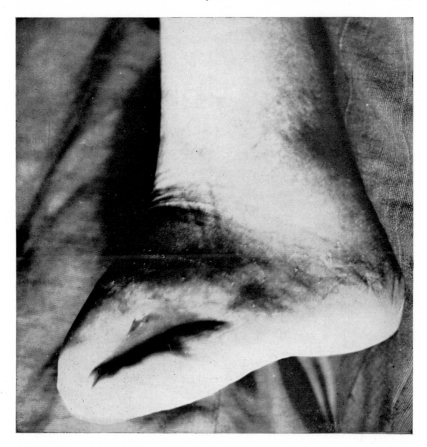

no reason to praise the surgeon who leaves him with a persistently painful stump.

REAMPUTATION

Reamputation for the purpose of obtaining a more satisfactory stump should not be done until all edema—which may persist for a long time—has subsided.

DRAINAGE

Even in clean amputations, a small soft rubber drain should always be inserted into each end of the incision. These drains prevent large hematoma formation. They should be removed 48 hours after the amputation. When infection is present, the wound should be left unsutured.

OPERATIONS ABOUT THE UPPER EXTREMITY

These operations, particularly amputations and disarticulations, should be most conservative. A stump of a finger is better than none at all. In amputations of the finger, place the scar on the dorsal surface of the affected member. In operations on the forearm, the same dictum holds true; save every inch of healthy tissue that you possibly can salvage. Following amputation of a finger, wherever possible, attach both flexor and extensor tendons to the proximal portion of the respective phalanx, the aim being to assure the patient control of the portion of the finger that remains. The removal of a metacarpal bone materially weakens the hand.

AFFECTIONS OF THE HIP JOINT

Operations About the Hip. To avoid errors in arthritis of the hip joint, it is of utmost importance that the type of involvement of the joint be ascertained in order to institute proper therapy and evaluate prognosis. Differential diagnosis here is of great importance. Pathologic dislocations are always a possibility. They are more frequent in the subacute and the chronic forms of joint affections than in the acute variety. Sudden dislocation may take place in a joint secondarily infected from a contiguous osteomyelitic focus. Calcareous

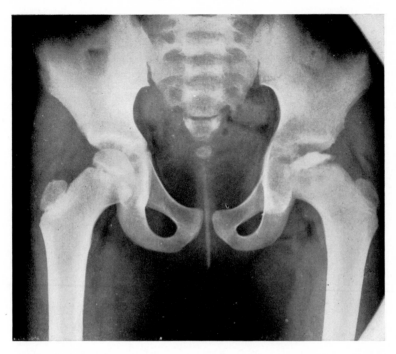

Fig. 108. Perthes' disease (osteochondritis deformans juvenilis). An 8-year-old girl, apparently in good health, fell and later complained of pain in the *knee*, which was treated by strapping, without relief. Six months later, following development of a definite limp, x-ray examination revealed the true condition. *Pain in the knee is often thus associated with hip-joint affections.*

bursitis or tendinitis may simulate arthritis. In osteochondritis of the hip the roentgenograms show characteristic findings. The clinical symptoms are similar to those of a chronic arthritis. In the former the joint cartilages are affected.

Diseases. Chronic arthritis, osteochondritis, sarcoma or osteitis of the upper portion of the femur are diseases of the hip joint (Fig. 108). Pain resulting from hip joint lesions such as osteoarthritis, slipped femoral epiphysis, Legg-Perthes disease or bone tumors is most often referred to the region of the knee. This often confuses the attending physician so that he may treat the normal knee and overlook or fail to diagnose the hip joint injury or disease.

LIGATIONS

INJURIES TO VESSELS

Gangrene of a lower extremity may occur after ligation of the external iliac artery. Paradoxically, it is less likely to occur after ligation of the common iliac artery as there is better collateral blood supply. Kümmell reported 55 ligations of the common iliac artery, with gangrene in only 4 instances. He cites Smith's statistics, which show that in 22 fatalities after ligation of the common iliac, there

was gangrene in but 3; while in 23 fatalities following ligation of the external iliac, gangrene was the cause of death in 11. Therefore, apart from functional disturbances, a fatal result from gangrene must always be considered a possibility in ligating the large vessels in the lower limbs. Ligation of the axillary artery is less dangerous, as far as necrosis of the upper extremity is concerned, than ligation of the brachial.

Arterial Contraction. After serious injury to arteries, the size of the affected vessels may be reduced and the pulse beat be suspended. Forgue and Aimé designate this condition "stupeur arterielle"; if the corresponding vein is intact, the arterial contraction usually relaxes within a few hours. During World War I, Fiolle observed that certain injuries of the arterial wall, consisting of a breech without bleeding, may occur; for these he coined the term "dry arterial wound."

In wounds of the volar arches, or in a region where collateral circulation is assured by adequate anastomosis, ligation of only the proximal portion of the principal distal artery is an error. Ligation of the radial, the cubital or the brachial arteries at the elbow is useless. The bleeding may be arrested only by ligating the brachial artery at the point of origin of

FIG. 109. Ischemic contracture of forearm resulting from constriction in treatment of Colles' fracture (constriction of only a few days duration).

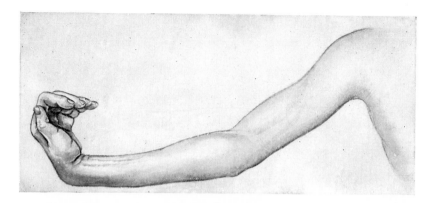

the profunda brachii or the so-called "point of Dubreuil."

Following injuries of the large vessels of the extremities, great care must be taken to avoid hemorrhage resulting from faulty ligation of both arteries and veins. The ligature must be placed in sound tissue, high on the retracted vascular stump.

If silk is used for ligature, it remains as a foreign body and may set up irritation. On the other hand, the rapid absorption of catgut may result in a late or secondary hemorrhage. Tight ligation of a vessel may cause injury to the intima and necrosis may follow. This danger may be minimized by a double ligature, but even this does not always give absolute security, particularly in septic wounds.

Aneurysm. Many skilled surgeons on occasion have mistaken aneurysm for abscess. This tragic error is even easier to commit when the aneurysm is complicated by local swelling.

Peripheral Vascular Disease. Despite the good results obtained by surgical intervention, it should be kept in mind that arteritis obliterans is of slow evolution and may yield to proper medical treatment. Arteritis in young patients and angiitis obliterans (Buerger's disease) may recede slowly.

Spasm or organic obstruction must receive consideration first. Depending on the existing conditions, the surgeon should decide what type of operation is indicated to relieve the condition (operation on the sympathetic nervous system, the endocrine glands or arteriectomy). Amputation may be avoided by relieving spasm. In any case, the acetylcholine test should be carried out. If intramuscular injections yield no results, a mechanical obstruction caused by arterial embolism prob-

ably exists, making intervention necessary. Anesthesia of the sympathetic lumbar nerves followed by an elevated skin-surface temperature indicates that vasodilatation of the arteries is still possible. Babinsky and Heits suggest placing the injured foot in a hot bath of 40° C. for 5 minutes. In the case of spasm, the skin becomes red and hot. In the case of an organic lesion, no change will be observed. Einar Key points out that it is very important and not always easy to distinguish embolism from thrombosis due to arteritis. Arteriography may be helpful.

Embolectomy. The removal of an embolus as well as a coagulum by operation has been performed hundreds of times since the first successful operation of Lahey. But Funk-Brentano pointed out that in order to be successful it must be performed within 10 hours after the onset of the trouble. Until fairly recently, operative intervention was resorted to when gangrene had already set in.

INJURIES TO NERVES

Radial Paralysis. When performing operations on the upper limb, remember that the middle third of the arm should be supported by a pillow on the flat surface of the operating table, instead of permitting it to hang, in order to minimize tension on the radial nerve and to avoid postoperative radial paralysis. For the same reason, tension on the nerves of the brachial plexus must be avoided. The median and the radial nerves may be injured during rough manipulation.

In the upper arm the radial nerve is involved in many fractures, the ulnar and the median nerves being traumatized much less frequently. These paralyses may cause perma-

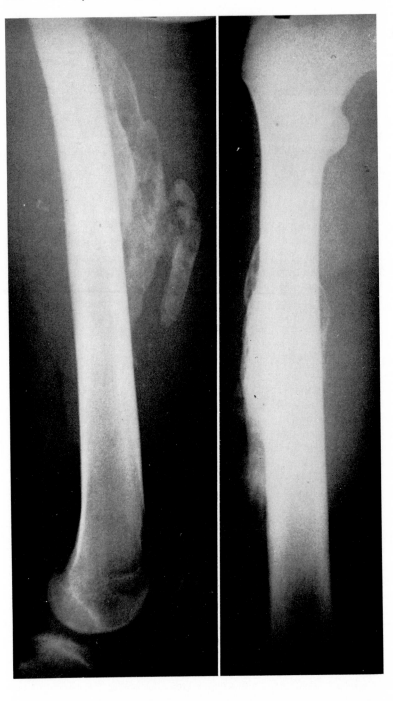

Fig. 110. Myositis ossificans which was erroneously thought to be sarcoma. (Compere, E. L.: S. Clin. North America 29:136)

nent contractures in the hand or the fingers. Injuries to the ulnar and the median nerves are more often encountered after fractures at the elbow and the wrist.

Paralysis Due to Ischemia of Muscles of Forearm. Ischemic paralyses of the muscles of the forearm result principally from injuries about the elbow, when the muscles are deprived of their blood supply. The obstruction to the circulation is often due to tight bandaging (Fig. 109), to an overflexed position of the elbow before reduction or to flexion of the

FIG. 111. Unilateral congenital dislocation of the hip in an adult.

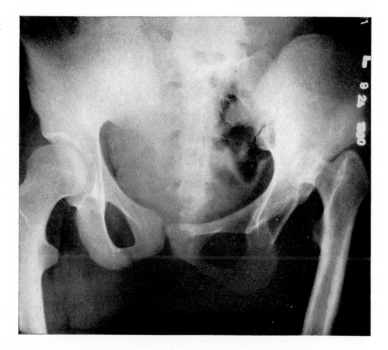

limbs when there is marked swelling (Page and Bristow). Pressure from a hematoma under the lacertus fibrosus can also cause ischemia and must be recognized and surgically relieved at an early moment. If there are signs of swelling, discoloration and pain, loosen all the bandages at once. Volkmann's ischemic contracture may result if these warnings are ignored.

Paralysis Due to Pressure on Nerves. Paralyses may also result from pressure on nerves by the ends of broken bones, from nerves caught between fragments of bone or from fibrous repair of torn muscles. The longer a paralysis which is due to an injured or severed nerve is allowed to remain untreated, the more difficult will be its operative treatment because of muscle atrophy, stiffness and contracture. The correction of a nerve injury should not be delayed longer than a few hours after the accident unless infection is present, then secondary suturing may be attempted a few months later.

In addition to the primary injury to nerves by contusion or by overstretching in the reduction of dislocations or in the treatment of fractures, nerves may be surrounded by callus formation. This complication is more common in shoulder and arm injuries.

Early Nerve Repairs. All injuries to nerves

should be repaired at the earliest possible moment (neurorrhaphy). In repairing a nerve, be sure that the skin cicatrix will not be directly over the sutured nerve. Do not crush the nerve with tissue forceps. Suture the epineurium, not the central substance. Avoid tension on the sutures. Hemostasis must be perfect.

DISLOCATIONS

Unreduced Dislocations. Errors are frequently encountered in the treatment of unreduced dislocations. The problems presenting themselves are sometimes extremely difficult. Attempts at reduction may be undertaken up to 2 months after dislocation. During the reduction it is an error to employ excessive force, thereby endangering the main blood vessels or the nerves. The greatest possible caution must be exercised when employing pulleys for extension.

Myositis Ossificans. A complication of excessive force in the reduction of an old dislocation is muscular injury, causing the condition known as myositis ossificans traumatica. More often this condition results from hemorrhage into a bruised or torn muscle, without fracture. This has been erroneously diagnosed and treated as a malignant bone tumor (Fig. 110).

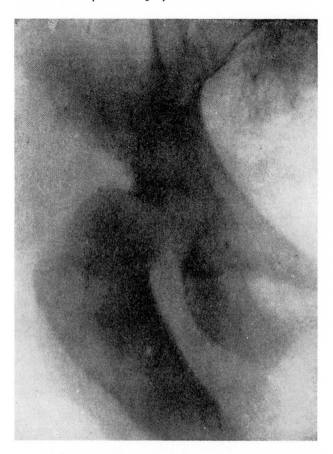

Fig. 112. Traumatic dislocation of the hip.

Period of Immobilization. A limb should not be immobilized for a long period after reduction of a dislocation. This leads to atrophy of the muscles and loss of function of the joints and of the limb. Early guarded active motion is desirable.

Dislocation of the Hip

In attempting reduction of a congenital (Fig. 111) or a traumatic dislocation of the hip (Fig. 112), the nerves, especially the sciatic nerve, may be injured by overstretching (Fig. 113).

Congenital Dislocations of the Hip. These should be recognized and treated during infancy. It will not help the physician's professional standing in his own community if he fails to discover it. Before an open operation is advised in these cases, one should try the bloodless reduction by the Lorenz technic. The earlier this is tried, the better are the results (50 to 90% cures). The operation is most successful during the first year. After the child has reached the age of 4 years, attempts at closed reduction should not be made.

Closed reduction is not free from such dangers as fracture of the shaft of the femur or injury to the epiphysis and the blood vessels. Open operation should be reserved for the older patient, and the results are not nearly so good as are those of closed reduction carried out during the first or second year.

Traumatic Dislocations of the Hip. These must be differentiated from bilateral coxa vara and epiphyseolysis. Complications of operative procedures are redislocation (recurrence), stiffness of the hip joint and aseptic necrosis. Occasionally, traumatic dislocation of the hip is bilateral. Always examine both hips for comparison.

Malingering and Hysteria. Do not be misled by malingerers or hysterical individuals who on many occasions have successfully simulated various surgical conditions. The aforementioned state should not be confounded with true hip lesions.

Reposition as well as diagnosis should always be confirmed roentgenographically.

Perivascular subinguinal hernia may follow forced reduction of the hip joint.

The femoral artery or vein may be injured in forced manipulations of the hip. *When faced with a combination of hip dislocation and thigh fracture,* the fracture should be set and immobilized in a favorable position first before the dislocation is reduced.

Dislocations of the Lower End of the Femur. These must receive prompt attention lest serious nerve and vascular trauma ensue. The sooner the dislocation is reduced the safer the limb will be.

Isolated Paralysis of the Peroneal Nerve. This may occur as a result of overstretching.

In 1909, Peltesohn collected from the literature 58 cases of nerve injuries in the reduction of hip dislocations. These included 26 cases of paralysis of the sciatic nerve, 12 of the peroneal and 3 associated with bladder and rectal complications. Although such paralyses commonly disappear under proper treatment, they may persist and be very troublesome to the patient.

INJURIES OF THE SHOULDER

Diagnostic errors are frequent in injuries of the shoulder (fractures of the tuberosity of the humerus; injuries to the glenoid cavity or to the neck of the scapula). One should be guarded in giving a prognosis; slight injuries here may be followed by serious consequences (persistent pain, reduced motion, atrophy, paresis). Make sure that the head of the humerus is not dislocated. X-ray examination should be made after every manipulation of a major joint because swelling may mask a dislocation.

Flatness of the Shoulder. In dislocations of the shoulder, flatness of the shoulder may be caused by an existing hematoma. Flattened shoulder may resemble a dislocation; it frequently occurs in fracture of the humerus with abduction.

Dislocation of the Shoulder. In a dislocation of the shoulder, the method of direct pull on the arm, with the physician's stockinged foot in the axilla, is dangerous only if the surgeon is rough or careless. Before and after reduction of the shoulder, an examination

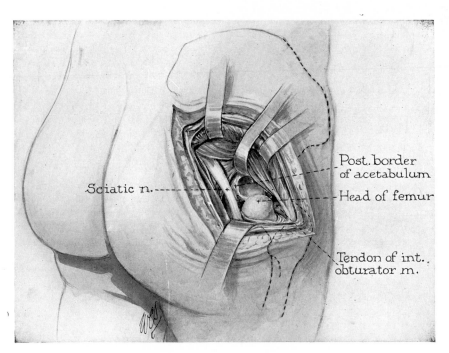

Sciatic n.

Post. border of acetabulum

Head of femur

Tendon of int. obturator m.

FIG. 113. Showing position of sciatic nerve in relation to posterior border of acetabulum.

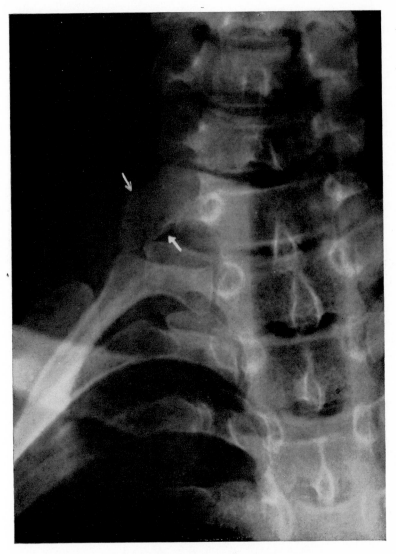

Fig. 114. Unilateral cervical rib—a fairly common anomaly. Its presence does not always explain clinical symptoms occasionally associated with it. In patient shown here, pain in right shoulder radiated into right arm and along third and fourth fingers (median nerve).

should be made to ascertain that the nerves are not injured.

Do not hastily give a favorable prognosis in acromioclavicular dislocations.

Cervical Ribs. When these produce symptoms which do not respond to conservative treatment, the rib should be removed. Scalenotomy affords only temporary relief (Fig. 114).

FRACTURE AND DISLOCATION OF THE ELBOW

These may go together. Thorough x-ray studies are necessary even after the fracture has been determined. Before attempting reduction, examine carefully the nerves and the

vessels for possible injury. Closed treatment is considered best here. Disturbances of the circulation and persistent hematoma are often concomitant with marked traumatism. Repeated x-ray examinations of the immobilized limb are necessary even after the disappearance of the edema (see Fig. 102).

Fractures and displacements about the elbow should rarely be subjected to plaster of Paris splints or bandages (Sir Robert Jones). It is dangerous to put a pad in the bend of the elbow before flexing it. By whatever method flexion is maintained, there are three important precautions to be kept in mind. First, there must be no interference with the blood supply of the forearm. Second,

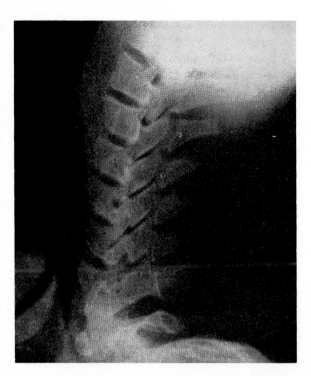

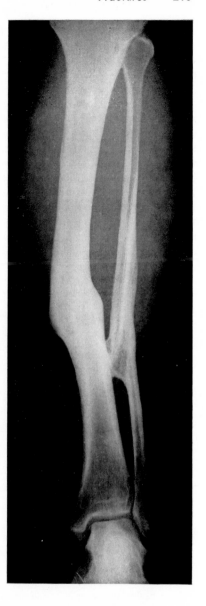

Fig. 115 (*Left*). Roentgenogram of normal cervical spine, lateral view. Note that anterior arch of atlas is in line with anterior border of rest of vertebrae; also, odontoid process immediately beyond anterior arch of atlas.

Fig. 116 (*Right*). Marked malalignment of fractured tibia and fibula.

the arm must be examined a few hours after it is put up and then daily for several days to make sure that there is no circulatory disturbance. Third, if the patient complains of pain, the bandages must be removed and readjusted.

DISLOCATION OF THE FOOT

From 30 to 50 per cent of the functional disabilities of the foot following dislocations could be prevented by prompt and proper treatment when the injury occurs. Do not omit roentgenographic investigation. Make sure that the conformation of the heel as well as the arch of the foot are properly restored and that the foot is in proper position.

FRACTURES

GENERAL CONSIDERATIONS

Fractures of the Cervical Spine. These may be overlooked. They are serious and may be followed by disastrous results (Fig. 115).

Errors. To avoid errors and complications in the treatment of fractures the following possibilities should be kept in mind:

1. Too long confinement in bed, particularly of elderly persons, may lead to hypostatic pneumonia or bed sores.

2. "Crutch paralysis" due to compression of the brachial nerves, especially the radial nerve, can be avoided by the use of properly constructed crutches. On appearance of the first symptoms of this troublesome complication, discontinue the use of the crutches.

3. Gangrene may result from (a) the immediate effect of the injury, (b) infection in

compound fractures, (c) errors in treatment, such as too tight bandaging, causing constriction of the vessels; acute flexion of a joint after bandaging (the bandage may injure the soft tissues); or pressure from a splint.

Unskillful and improper treatment of fractures is often worse than no treatment. Serious after-effects may follow from failure to attend to small details (Fig. 116). It does not suffice to relieve pain and swelling and provide for bony union. The functions of the muscles, the joints and the nerves must be maintained. A fracture may heal anatomically, but the functional value of the limb may be impaired permanently. Early and frequent passive and active movements should be instituted and

splints that unduly compress the muscles and the blood vessels avoided. This is especially important in the forearm. In applying splints, straps and bandages, every care must be taken to ensure that there is no undue compression. Any symptom of functional disability should be investigated immediately and remedied.

Insufficient Clinical Investigation. The first surgical error in dealing with a fracture is insufficient clinical investigation. As one surgeon has stated, the man who relies solely on roentgenograms to diagnose a fracture is allowing his faculties of observation to atrophy from disuse. However, whenever possible, it is always desirable to have roentgenographic corroboration of the existence of a fracture.

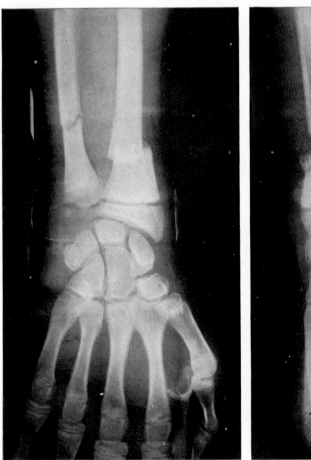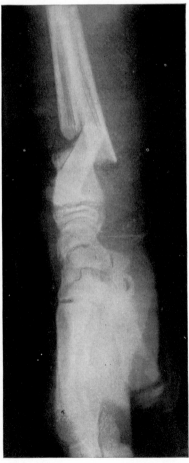

Fig. 117 (*Left*). Fracture of radius and ulna. Anterior view gives impression of good position of fragments.

Fig. 118 (*Right*). Same case as Figure 117. Lateral view shows the true condition.

Splints. It is a surgical error to employ any type of splint which does not allow access to the wound, in the case of an open fracture, for the purpose of inspection and dressing. For the lower limb, the Thomas splint is best, and for the upper limb a modified Thomas. However, it should be remembered that in the upper arm the position of extension which the splint maintains is liable to lead to subsequent limitation of movement of the elbow joint if kept up for more than a week or two.

Stereoscopic Roentgenograms. The results of manual reduction of fractures can best be interpreted by using stereoscopic x-ray plates. The use of a single plate is often misleading; one should always have anteroposterior and lateral views (Figs. 117 and 118).

For instance, if a needle is to be removed from the hand, one should endeavor to extract the foreign body under the fluoroscope. Images of broken needles on the flat x-ray plate are extremely misleading. If one is bent on avoiding errors and safeguarding the patient's interest, establish the position of the needle by x-ray stereoscopy.

Vascular Injuries. These are frequent in the reduction of fractures. Körte collected 44 cases of vascular injuries in the orthopedic reduction of shoulder fractures. The axillary artery was the vessel injured in the great majority of these. The injury to the limb was generally of long standing. The same danger exists in the reduction of old injuries elsewhere. Old age and arteriosclerotic conditions are predisposing factors.

Thrombosis and gangrene of the extremities may develop. Vascular injuries associated with fractures are encountered more frequently in the lower than in the upper limb, the femoral and popliteal vessels especially being involved.

Alignment. A good rule to remember in reducing fractures is that the upper fragment cannot always be brought into alignment with the lower, but one is usually successful in bringing the lower fragment into apposition with the upper.

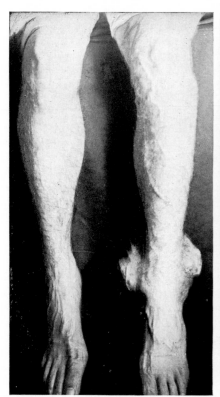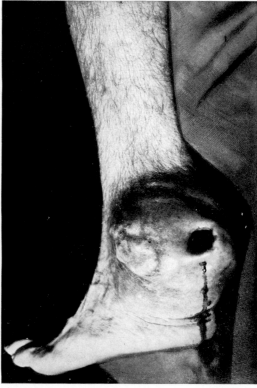

Fig. 119. Osteosarcoma developing on old, ununited fracture.

Complications. After reduction and immobilization of fractures, the physician should be on the lookout for complications. Before an open operation for fracture it is well to wait a few days, allowing the tissues to recover from the trauma incident to the accident. The more traumatized the tissues, the greater the indications for delay before reducing a fracture. Make sure that the vessels below the point of fracture have not been injured. Check the pulse. After extensive traumatic injuries of the limbs, early and thorough débridement (within 8 hours following the injury) will cleanse the traumatized area and often will save the limb.

FRACTURES WHICH DO NOT HEAL. Do not forget the Wassermann test and, if need be, examination of the spinal fluid in every case of fracture that fails to heal. In the case illustrated, months elapsed and the fractured leg did not heal. A Wassermann test showed the blood to be definitely positive. Intensive antisyphilitic therapy brought about osseous consolidation.

MALIGNANCY. Malignant degeneration cannot result from a fracture. In the case illustrated by Figure 119, a neglected simple fracture of the ankle resulted in an osteosarcoma that cost the patient's life. He came for relief too late, after metastases were implanted elsewhere in the body. The fracture may have occurred in this exact location because the bone was already weakened by the presence of a malignant lesion which had not previously made its presence manifest. A fracture which occurs at the site of a malignant lesion may incite the tumor to much more rapid growth and to earlier metastases.

FAT EMBOLISM. Small amounts of fat are carried into the circulation in every case of fracture. As a rule, this is of little consequence, but in an occasional case it may cause serious fat embolism.

Fat embolism may also appear after treatment for dislocations and fractures. There are two types: cerebral and respiratory. Fat embolism of the cerebral type commonly appears during the period of narcosis, while the respiratory type appears a few hours after waking from the anesthetic. Either type may follow even a very slight operation, such as a bloodless reduction of pes varus. This complication is most common in patients between 10 and 20 years of age. The best treatment appears to be the immediate use of saline solution. In all severe cases, fluids should be administered intravenously.

PULMONARY HYPOSTASIS AND DECUBITUS. Failures in the treatment of fractures often arise from lack of good nursing care. Protect the patient from lung complications, bed sores and pressure gangrene (air or water mattress). In elderly patients, be ever alert for hypostatic pneumonia, delirium, pseudarthrosis and decubitus.

SEQUESTRATION. This may occur in the canals produced by the nails used in the treatment of fractures by skeletal traction, necessitating secondary operations. Infection may appear, and in such event the nails or the plates should be removed forthwith and drainage instituted. There is a great need for proper care of the muscles in fractures. Early mobilization after fractures is followed by good results, especially in the function of the joints.

Tendon Suture. Primary suturing of a ruptured tendon should be done. Stitches should not be pulled so tight as to compromise the blood supply and cause secondary necrosis. Immobilize the joint above and below by the use of a plaster-of-Paris cast for 10 days. Then start *guarded active motion.*

Rupture of a Muscle. This should be diagnosed promptly and appropriate treatment employed.

Hemarthrosis. In repeated hemarthroses, think of hemophilia. Where intra-articular derangements are present by reason of repeated blood effusions into the joint, the roentgenogram will show a thickening of the capsule in the initial stages due to deposits of iron pigments. The presence of vacuoles in the epiphysis is also of diagnostic importance (Fonio).

SURGICAL TREATMENT

Open reduction and internal fixation affords perfect coaptation of fractures, but the results are not always satisfactory, and the procedure carries with it the danger of infection. However, in complicated fractures, the method shortens the time of treatment. On the other hand, consolidation is slower and many complications may occur (local infection, acute osteomyelitis, persistent osteitis, painful and exuberant callus, rarefaction of bones, pseudarthrosis, loosening of the fixation material, etc.). Statistics show that the results obtained by osteosynthesis are often inferior to those following closed methods. However, in evaluating the relative merits of open and closed methods of treatment, one must recall that usually only severe cases are subjected to open treatment; hence, statistical evaluations are of only relative value.

In operating the following precautions must be observed meticulously: strict asepsis; gentle handling of tissues; avoidance of injury to muscles, nerves, important blood vessels and bones; and thorough and adequate immediate postoperative immobilization. While bone consolidation may be retarded following operative procedures, the results, in the main, are satisfactory.

In 239 cases of osteosynthesis (30 to 40% were open fractures), Lambotte saw only 1 fatal case (due to tetanus) and 1 case requiring amputation. In other cases he obtained 90 per cent of either excellent or very good results, 60 per cent of complete restoration of function, while in 30 cases disability resulted in from 1 to 10 per cent. Carbonnel and Masse cite the following figures. Of 316 cases of all varieties of closed fractures since 1922, the closed treatment (241 cases) gave an average of 5½ months of temporary disability and 16.2 per cent of permanent partial disability. Osteosynthesis (75 cases) was followed by an average of 7 months of disability.

Osteitis Rarefaciens. On occasion the use of screws will cause osteitis rarefaciens. In applying mechanical retention devices (screws and plates), care should be taken that they do not exert too much pressure. In order to curtail infections, excessive denudation of bone should be avoided. Oxidation of metallic prosthesis as well as electrical reactions between 2 metals may cause phenomena of electrolysis. Wire sutures, hooks and similar devices are now rarely used. Screws and nails offer an excellent means of fixation. Plates are usually well tolerated, but they may cause osteitis or osteoporosis and often have to be removed.

Kirschner wires, Smith-Petersen nails, stainless steel, intramedullary pins, Duralumin and autografts have been added to the surgical armamentarium in the treatment of fractures.

In *open fractures* prompt cleansing of the affected region is imperative. Open reduction should be delayed except where closed reduction is impossible or where it is difficult to keep the fragments in proper coaptation. Avoid tight suturing of the wound; partial closure is often better. Immobilize the limb immediately and dress the wound only when indicated. External fixation is a good method, often yielding gratifying results.

Osteitis Delaying Solidification. This is the most important complication in osteosynthesis, it being responsible for delays and disability in from 50 to 80 per cent of the cases (Müller). Osteitis is likely to occur in open fractures even when these are not operated on. According to Charbonnel and Masse, this complication was observed in 17 per cent of the cases without osteosynthesis and in 16 per cent in which the operation was performed. When osteitis supervenes, remove the prosthesis promptly. Soft callus-causing deformities are also charged to the effects of metallic prosthesis. According to Fredet, Savariaud and Wiart, soft callus is observed in 50 per cent of the cases. On the other hand, Robineau believes that it may occur no matter what kind of treatment is employed. He attributes the complication to an infection during an operation.

If an osteosynthetic apparatus gives rise to considerable pain, it must be removed.

Infection and pseudarthrosis are the chief dangers in the operative treatment of complicated fractures. No completely detached pieces of bone or insufficiently nourished tissue should be left behind. The débridement of the wound should be as complete as possible.

Causes of Nonunion. Nonunion of fractures is not due, as many believe, to deficiency in systemic calcium or phosphorus (Henderson). Marked malposition or distraction of the fragments with, perhaps, intervention of muscle, inadequate fixation, the presence of a metal plate or other mechanical fixation appliance or injury to the surrounding tissues are the most common causes of nonunion (Fig. 120).

In the operative treatment of ununited fracture, complete exposure of the site of fracture is essential to success. The surgeon must have a full and free view of the conditions before he can decide how best to deal with them.

In a recent case under my observation, the patient, a woman, aged 40, a stenographer by

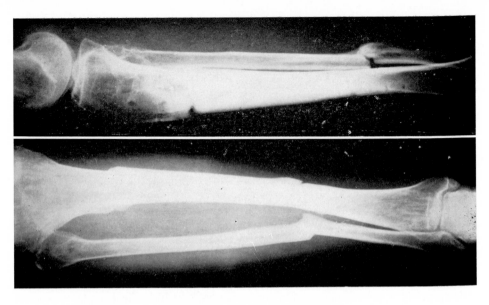

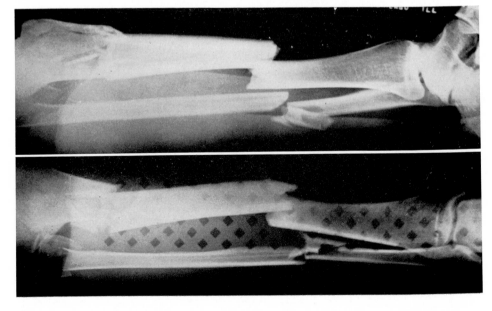

Fig. 120. (*Left*) These roentgenograms show a fracture of the right tibia with a detached fragment, representing more than the middle third and including the complete cortical circumference in one segment. It is a reasonable conclusion that the nutrient artery was either ruptured or entered the tibia above the proximal break, and that the middle fracture segment was nourished only by periosteal vessels. (*Right*) Fifteen months after injury, union has taken place. However, the segmental fragment has retained greater density than have the metaphyseal fragments, indicating aseptic necrosis. Although union has occurred, the fracture ends of the metaphyseal fragments are also of greater relative density than bone more distal to the fracture sites. (Compere, E. L.: J. Bone & Joint Surg. 31-A:47)

vocation, had sustained a fracture at about the middle of the left humerus, which had failed to unite following treatment. On operating, the radial nerve, greatly traumatized but not torn, was found interposed between the two fragments of bone. Primary union of the wound eventuated, but 5 months later bone consolidation was not yet complete, which demonstrates that a guarded prognosis should be given when operating on ununited fractures.

Proper Alignment. The great desiderata in

FIG. 121. Disastrous result of discontinuing immobilization too soon in comminuted fracture of the radius with dislocation of the wrist (*top*). Satisfactory reduction was obtained by skeletal traction with a threaded pin passed through 3 metacarpal bones and then incorporated in a plaster cast (*bottom, left*). When the pin was removed after 3½ weeks, position was lost and fracture healed with shortening of radius and deformity (*bottom, right*). Immobilization should have been continued at least 2 weeks longer. (Compere and Banks: Pictorial Handbook of Fracture Treatment, Chicago, Year Book Pub.)

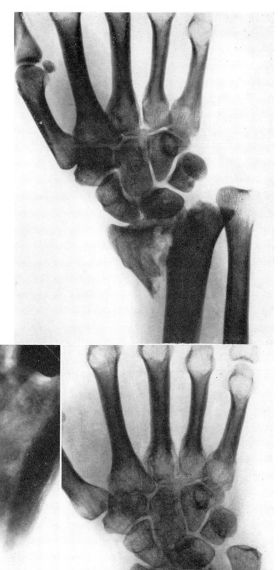

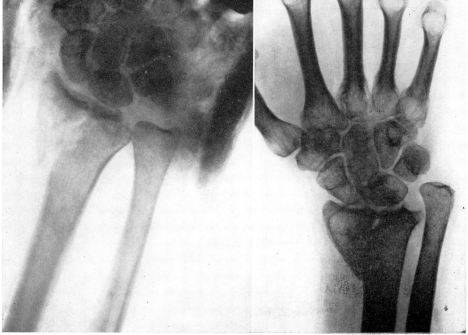

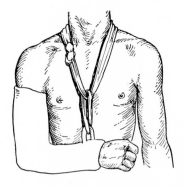

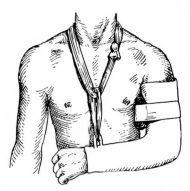

Fig. 122. The hanging cast for fractures of the humerus permits frequent exercises of the shoulder. This cast is an effective method for treating nearly all fractures of the humeral neck or the condyles. (Compere and Banks: Pictorial Handbook of Fracture Treatment, Chicago, Year Book Pub.)

Hanging cast.

Felt roll in position to correct medial displacement of lower fragment.

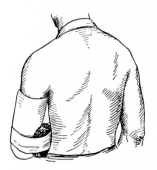

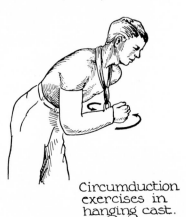

Sponge roll in position to correct lateral angulation.

Circumduction exercises in hanging cast.

the operative treatment of fractures are to avoid shortening due to overriding of the bony fragments and to prevent rotary distortion and angular deformity. A surgeon who has treated such a patient for fracture and obtained a very bad result will have in his community a permanent advertisement of his lack of skill. Contraction of important muscles and stiff joints will bring about the same result, in a lesser degree, although they are difficult to avoid in some cases.

FRACTURES OF THE UPPER EXTREMITY AND THE CLAVICLE

Fractures of the Vertebrae and the Jaws. Utmost care and vigilance is essential here (diagnosis, proper therapy and prognosis).

Fractures of the Wrist. These are often complicated by fractures of the radius. Dislocations and fractures of the carpal bones, sometimes difficult to demonstrate on roent-

genograms, should receive careful attention because complications are rather frequent. Comminuted fractures of the distal end of the radius require immobilization for 5 to 6 weeks (Fig. 121).

Fractures of the Metacarpals and the Fingers. These may lead to deformities such as permanent flexion of fingers, stiffness or ankylosis. The possibility of injury to nerves and tendons must be remembered in injuries of the fingers, the hand and the wrist (see Fig. 101).

Fractures of the Clavicle. There is always danger of injury to the subclavian vessels and the brachial plexus in fractures of the clavicle. In open operations these eventualities must be borne in mind. In the young, fractures of the clavicle are often subperiosteal and need no open interference unless this is especially indicated.

Disfigurement as a result of fractured clavicle is often an important consideration, particularly in women. It is an error not to apprise the patient of the possibility of such deformity. It is safeguarding the interest of both the patient and the surgeon to discuss the prognosis of closed and open reduction and immobilization of the fractured clavicle. Much misunderstanding and disappointment will be avoided by a frank expression of opinion in these cases. The conservative (closed) method should always be tried and given preference.

Dislocation of a Separated Head of the Humerus. This is difficult to ascertain. Where dislocation is evident, the fracture may be easily demonstrated.

Fractures of the shaft of the humerus are most safely treated by means of a hanging cast (Fig. 122). This simple, safe and effective method (Griswold reported 400 consecutive fractures of the humerus treated by this method without a single nonunion) is almost equally applicable for certain impacted fractures of the neck of the humerus and for

severely comminuted fractures of the humeral condyles.

Following traumatisms and dislocations of the shoulder, a thorough examination of the nerves and the blood vessels of the corresponding injured upper extremity should always be made.

Fracture of the Surgical Neck of the Humerus. In fracture of the surgical neck of the humerus the inferior fragment may be displaced upward and inward and thus subject the axillary vessels to injury. In closed fractures of the clavicle, the subclavian vein may be lacerated without being marked by pronounced symptoms.

Fractures of the Shoulder. Immobilization must be effective but not excessively prolonged after fractures of the shoulder because of the danger of adhesions and limited motion in the scapulohumeral joint. Atrophy of the muscles and stiffness of the elbow, the wrist and the hand may result. Exercises of shoulder motion should be started early (Fig. 122).

Carry out the reduction of a dislocated

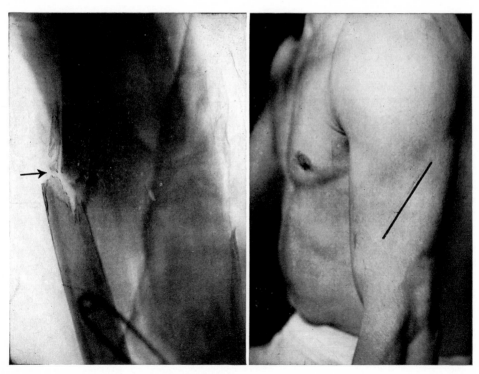

Fig. 123 (*Left*). Roentgenogram showing displaced fragments of fractured humerus which caused paralysis of radial nerve.

Fig. 124 (*Right*). Same case as Figure 123. Shows incision for exposure of radial nerve.

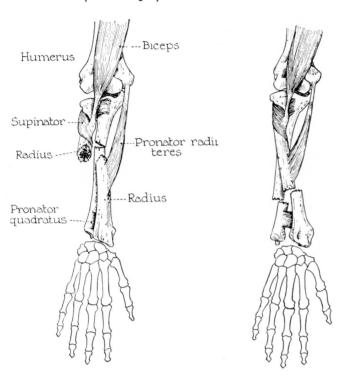

Humerus

---Biceps

Supinator---

Radius----

Pronator
quadratus ---

---Pronator radii
teres

----Radius

FIG. 125. Schematic diagram of the forearm muscles which influence the displacement or rotation of fragments in fractures of the radius and the ulna. (Compere and Banks: Pictorial Handbook Fracture Treatment, Chicago, Year Book Pub.)

shoulder according to roentgenographic studies. This is equally important during treatment of fractures of the humerus.

Complications in Humerus Fractures. Some authors believe that surgical intervention in fractures of the humerus is justified because of the frequency of structural interposition.

The possibility of injury to the radial nerve should be kept in mind in all fractures of the shaft of the humerus (Figs. 123 and 124). Always immobilize the forearm in fractures of the shaft of the humerus.

Complications of Forearm Fractures. Even in cases properly treated and carefully watched, fractures of the forearm may develop complications. Dislocations of the head of the radius are sometimes overlooked (see Fig. 102). The elbow joint and head of the radius should be carefully examined. It is well to remember that in simple fracture of the forearm the swelling rarely extends above the elbow. So-called hypertrophic callus may be mistaken for tumor.

Repeated x-ray examinations are necessary in the treatment of these fractures and dislocations in order to discover and remedy secondary displacement. The greatest difficulty lies in the proper reduction and immobiliza-

tion of fractures affecting the distal third of the bone; this also applies where the upper fragment is short (Fig. 125). Be sure to correct rotation so that the distal fragments are in the same degree of supination or pronation as are the proximal fragments.

Volkmann's Syndrome. This may occur even in properly treated cases and without plaster cast immobilization. Special care should be exercised in the presence of a large hematoma, contusion or compression of the nerves or the blood vessels. In the presence of cyanosis of the hand and the forearm, severe pain and marked edema, immediate surgical intervention to reduce the internal pressure, to evacuate clots and to liberate vessels and nerves is imperative.

Prevent secondary angulations and persistent stiffness of the fingers by proper therapeutic measures. Stiffness of fingers will not occur if the fingers are not included in the cast and the patient is compelled to exercise them while fractures are healing. Consolidation here is very slow (from 8 to 10 weeks in adults and 6 weeks in children). Keep fingers free and insist that the patient exercise them repeatedly every day.

Full flexion in reducing a fracture of the

elbow entails serious risk because of the swelling which commonly accompanies the injury and because a hematoma frequently forms under the deep fascia of the elbow. The forearm should be approximated to the arm, with the hand toward and touching the shoulder. Full flexion is also likely to impede the venous circulation and thus predispose to Volkmann's ischemia. Do not forget the close proximity of the ulnar nerve to the internal condyle.

Again, it is well to emphasize that early passive motion will prevent stiff joints. In fractures of both bones of the forearm, with marked displacement, impaired function is very likely to result. Open reduction and immobilization (mechanical) may assure better functional results.

Care of Joints in Long Bone Fracture. In extra-articular fractures, the function of the joint may be impaired by too long immobilization of the limb in plaster of Paris. Prolonged immobilization leads to stiffness, pseudarthrosis and loss of function.

FRACTURES OF THE LOWER EXTREMITY

Internal Fixation. Internal fixation of almost all fractures of the femur is now considered to be preferable to immobilization in a plaster cast. The *transcervical* or *subcapital* fracture is best treated by a Smith-Petersen 3-flange nail. The fracture at the *base of the femoral neck* or through the *trochanters* should be treated by a combination Smith-Petersen nail and a 6-hole plate. Fractures of the *shaft of the femur* are best treated by inserting an intramedullary rod and at the same time placing across the fracture line many 1 to 2-inch osteoperiosteal bone grafts obtained with an osteotome from the exposed femoral fragments.

After such internal fixation the patient can be gotten out of bed and into a wheel chair on the second day. If not too feeble, he may use a walker after 1 week. Pneumonia, cardiac decompensation and decubitus ulcers are very rare when this program is followed.

Complication of Internal Fixation. The following case demonstrates one possible complication of internal fixation of fractures of the hip.

Mrs. M. L., aged 50, was admitted to the Cook County Hospital on January 7, 1941, with a diagnosis of foreign body in the pelvis. The history of the patient revealed that she had been in the hospital from May, 1939, to January, 1940, suffering from a fracture of the left hip. She was operated on by an orthopedic surgeon for malunion of the fracture, and the fractured fragments were pinned with a flange in August, 1939. She left the hospital on January 3, 1940, and was to return in about a month because of nonunion. When she returned, it was found that she had a cardiac disorder which required attention, so she was advised to return 2 months later. She failed to return at the appointed time, remaining in bed at home because of pain in the left hip on motion. About November, 1940, she began to have pain again, as well as frequency of urination accompanied by burning and dribbling of urine. About the same time she began to complain of pain in the rectum. On November 8, 1940, she was operated on for a strangulated hernia. On December 11, the day before she was ready to leave the hospital, she requested that a roentgenogram be taken of her hip. It was discovered that the metal flange had worked its way into the pelvis. The pain in the left hip was so intense on walking that the patient remained in the hospital for the purpose of having the flange removed. These pains were accompanied by a bearing-down sensation in the rectum and the bladder, associated with pain on urination and defecation. The pain kept her awake at night, and she required sedatives. The x-ray report on January 17, 1941, read as follows: "Anteroposterior view of pelvis revealed the presence of a metal flange extending from the level of the left acetabulum upward and medially to the midportion of the true pelvis. The pointed end of the flange appears to be, stereoscopically, above and behind the urinary bladder in about the midportion of the true pelvis. There is subluxation present in the left hip, the femur being upward and laterally of the head of the bone showing decalcification and moderate absorption." At the end of January, 1941, an operation was performed by the same surgeon who introduced the flange from the pelvis. The operation consisted essentially of the following steps: Smith-Petersen incision; dissection to capsule of joint; incision of joint capsule; elements of fibrous union between the head of the femur and the femoral neck. Flange located and removed. Wound closed. The patient recovered.

Fractures of the Upper Thigh. Owing to the pull of the lateral muscles in fractures of the upper portion of the thigh, the fragments have a tendency toward lateral displacement. This must be corrected by putting the thigh in abduction, with slight flexion of the hip.

Surgical Differences Between Intracapsular and Extracapsular Fractures of the Neck of the Femur. There are important surgical differences between intracapsular and extracapsular fractures of the neck of the femur. In intracapsular fracture, callus formation fails in the great majority of cases, causing delay in bony union, with resulting pseudarthrosis. In the extracapsular fracture, there is likely to be a superabundance of callus, with resulting difficulty in movement. In the intracapsular fracture, necrosis of the head of the femur is not infrequent, and when this occurs extirpation becomes necessary, which carries with it all the possible dangers of an operation on the joint, including infection.

Extension-Traction of Fractures of the Lower Extremity. In these fractures *the skin* in the region of the head of the fibula and of the malleoli is subject to great pressure and should be protected with pads.

Fractures of the Thigh. Before any therapeutic measure is decided on in fractures of the thigh, the following must be clearly established: (1) site of the fracture, (2) the degree of lateral displacement, (3) the degree of shortening of the limb, (4) the extent of concomitant injury to the soft tissues, (5) the extent of the affected area, (6) the presence or absence of muscular interposition, and (7) the condition of the knee.

In examining the patient with hip disease, one should not fail to have the patient stripped and examine both hips simultaneously.

In hip injuries, never neglect thorough x-ray examination (front and lateral views). Sometimes, even after studying the roentgenograms, one may overlook existing fracture. The possibility of a spontaneous fracture of the upper portion of the femur must be considered in some cases (previous operation in some part of the body for carcinoma). In 15 pathologic fractures, Copeland found 13 to be due to metastases from carcinoma of the breast.

Fractures About the Knee. The knee joint structures are a site of predilection for osteomyelitis and sarcoma. Mistakes in diagnosis here are common.

In traumatisms of the knee, never rely on clinical manifestations alone: external signs may be relatively slight in serious injury. Again, the reverse may be true. Therefore, in knee injuries and injuries of the external meniscus, always make thorough x-ray examinations (stereoscopic studies).

In *fractures of the patella,* ask the patient to extend the limb actively in order not to overlook the possible existence of laceration of the quadriceps muscle.

Wounds of the knee may involve the joint. Thorough exploration is imperative. The possibility of the existence of a gonococcic arthritis or concomitant osteomyelitis should be kept in mind.

In suturing a fractured patella, strong wire should be used, and the sutures should pass through the cartilage. Silver wire may be too weak. Periosteal silk sutures of the patella are entirely insufficient. I have had a number of disappointing results where kangaroo tendon has been used in fractures of the patella, with marked separation of the fragments.

Suture of the patella under the strictest aseptic precautions is considered to be a safe method. But here, as in any surgical intervention in and about joints, danger of infection always looms as a possibility.

Circular osteorrhaphy tends to avoid many operative complications which may eventuate when a joint is deliberately opened and subjected to manipulations.

The usual technical errors in operations for fractures of the patella are insufficient apposition of bone fragments, remaining blood clots and incomplete freshening of the fractured bone surfaces to be apposed. Improper wiring may cause angular deformity. Stiffness of the knee, particularly in the aged and in patients suffering from various forms of arthritis, may follow prolonged immobilization. On the other hand, immobilization for too brief a period may be responsible for refractures, which are occasionally observed (according to some authors, in 8 to 10 per cent of the cases).

In intra- or para-articular fractures (condyles of the femur, tibia) hemarthroses are not infrequent. These may be followed by stiffness or restricted mobility of the affected joint. Exuberant callus is frequent. Prompt and proper orthopedic reduction and constant control are essential. Be on the alert and in these cases avoid such possible complications as genu varum, genu valgum or genu recurvatum. Surgical treatment is preferable, especially if there is marked displacement of the fractured internal tuberosity of the tibia. Fractures complicated with vascular lesions are particularly serious about the knee joint.

Arthritides of the knee may lead to much crippling, and a guarded prognosis should always be given.

In arthritis of the knee, exploratory puncture has its place, but some prefer arthrotomy (Forgue and Aimes). When arthrotomy of the knee is performed, the following precautions should be taken: ample incision, exploration of recesses, etc. Drainage of retrocondylar spaces is difficult and may require deep lateral incisions and on occasion even the resection of the posterior condyles of the femur (Läwen). In serious affections only timely resection may save the patient's life.

One of the most common complications of patellar fractures is retraction or atrophy of the quadriceps extensor muscle, and this should be guarded against by early massage and passive movements of the knee.

The bloodless methods of treating transverse fractures of the patella commonly lead to faulty consolidation of the upper fragment. In suturing a patellar fracture, any torn lateral ligaments should be included in the repair.

Owing to vulnerability to infection of the knee joint, the knife used to make the skin incision should not be used to open the joint. There is need for special surgical precautions about this point. Before closing the joint, following repair of a fractured patella, clear out the accumulated blood clots. If the best results are to be obtained, all strain should be kept off the fragments for 7 or 8 weeks, particularly in heavy individuals.

The most important sequel in resection of the knee is the resultant shortening of the limb, which may vary from 5 to 20 cm., in a growing child. The shortening may not always be due to the operation alone, as there is reason to believe that the tuberculous process itself may interfere with nutrition and affect growth. Resection should be avoided in a growing child. Another result of knee resection is contracture.

Fractures of the upper portion of the leg, particularly if extensive, may eventuate in circulatory disturbances and, finally, in gangrene. Pseudarthrosis and stiffness of the knee are frequent sequelae.

Fractures of the diaphysis of the bones of the leg, generally considered a simple condition, may frequently be followed by shortening of the limb, deviation of the axis of the leg or pseudarthrosis. Oblique or v-shaped fractures of the lower third of the leg are, on occasion, particularly troublesome. Dislocation may complicate the fracture. Successful reduction and good immobilization in these cases are often difficult. A projecting upper fragment, if improperly reduced and immobilized, may perforate the superimposed tegumentary structures. Deviation of the axis of the leg or other deformity may result. The rather frequent occurrence and persistence of trophic disturbances must be remembered (persistent edema, impeded circulation). In these cases bone consolidation sometimes requires from 3 to 6 months or even a year if the fracture is oblique or spiral. Therefore, besides correct reduction, proper traction and extended immobilization are imperative.

In fractures of the bones of the leg, it is always well to flex the knee, as this tends to overcome shortening. Shortening usually occurs when both bones of the leg are broken. Extension should never be so forcible as to separate the fragments, and the extension weight should be reduced as time goes on.

Pain in the tibia (nocturnal) should recall the possibility of syphilis.

Ulcers of the leg often offer diagnostic difficulties. Some so-called varicose ulcers prove to be of syphilitic nature. Antiluetic treatment should be instituted even when the serologic examinations are negative. Some cases prove to be of mycotic origin.

Fractures of the Ankle. A wrong diagnosis and improper treatment lead to unfavorable prognosis, functional disturbances, pain, deformity and stiffness. Make a thorough clinical and roentgenologic examination. Prevent ligamentary and tendinous adhesions.

Fractures of Toes. In some severe cases, in order to avoid deformity and stiff joints, a primary amputation or exarticulation may be advisable, as a better functional result will be obtained.

Fracture of Heel. In a fracture of the os calcis which involves the articular surface of the bone and causes distortion, if conservative measures of treatment are adopted, the functional result will almost certainly be unsatisfactory. In such cases operative treatment, either arthrodesis or even excision of the astragalocalcaneal joint, may on occasion be considered.

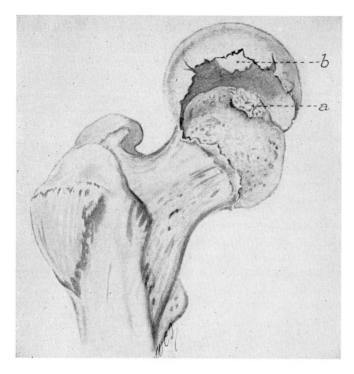

FIG. 126. Tuberculosis of the hip joint. (a) Tuberculous foci beneath the cartilage which has been elevated by subjacent suppuration. (b) Perforation of cartilage followed by infection of the hip joint.

In malleolar fractures there is great danger of the occurrence of flat foot.

The *manual reduction of a fracture of the tibia* should be carried out under a general anesthetic.

Rupture of the Bladder. In fractures of the pelvis, if there is blood in the urine, we must keep in mind the possibility of injury to the bladder and rupture of the urethra. If the latter is suspected, a metal catheter should not be used. If rupture of the bladder is suspected, it is advisable to inject some colloidal silver preparation and make a skiagram. If rupture is discovered, one should operate at once. Delays in making a diagnosis are dangerous.

JOINT INFECTIONS

The cardinal factors in diagnosing hip disease are limping, comparative position of the trochanters, Trendelenburg's sign, the position of the head of the femur and the comparative length of the lower limbs. The Nélaton line will aid in ascertaining the position of the great trochanter.

TUBERCULOSIS

In cases of tuberculous coxitis (Fig. 126) there is very little chance for diagnostic error,

but its early recognition is desirable for successful therapy. It must be differentiated from acute and chronic inflammatory conditions of the hip, from psoas contracture, bursitis, periarticular inflammations, epiphyseal detachment, fracture of the neck of the femur, coxa vara, Perthes' disease, tumors, hysteria, neuralgias and sacro-iliac slip. Patients less than 15 years old should be treated conservatively. Resection of a joint should only be a last resort in desperate cases.

Errors in diagnosis of bone and joint tuberculosis are very frequent. According to Forgue, do not depend primarily on radiologic signs of foci of infection; these may be delayed for several months. Study and evaluate clinical manifestations. In doubtful cases, only waiting will confirm the diagnosis. In the meantime, the patient must be at absolute rest and the affected limb rigorously immobilized. During the first 6 months the usual radiologic findings are decalcification of the affected epiphysis, narrowing of the intra-articular spaces and indistinct and irregular outlines of the joint cartilages.

Bone and joint tuberculosis are most frequently confounded with neuralgia, rheumatism, infectious arthritis and the so-called "growing pains" of adolescents. Čalvé has stated the belief that about 50 per cent of the cases of arthritis of the hip and knee joints may be of tuberculous origin.

To aid in the diagnosis of these conditions, laboratory examinations are essential (Bešredka's, skin reaction, cultures or injections of guinea pigs and other means of finding tubercle bacilli). In localized infections diagnosis is easier. In such cases the roentgenographic image shows stricter localization.

Before a joint is considered healed and movements of the patient allowed, pain must have disappeared and roentgenograms must show progressive recalcification and reconstruction of the cortex of the affected diaphysis.

The general condition of the patient must be improved (complete rest, nourishing food, vitamin D, cod liver oil, etc., climatic therapy and plenty of air and sunshine). Local treatment consists chiefly in prolonged absolute rest.

Surgical intervention should be resorted to, especially in children, only on strictest indications.

As already pointed out, haste at intervention in the beginning of the infection and in a rapidly evolving focus should be avoided whenever possible. Where the process of evolution of the infection is in an advanced stage, the focus of infection is well on the way to recalcification and the lesions are restricted. When the focus is localized and likely to be removed by surgical means, en bloc resection and excision usually yield excellent results, particularly in adults. Again, surgical intervention is justified only when such contemplated procedures as arthrodesis of an affected anatomic locality or a bone graft in Pott's disease offer reasonable assurance for success.

Roeder and Graffin point out that the best time for operation under such conditions is when the patient is afebrile and the appetite, sleep, weight and blood picture have much improved. Anemia, high leukocyte count and generally poor condition of the patient contraindicate operative intervention. In urgent cases operation should not be delayed. Under such circumstances, incision and drainage of "cold abscesses," excision or resection in secondary acute arthritis and amputation in fistualiza-tions with secondary septicemic conditions are the surgical methods usually resorted to.

Arthrotomy. In dealing with a tuberculous knee joint, arthrotomy has been, to a great extent, discarded, owing to the danger of fistula formation and secondary infection. Nevertheless, in discussing tuberculous knee joints, deQuervain stated that as good, or even better, results can be obtained from a well-conducted surgical operation as from conservative measures, such as heliotherapy, ultraviolet irradiation, etc. The latter measures bring about only temporary results—a "clinical latency"—not a cure. Operation, when successful, gives a definite cure.

From the economic standpoint, in the case of adults who have to earn their living and perhaps support a family, the time element is of great importance and in these cases operation is indicated. Resection of the joint, for many reasons, is the operation of choice. Opinions differ in regard to the removal of the patella, some believing it to be a choice location for tubercle bacilli; but if removed, there is very little protection of the knee joint from pressure, and necrosis may result from a tight plaster bandage placed over the joint.

TORTICOLLIS

The diagnosis of torticollis alone is not a sufficient criterion for the institution of treatment. Different types of torticollis will have to be distinguished, and each type requires its own treatment. While a muscular torticollis will require tenotomy of the sternocleidomastoid muscle, it would be entirely futile to perform this operation on a torticollis caused by a malformation of the cervical spine. Therefore, roentgenograms should always be taken. In the case of muscular torticollis, an open tenotomy should be performed. Subcutaneous tenotomy has been carried out with success but should be abandoned in most cases because the procedure is inaccurate and because there is the danger of severing the external jugular vein and the phrenic nerve. The decision as to which attachment of the sternocleidomastoid muscle should be severed depends entirely on the findings on physical examination. If satisfactory correction can be achieved without causing too great a bulging of the upper part of the affected muscle, it

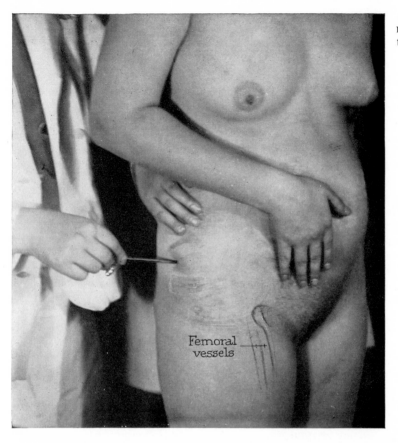

FIG. 127. Correct method of aspirating the hip joint.

Femoral vessels

will be sufficient to perform a lower tenotomy only, but it must be remembered that two attachments will have to be divided, namely, the clavicular and the costal attachments. If, on the other hand, the correction cannot be accomplished, or if the upper part of the sternocleidomastoid bulges considerably after correction, a double tenotomy will have to be done, that is, a tenotomy of the mastoid portion on one end and a tenotomy of the clavicular and costal insertion on the other end.

ASPIRATIONS OF JOINTS

Diagnostic and therapeutic punctures must be carefully executed, lest infectious material gain access to surrounding structures, with resulting contamination.

It is probably more important to prevent infection of the joint space in noninfectious conditions and superimposed infection in patients who already have an infection. For this reason rigid asepsis is necessary, and the needle should be inserted slanting toward the joint from a perfectly normal area of the skin.

Aspiration of the ankle joint should not be done on the inner side of the Achilles tendon, as the tibial artery or nerve may be injured by the needle. On the outer side of the Achilles tendon, the sheath of the peroneal tendon may be pricked by the needle, causing inflammation if the contents of the joint are infected.

The wrist joint can best be aspirated between the tendons of the extensor pollicis and indicis.

Aspiration of the hip joint is dangerous because of the possibility of traumatizing the femoral artery, which may result in the formation of an aneurysm. Palpation of the artery may not be easy when the joint and especially the iliac bursa are greatly swollen, with infiltration of the soft parts (Fig. 127).

In aspirating the knee joint for the withdrawal of exudate, the best place to insert the needle is in the spaces between the inner or outer edges of the patella, in the depression between the femur and the patella.

INFECTIONS OF THE HAND

The most common conditions which bring patients with hand lesions to the surgeon are the complications following infections arising out of simple injuries. Such infections should be treated from their very inception as serious surgical conditions. One should never temporize with them. Wherever indicated, the early adoption of hospital treatment will be found the best and, in the end, the most economic procedure.

If there is no immediate possibility of treating injuries of the hand thoroughly, the first thing to do is to ensure prompt and adequate hemostasis. Many complications may be avoided if proper therapy is instituted within the first 12 hours following the accident. To avoid the development of infection, promptly cleanse and excise all necrotic, soiled and suspicious tissues. Never suture the wound completely at this stage, because one can never be sure of the presence of remaining microorganisms lurking in the depths of the wound. It is safest to consider all traumatic lesions of the hand infected and treat them accordingly. If one is reasonably sure of the nonexistence of infection (6 or more hours after injury), all foreign bodies should be removed from the hand and the affected and devitalized tissues excised. In such cases local anesthesia should be used for injuries of the fingers and general anesthesia for complicated injuries of the hand. Explore the wound carefully; make sure that no tendons have been seriously injured.

The importance of the hand is so great in the economy of life and daily work that special precaution is necessary in all surgical manipulations connected with it. We must be sure that, following any operation on the hand, there will be no, or at least the minimum, interference with its function.

Kanavel, in his *Infections of the Hand,* stated that minor infections of the thenar space are often accompanied by marked edema on the dorsum. The diagnosis of pus in the thenar space is frequently erroneous, as the dorsal space is apparently involved. Edema on the dorsum is always greater than in the palmar aspect, even though a collection of pus may be in the latter region. A collection of pus is always accompanied by an indurated surface.

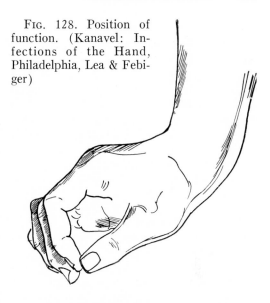

Fig. 128. Position of function. (Kanavel: Infections of the Hand, Philadelphia, Lea & Febiger)

Kanavel further stated that in hand infections the common habit of squeezing a wound or lesion to evacuate its contents cannot be condemned too strongly. An ample incision will be sufficient. Rubber tubes should not be inserted for drainage because of the danger of pressure necrosis; but if something must be used, let it be plain Vaselined rubber strips.

EVACUATION OF PUS

The great danger in infections of the hand is that the process may extend to the tendon sheaths. If possible, an incision to evacuate the pus must be made before this occurs.

In infections of the fingers, when the entire phalanx is involved, it is a technical error to make an incision on the palmar aspect, as this leaves a scar over the tactile part of the finger. The incision should be lateral and should not extend beyond the base of the phalanx, as it may result in tenosynovitis. Incisions should always be placed well to the side of a tendon; never incise over joints unless this is absolutely necessary.

In opening an abscess in the middle palmar space, guard important functional structures against injury and infection.

One of the most important factors in dealing with injuries of the hand, as pointed out by Kanavel, is that when placing the hand in a splint, it should always be put in the "position of function," even though the tendons are lost (Fig. 128).

AFTERCARE

In lesions of the hand which have been incised, Kanavel advised the use of hot, moist dressings during the first few days, as they relieve pain and wall off infection. They should not be continued for more than 48 hours since they tend to produce excessive granulation. The danger of systemic invasion over, passive and active movements should be initiated at once, that is, shortly after the primary incision, in order to prevent adhesions, particularly about the joints.

TENDON SUTURE

In wounds with injury to the tendons older than 4 to 6 hours, it is preferable to wait before suturing the tendons until the danger of infection has passed, approximately 2 or 3 days (Iselin). Sometimes injured tendons recover spontaneously.

Tendons should be respected and as much of the tendon as possible should be saved. Caution is advised when incising around nerve structures and important blood vessels. The surgeon must know the position of the tendon sheaths.

The functional result in injuries of the hand is of much greater importance than the esthetic appearance. Treatment is not evaluated by the number of fingers saved but by their functioning capacity. The thumb is the most important digit and deserves particular attention.

According to Forgue, if ligation of blood vessels, removal of segments of tendons, metacarpal bones or even fingers become unavoidable, it is best to intervene promptly in order to frustrate infection and to save all digits possible. Forgue admonishes further that it is an error to try to save fingers if many tendons are cut and metacarpal bones or phalanges are badly splintered. Here infection usually develops, and secondary amputation becomes imperative. Radical measures are preferable to superconservatism in obviously hopeless situations.

SECONDARY AMPUTATIONS

In 150 amputations, Dujardin-Beaumetz observed that a secondary amputation of one or more badly injured fingers greatly improves the total functional value of the hand. They also believe that, besides amputation of a hopelessly injured finger, it is also well to remove the head and forepart of the corresponding metacarpal bone.

The hand itself should be kept in dorsal flexion at the wrist, at an angle of 45°. The fingers should be in semiflexion, the thumb abducted from the flexor surface of the hand and rotated so that the flexor surface of the thumb is opposite the flexor surface of the distal phalanx of the index finger. Injured hands should never be permitted to be simply extended in dressings.

Injury to Radial Artery. When an infection of the hand has extended to the forearm, be careful, in incising, to avoid injuring the radial artery.

Secondary Hemorrhage. Occurring in the forearm after long-continued suppuration about the vessels, this nearly always involves the ulnar artery. In such a case the surgeon should not temporize but should incise and ligate the bleeding vessel.

LYMPHATIC INFECTIONS

I agree with Kanavel that the treatment of lymphatic infections of the hand is based on two principles—conservatism and conservation. Hot, moist dressings, applied voluminously, should be used until the infection is conquered. The Bier treatment is of some value in preventing rapid extension of the infection. Sulfa-drug therapy is, of course, indicated.

Incision in this type of infection is illadvised. The tendency of the surgeon to incise is due to his desire to "do something," rather than to an exact knowledge of what to do. Incisions should never be made unless there is an absolute certainty that an accumulation of pus is present. Here treatment of lymphatic infections differs from that of other infections of the hand and forearm.

TETANUS

While not so common now as formerly, tetanus is nevertheless liable to occur in extensive or even apparently insignificant injuries of the extremities complicated by infected open wounds. Prophylactic injections of antitetanus serum should invariably be given immediately in such cases. No matter how small the infection-atrium may appear, it is best to play safe.

GAS-BACILLUS INFECTION

One should always keep in mind the possibility of gas-bacillus infection. An open untreated wound of suspicious appearance should not be sutured because of the danger of infection.

X-RAY BURNS

Great care should be exercised in using x-rays for therapeutic purposes. If one is not certain about the technic, he should refer the patient to an expert. Figures 129 and 130 depict the hand of a patient who was referred to me for possible relief, following destruction of the tissues of the palm by the x-rays. As Figure 129 demonstrates, the treatment had destroyed the tissues down to the tendons. A series of skin transplants eventually cured

the patient. The results are not always so gratifying, however; x-ray burns are difficult to heal. Not infrequently there is more damage from roentgenotherapy than from the disease for which it is applied. It is wise to become expert in its use before attempting its application.

CARBOLIC ACID GANGRENE

In treating infections about the extremities, beware of carbolic acid (phenol) gangrene. It is well to remember that a 1 per cent solution of phenol, applied to the surface for 24 hours, may result in gangrene. Stronger concentrations act with proportionate rapidity in bringing about tissue destruction. V. Stapelmohr reports a case in which the application of a 5 per cent solution of lysol for 12 hours to the thumb of a 53-year-old woman resulted in gangrene of the thumb.

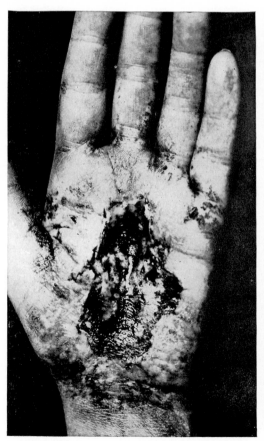 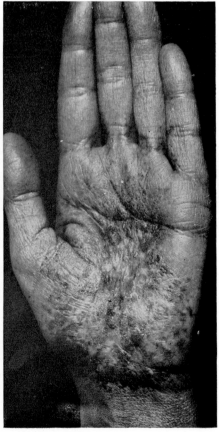

FIG. 129 (*Left*). X-ray burn of palm of left hand.
FIG. 130 (*Right*). Appearance of same hand 9 weeks later after skin transplantation.

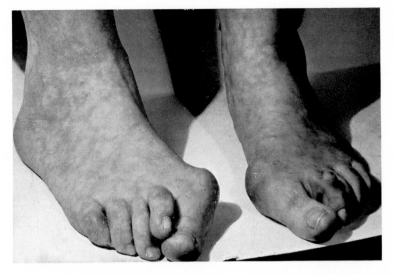

Fig. 131. Associated bunions and hammer toes.

DEFORMITIES AND LESIONS OF THE TOES

SYNDACTYLISM

Webbing of the toes should not be treated surgically until roentgenograms have been taken to determine whether or not there is a bridging of the bones of the webbed toes. Circulation should also be studied, and if the nails of the two toes have grown as one, it is best to consider a skin graft rather than a reconstruction operation.

POLYDACTYLISM

Here again, roentgenograms should be taken before any surgical operation is attempted in order to determine which is the normal toe and which is the accessory toe.

HAMMER TOES

The overriding toe does not usually respond well to operations designed for hammer toes. Amputation should be given consideration (Fig. 131).

PARONYCHIA

Paronychia of the great toe should not be treated as a minor affection. Never neglect to study the circulation of the lower extremity before performing any surgical procedure. The paronychia may be due to infection in a toe whose circulation is so impaired that healing cannot result favorably.

TUMORS

Tumors of the toes are only very rarely malignant; consequently, amputation of the leg or the foot, at the ankle, should not be done but merely amputation of the toe, if other forms of treatment do not yield the desired results.

HALLUX VALGUS

It is very important to differentiate a simple hallux valgus from a metatarsus primus varus because the latter requires an entirely different operative procedure. Distinction is possible only by x-ray studies; the history should prove the congenital nature of the latter deformity.

HALLUX RIGIDUS

Never operate before an x-ray study of both feet of the patient has been made in order to determine an existing tendency to osteoarthritis. If such tendency exists, refrain from surgical attempts at the joint unless a complete excision of the metatarsal head is contemplated.

OTHER DIAGNOSTIC AND THERAPEUTIC ERRORS IN SURGERY OF THE EXTREMITIES

NADELUNG'S DEFORMITY

It is generally believed that operation for

cosmetic reasons only should not be undertaken. The proper indication for surgical intervention should be the presence of marked pain and disability. It is also important to differentiate this deformity from a malunion of a Colles' fracture, which can be accomplished easily by taking a careful history, by examining both wrists and by taking roentgenograms of both wrists.

GANGRENE

One should not overlook the frequent occurrence of gangrene caused by metabolic diseases.

LIPOMA

It is to be remembered that not every tumor which is freely movable, globular in outline and apparently unattached to the surrounding structures is a lipoma. A patient was referred to me, by a man who is considered a good diagnostician, for the removal of a "lipoma" of the thigh. The physician was misled in this case by the clinical symptoms, for the tumor proved to be a fibrosarcoma.

INJURIES OF THE SEMILUNAR CARTILAGES AND LIGAMENTS

Diagnostic errors often arise in confusing "joint mice," Hoffa's disease, distortion, contusion, joint-fracture, tuberculosis, gonorrheal joint, rheumatism, gout, syphilis, arthritis deformans and arthropathia neuropathica of the knee joint, nutritional disturbances resulting in osseous pathology (Fig. 132), benign tumors of the skeleton (Fig. 133), developmental bone changes, such as "oyster-shell bone," osteoporosis, etc.

Osteomyelitis nonpurulenta, osteomyelitis sclerosans and bone abscess—all three can cause errors in diagnosis; they are sometimes diagnosed as "periostitis," tuberculosis, syphilis, etc., all of which must be differentiated.

ULCERS

It is important, for the purpose of treat-

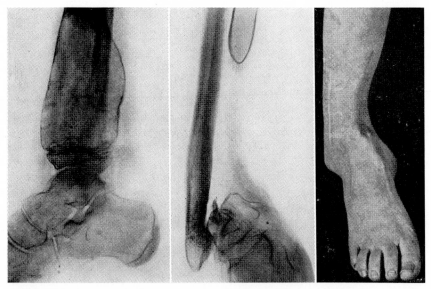

FIG. 132. A surgeon who was not competent to make a diagnosis from the roentgenogram and failed to do a biopsy before resorting to definitive surgery excised the distal half of the tibia of a 14-year-old girl because of a mistaken diagnosis of malignant tumor. A skilled roentgenologist or surgeon would recognize this as a benign bone cyst. Few qualified surgeons would do radical surgery without confirming the diagnosis by biopsy or exploration. Eight years after this needless mutilation, the 21-year-old patient, an attractive young woman, was still severely crippled. (Compere, E. L.: S. Clin. North America 13:1265)

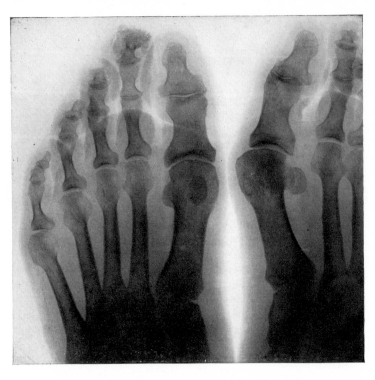

FIG. 133. Osteoma (benign) of terminal phalanx of toe.

ment, to distinguish between an ordinary varicose or simple ulcer of the leg and syphilitic, tuberculous or malignant ulcers. An effort should be made to differentiate early sarcoma from other swellings in the leg. One should exhaust all available diagnostic methods to arrive at a correct diagnosis.

Congenital Clubfoot

It is a great error to delay treatment beyond the earliest possible moment. Therefore, the obstetrician is the one who should encourage the parents to have treatment started the first day of life, and it is the duty of the pediatrician to see that the treatments are carried on until a final successful conclusion has been reached. Delay in treatment, therefore, is one of the most disastrous things that can happen to a child who has clubfeet.

Two types of treatment are in vogue, and both give good results, in most cases, if the details necessary are closely adhered to. The most frequently used treatment is that of plaster of Paris casts, which, for purposes of simplification, will be called treatment by immobilization, as contrasted with the Dennis Brown treatment, which will be called the treatment by mobilization.

The cast treatment is beset with many pitfalls. In general, it is unwise to leave the plaster of Paris casts on these deformed feet for longer than one week, unless one uses Dr. Kyte's method of wedge casting. The greatest error in this method is forcing the forefoot into a corrected position and forgetting the malalignment that usually exists between the calcaneus and the astragalus. Another error is to attempt to correct the equinus position too rapidly and without supporting the entire arch and sole of the foot. Placing the fulcrum of force too far anteriorly produces a rocker-foot, and this should be avoided. It is an error to stop treatment after the varus deformity has been eliminated. Overcorrection of the varus deformity to produce a valgus position is desirable; moreover, this correction is best accomplished before attempting to correct the equinus deformity. One great fault that occurs is the neglect of the surgeon to follow his talipes cases for a number of years after he has secured the initial correction. Nature has a tendency to reestablish the varus equinus deformity; therefore, constant treatment and supervision are necessary over a period of a number of years. This tendency to return to the varus equinus position can be minimized by the use of post-casting physical therapy.

In older cases, neglect to lengthen the Achilles tendon before attempting to correct the equinus position may cause rocker-foot. When the lengthening of the Achilles tendon is necessary, it should not be done by the usual tenotomy method, but by an open operation on the tendon, so as to avoid a complete separation of cut ends of the tendon, which will not grow together in the same manner as those tendons which have a sheath.

Avoid the Thomas wrench and other gadgets previously used for the forceful and rapid correction of the deformity, as these gadgets usually cause injury to the cartilage and the epiphyseal "anlages" of the bones of the foot, thus resulting in malformed bones and painful feet.

Pressure sores can occur when the cast method is used for correction; consequently, the toes of the foot must be constantly observed for circulatory disturbances. The general comfort of the child will also guide the surgeon.

Many operations for clubfoot in older patients have been designed but need not be discussed here.

FLATFOOT

In general, three types of flatfoot may be considered, namely, (1) flexible flatfoot, (2) spastic flatfoot and (3) rigid flatfoot.

Generally, when one is talking about flatfoot he is referring to the longitudinal arch of the foot. The greatest error is usually that of not recognizing the type of flatfoot that is present. The common type is that of flexible flatfoot, which usually does not require surgery. It can best be treated by supportive measures. In this type a usual error is to overlook the general health of the patient. The customary error in treating the rigid type is that of attempting to accomplish an end-result by supportive measures. Surgery is usually indicated in rigid flatfoot.

The spastic variety is usually confused with one of the other two, most often the rigid type.

HAMMER TOES

Removing callus formation in these deformities in the hope of correcting the pain which accompanies the deformity is useless. Tenot-omies of the extensor tendons will not cure the condition. It is an error to amputate the second toe for this deformity because many complications can arise following such an operation.

Differentiate ingrowing toenail from paronychia and subungual exostosis and osteomyelitis of the distal phalanx.

JOINT INFLAMMATION

Inflammation of joints results in frequent errors. There are many conditions (skin infections, erysipelas, gonorrhea, etc.) which may lead to inflammation of the joints. It is important that the physician should guard against possible complications. Be particularly on guard in infected fractures.

PAIN IN FOOT AND HEEL

Pains in the foot and heel region are often due to calcaneal and other bone spurs, which are quite frequently observed (in about 10 per cent of patients). They may follow periostitis, bursitis, traumatism, rheumatism or gout (roentgenograms will show them).

KOHLER'S DISEASE

This is frequently observed in children up to the fifth year and leads to diagnostic errors. It is observed in the scaphoid or in the second and third metatarsals and may be confused with tuberculous or other bone disease.

CHARCOT'S JOINT

No matter how desperate this condition may appear to be, always try antisyphilitic treatment. A man, aged 46, was sent to me with a diagnosis of Charcot's ankle and a request to amputate the limb. Antisyphilitic treatment was tried, and the results were striking.

FRAGILITAS OSSIUM

This calls for a guarded prognosis.

Figure 134 is a roentgenogram of the pelvis of a child before ossification is completed. The uninitiated in x-ray interpretations may err in interpreting a normal epiphyseal line for a fracture. Such an occurrence is not at all infrequent.

ICE AND HEAT

Applications of ice and heat should be made only with thorough supervision as to the in-

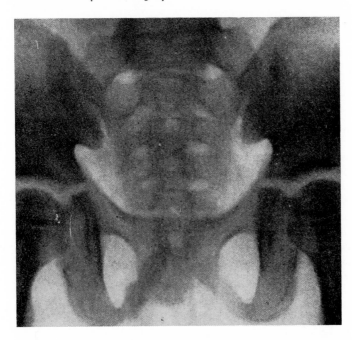

FIG. 134. Errors in diagnosis can result from misinterpretation of normal epiphyseal lines.

tensity of the medium and the length of the application.

COLD ABSCESS

Do not open a cold abscess. Fistula is likely to follow. Such abscesses are usually tuberculous in nature and can be treated more effectively by aspiration, thereby circumventing the formation of fistulas.

OSTEOTOMY

Remember that although, as a rule, there is no danger in performing an osteotomy in healthy bone, there is always the risk of wound infection. In an osteotomy of the upper portion of the femur there is risk of infecting the hip joint.

It is an error to use the osteotome as a lever to complete the fracture of a partially cut bone, for its cutting edge is likely to break. Care must also be exercised not to injure the soft tissues with the edge of the osteotome.

TETANUS

Königsweiser, in 1926, reported three fatal cases of tetanus following aseptic conditions on the plantar surface of subjects going barefoot. Derocque, in 1929, placed on record two more cases.

Case Report. In the first case, an arthrodesis for clubfoot was performed on May 6, the patient being a woman, aged 22. The first dressing was on the fifth day, when the wound seemed to be in good condition. Two days later there was slight trismus, which increased, with marked stiffness of the muscles of the neck; the other muscles, especially of the limb operated on, were not involved. There were no spasms and no rise in temperature. Subcutaneous injections of 150 cc. of tetanus serum were administered, but death occurred 9 days postoperatively, 36 hours after onset. The operative wound was always healthy, with no gangrene. Derocque did not believe the catgut was at fault, for it was from the regular supply of the hospital. The patient lived in the country, and it is very likely that she had walked in infected soil, had become inoculated, and the germs soon were beyond the reach of the most careful cleansing and applications of iodine.

The second case was that of a man, seriously ill, who was admitted to Derocque's service two days before death. In that case the tetanus came on after removal of a corn by a colleague whose surgical education guaranteed operative asepsis. Derocque has suggested that before undertaking any operation, even aseptic, on the foot, it may be well to give a preventive dose of antitetanus serum, especially for patients living in country districts.

Prophylaxis. Stolze discusses prophylaxis from a clinical and medicolegal standpoint. He states that, during the war, neglect to give a prophylactic injection was looked on as a technical error. The present teaching differs but slightly. While it is true that all wounds may be infected, those soiled by earth, animal or human excreta and any wounds in subjects walking barefoot are especially suspicious. In operative wounds, one should note those involving the bowel, the contents of which are likely to contain bacilli from raw vegetables, contacted in turn from manure. On the other hand, war wounds sustained in Africa seem to have rarely been followed by tetanus, and this complication grows less frequent in mines as horses are eliminated. Tetanus is quite exceptional after wounds with splinters or needles. Industrial wounds and those acquired in city life rarely are complicated by tetanus, an exception being made of butchers and those similarly occupied.

Stolze emphasized that an injection of serum protects against tetanus, provided it is made promptly. His studies were made at the Poliklinik where, from 1910 to 1928, some 10,800 accident cases were cared for. In a series of 1,277 in 1920, serum was given at once to 665 patients. Of 600 industrial accidents, principally from presses and lathes, 210 patients received no serum. All patients injured in the town itself received serum, and also those injured by automobiles. Some 9 per cent developed "serum disease," and 3 per cent had to stop work because of general urticaria. Three subjects had anaphylactic shock. No instance of tetanus developed in the 3,900 individuals receiving no serum, nor in those receiving serotherapy, but the inconveniences of the latter were such that this measure should not be resorted to indiscriminately. In some cases the injection must be repeated.

Murphy often referred to the prophylactic use of serum and also emphasized the need of efficient local measures.

Calvin and Goldberg report some rather startling findings regarding the prognosis in tetanus. They found that the mortality from tetanus at the Cook County Hospital had not decreased for a period of 15 years, despite the fact that in the last 5 years larger amounts of antitoxin were used and it was more often given intraspinally. A larger number of cases occurred between the 10- and 15-year period than in any other 5-year period, and the smallest number between 1 and 5 years. The mortality was lowest in the period between 5 and 10 years, 34 per cent, and highest between 1 and 5 years, 83 per cent. Tetanus was five times as common in males, and this proportion applied also to children. Following gunshot and powder wounds the mortality was 93 per cent; following lacerations, 44 per cent; and following puncture wounds about midway between. Tetanus following wounds about the head and face was not more fatal than following wounds of the limbs. The incubation period in 56 per cent was less than 10 days, the maximum on the fifth to the seventh day. The mortality in cases having an incubation period under 10 days was 84 per cent, whereas in those with an incubation period of 14 to 21 days it was 25 per cent. The deaths were more numerous on the second and third days of the disease and decreased rapidly thereafter. If a patient survived the first 3 days, the chances of ultimate recovery were much greater.

The available evidence in these cases as to the value of antitoxin does not justify any assertion that its use appreciably affects the character of the mortality, whether the serum is given intraspinally or intravenously or both, whether large doses are given or not or how early they may be given.

The old method of intracranial injection of serum has been revived in Germany. A trephine opening is made over the parietal area, and puncture of the cisterna magna without trephining had been used successfully a few times. At Wendel's clinic, according to Lehrnbecher, another success was obtained.

Case Report. A woman, aged 33, while scrubbing a floor, ran a splinter under a thumbnail. She pulled out part of it at once, and the rest was extracted by a physician some 3 hours later. By that time the thumb was swollen and painful with lymphangitis. Trismus appeared on the ninth day, March 19. By the next day tetanus was present, and an intraspinal injection of 100 units, under Avertin narcosis, was given. The wound was cleansed and still another fragment removed. On March 21, another spinal injection of 100 units was given, with no change in the condition. On the same evening cisternal puncture was performed, with the injection of 20 units. On March 22, she received 100 units intraspinally; on the following day, 200 units intravenously; and on the same evening the cisterna was repunctured, 30 cc. of cerebrospinal fluid removed and 100 units injected. Some improvement was noted the next day and 300 units were given, 100 intraspinally and 200 intravenously, and more Avertin was administered. The improvement continued, and the patient was out of danger early in April.

While the success in this instance was believed due to the puncture of the cisterna, it seemed uncertain, since the author stated that the patient received a total of 35.7 Gm. of Avertin, 1,900 cc. of magnesium sulfate, 1,660 units of serum (only 120 into the cisterna) and 30 cc. of Pronestyl.

Harris reports the case of a man, aged 45, who received a total of 180,000 units intraspinally, intravenously and intramuscularly! He made a complete recovery, with no resulting disability. The recovery was hastened by diathermy and massage for the general muscular soreness. It was noted that this man had been under the care of his family physician for several days before coming to the hospital. The doctor had expressed the opinion that the patient was "probably having a little touch of lockjaw" and was using liniment externally and epsom salts internally while waiting to make a positive diagnosis.

Lindemann, at Anschütz' clinic, reports that Avertin was used successfully in curing tetanus.

Case Report. A youth, aged 18, had sustained a puncture on the right dorsum from a nail 9 days before. An intraspinal injection of 100 units was given, also injections of magnesium sulfate and morphine-scopolamine. There was no definite effect after 4 days, and contractions of the respiratory muscles began. Then an enema of 6.5 Gm. of Avertin (0.1 Gm. to each Kg. of weight) stopped the spasms for 4 hours. The Avertin was continued until the ninth day, when spasms and trismus had disappeared. In all, 65 Gm. were given, in 10 enemas. After each injection the spasms stopped for 2 to 4 hours, lessening the danger of asphyxia and permitting feeding.

However, this plan fails in very serious cases. In a case of fulminant puerperal tetanus, death ensued despite hysterectomy and Avertin.

Beaulieu has announced the successful use of serotherapy.

Case Report. The patient was a woman, aged 36, who was seen 4 days after the onset of trismus. The atrium was not found at first. There were a few slight scratches that had been sustained during gardening but they had healed. Finally, an ingrowing toenail on the left big toe was discovered, and it was learned that a fortnight before this it had become red and discharged pus for a short time. This was believed to be the portal of entry, for the patient lived in the country and often went into her garden with light slippers on. She recovered after receiving a total of 650 cc. of serum, in doses of 50 to 100 cc.

MYOGELOSIS

Many errors are committed daily in the diagnosis and treatment of diseases of the muscular system. Such conditions as lumbago, myalgia, the arthritides and so-called rheumatic affections are usually due to a condition described by Max Lange as myogelosis. This condition arises from pathologic changes in the muscles and readily yields if the etiologic factor is ascertained and proper therapy is instituted.

OSTEOMYELITIS

ACUTE OSTEOMYELITIS

Do not attempt to diagnose an early osteomyelitis by the use of roentgenograms; these will give disappointing results here.

Avoid operation in the acute stage. It only spreads the disease or kills the patient. Use one of the sulfa compounds, orally if possible, otherwise intravenously.

In prolonged drainage in an osteomyelitic area there is danger of erosion of the vessels by the drain.

Complications. In an extensive removal of necrotic bone in osteomyelitis, the possibility of fracture should be remembered and guarded against.

In extensive osteomyelitic processes involving the femur or the humerus, the risks of shortening or deformity are very great.

In obscure fevers, particularly in children, always think of the possibility of acute osteomyelitis. Treat it promptly; surgically.

To rule out osteomyelitis, although no definite bone localization exists, blood culture should always be resorted to.

Secondary osteomyelitic septicemia does not

offer great diagnostic difficulties because of an already existing focus of infection. The sudden onset of pain and strict localization are characteristic symptoms of osteomyelitis.

In the further evolution of the condition, the affected limb becomes intensely swollen, edema of the skin develops, the glistening surface and dilated veins display the entire picture, giving the impression of a deep lymphangitis, which, however, is rare. Error may be avoided by careful scrutiny of the underlying bone. Adenopathy, while a symptom of lymphangitis, is rarely seen in osteomyelitis. During the first ten days after the beginning of the infection, roentgenograms usually do not show any characteristic lesion. Nevertheless, one should always think of a possible osteomyelitis. M. Faivre calls attention to a strictly localized subarticular edema, revealing clear-cut outlines of the soft tissues on the roentgenogram. Later the roentgenogram may show evidences of involvement (decalcification of the metaphysis, periosteal changes).

In treating an established osteomyelitis, one should not use a sharp spoon or a curet to remove the suppurating medulla, as it is likely also to remove osteogenetic portions of the medulla which have escaped suppuration. No bone should be removed unless for the purpose of ample drainage; on the other hand, removal of all devitalized tissue must be complete, otherwise sinuses may result.

Necrotic Bone. Definitely necrotic bone should be removed before it degenerates into a true sequestrum, that is, before the dead portion has become locked in and buried by newly formed periosteal bone (involucrum). The best time to remove necrotic bone is while the periosteum is still soft and plastic.

Juxta-articular pain often leads to error. Osteomyelitis may be mistaken for acute articular joint rheumatism (Fig. 135). The differential diagnostic points between phlebitis and osteomyelitis should be kept in mind, lest errors lead to serious consequences. Patients giving a history of trauma should be thoroughly scrutinized.

In nurslings the possibility of pseudoparalysis of Parrot should be taken into consideration.

Osteomyelitis may sometimes be mistaken for bone tumor and vice versa. X-ray examination is not always conclusive.

Osteomyelitis may initiate peripheral neoplastic changes due to a reaction of the periosteum similar to those observed in periosteal sarcoma. Biopsy is essential here.

Cortical osteitis of the diaphysis (Lériche and Baur) affects adults. It causes pains in the large bones (femur, humerus), tumefaction and slight rise of temperature. X-ray examination shows a cortical swelling and periosteal reaction. This form of bone pathology is similar to Ewing's tumor but develops in the metaphysis.

The site of osteomyelitic foci may cause diagnostic errors. When localized in the skull or in the spine, possibility of meningitis or typhoid should be kept in mind.

The chronic forms of osteomyelitis may be mistaken for Pott's disease; there are no clinical or radiologic signs distinguishing one from the other. Aspiration and examination of the pus, using aseptic precautions, are the diagnostic guides at our disposal (M. and R. Sieur).

Large swellings in the axilla may be mistaken for acute osteomyelitis of the humerus,

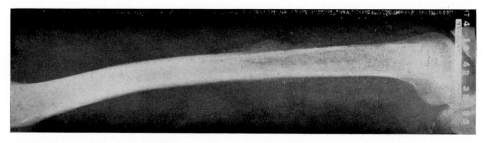

Fig. 135. Original diganosis in this case was acute rheumatic arthritis of knee, activated by a fall. Six weeks after onset, re-examination by x-ray revealed the true condition—acute osteomyelitis of the femur.

osteomyelitis of a rib or a simple inflammation of the axillary soft tissues.

Osteomyelitis of the hip is difficult to diagnose. It occasions an acute arthritis, the general symptoms of which mask the true pathology, particularly in nurslings. In enfeebled subjects it may be mistaken for coxalgia. The seat of pain must be carefully noted and the affected joint immobilized.

In osteomyelitis both undue abstention or too early intervention may be dangerous! Acute osteomyelitis is usually considered to be the result of a localized staphylococcic septicemia, and intervention during the septicemic stage is preferably avoided. It is different when the process is localized. The resistance of the organism against general infection should be fortified by all possible means.

Septicemia may also follow bone infection. In such cases abstention may lead to new focal localizations or even death. On the other hand, prompt intervention may not only be useless but also dangerous and may increase the death rate. Out of 15 children promptly operated on by Leveuf, 8 died; among 16 patients not undergoing operation, only 1 death occurred.

Crossen's statistics in this connection are illuminating: 26 per cent died after prompt operation, 15 per cent after delayed intervention. Death rates of early operation were: 39 per cent during the first 4 days, 35 per cent during the first week, 3 per cent during and 15 per cent after the second week. In 46 cases treated by simple incision, the death rate was 5 per cent. In 39 cases of bone-trephining operations the mortality rate was 40 per cent, and in exenteration operations 35 per cent. Many surgeons prefer to intervene promptly because of the danger of serious complications. Even in properly treated cases, osteomyelitis still yields a high death rate: 15 deaths and the necessity of 5 amputations in 94 cases (Ingelrans); 11 deaths in 59 cases (Sorel); 16 deaths in 72 cases (Boppe).

The prognosis at the beginning of the infection should always be guarded. In treating these cases the limb should be immediately immobilized in a fenestrated plaster cast, allowing easy access to the focus of infection. The general condition of the patient must be carefully watched and supported to resist the infection. If the evolution of the infection is favorable, intervention should be delayed. If it becomes progressively worse, operation at first should be limited to a withdrawal of pus localized under the periosteum. Then trephining may be done if the bone appears blanched and does not bleed and if the temperature is still high (Ombrédanne).

However, early in the infection, resection is rarely advocated. On occasion such procedure may appear to be justifiable, particularly in extensive necrotic processes of the diaphysis in which complications appear to be probable (Mathieu). On the other hand, the operation may become imperative when the bone is denuded, its marrow infected with marked suppuration; here prompt intervention is indicated.

General Care. Avoid massage and active use of the involved limb. Immobilize. Do not neglect general supporting measures. Resort to these as in any other acute infection: fluids, bed rest, nutritious diet, sedatives, blood transfusions and plasma infusions.

CHRONIC OSTEOMYELITIS

There is some debate as to whether or not a sequestrum should be removed and, if so, when.

Sequestrectomy. This should be done whenever there is sinus formation. Most surgeons believe a sequestrum should be removed as soon as the patient's general condition will permit.

Never neglect to use adequate mechanical support for external immobilization after extensive sequestrectomy.

Postsequestrectomy Treatment. There are two schools of thought as to postsequestrectomy treatment. One advocates the Orr method, and the other may be said to include all other methods, such as the maggot treatment, the use of Dakin's solution for irrigations, the packing with sulfa drugs and tight closure and the aluminum-potassium-nitrate method.

The Orr method is the simplest and cheapest, but withal the most odoriferous. A criticism of the Orr (bacteriophage?) method of treatment is that it leaves a quantity of scar tissue which interferes with functioning.

Baer's maggot treatment has been reported upon favorably as being a useful adjunct in the surgical treatment of chronic osteomyelitis.

In small hospitals, however, the breeding and care of sterile maggots is impractical, and their purchase is rather expensive. Moreover, the permanency of the results obtained by this method cannot yet be reported upon unequivocally.

Excellent results have been obtained with *the aluminum-potassium-nitrate method* in chronic infective suppurative processes, especially of bones. In the old cases, where surgical treatment is likely to be a failure, the results gained by the application of this compound are excellent. The compound is not an antiseptic but acts as an accelerator of bacterial growth, which at the same time lowers the virulence and the vitality of the organisms and increases the normal resistance of the body. In a series of 116 cases reported, over 75 per cent of the patients became ambulatory and able to pursue their vocations, coming to the clinic only for dressings, in contrast with the results of the radical surgical procedures of the past. Typical reactions from aluminum-potassium-nitrate applications over osteomyelitic foci are shown in Figures 136 and 137. Long hospitalization and later invalidism, with its attendant expense and discomfort, are eliminated. This aluminum-potassium-nitrate compound should certainly be given a trial when other methods of treating osteomyelitis and similar chronic suppurations have proved to be unsuccessful.

VARICOSE VEINS

Surgical Treatment

One of the principal reasons of failure in the surgical treatment of varicosities in the limbs is the lack of proper examination before

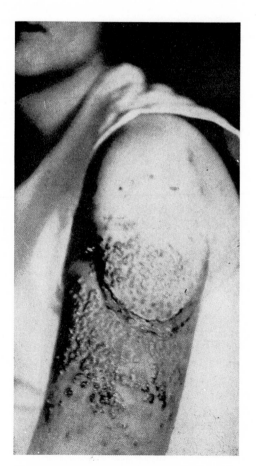

Fig. 136. Cutaneous reaction to application of aluminum-potassium-nitrate over affected area.

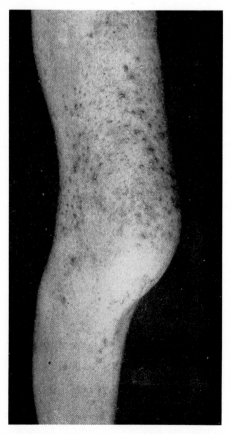

Fig. 137. Cutaneous reaction to application of aluminum-potassium-nitrate.

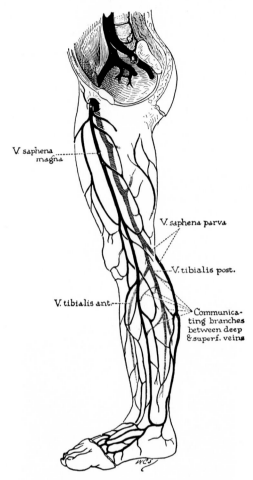

V. saphena magna

V. saphena parva

V. tibialis post.

V. tibialis ant.

Communicating branches between deep & superf. veins

FIG. 138. Distribution and intercommunication of the deep and the superficial veins of the lower extremity. Solid black denotes the superficial vessels and anastomotic branches. Cross lines indicate the deep veins. Note the presence of communicating branches between the deep and the superficial veins. (F. V. Theis)

intervention. It is absolutely necessary to have a clear picture of the circulatory condition of the limb in order to be able to select the proper kind of treatment. It is also important to consider the condition of the overlying skin to avoid complications.

Surgery is frequently quite unsatisfactory in its results and occasionally is attended by serious complications. Ligation of the internal saphenous vein, in Scarpa's triangle for in-

stance, may be followed by thrombosis of the femoral vein. To guard against this as far as possible, even the mildest infection should be avoided, and the ligatures should be applied low in the thigh (Fig. 138).

When varicose veins are accompanied by varicose ulcers, special precautions are necessary to avoid septic phlebitis following operation.

The most common disappointment in the surgical treatment of varicose veins is recurrence, which is especially liable to occur when the deep-lying veins are involved. McPheeters has stated that in 6,771 surgically treated cases there was a recurrence of 19.22 per cent after 5 years. This figure, the author feels convinced, is much below the average. The experience of most surgeons is that in the majority of cases in which the deep veins are involved there is recurrence within a few years following surgical intervention, although the immediate effect of the removal of surface veins is very good.

Pulmonary embolus is another danger, but this is not frequent. In McPheeters' series there were 35 deaths from this cause and 28 nonfatal cases.

TREATING VARICOSE VEINS BY THE INJECTION METHOD

Injection treatment offers good results in selected cases. This treatment, however, is applicable to superficial dilatations only. One of the dangers connected with it appears to be the possibility, in the hands of inexperienced surgeons, of depositing sclerosing solution outside the vein—thus producing an inflammatory necrosis and sloughing. It is necessary to guard especially against injecting a vein which shows thrombophlebitic involvement as an embolism or exacerbation of the process may result.

Pulmonary embolism following this method, while possible, is rare. I had a patient under my care at the hospital in whom a serious thrombophlebitis resulted following the injection treatment of varicose veins of the right leg. The thrombotic involvement extended upward along the internal saphenous vein, nearly reaching Poupart's ligament. The patient had been at the hospital over two months, but the thrombotic process, while apparently localizing, was still threatening, as evidenced by occasional flare-ups (rigors, high fever, etc.).

The commonly used technic of bandaging an injected part tightly interferes with the physiologic results because the lumen of the vessels is at least partially collapsed.

Sclerosing Solution. Care has to be taken in selecting a suitable sclerosing solution. Sodium chloride and sodium salicylate should be avoided because severe venospasm may precipitate an attack of angina pectoris. Furthermore, the rapidly formed thrombus has a greater tendency to soften and to be absorbed subsequently and thus allow a recurrence of the varices. Hypertonic sugar solution would be ideal for the purpose, but, as it has to be injected in a bloodless area in order to avoid dilution, the technic appears to be too difficult. In our experience, sodium morrhuate appears to be preferable to any other sclerosing agent.

Test of Venous Circulation. Vein ligation should never be done without previous investigation of the venous circulation in the affected extremity. Keep always in mind that varicosities of the superficial veins may be a symptom of an occlusion of the deep veins. In this case, ligation of the saphenous vein may be followed by disastrous results.

From a prognostic as well as from a therapeutic point of view, it is important to ascertain whether the deep veins of the leg are affected. Trendelenburg's sign will aid in ascertaining whether the large or the small saphenous group is involved. It is depicted in Figures 139 and 140 and its technic pointed out in the legends.

If the valves in the communicating veins do not function (Perthes' test), high ligation of the saphenous vein alone will be useless and should be accompanied by low ligation at the femoral condyle or even by low injections.

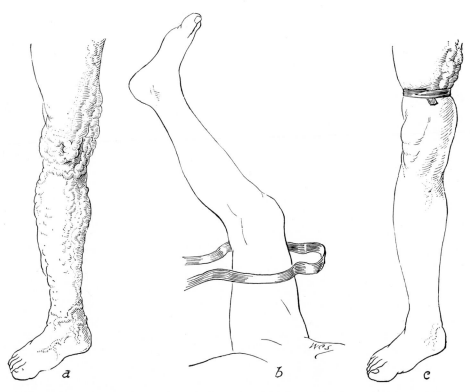

Fig. 139. Tourniquet test. (a) Limb depressed—varicosities dilated. (b) Limb elevated and tourniquet applied—varicosities collapsed. (c) Limb depressed without refilling of varices below the constrictor. This indicates that the varicosities are due to the hemodynamic reflux from incompetent valves in saphenous vein. (F. V. Theis)

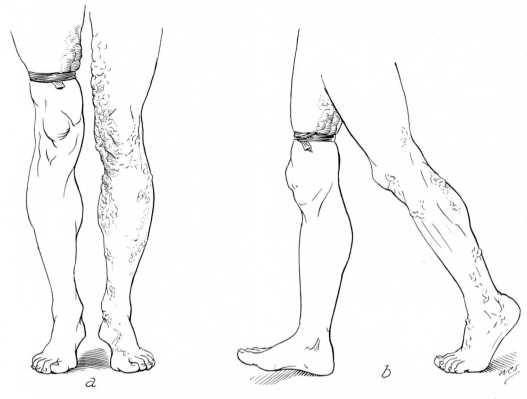

FIG. 140. Tourniquet applied while patient is standing. (a) Active movement of the calf muscles in rising on the toes empties the superficial varices by forcing the blood through the communicating veins into the deep veins. Patency of the deep veins is thereby established. Competent valves in the communicating branches prevent a reflux. Removal of the constrictor is followed immediately by refilling of the veins due to the reverse flow in the saphenous veins. (b) Active walking is more effective in forcing the blood through the communicating veins. (F. V. Theis)

Ligation alone is insufficient because recanalization may occur. Therefore, a part of the affected vein, at least one inch long, should always be removed.

Principles of Injection Method. F. V. Theis points out that thrombosis within the varices is the primary object and basis of the obliteration. In general, three factors favoring the formation of thrombi within the veins are concerned: (1) changes in the rapidity of the flow of blood; (2) changes in the qualitative and quantitative condition of the blood itself; (3) changes in the walls consisting of a loss of endothelium. The first factor is subject to our control and is employed when one resorts to ligation of the veins, but where a thrombus occurs in a stagnant stream there is a mini-

mum fixation to the vessel wall and emboli may develop. Postoperative thrombosis of the veins of the lower extremities is likewise attributed to a slowing of the blood stream. The lack of fixation makes it a very dangerous occurrence. The second factor, as to the qualitative and quantitative regulation of the state of the blood, is not within the scope of our local consideration. The third factor is the only controllable, safe and reliable measure at our disposal. Accordingly, various noncoagulating chemical irritants are successfully employed to damage sufficiently or destroy the endothelial lining of varicosed veins to set in motion the physiologic process of obliteration.

Following the injection of the chemical irritant, circulation is re-established in the vessel.

Gradual deposition of the cellular elements of the blood stream takes place on the damaged intima, with resulting thrombus formation. The character of the thrombus varies according to the swiftness of the circulating blood as well as the rapidity of the developing clot. The ultimate permanent result of the injection treatment depends on the type of thrombus obtained.

According to Kaufman, "the integrity of the wall of the vein is essential for organization of the thrombus." This accounts for recurrence of the veins in postoperative thrombosis and in extensive thrombosis following ligation or injection of chemical irritants. Recurrences are infrequent at the site where the intima is adequately injured by chemical irritants and a selective thrombus originates. When they do occur it is probable that only a part of the circumference of the intima is adequately destroyed. It must be kept in mind that a rapidly occurring obliteration is less selective than a slowly forming one. With the quinine and urethane solution the vein becomes hard within 10 to 15 minutes, irrespective of the activity of the patient. With the sugar solutions, complete thrombosis may occur within 4 to 6 hours or more. In view of the numerous recurrences following the quinine solution, and the usual lack of recurrences when the sugar irritant is used, Theis feels that the latter assures a more selective character of the primary obliteration. Following injection of the sugar solution, the patient should be encouraged to avoid the reclining position for at least 8 hours. The use of a tight bandage or adhesive strapping after injection interferes with the physiologic results, because the lumen of the vessels is at least partially collapsed and the circulation consequently delayed.

In determining the most effective means of damaging the intima, one should take into consideration the safety, controllability and reliability of the chemical irritants of the noncoagulating elements to be used. The powerful action of hypertonic sodium chloride, sodium salicylate, quinine and urethane, mercuric chloride and other solutions commonly advocated is attested by destructive tissue reaction when a small amount escapes perivascularly. The tortuosities and sacculations of the varices make this a common occurrence even with the most skilled technic. The necrosis produced by a small quantity of the solution in the perivascular tissues frequently requires months to heal. Sodium chloride and sodium salicylate may also cause such a severe venospasm as to simulate an attack of angina pectoris. The resulting thrombus has a greater tendency to soften and by subsequent absorption result in a recurrence of the varices. The less destructive irritation of the hypertonic sugar solutions produces neither necrosis nor venospasm when, accidentally, it escapes into the tissues. The sugar solutions ordinarily used require prolonged action on the intima in their undiluted concentration. Dilution of injected solutions by blood accounts for most of the reported unreliability of the sugar irritants, and a bloodless area is difficult to obtain. With the stronger and more destructive chemicals, momentary action of the solutions diluted with blood usually produces sufficient intimal damage for thrombosis to follow. Only 1 or 2 cc. of the quinine and urethane injected into a vein partially filled with blood is usually active enough to injure the intima adequately. The coincident danger of necrosis and severe venospasms, as well as the physiologically inferior quality of the resulting primary obliteration, should make one hesitate to employ the stronger irritants routinely.

For the most part, the diverse methods suggested for emptying the groups of veins in order to obtain a bloodless area are impracticable. To obtain this essential of a bloodless area, Theis has adopted the use of a specially designed varicose vein occluder. Sufficient pressure uniformly applied around the ring unquestionably occludes the main stem of the vessel as well as all superficial ramifications within the area. This is accomplished by two means—by direct pressure of the metal ring of the occluder on the skin and transmission through the subcutaneous tissues to the veins, and by the resulting increased tension of the tissues further compressing and collapsing the vessels. Under no circumstances should pressure be applied prior to the introduction of the needle into the vein. This precludes the use of a self-retaining instrument where preliminary pressure is to be applied by fixation of the instrument.

Technic of Injection Method. Routine histories and complete physical examinations establish the fact that no contraindication is present.

With the patient standing, the course of the varices to receive the injection is indicated with Mercurochrome. Then, in the recumbent position, with sterile towels the field is laid out and cleansed with alcohol. A 10-cc. syringe filled with a 60 per cent levulose dextrose (invert sugar) is attached to a special two-way stopcock adapter. In the upright position the adapter is filled, and then the stopcock is turned so that the solution flows back by gravity to fill the side arm and a drop escapes. This may have to be repeated in order to fill the adapter solution completely. The short bevel 24-, 25- or 26-gauge needle is then attached. The 60 per cent sugar solution readily flows through the small caliber needles. The assistant holds the occluder over the veins without pressure and the needle is inserted into the vein. With the stopcock adjusted to the side-arm, the moment the needle enters the lumen of the vein the last drop of sugar solution in the side-arm escapes. With the least manipulation or delay, the surgeon is assured that the vein has or has not been entered without waiting for the actual blood to be seen. The vein having been entered, the assistant gently but firmly applies pressure to the occluder, with consequent isolation of the area from the adjoining vessels. The tension of the tissues forces the remaining blood through the side-arm. Continued flow indicates the presence of a deep communicating branch within the area, and a bloodless area is therefore unattainable. Shifting of the occluder usually is sufficient to avoid the branch, and a bloodless area for injection is obtained. By simply turning the stopcock straight, the undiluted solution is injected into the vein. Continued pressure on the occluder is maintained for five minutes; consequently, uniform destruction of the endothelium occurs. Back pressure from the distended veins almost always forces some of the solution through the needle-puncture hole. Under no circumstances has perivascular escape of the solution given greater distress than a few moments of burning sensation. Overdistention of the tissues by perivascular injection should be avoided, but in no instance has Theis seen a slough following the use of sugar solution.

Occasions arise, due to numerous communicating veins, which make it impossible to obtain a bloodless area. Where reactions fail to occur with the sugar solutions, one must resort to hypertonic sodium chloride. Routinely, the 60 per cent levulose dextrose solution (invert sugar) is the most satisfactory and the safest solution to use. A 50 per cent dextrose solution may be used but is more viscous and less efficient in producing the necessary intimal changes.

Recurrence Following Injections. Howard, Jackson and Mahon of San Francisco have made an extensive study of the pathologic nature of the recurrence of varicose veins following treatment by the injection method. A critical survey of the end-results of their treatment for a 3-year period revealed a startling percentage of recurrences. In a series of 66 cases, recurrence was observed a year or more after thrombosis in 52 patients. The wave of enthusiasm that several years ago greeted the treatment of varicose veins by the injection of sclerosing agents gave the method an impetus that has not been justified by the ultimate results, and it is becoming increasingly evident that a more careful elimination of unsuitable cases and a return to surgical procedures combined with injection of sclerosing agents is necessary to obtain satisfactory and more permanent results.

Complications. Many complications were encountered in their series. Periphlebitis, apparently more alarming and painful than dangerous, occurred in 18 cases. Rest in bed with compresses and elevation of the legs brought relief, but the process often lasted from 3 to 4 weeks before subsiding.

Sloughs were produced by perivenous injection or leakage along the needle track in 11 cases. Separation of the slough took place in from 3 to 4 weeks, and for complete healing from 8 to 10 weeks were necessary.

Nonfatal pulmonary embolism with frothy, bloody expectoration, pleural pain, physical and roentgenographic signs of consolidation of one lobe of the lung occurred in one person. Another patient received 4 injections resulting at one point in slough from extravasation into the tissues.

The results of their follow-up examinations with the microscopic studies of therapeutic thrombosis convince them that incompetent treatment by injection unaided by ligature, excision or stripping of main venous channels and perforating veins will ordinarily not serve to obtain permanent cure in cases of varicose veins. The few isolated cases of dilated single veins with competent valves are the exception.

Treatment of Choice

The most successful treatment of varicose veins by the methods available at the present time is by operation with removal of the saphenous segment from the fossa ovalis to the knee and eradication of the dilated veins below this point at a time when the valves are still competent and ulceration, eczema and edema are yet undeveloped. For permanent results such a procedure can have no substitute. Incomplete measures, such as ligation, ligation with excision of small vein segments or multiple small incisions, have been proved to be unsatisfactory.

Selection of Treatment

The majority of sufferers from varicose diseases are small-wage earners or overworked housewives whose family resources prevent hospitalization and means of care for their children while under treatment. The economic factors do, and will, frequently determine the available method of treatment. In this particular situation the treatment of varicose veins by injection has proved to be of real value in obtaining relief from suffering and in maintaining ability for productive labor. With the attitude of adopting the best available method to the particular case under the economic circumstances, and using the method of complete operation when possible, these investigators suggest the following indications:

1. When single or isolated dilated vein segments exist in the presence of completely competent valves, symptoms are rarely present. Persons presenting themselves for treatment of such varices do so mainly for cosmetic reasons. Treatment by injection may be employed entirely.

2. If the patient has moderate dilatation or tortuosity of the saphenous system, provided that the valves are competent, interruption of the venous continuity at the saphenous opening, with injection into the veins below, may be carried out. The interruption of the venous flow may be by ligature with excision of a segment of the vein

under local anesthesia, and the treatment may thus be entirely ambulatory. Such a procedure has been successfully carried out by DeTakats with promise of lasting results. Tavel utilized this method in 1905 and noticed that in 7 of 25 cases spontaneous thrombosis occurred distal to the ligature, and apparently permanent cure resulted. Instead of making an injection into the veins distally after an interval of several days following the high excision, as is usually done, one may make the injection into the veins in the wound at the time of operation.

It should be emphasized that ligature and excision should be done at the fossa ovalis, and all tributary vessels emptying into the saphenous vein at this point should be ligated and cut across as well. A double saphenous vein may be present in the thigh, and mid-thigh ligation of a single vein may fail to give additional benefit. The group of superficial tributary vessels emptying into the saphenous vein at the saphenous opening are known to have caused recurrence by opening up of collateral channels following operative excision when these tributary veins were not ligated.

Perhaps a more permanent way of interrupting the back pressure would consist in stripping the saphenous veins from the femoral opening to the knee and making the injection into the veins below this point. The procedure need not necessitate prolonged hospitalization. As DeTakats pointed out, the endeavor is to prevent thrombosis and consequent embolism from the deep and proximal veins by early mobilization.

3. When varicose veins are accompanied by incompetency of both saphenous and perforating valves, the complete operation of stripping with excision should be carried out at the expense of temporary loss of time from employment. It is in this type of case that it is felt recanalization will occur in spite of complete and repeated thrombosis, and that complete interruption of the continuity of the vein is necessary. Injection into the isolated vein segments may follow such an operation.

4. Those persons are poor subjects for operation who have long-standing varicosities with incompetency of both sets of valves and who have extensive chronic ulceration, eczema and a hard, brawny lymph edema approaching the elephantoid condition. The swollen, indurated tissues of the leg hide numerous venous channels and dilated perforating veins which are extremely difficult to eradicate, and in this type of patient the operative results are not brilliant. Such patients are considerably improved but not cured by injection. Injection should be supplemented by the use of sulphurated zinc paste stockings, rest in bed and elevation or skin grafting to hasten healing of

ulcers. The edema subsides remarkably but not completely, even under ambulatory treatment, and with the subsidence of the edema the hidden veins become visible or palpable and can be treated by injection. With recurrence of varicose veins, such a patient must receive another injection to hold the improvement gained.

5. Following apparently complete operative excision, varicosities sometimes make their appearance. When this occurs, the new veins are irregular in their distribution and in their connection with the deep set and offer a considerable obstacle to complete re-excision. This type of vein may be properly treated by injection, which will probably have to be repeated.

In summarizing their findings, the authors state that in the 66 patients treated for varicose veins by the injection of 20 per cent sodium chloride, they have been able to re-examine 49 a year or more after treatment.

Forty-eight of the 49 patients showed recurrence of their previously thrombosed veins. Four additional patients were known to have had early recurrence but could not be located after a year.

The recurrence rate was 79 per cent of all patients treated, or 98 per cent of all those they had followed a year or more.

In contrast, 49 had partial or complete relief from symptoms attributed to the varicosities, 28 of these patients being completely relieved from all symptoms.

Recurrence of veins thrombosed by injection was found to take place by recanalization, a natural pathologic response to thrombosis. The interruption of the continuity of the vein by excision, especially in the presence of incompetent saphenous or perforating valves, is held to be vital in securing more permanent results.

S. A. MACKLER, M.D.

12 The Pleural Cavity, the Mediastinum and the Lungs

INTRODUCTION

It is perhaps platitudinous to remark that an understanding of the physiology of the thorax is of fundamental importance before undertaking surgical treatment. Nevertheless, it was lack of such knowledge that retarded the development of surgical treatment of this body cavity until well past the time when operative technics in other regions had matured. As a result of the work of Pasteur and Lister, and an understanding of the bacteriologic nature of infection, surgical exploration of the greater part of the human anatomy progressed with rapidity and success, but the thoracic cavity persisted in repulsing surgical intrusion. Except for the drainage of empyema, as mentioned by Hippocrates, operative procedures within the thorax entailed a prohibitive mortality.

It was evident that the difficulty arose immediately on opening the pleural space, but the nature of the derangement in intrathoracic physiology created by such an open pneumothorax eluded solution for many years. It was not until 1918 that a basic concept was gained, as a result of the observations of Evarts Graham[1] and his refutation of many prevalent misconceptions.

The thorax differs from other body cavities in that it maintains an internal state of suction or negative pressure. This is conditioned by the changes in intrathoracic volume consequent to the respiratory movements of the thoracic wall and the diaphragm, and by the eternal centripetal recoil of the lungs away from the parietes. When a breach is made in the hermetic seal of this space, whether due to trauma or under conditions of asepsis and hemostasis, the state of vacuum is lost, and the intrathoracic pressure on the affected side approaches that of the surrounding atmosphere. There results therefrom a series of consequences which, if uninterrupted by closure of the defect, will terminate fatally. It is a combination of these factors, rather than a single effect, which ultimately culminates in a fatal issue.

The following are the pathologic processes resulting from an open pneumothorax. For the purpose of simplicity, these effects are considered as a result of a large open pneumothorax, such as a thoracotomy wound.

1. Collapse of the Ipsolateral Lung. It is obvious that as a consequence of the loss of negative tension, the lung collapses in its new environment of atmospheric pressure. The power of elastic recoil is no longer overcome by the suction effect of subatmospheric tension, and its force of contractility is now free to act without impediment. The body thus suffers the physiologic loss of one lung, or about one half its respiratory capacity.

Sufficient respiratory function can be maintained by a single lung because it is endowed with an adequate reserve capacity. However, additional respiratory and circulatory burdens accrue. It is these additional derangements which were obscure to the pioneer surgeons and remained enigmatic until the first quarter of this century had passed.

2. Compromise in Capacity of the Contralateral Lung. The mediastinal septum, if unaffected by previous disease processes, is a mobile structure, and its position in the midline is subject to change. In the intact chest, the negative forces of one pleural space are negated by a similar negative pressure on the opposite side, hence there is no variation of the mediastinum from its usual midline position. However, in the presence of an open pneumothorax, this surface of the mediastinum is now exposed to atmospheric conditions, while the obverse surface is subjected to the influence of subatmospheric pressure. Therefore, the septum becomes dislocated into the intact hemithoracic space. The lung of the uninvolved side then becomes crowded, and its ventilatory capacity is compromised by confinement of space.

3. Compromise in Ventilatory Ability of the Contralateral Lung. The ability of a lung to expand depends on the developing negative pressure which sucks the lung out, as it were, during inspiration. Any enfeeblement of this force of negative pressure reflects in a poorer state of pulmonary ventilation. Although the pleural cavity on the side opposite to that containing the open pneumothorax remains anatomically intact, it nevertheless suffers an impairment in its negative-pressure-producing ability. This follows as a result of substituting one rigid side of the intact thoracic space with a flaccid one. The mediastinum now presents as a wall of the chest, one side exposed to environmental pressure conditions (via the hemithorax containing the open pneumothorax), while the obverse side faces upon a space in which a negative pressure is retained. If, in analogy, one considers a set of bellows in which one wall is replaced with a flaccid sheeting, the capability to generate suction here is far less than that of a bellows with intact, rigid walls, inasmuch as a great amount of negative tension is dissipated by sucking in its own wall.

4. Pendular Air Phenomenon (Pendelluft). In normal inspiration, an approximately equal quantity of air is aspirated through each bronchus as a result of bilaterally equal negative pleural pressures and equal luminal diameters. During expiration, the same situation obtains in expulsion. However, in the presence of a large open pneumothorax, the bronchus on the affected side is no longer a functioning tube but exists as an appendage, so to speak, attaching an atelectatic lung to the remaining dynamic tracheobronchial tree. During inspiration, the residual air retained within the inert bronchus is aspirated across the carina to the other bronchus, along with inspired tracheal air from the outside. In expiration, as air is expelled, a similar quantity again retraces its pathway across the carina to fill the lumen of the inert bronchus. Although the amount is small, this to-and-fro transportation of air

serves no useful respiratory purpose but only vitiates the inspired environmental air.

5. Effects on Circulation. All structures within the thoracic cavity exist in an environment subatmospheric in tension, which rhythmically heightens and falls with the respiratory movements. This applies to the extrapleural organs as well as to the lungs. The play of the forces of pressure on such organs may be demonstrated by observation of the esophageal lumen during an esophagoscopy. There occurs a rhythmic widening and narrowing of the lumen, consonant with inspiration and expiration. With inspiration, the increased intrathorax negative pressure playing on the esophageal walls sucks them out, to increase the luminal diameter. In expiration, as the negative tension falls, the walls are released to fall together, thus obliterating the lumen. These same forces operate on the large veins and, by such a milking action, effect venous return to the heart. Thus, an open pneumothorax not only destroys the internal negative pressure but materially reduces the effectiveness of such action on venous flow. Furthermore, dislocation of the mediastinum adds to the impediment of venous return. In addition to total displacement of the mediastinum toward the intact hemithorax, a rhythmic, lateral oscillation (flutter) occurs with the respiratory movements, toward the unaffected side in inspiration (by increasing negative pressure here) and back toward the opposite side in expiration. The greater the dislocation of the heart, the greater the interference with atrial filling. Inasmuch as there are about 4 heartbeats per respiratory cycle, each diastole will receive varying quantities of venous blood, depending on the station of mediastinal displacement at that phase of respiration.

The fatal issue resulting from an unattended open pneumothorax is thus the consequence of multiple physiologic disturbances rather than that of a single derangement. As stated previously, for the purpose of simplicity, these have been described as effects of a large, open pneumothorax, such as a thoracotomy wound. However, an opening in the chest is not *necessarily* lethal. There is a direct ratio between the size of the open pneumothorax and the effects therefrom; the smaller the opening, the greater the capability of toleration. This is so because the hemithoracic bellows, although breached, is still capable of creating suction on inspiration, although its ability is impaired by the presence of the opening. There now exists a competition between the expanding lung as it is drawn out by the inspiratory negative pressure and the simultaneous rush of air drawn in through the wound. The greater the opening, the less capable is the chest of developing suction, until such time as the wound reaches a size so large that the production of any suction on inspiration is impossible and the pleural space remains constantly at atmospheric pressure. Once the wound is occluded, there no longer exists a competition between lung and atmosphere for the developing suction, and its entire force now may be utilized for expansion of the lung.

Although the pioneer thoracic surgeons lacked detailed knowledge of the effects of an open pneumothorax, gross observations showed that the lung collapsed soon after opening the chest, followed shortly by symptoms of asphyxia. Based on the logic that this was due to violation of the hermetic seal of the chest cavity, with subsequent loss of negative pressure, investigations were conducted to determine the action of the lung when exposed to an external environment where the tension was artificially reduced so as to resemble closely that within the thorax.

Following these experimental procedures, initiated by Sauerbuch[5] in 1903, there evolved the "negative-pressure chamber," a device whereby the operating chamber was maintained under subatmospheric conditions by means of suction pumps. However, the patient's head was exteriorized through a cuffed aperture to the outside, so that while his torso was exposed to negative-pressure conditions, he breathed the normal atmosphere. Thus, when subjected to a thoracotomy, a pressure differential was maintained between the internal and the external surface of the exposed lung throughout the duration of the procedure. The chamber is of historic value only, but its importance rests upon the fact that for the first time it was possible to maintain successfully a large thoracotomy wound for a sufficiently extended period of time to permit surgical exploration.

The negative-pressure chamber was later superseded by today's method, *positive-pressure anesthesia*. By means of the endotracheal tube—in effect, an anatomic external prolongation of the trachea—direct control over intrapulmonic pressure is possible. By maintaining anesthetic gas-oxygen pressure to a degree slightly above that of the atmosphere, the surgically exposed lung may be kept in a state of inflation. Indeed, it may be partially or wholly compressed by manual retraction, exerting a pressure just exceeding that maintained in the tracheobronchial tree, to obtain greater freedom in surgical exploration. The opposite, unexposed lung carries on with respiration and resists atmospheric compression transmitted by way of the mediastinum because of the maintained intrabronchial and intrapulmonic pressure.

SURGERY OF THE PLEURAL CAVITY

An elementary principle governs the treatment of all forms of thoracic disease, trauma or the postoperative state. Simply stated, this avers that anatomic structures should be made to resume their normal configuration and spatial relationships after being deranged. The pleural cavity is particularly prone to accumulate collections of fluid, blood, pus or air. Such collections forming within it occupy space at the expense of the lung and must be evacuated to allow the compressed lung to expand to reoccupy the space it formerly possessed. This may be done, in most instances, by simple thoracentesis, using needle and syringe. When persistent reaccumulation occurs, or when thoracentesis is not suitable because of the consistency or the quantity of the material, a more permanent type of drainage is required.

It is obvious that evacuation cannot be accomplished by the insertion of a simple drain, as in the abdominal cavity, for the aperture so created as a means of exit would also serve as an avenue of entrance for air, and one would have, in essence, an open pneumothorax. The ill-effects of such an opening would outweigh by far the good accomplished by decompression. Such derangements in thoracic physiology consequent to an open pneumothorax are precipitated when the condition of the intrathoracic tissues is in a normal state of health. Where there has existed previous inflammation, the stated situation no longer

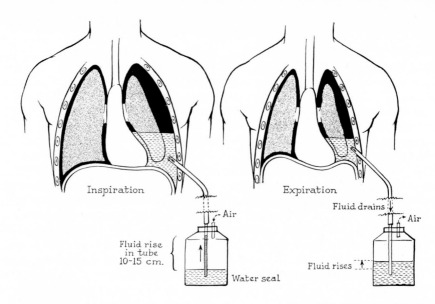

Inspiration

Expiration

Fluid drains

Air

Fluid rise
in tube
10-15 cm.

Water seal

Fluid rises

Air

Fig. 141 (*Top and bottom*). The
water-seal system for drainage of the
pleural cavity. (Zimmerman and
Levine: Physiologic Principles of
Surgery, Philadelphia, Saunders)

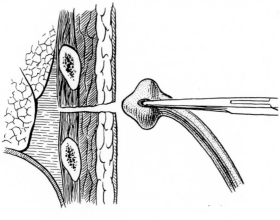

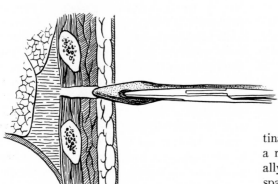

obtains. Here there may be complete absence
of the pleural space due to fusion of the parietal and the visceral surfaces, and the lung is
prevented from collapsing because of fixation
to the inner surface of the thoracic cage. Moreover, inflammatory thickening of the mediastinal pleural surfaces and structures results in
a rigid, true mediastinal septum, architectur-
ally compartmentalizing each hemithoracic
space so that they now become functionally,
as well as anatomically, independent units,
and physiologic derangements of one plural
cavity are no longer transmitted to the other
via a yielding mediastinum.

This does not imply that one must refrain
from attempting to empty the pleural cavity
until the stabilizing effects of inflammation
have been brought about. Indeed, early and

complete emptying of the space to re-expand the lung rapidly to its previous anatomic state of inflation is the basic consideration. However, this must be accomplished in a "closed" manner by providing a one-way route of exit for the intrapleural collection but denying entry to atmospheric air.

The "water seal" or "water trap" provides such closed drainage from the pleural cavity by means of a snugly fitted intercostal tube connected to a length of hollow glass tubing reaching below water level (Fig. 141). In inspiration, the rise in intrathoracic negative pressure sucks water, instead of air, up into the system, but this effort rarely exceeds the force to raise a column higher than 15 cm. It is apparent that caution must be observed to ensure that the water bottle remains well below 15 cm. from the level of the chest to prevent aspiration of water. To safeguard against such an accident, it is the rule to fix the bottle to the floor at the bedside. When this system of drainage is established in the operating room, as is routinely customary following thoracotomy, it is essential to make sure that the rubber tubing is well occluded by clamps before the bottle is elevated, preparatory to transporting the patient. Avoid the error of removing the clamps before the bottle is placed on the floor, well below the level of the chest. Another matter requiring careful supervision is the manner in which the tubing is connected to the water bottle. By mistake, the rubber tubing may be applied to the short segment of glass tubing instead of to the length reaching below the water level. The patient will have, in effect, an open pneumothorax as a cause of his immediate postoperative difficulty, which enlists frantic but fruitless attempts at correction by tracheal aspiration, oxygen administration and other nonpertinent measures. A *quick, precautionary, inspecting glance will prevent such an anxious situation*. The attachment, care and regulation of the water-seal drainage system is a function of the medical house staff; this duty should not be relegated to the nursing personnel.

The last 5 years have witnessed a steady but persistent increase in the number of cases of empyema in infants and children. In a large proportion of these cases, it has been possible to incriminate the *Micrococcus pyogenes* (*Staph. aureus*) or other antibiotic-resistant organisms. Nevertheless, even in patients harboring organisms sensitive to antibiotics, accumulations within the pleural space demand the application of the elementary surgical principle for the care of the pleural cavity, namely, *decompression*.

Technic of Decompression

Localization and determination of the nature of the collection is first accomplished by needle aspiration, and if the accumulation is small, repeated thoracenteses may suffice for treatment. In most instances, however, this will be found to be ineffectual, and a more adequate means of maintaining an empty pleural cavity becomes necessary. Closed drainage by catheter and water seal usually suffices. Under local anesthesia, a small incision is made over the appropriate region, and a pointed hemostat is insinuated to the pleura by repeatedly spreading a channel through the intercostal musculature. A blunt-nosed catheter (Pezzer), stretched over a forceps, is then introduced into the pleural cavity through the prepared passage (Fig. 141) and quickly connected to the water-seal system. The simplicity of this method recommends it over that of trocar introduction. Further, by creating a passage through the intercostal musculature by blunt separation, advantage is taken of the cross-direction in which the fibers of the internal and the external intercostal muscles run, so that these act in a sphincterlike manner on the tubing. This eliminates sucking around the tube, particularly in regions where the overlying tissues of the chest cage lack depth, as in the midaxillary line. The flange permits the catheter to be brought flush to the inner thoracic wall. This not only helps in preventing accidental withdrawal but also, with the infant or child, gives certainty to its position within the chest. The midaxillary line, at the horizontal level of the nipple, is the most advantageous region for the introduction of a catheter, if previous exploration with a needle indicates that the collection may be reached here. This location is also most suitable for thoracentesis because the procedure can be performed with the patient in a reclining and restful position.

Adequate drainage may be obstructed by

flocculent material or by the inspissated character of the pus itself. A solution of streptokinase-streptodornase may be used to advantage to thin the accumulation. The solution is instilled into the chest cavity through the catheter. The catheter is clamped close to the thoracic wall, and the solution is injected by needle into the tubing. The catheter should remain occluded for several hours to permit effective enzymatic fibrinolysis. It is usually necessary to repeat the procedure on successive days. If, in spite of such energetic measures employed over a sufficient period of time, the condition shows little response clinically or roentgenographically, it is preferable to perform a thoracotomy and decortication to salvage the lung. This is better than establishing open drainage by rib resection, provided that the empyema has not been present for such a chronically extended period of time as to nullify in advance the possible success of a decortication.

Persistent reaccumulation of fluid (transudates) in the chest likewise indicates the use of closed drainage for the benefit of continuous decompression. By denying the material any possibility of accumulating, empyema formation will be thwarted, in spite of the presence of an infectious process, as in pneumonitis and pleuritis. The fear of introducing infection by the catheter is ill-founded, particularly with the use of antibiotics, and the advantage gained by preventing any stagnant collection, the incipient stage of empyema, more than offsets this remote possibility. To be sure, removal of the tube is to be affected expeditiously, when it is felt that no further accumulation is likely and that adherence of the pleural surfaces is in progress, usually 7 to 10 days.

SURGERY OF MEDIASTINAL TUMORS

Space forbids an inclusive discussion of the various tumors and cysts which affect the mediastinum. Suffice it to say that for diagnostic purposes the mediastinum is arbitrarily divided into compartments because most tumors show a site of predilection in which to appear (Fig. 142). Briefly stated, the three most common new growths are the lymphomas (lymphosarcoma, Hodgkin's), the teratoid tumors (dermoid and teratoma) and the primary nerve tumors (neurofibroma, neuroblastoma, ganglioneuroma, etc.). The first two occur within the anterior mediastinal compartment, the third group in the posterior compartment. In addition to these two designated sections of the mediastinum, a third region is of diagnostic significance. This is the mid-mediastinal zone. Bronchiogenic cysts, arising from one of the main bronchi or from the bifurcation of the trachea, occupy this area and not only retain an intermediate position in the anteroposterior diameter but also extend to reach either the superior or the inferior limit of the mediastinum.

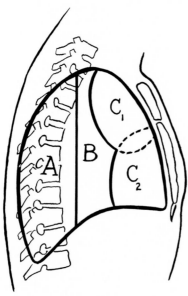

Fig. 142. Artificial compartmentation of the mediastinum, showing sites of predilection of tumors. (A) Posterior mediastinum: tumors of neurogenic origin (neurofibroma, ganglioneuroma, etc.). (B) Bronchogenic cyst, enterogenous cyst (inferior portion). (C) Anterior mediastinum: dermoid and teratoma (C_1 and C_2), lymphoma and thymoma (C_1), pericardial cyst and hernia foramen of Morgagni (C_2).

DIFFERENTAL DIAGNOSIS

Although the preoperative conjecture as to the nature of the tumor is based primarily on its location in the mediastinum, other clues may afford helpful information. Roentgenographically, a thin rim of calcification at the margin of a round density in the anterior mediastinum is strongly suggestive of a *dermoid cyst*. This is frequently misinterpreted as a "vascular" or "aneurysmal" mass because of the calcific rim. The dermoid cyst is filled with an oil and water emulsion, comprised of secretions from sebaceous and sweat glands. If the patient is kept sitting quietly in an upright position for a period of time sufficient to allow the components of this emulsion to separate, a roentgenogram may show the oil-fluid level within the mass. This is sometimes mistaken for an abscess cavity. Fats and oils are radiolucent, hence the zone of "highlight" above the fluid level, water being relatively opaque to roentgen rays.

Tomograms, or an overexposed film, will sometimes reveal the density of a tooth or a toothlike structure within a teratoma. Vigorous (transmitted) pulsation of a mediastinal mass excludes aneurysm from differential consideration, whereas immobility may indicate an aneurysm. This seemingly contradictory statement is true, because luetic aneurysms, as a result of periarteritis, are adherent to surrounding structures, whereas true tumors are free of any pre-existing inflammation and freely respond to the transmitted pulsation of aorta or heart.

A mass projecting into the left hemithorax, if considered to be an aneurysm, must be situated in the posterior mediastinal compartment on lateral roentgenographic examination, the position of the aorta. When projecting into the right hemithorax, the considered "aneurysm" must be situated in the anterior mediastinum, the position of the ascending aorta. Densities in association with the heart shadow may be pericardial cysts or diverticulae. Confirmation is sometimes possible by fluoroscopic examination, if it is noted that the mass tends to gravitate with changes in body position. Such cysts are thin-walled and lax, and the contained watery fluid may alter its position to a degree sufficiently great to be detected when the position of the body is changed from the horizontal to the vertical.

Tumors of lymphomatous origin are usually radiosensitive, and if the diagnosis cannot be confirmed histologically by lymph-node biopsy, together with examination of sternal marrow or peripheral blood, its response to a test dose of irradiation affords a presumptive diagnosis. Approximatly 750 r.u. in divided doses over a period of 1 week to 10 days should result in an unequivocal reduction in the size of the mass. Such sensitivity to irradiation is taken as diagnostic evidence of the lymphomatous nature of the tumor, and irradiation, rather than surgery, is the indicated treatment. Persistence in irradiating a mass, unresponsive to a prior diagnostic test dose, is a very grave error, as the difficulty of ultimate surgical extirpation will be compounded.

Surgical extirpation is the recommended treatment for intrathoracic neoplasms, with the exception of radiosensitive lymphomas, because of compression of adjacent vital structures and because of malignant degeneration. Erosion into the lung by chronic compression of an adjacent mediastinal tumor is not unusal. With the development of a communication between the two structures, the contents of the tumor may be evacuated in intervals via the tracheobronchial tree. Cough productive of detritus and hair is diagnostically significant of such a union with a teratoid growth. Conversely, the flora of the pulmonary passageways gains access to the neoplasm, with consequent infection. Excluding lymphomas, tumors of neurogenic origin have the greatest incidence of malignant degeneration. Metastatic dissemination is rare, but its malignant manifestation is marked by local recurrence and invasion.

CYSTIC TUMORS

Sometimes these may be fused so inextricably to adjacent vital structures that complete extirpation is an impossibility. In anatomic regions other than the thorax, such a situation may be countered by the method of marsupialization. As a rule, such a stratagem cannot be adopted in the chest because of the unyielding nature of the thoracic wall and the difficulty in maintaining an airtight closure between the exteriorized segment and the apposed thoracic wall, in constant motion. Here, then, the cyst should be opened, its contents evacuated, and as much as possible of the freed wall excised. The epithelial lining of the retained portion should be destroyed, either by stripping it from its fibrous shell or simply by abrasion with a dry sponge. Destruction of the epithelial surface with chemical agents, such as silver nitrate, has been abandoned because of persistently reaccumulating postoperative effusions.

THE ESOPHAGUS

The esophagus, a member of the mediastinal septum, is frequently involved in disease processes requiring surgical treatment.

Carcinoma. Perhaps the most common condition in the adult is primary *carcinoma*. Unfortunately, with the exception of lesions occurring at the lower end, the rate of resectability is extremely low. Because of the involvement of contiguous vital structures (bronchus and aortic arch), extirpation of the diseased segment frequently cannot be accom-

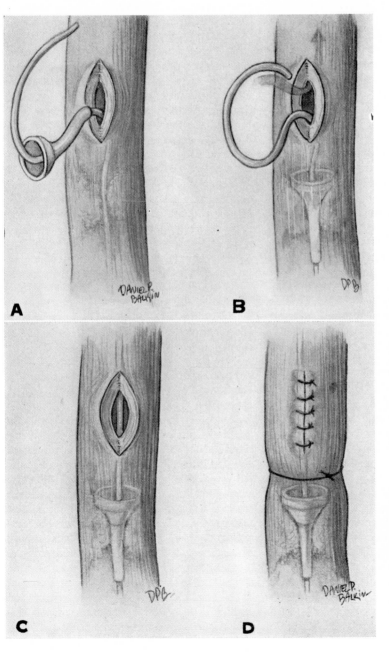

FIG. 143. (A) A Levin tube has been passed through the carcinomatous region to the stomach via an esophagotomy. An esophageal tube or prosthesis has been threaded over the Levin tube. (B) Using the latter as a guide, the prosthesis has been pressed through the obstructed segment; its cuff rests on the tumor mass, preventing complete passage. (C) The proximal end of the nasogastric tube has been directed to the mouth. (D) The esophagotomy has been closed. (Mackler and Mayer: J. Thoracic Surg. 28:431)

plished, even for the sole purpose of palliation of obstruction without the prospect of cure. The esophagus, particularly in the upper region, does not lend itself to short-circuiting procedures to bypass the obstructed site, as does the lower alimentary tract.

When confronted with such an operative situation, the surgeon usually has one of three choices: (1) doggedly to attempt to extirpate the segment and perform an esophagogastrostomy for the purpose of palliation; (2) to abandon any further intrathoracic surgery and perform a gastrostomy or jejunostomy; or (3) simply to close the chest and permit the disease to run its unaltered course. The first choice carries with it a prohibitively high mortality rate (well over 40%); the second necessitates another operative procedure, notwithstanding the added surgical risk and its undesirability from an esthetic standpoint; the third engenders a feeling of frustration and helplessness.

A procedure which would permit food to pass through the site of carcinomatous obstruction would solve the problem of palliative alimentation in the face of ineradicable disease. This may be achieved by inserting an intraluminal tube (Fig. 143) through the site of carcinomatous obstruction, leaving it permanently in place.[2] An artificial lumen is thus constantly maintained in spite of the continued growth of the tumor. The tube should be surgically inserted at the time of thoracic exploration if it has been determined that resection of the esophagus is neither feasible nor desirable.

Spontaneous Rupture. Although reputedly a rare condition, spontaneous rupture of the esophagus has been reported increasingly within the past decade. It seems probable that a lack of clinical awareness of the condition has been responsible for the rarity of reports of the accident in the past. It occurs, in most instances, following prolonged or forceful vomiting and is characterized by a sudden splitting apart of the wall of an apparently normal esophagus, with the escape of gastric content into the mediastinal space. The defect appears as a longitudinal rent through the whole thickness of the wall of the esophagus and is almost invariably located in the left lateral wall at the lower end, approximately 1 to 2 inches above the cardia.

Many explanations have been proposed as to the etiology of spontaneous rupture of the esophagus. However, it seems most likely that the rupture is a result of the transmitted force of ejected gastric content due to an abrupt rise in intra-abdominal pressure.[3] Rupture has been reported as occurring following blunt trauma to the abdomen, while straining at defecation, after lifting a heavy weight, during a convulsive seizure and in the labor of childbirth. However, the most common cause of

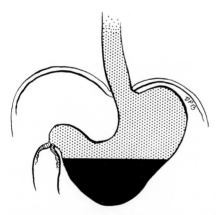 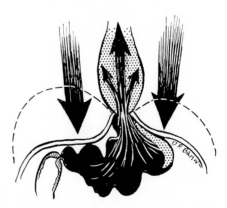

Fig. 144. Diagrammatic representation of the mechanism of vomiting. (*Left*) Inhibition of tone and flaccid relation of the cardiac pouch and sphincter of the stomach. (*Right*) Sharp contraction of the diaphragm and abdominal muscles with resultant compression of the stomach and forcible ejection of its contents into the esophagus. (Mackler, S. A.: Surg., Gynec. & Obst. 95:345)

an abrupt rise in intra-abdominal pressure is the act of vomiting.

VOMITING. Vomiting is a series of co-ordinated reflexes, the expulsive force being supplied, however, by convulsive abdominal compression and not, as might be supposed, by antiperistaltic activity of the esophageal tube. Indeed, the role of the esophagus and that of the stomach are purely passive in nature. A deep contraction occurs in the region of the incisura, clamping shut the pyloric end of the stomach. The upper portion of the stomach or cardiac pouch and the cardiac sphincter undergo complete relaxation. Prior to the commencement of vomiting, the reduction in gastric tone is such that the stomach drops several inches in the abdominal cavity, as seen roentgenographically. The esophagus, too, is relaxed throughout. The hyoid bone and the larynx are drawn and held forward, thus enlarging the opening of the pharyngo-esophageal region to allow free exit for the stomach contents. A sudden increase in the intra-abdominal pressure is then effected by a sharp descent of the diaphragm and con-traction of the abdominal muscles. The dilated, patulous stomach is now subjected to a strong compressive force, and the gastric content is forcefully ejected through a re-laxed cardia into the esophagus (Fig. 144).

Following the tear, the liquid, the solid and the gaseous contents of the stomach escape into the mediastinal space, where the gas rapidly ascends to reach the tissue spaces of the neck. The *crepitus* of subcutaneous em-physema is detectable clinically at the base of the neck within the first hour after the acci-dent. Later, in 8 to 12 hours, the digestive action of the liquid content will erode through the mediastinal pleura to evacuate itself into the left pleural cavity, manifested clinically as a *hydropneumothorax*.

CLINICAL PICTURE. In the lower sternal region, the patient experiences severe pain which radiates to the back during or shortly after severe or protracted vomiting. The pain is usually accompanied by signs of collapse. Because of simultaneous abdominal tenseness or rigidity, the usual diagnosis is that of perforated peptic ulcer, and it is only when this has been excluded by an exploratory laparotomy that the true condition may be-come evident. However, the appearance of interstitial emphysema at the base of the neck is a sign of diagnostic significance and constitutes sufficient evidence for a diagnosis of spontaneous rupture of the esophagus and an indication for a left thoracotomy.

DRAINAGE OF THE MEDIASTINAL SPACE

Although no longer as common a procedure as in the pre-antibiotic era, nevertheless drain-age of the mediastinal space is required on occasion. Two means of approach are possible: via the neck and the superior thoracic strait for the upper mediastinal space, or by way of the posterior thoracic wall for the lower re-gions of the mediastinum. The first approach is made by a cervical incision along the an-terior border of the sternocleidomastoid muscle to the sternal notch. The muscle is retracted, and the sternothyroid and the sternohyoid muscles are separated in the paratracheal re-gion, in the direction of the incision. A spread-ing forceps continues the dissection, separating the trachea medially from the palpably pul-sating carotid artery, laterally, to reach the fascial plane in front of the bodies of the cer-vical vertebrae. The finger is then guided along the anterior surfaces of the vertebrae until it reaches the superior mediastinum in this com-mon fascial space with the neck.

The lower mediastinum is approached by resecting short posterior segments of two or more ribs, close to their transverse processes, and dividing the intercostal bundles to lay bare the posterior aspect of the parietal pleura. The pleura is gently reflected from the lateral surfaces of the vertebral bodies to reach the mediastinal space. Great care must be exer-cised to safeguard the pleura and keep it intact while stripping it from the parietes and verte-bral bodies. If it is torn, a simple drain cannot be used for the mediastinal space; the entire procedure must be abandoned, because the retropleural wound now communicates with the pleural cavity, and to persist with simple drainage would be to maintain a sucking wound or open pneumothorax. Except in infants and children (as in surgery for tracheo-esophageal fistula and atresia), it is virtually impossible to gain access to the mediastinum by the retropleural pathway without injury to the transparent pleural membrane. This is par-ticularly true when separation is attempted over the surface of the length of the azygos

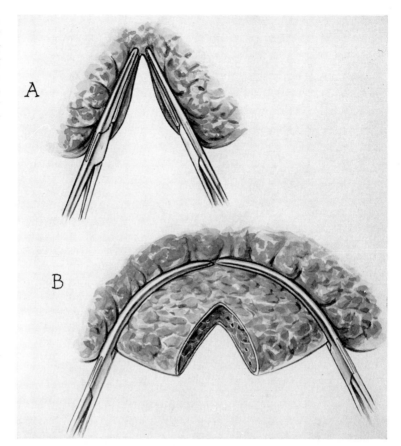

vein on the right or the surface of the aorta on the left. For this reason, the retropleural route has now been abandoned, the mediastinum being approached directly via the transpleural route.

A routine thoracotomy exposes the mediastinal pleura, which then is incised widely to open the mediastinal compartment. This is left widely open so as to drain into the pleural cavity, which, in turn, evacuates to the outside by closed drainage.

The common indication for mediastinal drainage is perforation of the esophagus, usually the result of an error during instrumentation. If it can be ascertained that the perforation is small, resulting from inadvertent manipulation of a fine bougie, conservative management with vigorous antibiotic therapy, defunctionalization of the esophagus and simple closed drainage of the pleural space—if necessary—may suffice. However, if it seems probable that the trauma is greater, and is a

rent rather than a small perforation, it is more cautious to expose the region surgically, affording wide drainage of the mediastinum. Otherwise, in spite of defunctionalizing the esophagus by means of intravenous feedings or an indwelling nasogastric tube, leakage of esophageal secretion and saliva will accumulate and spread within the mediastinal compartment. The defect may be repaired if it is readily accessible and of recent origin.

SURGERY OF THE LUNG

The last decade has witnessed an increase in the treatment of pulmonary disease processes by surgical excision. With the help of antibiotics and modern anesthetic technics, the magnitude of the extirpative procedure is dictated more by an awareness of the patient's pulmonary reserve than by the disease process itself. Resective operations range from the conservative "wedge" excision to pneumonectomy.

WEDGE RESECTION

The wedge resection removes the smallest possible amount of uninvolved pulmonary tissue because the dissection follows only the perimeter of the lesion and is not influenced by the pattern of lobular anatomy. Therefore, lesions subject to this method of extirpation must be well localized, not too extensive and situated in the more peripheral aspect of the parenchyma. Those situated close to the hilar structures necessitate anatomic dissection. The wedge technic is used most commonly in resecting the "coin" lesion. As in tumors of the breast, if gross or immediate microscopic examination indicates a benign condition (granuloma, hamartoma, bronchiogenic cyst, etc.), further surgery is usually unnecessary, wedge resection sufficing. However, if the lesion is found to be malignant, a more radical extirpative procedure is indicated, and a pneumonectomy or a lobectomy should then be done.

There are numerous technics for performing the wedge resection, but the most common is that whereby the lesion is excised from between two clamps. While simplicity is the virtue of this procedure, it is countered by the disadvantage that following the excision, the lung tissue caught between clamps is oversewn while completely airless. When the lung is ultimately expanded, this area remains indented and puckered as the adjacent tissue inflates (Fig. 145 A). To obviate this, the following method has been devised. Two curved, unshod Doyen intestinal occluding forceps are applied so as to encircle the involved zone well proximal to the lesion itself. This temporarily isolates the area from its vascular supply, permitting unimpeded enucleation of the lesion (Fig. 145 B). Many empty, nonbleeding vessels may be seen as they are cut across. These are ligated as the excision proceeds, *before they are permitted to retract into the parenchyma*. On completion of the dissection, the clamps are tentatively released and the remaining bleeding points individually sutured. The utilization of intestinal forceps as a temporary occluding device does no harm, as they compress rather than crush the pulmonary tissue. On removal, there remains no telltale mark at the site of application. The two adjacent raw lung surfaces are now apposed with interrupted sutures in the depths of the wound and along the visceral surface. This technic results in the least possible amount of puckering because hemostatic control is accomplished at multiple individual sites rather than by gross inclusion of all tissue within a running suture.

SEGMENTAL RESECTION

This involves removal of the smallest surgical anatomic unit. It is not within the scope of this presentation to detail the surgical anatomy or technic, but rather to stress those features of importance. The dissection commences at the hilum, and the appropriate segmental artery and vein are interrupted. The segmental bronchus is then isolated and divided, and the distal portion is used as an anchor or stem in extirpating the lobule. There is no anatomic demarcation or septalization of the parenchyma between adjacent segments, but the distal bronchial stalk helps to guide the fingers in "peeling out" the structure (Fig. 146 A). The separation is accomplished almost solely by finger dissection, as the normal pulmonary parenchyma is fragile and yields readily before the probing fingers. The diseased tissue has not the same spongy, yielding character of the normal parenchyma, and this also helps in guiding the extirpation. The only other impediment encountered by finger dissection is the intersegmental veins. These will be felt as firm, stringlike structures traversing the parenchymal tissue. If the dissection is momentarily discontinued to divide and ligate these vessels, possibly 6 to 10 in number, little else will be found to be necessary for hemostasis on completion of the enucleation.

The *bronchial stump* is treated in the usual manner (see Pneumonectomy) and sutured with interrupted fine silk. The ends are left long and, after completion of the bronchial closure, are re-threaded and used to bury the stump in the adjacent pulmonary tissue (Fig. 146 B). The opposing raw surfaces are then approximated.

LOBECTOMY

The lobe is the next largest anatomic unit which is subject to excision. Although pneumonectomy is the classic radical procedure of choice in the eradication of carcinoma, a lobectomy frequently is selected as the indicated method of extirpation. The choice is dictated by the patient's state of pulmonary reserve. It is wiser to limit the nature of the excision when it is felt that the reserve capacity of the remaining lung is inadequate to meet the required respiratory need and that immediate postoperative survival might only be followed by a state of chronic respiratory insufficiency and *cor pulmonale*.

This does not mean that one must compromise the established principles of surgery for carcinoma. Lobectomy may be performed with the anticipation of cure if the hilum is free of involved lymph nodes, or if such nodes are present and others draining the site of cancer are free of metastatic disease.

In performing lobectomy, it is desirable first to interrupt the arterial supply. The vascular reservoir of the lung is huge and readily adapts itself to vast changes in circulatory volume. Hence, occlusion of the venous exit prior to dividing the arterial inflow permits pooling of large quantities of blood in the capillary bed. The lobe, on removal, is boggy and heavy with trapped blood, which is lost to the general circulation. Gross estimates of the quantity of blood thus trapped and removed with the lobe measure from 200 cc. to 350 cc. more than when the artery has been divided primarily. Initial arterial ligation is technically feasible in all lobes, with the possible exception of the right upper lobe, where the apical segment of the superior pulmonary vein occasionally may interfere with adequate exposure of the main artery.

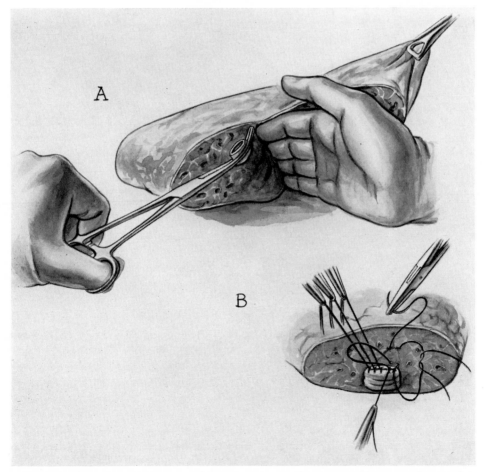

Fig. 146. Segmental resection. (A) Distal portion of isolated segmental bronchus used as a guide in extirpating the lung segment. (B) Method of "burying" the remaining bronchial stump in adjacent pulmonary tissue.

Transection of the bronchus and closure of the stump is performed in the manner described for pneumonectomy. In situations where the stump cannot be buried adequately, it is necessary to cover it with a pedicled pleural flap. In dealing with the lower lobe, particularly on the right, the bronchus is severed at its two major divisions, the basilar bronchus and the dorsal segmental bronchus, thus leaving a stump with two sutured orifices. The purpose in so treating the bronchus is to prevent encroachment on the orifice of the middle lobe. If the lower lobe were to be removed by a single transection, it would be necessary to cut across the bronchus in an oblique plane to avoid injury to the bronchus of the middle lobe (Fig. 147). Such a tangential incision not only makes a larger opening, but also sutures at the medial angle would impinge closely on the middle-lobe orifice, which might become temporarily compromised by postoperative edema. On the left side it is usually possible to remove the lower lobe by a single transecting incision through the bronchus. However, in situations where the bronchus of the superior segment originates so high that its location is opposite the upper-lobe orifice, the lower lobe is dealt with as on the

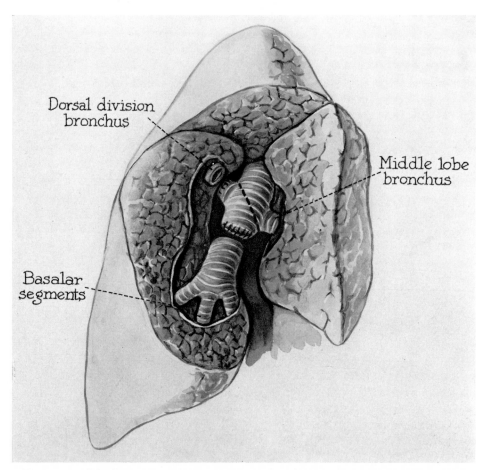

FIG. 147. Right lower lobectomy, showing related bronchial anatomy and sites of amputation. Amputation by a single incision necessitates cutting on the bias (dotted line), with the following disadvantages: (1) excessively large orifice to suture, (2) transection of multiple cartilages, (3) danger of compromising middle lobe orifice with the suture line.

right, namely, transection and suture of the bronchus of the superior and of the basilar segments as individual components.

To Rudolf Nissen[4] belongs the credit of having been first to perform lobectomy.

PNEUMONECTOMY

The lung was excised successfully for the first time in 1933. Since then pneumonectomy has become a common surgical procedure for the eradication of pulmonary disease processes. In the early developmental years, the mortality rate was formidable. The majority of fatalities occurred during the early postoperative period, usually between the fifth and tenth postoperative day, and the common cause was the appearance of a fistula in the bronchial stump. That this dreaded complication was both frequent and mortal is attested by the numerous technics described for closure of the stump. Fortunately, this is now an uncommon complication. The error responsible for development of these fistulae was a lack of appreciation of the nature of healing of the bronchial stump.

The healing ability of the larger bronchi is notoriously poor because of lack of adequate blood supply. Although large bronchial vessels may be found coursing on the exterior, producing brisk bleeding when transected, nutrient capillaries supplying the cut tissue surfaces are inadequate because of the cartilaginous nature of the bronchus. The older the bronchus, the greater the calcification of its cartilaginous structure and the more inadequate the nutrient blood supply. In addition, the very structure of the bronchus, as designed by nature, is to maintain a patent passageway. This ability to resist obliteration of its lumen by the springlike action of the cartilages tends to impose a state of tension on the occluding sutures. Thus, if the bare, sutured stump were left to protrude into the free pleural space, a fistula would be the expected consequence as the sutures start to cut through about the fifth postoperative day, and as the suture holes enlarge, not only does air escape but also the bacterial flora of the bronchial passages escape to compound the insult.

Safeguards against such accidents are proper attention to the preparation and the closure

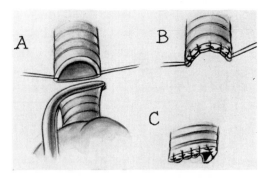

FIG. 148. Method of bronchial amputation and closure. (A) Guide sutures alone stabilize the proximal stump. The clamp with crushed bronchus is on the portion to be extirpated. (B) Mucosa is "folded in" and sutured to conform with the cartilaginous arch. (C) A poor bronchial stump, with inclusion of a "cracked" and infolded cartilage ring in the suture line. This results from improperly placed stay-sutures and clamp prior to amputation.

of the bronchial stump which will avert the development of a fistula. The primary consideration, which must be enforced without compromise, is to ensure that the stump is adequately covered with viable tissue. This permits the organization and the early union of such tissue over and to the raw surface of the stump, prior to its anticipated loss of integrity. It is during this "period of grace," the first 4 to 5 postoperative days, that such tissue union must occur to prevent the escape of bronchial contents through enlarging suture holes and gaping stump aperture, which otherwise would follow.

In performing a pneumonectomy, the bronchus is prepared and cut with the objective of having the stump buried within the mediastinum. This is accomplished more easily on the left side because the arch of the aorta forms a natural recess into which the stump may retract if cut sufficiently short. On the right, there is no such easily available structure for protection, and the length of this bronchus is so short that its stump will not retract naturally into the mediastinum. This condition must be kept in mind as the dissection is begun so that an adequate portion of mediastinal pleura may be conserved to cover over the bronchial stump. This will be a safeguard when sufficient adjacent tissue is lacking. A pedicled flap of parietal pleura can then be dissected and made to cover the free stump.

Treatment of the Bronchial Stump. Prior to preparing the stump, the lung is usually first removed by transecting the bronchus well distal to this site. The bronchus then may be retransected at a point of election without the impediment of the bulky lung mass. To minimize trauma of the cut end of the bronchial stump by repeated instrumentation with tissue forceps, a stay suture is placed at either end of the anticipated ostium. A clamp then occludes the bronchus just distal to the line of section and is used to guide the scalpel in a clean, transecting stroke across the bronchus (Fig. 148 A). The stay sutures alone stabilize the stump, as interrupted silk sutures are inserted to close the orifice. A suture through the center is placed first to reduce oxygen-gas loss as rapidly as possible. The membranous portion of the bronchus should "fold in" to meet the cartilaginous ring, thus reducing to a minimum the amount of tension placed on the suture line (Fig. 148 B). This must be considered in advance when originally positioning the stay sutures and the guiding clamp. It is an error to infold a margin of the cartilaginous ring (Fig. 148 C), as it subjects the suture here to undue tension.

On completion of the procedure, there is left a large vacant space formerly occupied by the lung. The treatment of this space has been the subject of much controversy. Following any other intrathoracic procedure, every effort is made to decompress adequately the pleural cavity of accumulating air or fluid, allowing the remaining lung to expand without compromise. However, following a pneumonectomy, there is no pulmonary tissue left to occupy the space. In contrast, an undrained and intact thoracic cavity is desired here to retain the accumulating fluid so as to fill this empty space. It will fill with a serosanguinous fluid, reaching its capacity in approximately 5 days. During this time it is desirable to withdraw the retained air at intervals, thus not only permitting a completely fluid-filled cavity but also preventing dislocation of the mediastinum to the opposite side. It is sometimes necessary to withdraw several hundred cubic centimeters

of fluid as well, if overproduction causes the mediastinum to encroach on the space of the opposite lung. After 2 weeks, absorption of the fluid starts, and the hemithorax becomes progressively smaller as the heart and the mediastinum are drawn in the opposite direction to help occupy this cavity. As shrinkage continues, the intercostal spaces narrow, and the diaphragm is elevated as high as the third anterior intercostal space. On the left side, gastro-intestinal symptoms frequently are manifested as a result of such marked dislocation of the stomach and the splenic flexure of the colon into the region of the left hemithorax. The residual fluid ultimately becomes organized.

The development of a fistula may be suspected when, on or about the fifth postoperative day, coughing sets in. This is associated with change in position, that is, it is induced by postural change from the upright to the supine or, particularly, when the patient turns to lie upon his unoperated side. The accumulation within the vacant pleural space then trickles by gravity through the fistulous opening into the tracheobronchial lumen and is expectorated as a pink or red semiliquid material, similar to that which may be aspirated from the thorax by thoracentesis. The appearance of a fistula necessitates complete evacuation of the hemithoracic space to relieve the patient of the fatiguing burden of emptying it himself via the bronchus by a constant, harassing cough. Inability to keep the bronchial passages clear of this persistent seepage, because of fatigue or loss of vigilance of the cough mechanism, ultimately results in aspiratory pneumonitis of the remaining lung. Emptying the thoracic space by closed drainage also removes the retained fluid from the contaminating presence of the bronchial flora and thus prevents it from becoming purulent. In addition, a catastrophic occurrence may be averted, because, should the stump suddenly become widely patent by the sloughing through of a suture, the entire content of the space, if unemptied, might instantaneously flood the tracheobronchial tree, with rapid asphyxia as a consequence.

Definitive treatment of the fistula by reoperating to expose and resuture the bronchial stump is an error, because if the original preoperative preparation were made properly, under circumstances favoring the best technical conditions, yet without success, a second try, under circumstances less fortuitous and with tissues contaminated and indurated, would be still less likely to succeed.

Obliteration of the empty space is now the desired goal, and this may be accomplished by a thoracoplasty or by extraperiosteal *plombage.** In the presence of overt infection (empyema), thoracoplasty is the preferred procedure. Not only will obliteration of the space diminish or avert an empyema, but also the approximation of tissues promotes effacement of the fistula.

* The surgical operation of filling an empty space in the body with inert material.

REFERENCES

1. Graham, E. A., and Bell, R. D.: Open pneumothorax; its relationship to the treatment of empyema, Am. J. M. Sc. **156**:839, 1918.
2. Mackler, S. A., and Mayer, R. M.: Palliation of esophageal obstruction due to carcinoma with a permanent intraluminal tube, J. Thoracic Surg. **28**:431, 1954.
3. ———: Spontaneous rupture of the esophagus; an experimental and clinical study, Surg., Gynec. & Obst. **95**:345, 1952.
4. Nissen, R.: Extirpation eines ganzen Lungenfluegels (extirpation of an entire lobe of the lung), Zentralbl. Chir. **58**:3003, 1931.
5. Sauerbuch, F. (Quoted by Meyer, H. W.): History of negative differential pressure chamber, J. Thoracic Surg. **30**:114, 1955.

ARTHUR VINEBERG, M.D.,* OSMAN GIALLORETO, M.D.,†
AND JULES LABERGE, M.D.‡

13 Cardiac Surgery

Surgery of the human heart, like the development of atomic power, represents centuries of human study and effort. Both are symbols of our highly developed Western civilization. Our scientists have released the tremendous power locked in the atom—our physicians have laid bare the human heart.

Over 300 years ago, it was discovered that the human heart could be wounded without fatal outcome. During the intervening years, however, little progress had been made in cardiac surgery until comparatively recently. In the past 10 years, aided by the developments in anesthesiology and thoracic surgery, cardiac surgery has emerged as an independent specialty. Operations on the human heart are no longer considered to be highly experimental and dangerous but are being performed daily throughout the world. Thousands of formerly crippled cardiac patients have experienced great benefit as the result of cardiac surgery. However, this state of affairs has not been achieved without many mistakes and at the cost of many lives. Numerous white crosses mark the paths of those surgeons who have been in the forefront of development in this field, and a great number of those deaths could have been avoided.

In this chapter it is our intention to point out the errors which may occur in the diagnosis and the treatment of cardiac diseases which may be helped by surgery. No attempt will be made to give technical details, since this is not intended as a textbook of cardiac surgery. Instead, wherever possible, safeguards in the handling of cardiac surgical cases will be pointed out. In the diagrammatic representation of the pathology of each lesion, only defects or diseased areas are shown.

ORGANIZATION OF A CARDIAC SURGICAL UNIT

Organization of a cardiac surgical unit is

absolutely essential for the successful completion of surgical procedures on the human heart. There is no field of medicine and surgery in which success is so dependent on the combined efforts of a number of people working as a team in a well-equipped hospital center. It is a grievous error to attempt such work in hospitals not properly organized and equipped to handle such patients. Thus we find certain minimum requirements, namely, (1) a thoracic unit, a recovery room and special nurses; (2) experienced cardiologists and at least two cardiac surgeons; (3) complete diagnostic x-ray and cardiac catheterization facilities. Experience in medical cardiology or pulmonary surgery does not qualify such personnel to handle surgical heart problems.

It is necessary for those who contemplate cardiac surgery to have special training. There are many hundreds of expert thoracic surgeons throughout the country, most of whom think that their training qualifies them to operate on the heart. Nothing is further from the truth. The anatomy, the physiology and the pathology of the human heart are extremely complex and must be learned. It is not always possible for an experienced cardiac surgeon to prevent a pupil from making a mistake. The comparatively simple and standardized procedure of mitral commissurotomy is perhaps the best example of this. The left atrium tolerates only one finger at a time! The teacher may feel the mitral valve before and after commissurotomy, but he cannot see or feel what the pupil is doing until after it has been done. Only the finger in the atrium knows! Inexperienced fingers need practice in the beating hearts of animals and in the autopsy room. The performance of an intracardiac procedure on a pathologic specimen helps to orient the inexperienced surgeon. The result of the technical procedure is easily checked. It is far better to make an error on a pathologic specimen than to find it out in a specimen produced as the result of a mistake made in

* Director, Department of Cardiology, Royal Victoria Hospital, Montreal.
† Cardiologist, Montreal Institute of Cardiology.
‡ Radiologist, Montreal Institute of Cardiology.

the operating room. Finally, the experienced cardiac surgeon, before repeating a new technic or initiating a new procedure in man, must prove that the technic works well in the laboratory animal. It is true that what works in an animal may not work in man; on the other hand, it is much more likely that what does not work in an animal will not work in man.

SELECTION OF PATIENTS FOR CARDIAC SURGERY

Our thinking concerning the selection of patients for cardiac surgery should be based on the same principles that have been followed by the general surgeon for many years. Surgery rarely cures disease, but it does relieve mechanical abnormalities caused by disease or physical forces. Thus, the first consideration in the selection of a patient for a heart operation is whether there is a mechanical condition present within or around the heart which could be relieved by surgical intervention. It is an error to assume that cardiac surgery is indicated under such conditions unless the patient has failed to respond to adequate medical treatment and unless his future, by medical treatment alone, is poor. The presence of either mitral stenosis or coronary artery disease is not, in itself, an indication for surgical interference, any more than the presence of a duodenal ulcer, per se, is an indication for gastrectomy. The condition must create subjective and objective evidence that it is causing, or may cause, disability before surgical interference is justified. The next important consideration, which is weighed far too infrequently, concerns mortality and morbidity. A surgical procedure that carries a mortality of 20 to 25 per cent can hardly be justified unless a high percentage of those who survive are greatly benefited and unless such patients were disabled or going downhill at the time of consideration for surgery. Cardiac surgical procedures which have not been proved clinically or in the laboratory must be avoided.

Bad-Risk Patients

It is questionable whether extremely bad-risk patients should be subjected to an elective cardiac operation. The answer to this query rests on the extent of irreversible or irreparable disease that exists. Certainly, experience

has shown that chronic left ventricular failure rarely can be reversed, the same being true of irreversible serious pulmonary arteriolar or liver changes. Correction of mechanical cardiac defects in such cases, although successful technically, is usually attended by a high mortality and a small percentage of patients who are improved. Likewise, the presence of serious associated diseases, such as essential hypertension, general arteriosclerosis, blood dyscrasias, etc., are contraindications for cardiac surgery.

Importance of Accurate Diagnosis in Selection of Patients for Cardiac Surgery

Before cardiac surgery is attempted, a most complete evaluation of the patient must be made. This includes a thorough understanding of the patient himself, as well as his heart. It is useless to correct a cardiac condition in a patient who is mentally incompetent or in one who is going to die from leukemia. The importance of accurate diagnosis of the cardiac condition and its sequelae cannot be stressed too strongly. Hundreds of cardiac operations have been performed in the past without benefit to the patient because of incomplete awareness of other existing pathologic conditions.

PREOPERATIVE CARE

The preoperative and postoperative responsibility of the nursing team in charge of cardiac patients is great. Errors of omission may result in serious complications and even death following operation. Failure to measure correctly fluid intake and output, weight and salt consumption could mislead the surgeon into thinking that the patient was ready for surgery when actually there was still too much fluid in the body, particularly in the lungs. Total blood volume should be within 15 per cent of normal; mortality is higher in the presence of an elevated blood volume. Accurate blood pressure measurements taken preoperatively indicate the average blood pressure for that individual and serve as a guide for postoperative care.

THE EFFECT OF FEAR AND EXCITEMENT

Idle gossip concerning the progress of other patients may disturb the patient who is about to undergo heart surgery. Confidence is essential in order to allay fears. The excitement caused by a visitor before or after operation may cause complications or even death. The effect of excitement on patients with coronary artery disease is well known. Cases of mitral stenosis have been known to go into pulmonary edema following or during the visit of a loved one, particularly shortly after surgery. It is an error to permit visitors too early after operation. Our nurses have been instructed to allay the patient's fears prior to operation as much as possible. In order to avoid any unnecessary waiting period in the operating room, our patients never leave the ward until called for by the anesthetist.

During the postoperative period there is probably no group of cases where so much depends on intelligent nursing care.

POSTOPERATIVE CARE

Maintenance of a functionally adequate blood pressure is important after any operation to prevent irreversible shock and damage to heart, brain, liver and kidneys. The mistake that is made most frequently is failure to recognize that the safe functional level of blood pressure varies from patient to patient. Thus the maintenance of blood pressure at a set arbitrary level may keep one patient alive and result in the death of another. The preoperative blood pressure measurements act as a guide for each patient, and all efforts must be made to keep postoperative blood pressure levels as close as possible to the preoperative levels.

Administration of parenteral fluid, again, should be based on the daily intake of the patient preoperatively. Cardiac drugs should be given intramuscularly until it is certain that the gastro-intestinal tract is functioning well. It is an error not to check electrolytes.

In the following pages, various types of cardiac conditions which can be treated by surgery are outlined, particularly from the viewpoint of error in diagnosis and treatment and in regard to safeguards which may be taken to avoid such errors. These conditions may be divided into *congenital* and *acquired* cardiac lesions.

PATENT DUCTUS ARTERIOSUS

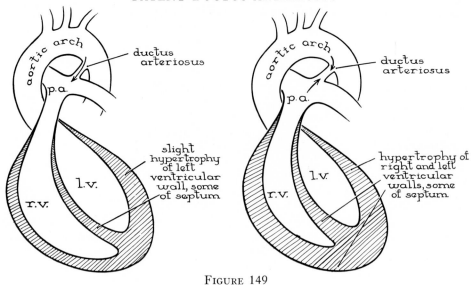

FIGURE 149

UNCOMPLICATED

History: Patent ductus arteriosus is an acyanotic disease compatible with normal physical development and relative longevity. Often the symptoms are limited to exertional dyspnea, which may be slowly progressive, terminating in heart failure.

Diagnosis: There is a characteristic systolic-diastolic continuous murmur heard in the 2nd or 3rd left intercostal space.

PULMONARY HYPERTENSION

History: Increasing pulmonary pressure is not well tolerated, resulting in accentuation of symptoms. Dyspnea is more pronounced, and progress of the disease is faster. Once the increasing pulmonary pressure reaches the systemic level, the shunt becomes mixed or reversed from right to left. When the latter occurs, there is cyanosis in the lower part of the body and occasionally clubbing of the toes.

Diagnosis: The continuous systolic-diastolic murmur is still present, but when the pulmonary artery pressure is sufficiently elevated, the diastolic component is reduced or disappears.

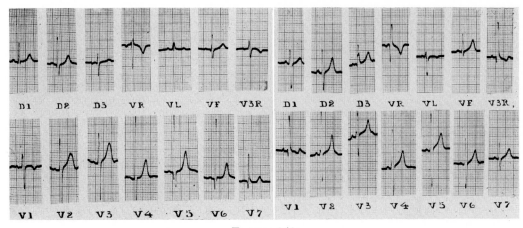

FIGURE 150

(*Left*) UNCOMPLICATED. This may be normal or show slight left ventricular hypertrophy.

(*Right*) PULMONARY HYPERTENSION. This shows balanced or right axis deviation with right or combined ventricular hypertrophy.

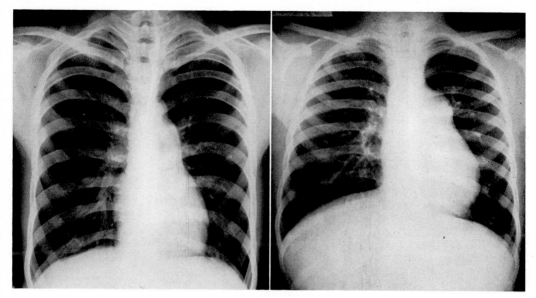

FIGURE 151

UNCOMPLICATED

Postero-anterior Roentgenogram: The heart size may be normal but is usually slightly or moderately increased. The pulmonary arch is prominent and is often confluent with the aortic arch. The pulmonary vessels show a variable degree of enlargement. The ventricular mass is increased, most often due to enlargement of the left ventricle. Enlargement of the left atrium occasionally may be seen in the right oblique projection.

Fluoroscopy: The pulsations of the pulmonary arteries are usually increased.

PULMONARY HYPERTENSION

Postero-anterior Roentgenogram: The heart size is increased. The pulmonary arch is markedly enlarged. Both ventricles are increased in size, right ventricular hypertrophy being more prominent.

Fluoroscopy: The pulsations of the pulmonary arteries are usually very slightly increased.

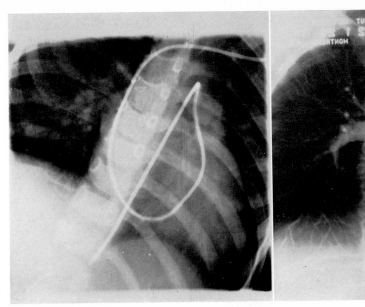

FIGURE 152

UNCOMPLICATED	PULMONARY HYPERTENSION
Spot Film and Catheterization: When the catheter passes through the ductus into the aorta it takes the form of the Greek letter Phi ϕ suggesting the diagnosis.	*Selective Angiocardiography:* Radiopaque substance is injected into the right ventricular outflow tract.
	Anteroposterior Roentgenogram: Shows the dye entering the huge pulmonary trunk and the main branches, with simultaneous injection of the descending aorta through the ductus. No opacification of the aortic arch proximal to the ductus.

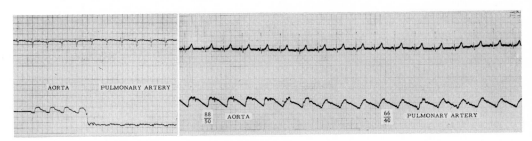

FIGURE 153

UNCOMPLICATED

Pressure Curves: The pressure drops suddenly from systemic levels to normal pulmonary artery pressures as the catheter is slowly withdrawn from the aorta through the ductus into the pulmonary artery. Oxygenated blood is present in the pulmonary artery.

Errors in Diagnosis: The characteristic systolic-diastolic murmur of ductus arteriosus may be present in (1) aortic pulmonary fistula, (2) truncus arteriosus, (3) ventricular septal defect with aortic insufficiency, (4) ruptured sinus of Valsalva. Careful catheterization studies, with angiocardiography when necessary, will establish the correct diagnosis.

PULMONARY HYPERTENSION

Pressure Curves: The elevated pulmonary artery pressure results in diminution or disappearance of the pressure gradient between the pulmonary artery and the aorta. Oxygenated blood is less likely to be obtained from the pulmonary artery. Oxygen saturation of aortic blood may be lower than normal, and there is a difference in O_2 saturation in the brachial artery and the descending aorta.

SURGERY OF DUCTUS ARTERIOSUS

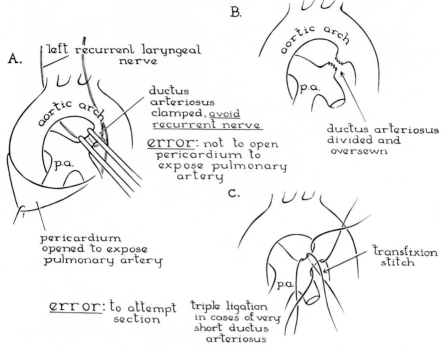

A.
left recurrent laryngeal
nerve

aortic arch

ductus
arteriosus
clamped, avoid
recurrent nerve

error: not to open
pericardium to
expose pulmonary
artery

p.a.

pericardium
opened to expose
pulmonary artery

error: to attempt
section

B.

aortic arch

p.a.

ductus arteriosus
divided and
oversewn

C.

transfixion
stitch

p.a.

triple ligation
in cases of very
short ductus
arteriosus

FIGURE 154

This persistent communication between the aorta and the pulmonary artery may be interrupted by cutting the ductus across or by ligating it. Transection of the ductus is preferable. If this appears to be technically difficult, triple ligation is advisable.

In both procedures it is dangerous not to obtain good exposure of the pulmonary artery by opening the pericardium, and to obtain satisfactory mobilization of the aorta. Tears in the pulmonary artery or the aorta may thus be controlled more easily.

Careful isolation of the left vagus and the recurrent laryngeal nerve avoids left vocal-cord paralysis.

In spite of the most careful preoperative diagnostic investigation, errors can be made, and the ductus may be needed to compensate for other congenital defects. In such cases its closure is dangerous. A trial period of temporary occlusion is necessary before definite occlusion of the ductus is performed.

COARCTATION OF THE AORTA

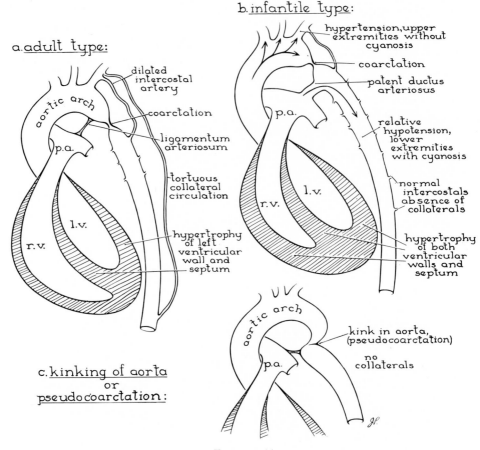

b. <u>infantile type</u>:

hypertension, upper
extremities without
cyanosis

coarctation

patent ductus
arteriosus

relative
hypotension,
lower
extremities
with cyanosis

normal
intercostals
absence of
collaterals

hypertrophy
of both
ventricular
walls and
septum

a. <u>adult type</u>:

dilated
intercostal
artery

coarctation

ligamentum
arteriosum

tortuous
collateral
circulation

hypertrophy
of left
ventricular
wall and
septum

aortic arch

p.a.

l.v.

r.v.

p.a.

l.v.

r.v.

c. <u>kinking of aorta</u>
or
<u>pseudocoarctation</u>:

aortic arch

p.a.

kink in aorta,
(pseudocoarctation)

no
collaterals

FIGURE 155

A. ADULT TYPE

History: This condition is generally well tolerated, with minimal symptomatology until maturity. Elevation of the blood pressure in the superior part of the body produces symptoms which are similar to those seen in essential hypertension. Cerebral, coronary and other vascular accidents occur, as well as left ventricular failure.

Diagnosis: Young subjects have upper extremity hypertension and decreased blood pressures in the lower extremities, with a weak and delayed femoral pulse. Enlarged intercostal arteries can be felt in the back.

Murmur: A systolic murmur is present in the 3rd left intercostal space anteroposteriorly, with wide distribution, depending on the extent of collateral circulation.

B. INFANTILE TYPE

History: In the infantile type the coarcted segment is longer, and there is a patent ductus arteriosus distal to it which prevents the development of collaterals. It is generally associated with other congenital lesions which cause early death. Patients with the infantile type of lesion rarely live long enough for surgical correction.

Diagnosis: There is upper extremity hypertension with normal pressures in the lower extremities; there is slight cyanosis of the lower part of the body and the lower extremities which may be masked by general cyanosis caused by other associated congenital lesions.

Murmur: There may be various auscultatory signs. A systolic-diastolic murmur may be heard at the 3rd left intercostal space. More often a systolic murmur alone is heard in the same region and at the back, as in the adult type of coarctation.

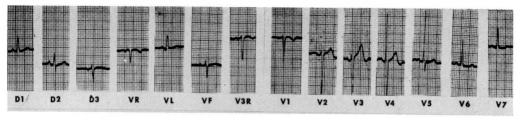

| D1 | D2 | D3 | VR | VL | VF | V3R | V1 | V2 | V3 | V4 | V5 | V6 | V7 |

FIGURE 156

ECG. ADULT TYPE: This may show left ventricular hypertrophy or may be normal. There is nothing characteristic in the ECG of the infantile type, due to frequent association with other congenital lesions.

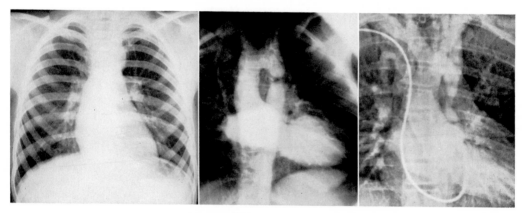

FIGURE 157

(Left) ADULT TYPE

The aortic arch is deformed and may show interruption of continuity. The left ventricle is enlarged, and when there is severe coarctation there is notching of the ribs.

Fluoroscopy: Poststenotic dilatation, when it occurs, displaces the barium-filled esophagus anteriorly, which is clearly seen in the oblique position.

Errors in Diagnosis: Coarctation can exist with normal or slight elevation of the systemic blood pressure. Failure to take the lower extremity blood pressures in young subjects with hypertension may lead to the diagnosis of "essential hypertension" when, in effect, the elevated blood pressure is due to the coarctation.

(Center and right) ANGIOCARDIOGRAPHY

(Center) Case 1. Short narrow constriction of aorta.

(Right) Case 2. Long constriction of aorta. Selective angiocardiography as well as retrograde aortography satisfactorily visualized the coarcted segment.

Kinking of Aorta: Kinking of the aorta may simulate true coarctation. Angiocardiography shows sinuosity of the aorta without coarctation.

SURGERY OF COARCTATION OF THE AORTA

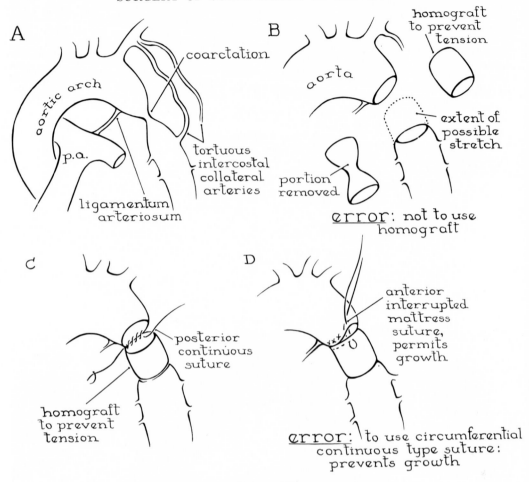

FIGURE 158

ADULT TYPE

The area of aortic narrowing is usually distal to the ductus arteriosus or the ligamentum arteriosum. In the adult type of coarctation this may be a long or a short segment. The operation is long and tedious due to many dilated chest wall vessels.

It is wise to perform this operation with two surgical teams, so that a fresh team actually does the resection of the narrowed aortic segment and the subsequent anastomosis. Careful mobilization of the aorta above and below the coarctation is obligatory. Failure to use an homologous or plastic graft may lead to a torn aorta due to tension on the suture line. When a continuous suture is used, it should anatomose only half the circumference of the vessel. The use of interrupted mattress sutures on the second half permits expansion during growth.

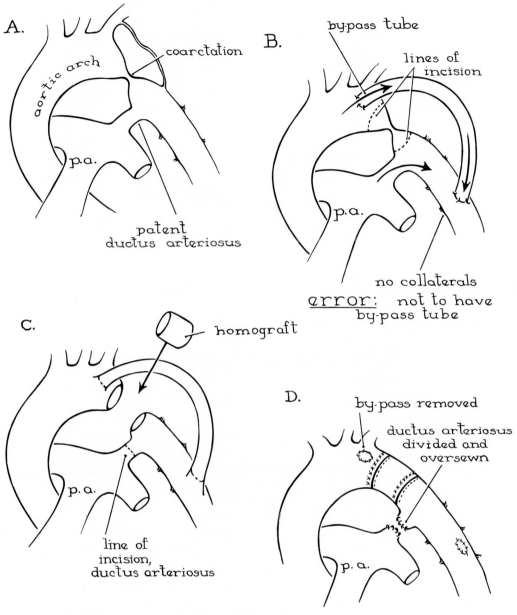

A. aortic arch

coarctation

p.a.

patent
ductus arteriosus

B. by-pass tube

lines of
incision

p.a.

no collaterals

<u>error</u>:   not to have
by-pass tube

C. homograft

p.a.

line of
incision,
ductus arteriosus

D. by-pass removed

ductus arteriosus
divided and
oversewn

p. a.

FIGURE 158

INFANTILE TYPE

In this comparatively rare condition, the coarctation is proximal to an open ductus arteriosus. Blood reaches the lower part of the body through the ductus arteriosus, so that no collaterals develop to bridge the area of coarctation.

A serious error may result if provision is not made for oxygenated blood to reach the aorta distal to the coarctation during resection, resulting in kidney, liver and spinal cord damage. The use of a bypass graft or extracorporeal circulation to supply the lower extremities with oxygenated blood during coarctation resection prevents these complications.

PULMONIC STENOSIS

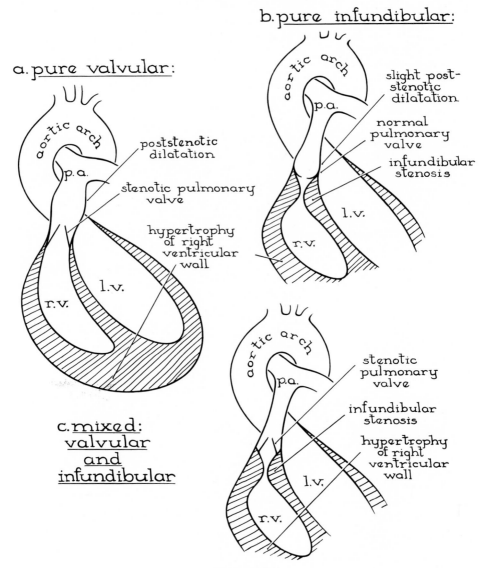

a. pure valvular:

poststenotic
dilatation

stenotic pulmonary
valve

hypertrophy
of right
ventricular
wall

l.v.

r.v.

b. pure infundibular:

slight post-
stenotic
dilatation

normal
pulmonary
valve

infundibular
stenosis

l.v.

r.v.

c. mixed:
valvular
and
infundibular

stenotic
pulmonary
valve

infundibular
stenosis

hypertrophy
of right
ventricular
wall

l.v.

r.v.

FIGURE 159

A. PURE VALVULAR

History: With the improvements in diagnostic technics, this lesion is detected more frequently. It is compatible with normal physical development. Symptoms are limited to progressive exertional dyspnea and palpitations; right heart insufficiency may develop.

Diagnosis: A harsh systolic murmur is heard in the 2nd left intercostal space, often accompanied by a corresponding thrill. The 2nd pulmonary sound is faint or absent.

B. PURE INFUNDIBULAR

History: Isolated infundibular stenosis is very rare. The symptomatology is the same as in the valvular type.

Diagnosis: There is a harsh systolic murmur heard in the 2nd left intercostal space, as in the pure valvular type. The presence of a well-defined second sound is suggestive of an infundibular lesion.

ECG: The same as in pure valvular stenosis.

C. MIXED VALVULAR AND INFUNDIBULAR STENOSIS: Definitive diagnosis is possible only by catheterization.

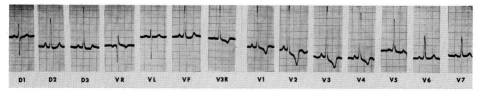

FIG. 160. ECG. *Pure Valvular:* Right axis deviation and marked right ventricular hypertrophy with systolic overload.

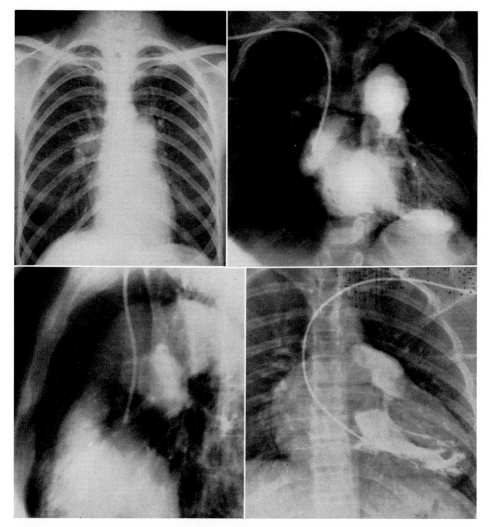

FIG. 161 (*Top, left*). Postero-anterior roentgenogram. The cardiac volume is slightly or moderately increased, with evident right ventricular hypertrophy. The pulmonary arch is prominent, and the peripheral pulmonary vessels are of diminished caliber. The pulmonary hypovascularity causes increased translucency of the lung fields.

FIG. 162 A (*Top, right*). Angiocardiography: antero-posterior roentgenogram showing post-stenotic dilatation.

FIG. 162 B (*Bottom, left*). Angiocardiography, lateral view. The pulmonic stenosis may be clearly demonstrated by a lateral angiocardiographic view.

FIG. 163 (*Bottom, right*). Angiocardiography. Infundibular pulmonic stenosis.

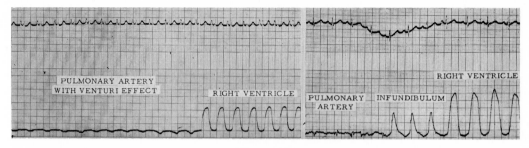

FIGURE 164

Catheterization Data: (*Left*) Pure Valvular Stenosis. Withdrawal of the catheter from the pulmonary artery into the right ventricle is associated with a sudden rise of the systolic pressure to a level which remains the same in all parts of the right ventricular cavity. (*Right*) Mixed Valvular Stenosis. There are two systolic pressure rises: (1) between pulmonary artery and infundibulum; (2) between infundibulum and right ventricular cavity.

Errors in Diagnosis: Failure to recognize the presence of infundibular narrowing in pulmonary valvular stenosis may lead to serious surgical error. It is an error to operate on a case of pulmonary stenosis without complete preliminary hemodynamic studies, and, when necessary, selective angiocardiography.

operative treatment: pure valvular

1. direct open:

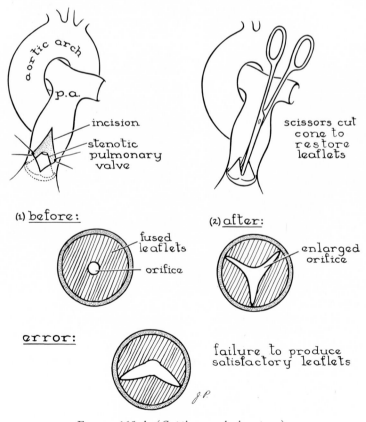

FIGURE 165 A (*Caption on facing page*)

II. direct closed:

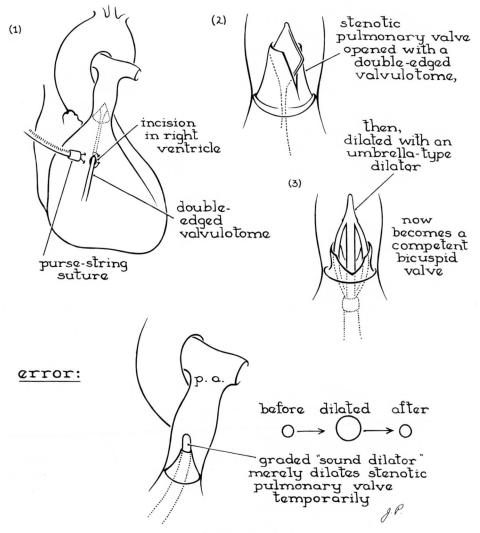

(1)

incision
in right
ventricle

double-
edged
valvulotome

purse-string
suture

(2)

stenotic
pulmonary valve
opened with a
double-edged
valvulotome,

then,
dilated with an
umbrella-type
dilator

(3)

now
becomes a
competent
bicuspid
valve

error:

p. a.

before dilated after

graded "sound dilator"
merely dilates stenotic
pulmonary valve
temporarily

FIGURE 165 B

In these cases the only point of pulmonic stenosis is at the pulmonary valve. This may be corrected by

I. *Direct Approach (Open)* through the pulmonary artery. Hypothermia or the pump oxygenator permit direct visualization of the pulmonic valve. Failure to create satisfactory valve leaflets results in pulmonary valve insufficiency.

II. *Direct Approach (Closed)* is through the right ventricle, in which case the stenotic pulmonary valve is blindly cut or dilated. After passage of the valvulotome, pressures taken in the right ventricle and the pulmonary artery indicate the extent to which the pulmonary valve has been opened. It is an error to discontinue valvulotomy until the right ventricular and the pulmonary artery pressures have been equalized.

operative treatment: infundibular

I direct closed: (unsatisfactory operation)

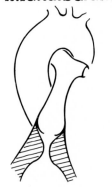

normal
leaflets

infundibular
stenotic portion
removed by
punch forceps

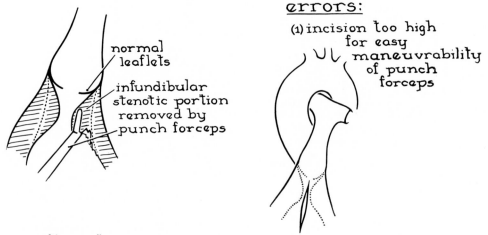

errors:

(1) incision too high
for easy
maneuvrability
of punch
forceps

(2): insufficient
removal of
infundibulum:

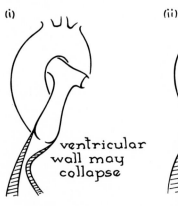

(3) removal of too much infundibulum:

(i)

ventricular
wall may
collapse

(ii)

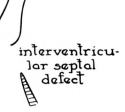

interventricu-
lar septal
defect

FIGURE 166 A

Infundibular pulmonic stenosis rarely occurs alone. It is usually present in combination with pure valvular stenosis or tetralogy of Fallot. There are 3 surgical approaches for correction of infundibular pulmonary obstruction.

I. DIRECT (CLOSED). This method, devised by Brock, is most unsatisfactory. There are errors involved in the technic which are difficult to avoid. Insufficient removal of the infundibular obstruction may occur in some cases. In others, too much of the infundibular wall is removed, so that the remaining wall falls into the outflow tract of the right ventricle, causing as much or more obstruction as the original lesion. Sometimes, by accident, part of the interventricular septum is removed, producing an interventricular septal defect.

(Continued on facing page)

II. direct open:

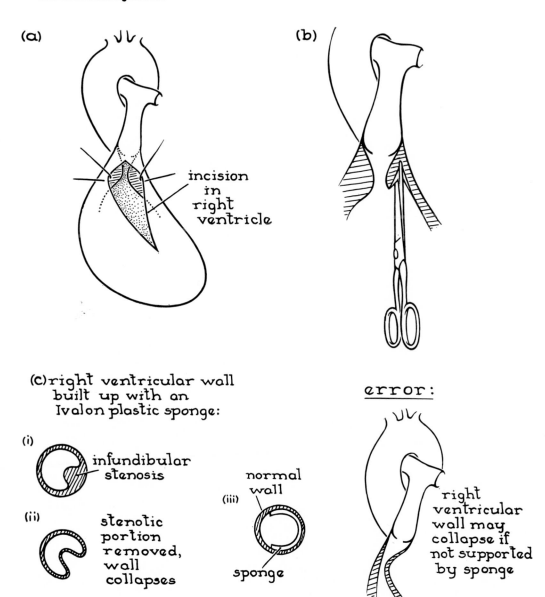

(a)

incision
in
right
ventricle

(b)

**(c) right ventricular wall
built up with an
Ivalon plastic sponge:**

(i) infundibular
stenosis

(ii) stenotic
portion
removed,
wall
collapses

(iii) normal
wall

sponge

error:

right
ventricular
wall may
collapse if
not supported
by sponge

FIGURE 166 B

II. DIRECT (OPEN). This is the method of choice. The approach is through the outflow tract of the right ventricle. It is an error to attempt this procedure under hypothermia, because the hypothermia does not permit sufficient time for the reconstruction of the infundibular area after the excess tissue has been removed. Infundibular stenosis is handled best by using the pump oxygenator which permits of an open, dry heart for as long a time interval as is required.

Bypass Operations. In these operations no attempt is made to relieve the primary lesion; instead, systemic blood is shunted into the pulmonary artery by anastomosis with the subclavian artery or the aorta. The treatment of pulmonic infundibular stenosis with or without pulmonary valvular stenosis by such means is a serious error (see tetralogy of Fallot).

tetralogy of fallot

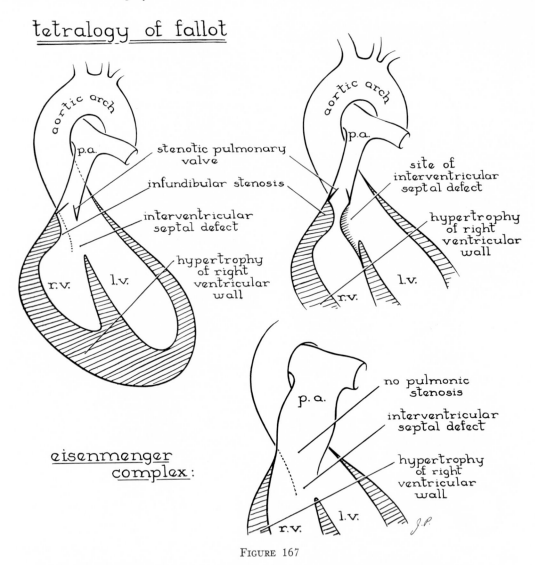

aortic arch

p.a.

stenotic pulmonary valve

infundibular stenosis

interventricular septal defect

hypertrophy of right ventricular wall

r.v.   l.v.

aortic arch

p.a.

site of interventricular septal defect

hypertrophy of right ventricular wall

l.v.

r.v.

eisenmenger complex:

p.a.

no pulmonic stenosis

interventricular septal defect

hypertrophy of right ventricular wall

r.v.   l.v.

FIGURE 167

TETRALOGY OF FALLOT

History: This is the most frequent congenital cyanotic lesion compatible with normal development. There are 2 primary anatomic anomalies: (1) infundibular stenosis and (2) overriding of the aorta. Both are associated with ventricular septal defect and right ventricular hypertrophy. These lesions give rise to the characteristic symptomatology of the disease—dyspnea, cyanosis, clubbing of the fingers and squatting.

Diagnosis: Cyanosis and clubbing of the fingers are constant. A harsh systolic murmur of maximum intensity is heard in the 4th left intercostal space. The second pulmonary sound is difficult to hear.

EISENMENGER COMPLEX

History: This is not as frequent as tetralogy of Fallot. Cyanosis appears later in life. The anatomic lesions are the same, except for the absence of pulmonary stenosis; consequently, the hypertension present in the right ventricle is commonly transmitted to the pulmonary arterial tree.

Diagnosis: Characteristic symptomatology: (1) late cyanosis, (2) clubbing of the fingers, (3) dyspnea, as in tetralogy of Fallot, but the second pulmonic sound is accentuated.

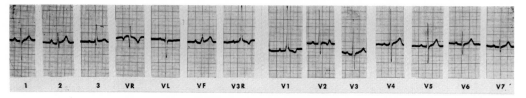

FIG. 168. Tetralogy of Fallot.

ECG: This shows right axis deviation and right ventricular hypertrophy. The ECG in Eisenmenger's complex is practically the same.

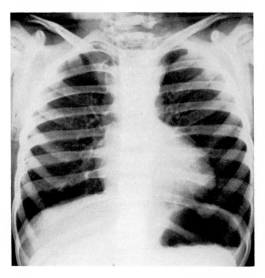

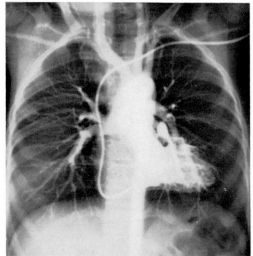

FIG. 169 (*Top, left*). Tetralogy of Fallot. Postero-anterior roentgenogram shows (1) concavity of the pulmonary segment, (2) right ventricular hypertrophy—apex elevated, (3) decreased vascularity of pulmonary field.

FIG. 170 (*Top, right*). Tetralogy of Fallot. Angiocardiogram showing simultaneous visualization of pulmonary artery and aorta, contrast media being injected directly into the right ventricle.

FIG. 171 (*Bottom*). Trilogy of Fallot. Postero-anterior roentgenogram showing increased heart size, with prominent right ventricle and atrium. Pulmonary vascularity decreased.

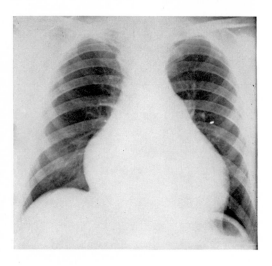

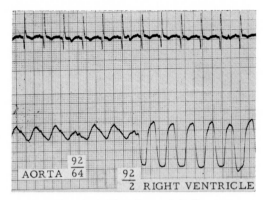

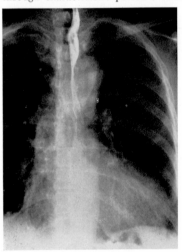

AORTA 64 92 / 2 RIGHT VENTRICLE

FIG. 172. Tetralogy of Fallot.

CATHETERIZATION:

Slow withdrawal of the catheter from the pulmonary artery into the right ventricle detects through characteristic pressure changes the presence of pulmonary stenosis and often indicates the type of stenosis. The catheterization of the aorta through the right ventricle proves the presence of overriding of the aorta.

ERRORS IN DIAGNOSIS:

1. Tetralogy of Fallot may exist with normal heart contour and even with a prominent pulmonary arch as in pulmonic stenosis and atrial septal defect. In such cases the pulmonic vascularity is close to normal. The cyanosis usually present may be slight and sometimes absent (Pink Fallot).

2. A large heart which may be confused with atrial septal defect and valvular pulmonic stenosis.

3. Truncus arteriosus is difficult to differentiate from the severe forms of tetralogy.

4. It is important to assess whether the pulmonary artery is patent or atresic and if there is a patent ductus arteriosus.

5. Complete hemodynamic studies and angiocardiography are essential to establish a precise anatomic diagnosis in each case.

FIG. 173 (Left). Truncus Arteriosus. Postero-anterior view. Concavity of pulmonary segment is exaggerated. Pulmonary arch is absent. Vascularity is often asymmetrical.

FIG. 174 (Bottom). Truncus Arteriosus. (Left) Angiocardiogram shows a large arterial vessel arising from the base of the truncus, with absence of the pulmonary trunk. Other bronchial arteries arise from the descending common trunk. (Right) Lateral view of angiocardiogram.

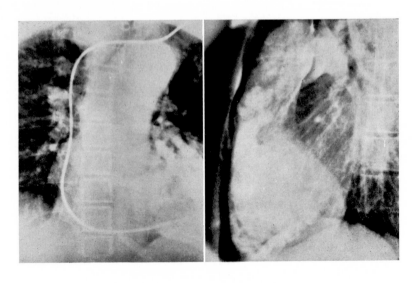

OPERATIVE CORRECTION OF TETRALOGY OF FALLOT

infundibular pulmonic stenosis and tetralogy of fallot
by-pass operations: blalock-taussig

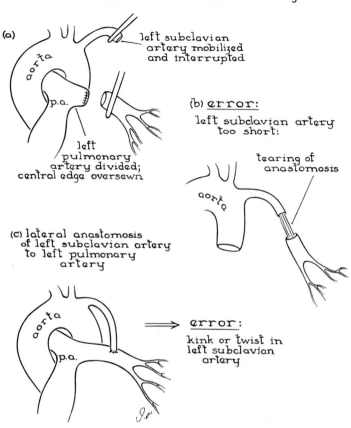

FIGURE 175

The tetralogy of Fallot presents defects which require correction. These are pulmonic valvular stenosis, pulmonary infundibular stenosis, interventricular septal defect and aortic overriding. There are two surgical approaches.

I. DIRECT—OPEN HEART. Using the pump oxygenator, the pulmonic and infundibular stenosis may be removed and the interventricular septal defect closed (see Interventricular Septal Defect). Errors may be made in the treatment of pulmonary valvular and infundibular stenosis, as well as in the closure of interventricular septal defects, and must be avoided. Since mortality is high in the treatment of tetralogy of Fallot by using the pump oxygenator, it is considered by some to be an error to attempt treatment of this lesion by the direct approach.

II. BYPASS OPERATION. BLALOCK-TAUSSIG PROCEDURE. In this procedure, the subclavian artery rising from the innominate artery is anastomosed to the pulmonary artery, thus introducing arterial systemic blood beyond the point of pulmonic stenosis.

Errors. Four major technical errors must be avoided:

1. Use of the wrong subclavian artery. Use of the subclavian artery rising from the innominate artery causes less angulation; therefore, the operation should be done on the side opposite to the aortic arch.

2. Tension on the anastomotic line due to a short subclavian artery may result in tears.

3. The subclavian artery during anastomosis may twist and kink.

4. If the vessels are not equal in size, end-to-end anastomosis may result in a constricted lumen at the point of anastomosis. In such cases, end-to-side anastomosis should be done.

by-pass operations: potts-smith

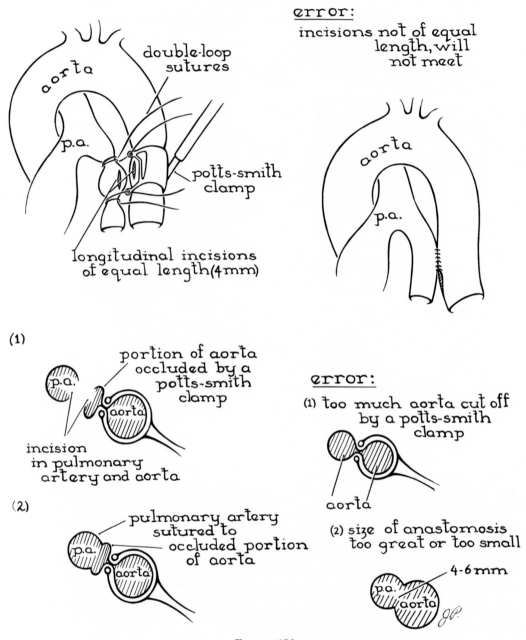

error:
incisions not of equal
length, will
not meet

aorta

double-loop
sutures

p.a.

potts-smith
clamp

longitudinal incisions
of equal length(4mm)

aorta

p.a.

(1)

portion of aorta
occluded by a
potts-smith
clamp

p.a.

aorta

incision
in pulmonary
artery and aorta

error:

(1) too much aorta cut off
by a potts-smith
clamp

aorta

(2)

pulmonary artery
sutured to
occluded portion
of aorta

p.a.

aorta

(2) size of anastomosis
too great or too small

4-6mm

p.a.

aorta

FIGURE 176

Side-to-side anastomosis between pulmonary artery and descending aorta.
ERRORS:
1. Too many intercostals may be tied in freeing the aorta and may damage the spinal cord.
2. Too much of the aorta may be cut off in the placement of Potts's clamp.
3. Opening between the vessels may be too small or too big—ideal is 4 to 6 mm.

truncus arteriosus

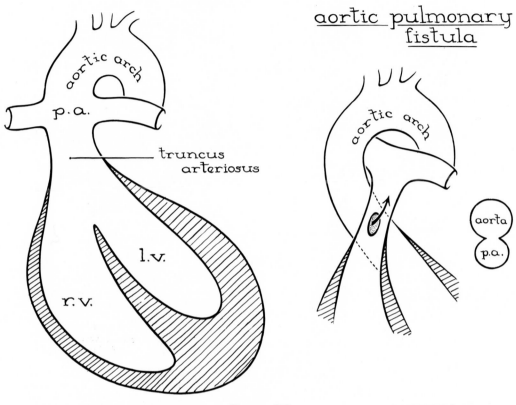

aortic pulmonary fistula

FIGURE 177

atrial septal defects

b. ostium primum:

a. ostium secundum

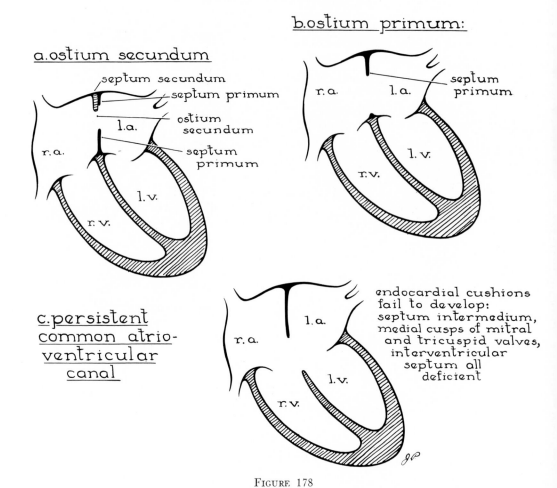

FIGURE 178

A and B. *Atrial septal defect* (*ostium primum and secundum*) is an acyanotic disease compatible with normal physical development and relative longevity. For a long time the symptoms are limited to exertional dyspnea and palpitation.

Diagnosis: A soft systolic murmur localizes to the 2nd or the 3rd left intercostal spaces.

C. *Persistent common atrial ventricular canal.*

History: This peculiar and complex congenital lesion is compatible with normal development; it is not as well tolerated as the pure form of atrial septal defect. Exertional dyspnea appears early and is often associated with palpitation.

Diagnosis: Murmurs—a soft systolic murmur localized to the 2nd or the 3rd intercostal space, with a louder systolic murmur in the 4th left intercostal space, as in ventricular septal defect. When the mitral valve is involved, a systolic murmur can be heard at the apex, as in mitral insufficiency.

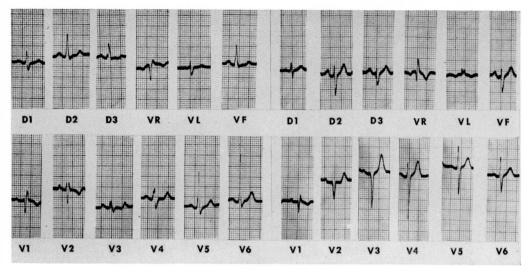

FIGURE 179

Atrial Septal Defect (Ostium Primum and Secundum).

ECG may be normal or show right axis deviation with incomplete right bundle branch block.

Persistent Common Atrial Ventricular Canal.

ECG shows incomplete right bundle branch block with left axis deviation.

Vectocardiogram is likewise characteristic and shows a significant levorotation in the frontal plane.

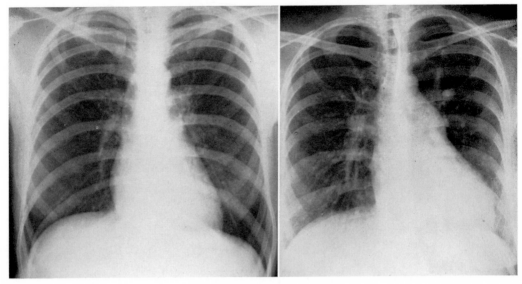

FIGURE 180

Simple atrial septal defect. Postero-anterior roentgenogram shows little or moderate heart enlargement: prominent pulmonary arch with increased pulmonary vasculature.

Fluoroscopy is essential for the diagnosis, revealing increased pulsations of the pulmonary arteries and varying degrees of right ventricular enlargement.

Common atrial ventricular canal. Enlargement of the heart is more pronounced than in pure atrial septal defect. Right and left ventricular enlargements are present.

Fluoroscopy shows increased pulsation of pulmonary arteries.

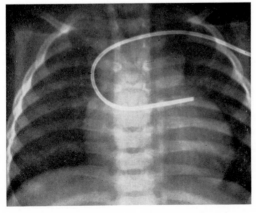

FIGURE 181

CATHETERIZATION:

Ostium Secundum. Catheter has been passed into the left atrium through the defect in the upper part of the septum.

Ostium Primum. Catheter passes through a defect in the lower part of the septum into the left atrium.

Common Atrial Ventricular Canal. The catheter may pass into the left atrium and ventricle. During withdrawal from the left ventricle, the catheter may drop directly into the right ventricle because of the presence of a ventricular septal defect.

Errors in Diagnosis. Differentiation between pure atrial septal defects and common atrial ventricular canal is essential and can be accomplished satisfactorily in the majority of cases with the aid of electrocardiographic and vectocardiographic studies.

open operative treatment:

gross-well technic

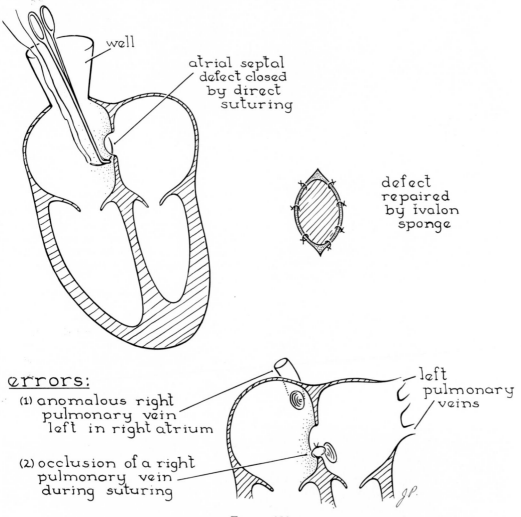

well

atrial septal
defect closed
by direct
suturing

defect
repaired
by ivalon
sponge

errors:

(1) anomalous right
pulmonary vein
left in right atrium

(2) occlusion of a right
pulmonary vein
during suturing

left
pulmonary
veins

FIGURE 182

In the closure of an atrial septal defect there are 3 serious errors that can be made.

1. The choice of a surgical procedure which does not permit sufficient time for unhurried careful septal closure. This is particularly true when hypothermia is used. It is preferable to use the Gross-well technic or extracorporeal circulation, both of which methods permit unhurried exploration of the defect and of the pulmonary veins. In this way, correction of the defect is possible, as well as correction of anomalous pulmonary venous drainage.

2. Closure of a large defect by sutures alone. The sutures may tear out. Large defects should be repaired by inserting a piece of Ivalon sponge.

3. Anomalous pulmonary venous drainage must be corrected so that all pulmonary veins drain into the left atrium.

INTERVENTRICULAR SEPTAL DEFECTS

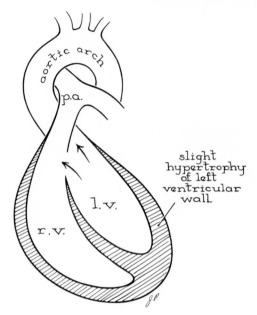

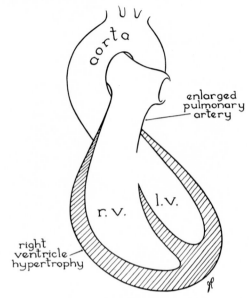

FIG. 183 (*Left*). UNCOMPLICATED.

History: This acyanotic type of congenital malformation is compatible with normal development and longevity. There is a slight degree of dyspnea which may increase, depending on the size and the position of the defect.

Diagnosis: Murmurs—a harsh systolic murmur, which radiates in all directions, is heard in the 4th left intercostal space. Occasionally, a diastolic murmur may be heard at the left border of the sternum when there is an associated anomaly of the aortic leaflets.

(*Right*) *With pulmonary hypertension*. Diagram shows hypertrophy of the right ventricle and enlargement of pulmonary artery. Sections of pulmonary arterioles show hypertrophy of media, intimal proliferation and narrowing of lumen of vessel.

History: Lesion is not as well tolerated as simple interventricular defect. Dyspnea develops early and is progressive. With increasing pulmonary hypertension, the left-to-right shunt through the interventricular defect may reverse, and cyanosis may develop. Consequently, the onset of cardiac insufficiency is accelerated and becomes irreversible.

Diagnosis: Same systolic murmur, with an accentuated second pulmonary sound.

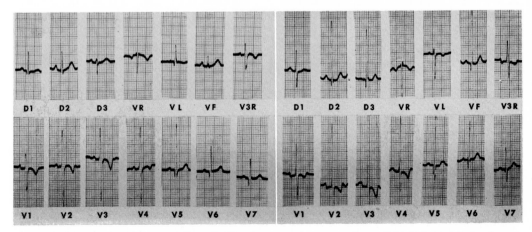

FIG. 184. ECG (*Left*) Uncomplicated. May be normal or may show slight left ventricular hypertrophy. (*Right*) With pulmonary hypertension. Shows right or combined ventricular hypertrophy.

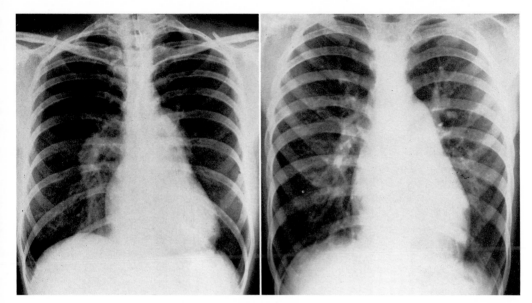

FIGURE 185

Postero-anterior roentgenograms. (*Left*) *High interventricular septal defect.* Heart size and shape are sometimes within normal limits. Often left ventricular enlargement is present.

Fluoroscopy: Some degree of increased pulmonary artery pulsation—slight or moderate.

(*Right*) *With pulmonary hypertension.* The heart is moderately or sometimes greatly enlarged, with prominent pulmonary arch and increase in the size of the main pulmonary artery branches.

Fluoroscopy: Increase in the ventricular mass, both right and left ventricles being enlarged.

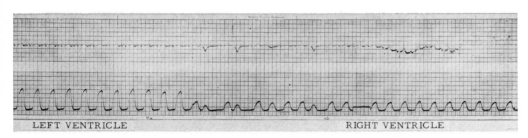

LEFT VENTRICLE   RIGHT VENTRICLE

FIGURE 186

Catheterization: Rarely, the catheter is threaded through the interventricular septal defect. Gas analysis detects arterial blood in the right ventricle. When the pressure in the right ventricle rises secondarily to pulmonary artery hypertension and reaches the systemic pressure levels, there is diminution of oxygen saturation in the peripheral arterial blood. Cine-angiocardiography may be useful to detect the shunt. The dye dilution curve is the method of choice.

Errors in Diagnosis: (1) Failure to detect pulmonary hypertension; (2) in the presence of sufficiently high pulmonary artery hypertension, a lung biopsy to show the extent of pulmonary arteriolar narrowing is essential; (3) the Eisenmenger complex may be overlooked.

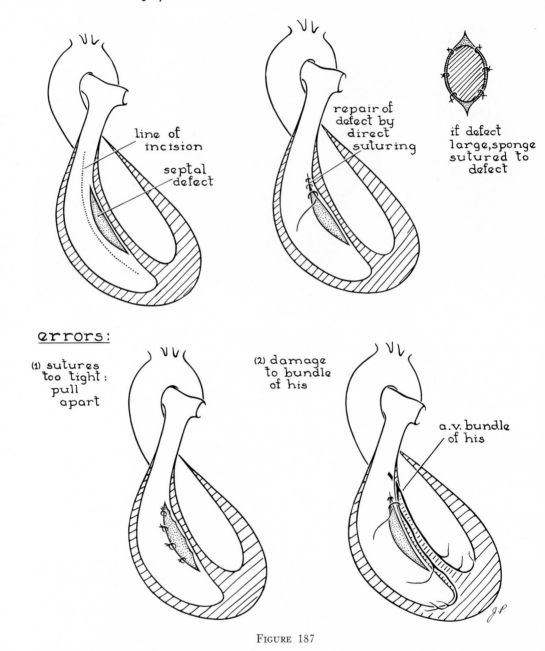

line of
incision

septal
defect

repair of
defect by
direct
suturing

if defect
large, sponge
sutured to
defect

errors:

(1) sutures
too tight:
pull
apart

(2) damage
to bundle
of his

a.v. bundle
of his

FIGURE 187

DIRECT APPROACH: There are 2 methods which permit direct visualization of the lesion: (1) hypo-thermia and (2) the use of extracorporeal circulation.

1. Under *hypothermia* it is possible to occlude the superior and the inferior vena cava and the azygos vein, which results in a heart empty of blood. The right ventricle is incised, and an attempt is made to correct the interventricular septal defect. Unfortunately, too short a time is available under hypothermia to permit accurate evaluation and careful correction of the lesion. Therefore, it is an error to attempt to repair an interventricular septal defect under hypothermia.

(*Continued on facing page*)

FIG. 187 (*Continued from facing page*)

2. *Extracorporeal circulation*, frequently referred to as "the pump oxygenator," is an apparatus which replaces both heart and lungs, permitting all blood to be drained from the heart through cannulae placed in the superior and the inferior vena cava, respectively. These cannulae collect the venous blood and convey it to a container where it is oxygenated. The oxygenated blood is returned to the patient by means of a pump which sends it through a cannula placed either in the subclavian or the femoral artery; in this manner the heart is emptied of all blood except when it is driven through the coronary and the bronchial arteries by the pump oxygenator. The patient is kept alive by the artificially oxygenated blood pumped through his arterial system during the bypass of heart and lungs. With this technic the right ventricle may be opened for a considerable time, during which a careful repair of the interventricular septum may be carried out in an unhurried and accurate manner. The extracorporeal circulation is extremely complicated, and the errors which may be made are far too numerous to be considered in this chapter.

Errors: The major errors are (1) failure to recognize the presence of other congenital anomalies which may contraindicate closure of the interventricular septal defect and associated severe pulmonary hypertension; (2) the defect is too large to close with sutures alone, which may pull out; in such cases, Ivalon sponge should be used; (3) sutures may catch or pull on the bundle of His, resulting in heart block; (4) failure to use a pacemaker by placing a wire in the wall of the right ventricle when bundle branch block develops.

PERICARDIAL EFFUSION—CARDIAC TAMPONADE

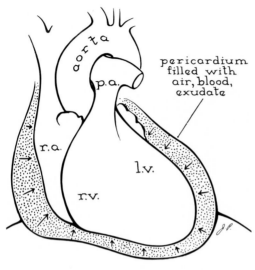

FIGURE 188

History: This occurs when fluid accumulates rapidly in the pericardial cavity, resulting in a sudden rise of intrapericardial pressure. This interferes with diastolic relaxation of the heart and filling of its cavities. The persistence of the condition leads to severe shock and may end in cardiac arrest. The following conditions which lead to rapid pericardial effusion with cardiac tamponade are:

1. Cardiothoracic trauma, direct or indirect (hemopericardium)

2. Rupture of the heart wall secondary to myocardial infarction (hemopericardium)

3. Postoperative complications of cardiac surgery

4. Acute pericarditis with effusion

5. Tumor—primary or metastatic

Symptoms: Dyspnea, orthopnea, rapid onset of shock.

Diagnosis: A rapid small paradoxical pulse, with a low systemic blood pressure and an elevated venous pressure, characterizes this condition.

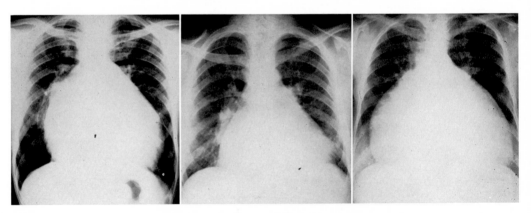

FIGURE 189

Postero-anterior roentgenograms. (*Left*) Showing a large heart with widened waist. The cardiac shape suggests the presence of pericardial effusion, which may or may not cause cardiac tamponade. (*Center*) Shows enlargement of heart of unknown origin without pericardial effusion. (*Right*) Shows large heart with undetected valvular disease with pericardial fluid.

Fluoroscopy: The cardiac shadow is increased and often shows the typical shape of a large pericardial effusion, with widening of the waist of the heart and with an acute cardiophrenic angle. The most characteristic sign of cardiac tamponade is that of a hypodynamic or an adynamic heart. However, this sign is not pathognomonic unless other signs are present.

Errors in Diagnosis: This condition must be differentiated from (1) a large heart of unknown etiology and (2) cardiomegaly due to undetected valvular disease in its terminal stage.

Study of the circulation time may aid in the diagnosis. It is normal in cases with acute cardiac tamponade and delayed in the presence of myocardial insufficiency.

aspiration treatment

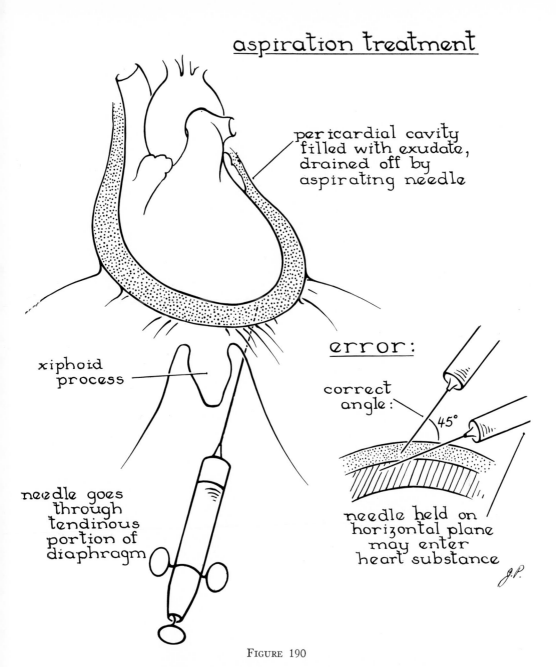

pericardial cavity filled with exudate, drained off by aspirating needle

xiphoid process

needle goes through tendinous portion of diaphragm

error:

correct angle:

45°

needle held on horizontal plane may enter heart substance

J.P.

FIGURE 190

PERICARDIOCENTESIS. Aspiration of fluid from the pericardial space is imperative to establish the character of the fluid and to relieve cardiac tamponade. Penetrating heart wounds should be treated by one pericardial aspiration of hemorrhagic fluid. Failure to improve is then an indication for operative closure of the heart wound. It is an error to wait if tamponade recurs after pericardiocentesis. Nonpenetrating heart injuries should be treated by repeated pericardial aspirations of the serosanguineous fluid.

PERICARDIOSTOMY. Purulent pericardial effusion requires open pericardiostomy by resection of the left 7th costal cartilage. The opening in the pericardial sac should be at the level of the diaphragm. Digital exploration of the pericardium is indicated, both anteriorly and posteriorly, to break down adhesions gently. However, it is an error to attempt to tear free adhesions, as this may result in fatal hemorrhage. Soft irrigating tubes should be placed high up in the anterior and posterior pericardial sac for daily irrigation. The pH of the irrigation fluid should be as nearly neutral as possible to avoid ventricular fibrillation. It is an error to remove these tubes too quickly.

CONSTRICTIVE PERICARDITIS

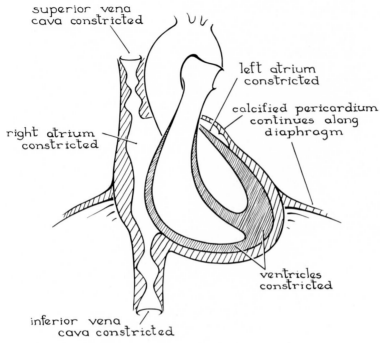

superior vena cava constricted

left atrium constricted

calcified pericardium continues along diaphragm

right atrium constricted

ventricles constricted

inferior vena cava constricted

FIGURE 191

History: This is usually a late manifestation of a progressive disease of the pericardium, often of tuberculous origin. The resultant fibrous tissue interferes with cardiac function, and there is impairment of adequate diastolic filling and systolic ejection.

In the early stage of the disease the patient may be asymptomatic or may complain of slight dyspnea and asthenia. Later, there are signs of venous stasis, the jugular veins are distended, and the presence of hepatomegaly with ascites gives the patient a characteristic batrachian appearance.

Diagnosis: There is an elevated venous pressure with a paradoxical pulse. On auscultation a third diastolic heart sound may be heard.

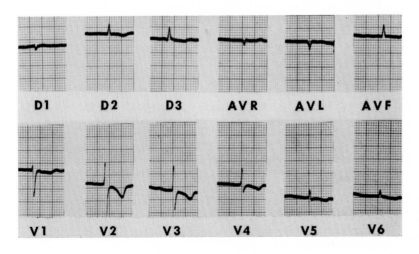

D1   D2   D3   AVR   AVL   AVF

V1   V2   V3   V4   V5   V6

FIGURE 192

ECG shows low voltage in all leads and flattened, irregular T waves.

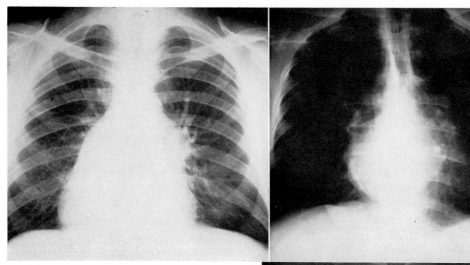

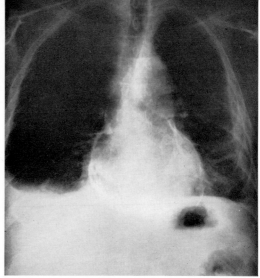

FIGURE 193

Postero-anterior roentgenograms. (*Top, left*) Case of constrictive pericarditis. No evidence of calcification seen. *Note* the irregularities in cardiac contour. (*Top, right*) Same patient, with appropriate penetrated chest film showing calcification along the left lower pericardial border. (*Bottom, right*) Typical case of constrictive pericarditis, showing typical extensive calcification.

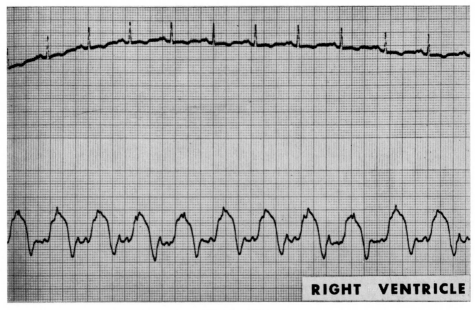

RIGHT VENTRICLE

FIGURE 194

Cardiac Catheterization: The right ventricular diastolic pressure is elevated. The morphology of the curve is peculiar, with an early diastolic dip followed by a high diastolic plateau. The pulmonary wedge pressure may be increased when the constriction involves the left side of the heart.

Errors in Diagnosis: The absence of pericardial calcification in the presence of other signs of constrictive pericarditis suggests the possibility of endocardial fibrosis. The differential diagnosis is very difficult and sometimes impossible. The presence of eosinophilia may suggest the diagnosis of a particular myocardial fibrosis (Loeffler). In such cases the final diagnosis may be made only by cardiac exploration and myocardial biopsy.

operative treatment:
pericardectomy

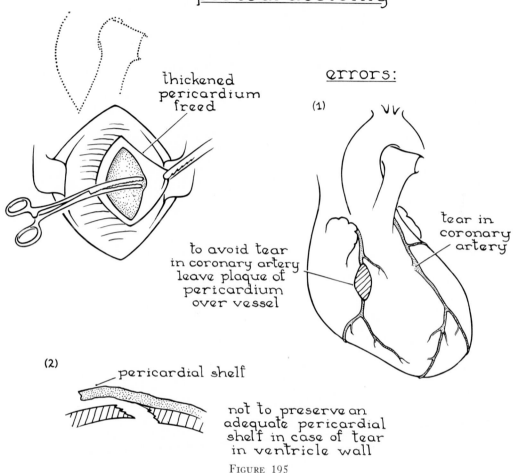

thickened
pericardium
freed

errors:

(1)

tear in
coronary
artery

to avoid tear
in coronary artery
leave plaque of
pericardium
over vessel

(2)

pericardial shelf

not to preserve an
adequate pericardial
shelf in case of tear
in ventricle wall

FIGURE 195

PERICARDECTOMY OR CARDIAC DECORTICATION.
Objective: To free the venae cavae and the heart chambers of their constrictive, thickened pericardial encasement by sharp and blunt dissection.
Errors:

1. To free right side of heart first, which permits too much blood to reach an encased left ventricle.
2. Decortication of the atria is dangerous because of the likelihood that hemorrhage will occur due to their thin walls.
3. To remove plaques over coronary arteries unless constrictive bands cause mitral or tricuspid insufficiency.
4. Not to free completely the superior and the inferior venae cavae and the diaphragm along with the posterior surface of the left ventricle.
5. Not to leave a ledge of calcific pericardium at all times which can be sewed back over any hole accidentally made through the ventricular wall or the atrial walls.
6. If, rarely, the condition is that of endocardial fibrosis, and if there is no outer constricting encasement, it is important to take a muscle biopsy by amputating the left or right auricular appendage to confirm the diagnosis.

MITRAL STENOSIS AND PURE PULMONARY HYPERTENSION

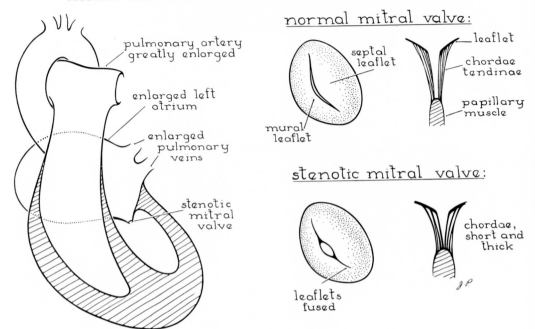

normal mitral valve:

pulmonary artery greatly enlarged

enlarged left atrium

enlarged pulmonary veins

stenotic mitral valve

septal leaflet

mural leaflet

leaflet

chordae tendinae

papillary muscle

stenotic mitral valve:

leaflets fused

chordae, short and thick

FIG. 196. Mitral Stenosis.

History: Pure, tight mitral stenosis is incompatible with a normal life span. It causes elevated pulmonary, venous and arterial pressures which are responsible for the symptomatology and the physical signs. Asthenia and exertional dyspnea, plus nocturnal dyspnea and hemoptysis, are relatively early manifestations of mitral stenosis. Auricular fibrillation occurs in the more advanced stages of the disease. Right ventricular insufficiency with hepatomegaly and edema of the lower extremities are signs which appear in the more advanced stages.

Diagnosis: Auscultation—the first sound at the apex is loud and snapping. The second sound is reduplicated. The most characteristic signs are those of a presystolic murmur and a localized apical diastolic rumble. The second pulmonary sound is loud and sometimes reduplicated.

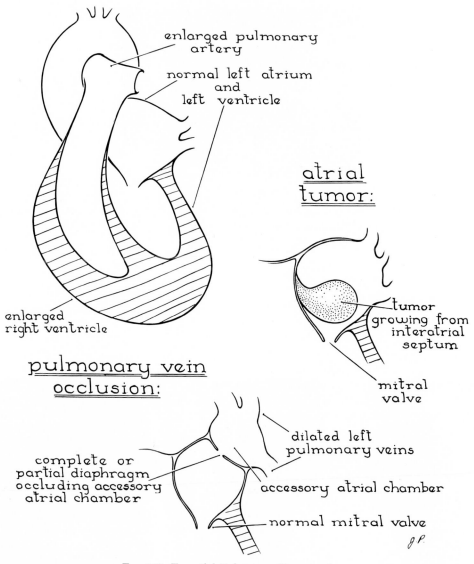

enlarged pulmonary
artery

normal left atrium
and
left ventricle

atrial
tumor:

enlarged
right ventricle

tumor
growing from
interatrial
septum

mitral
valve

pulmonary vein
occlusion:

dilated left
pulmonary veins

complete or
partial diaphragm
occluding accessory
atrial chamber

accessory atrial chamber

normal mitral valve

FIG. 197. Essential Pulmonary Hypertension.

History: This is a disease of unknown etiology. The symptoms of asthenia, exertional dyspnea and nocturnal dyspnea occur in the same manner as in mitral stenosis. Right ventricular insufficiency may develop, with all its associated signs and symptoms.

Diagnosis: The pulmonary second sound is loud and sometimes is reduplicated.

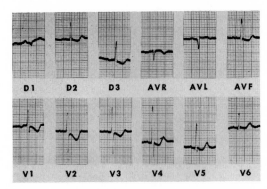

FIGURE 198

ECG. Mitral stenosis. There is a tendency to right axis deviation. The signs of left atrial dilatation appear frequently and are often associated with right ventricular hypertrophy.

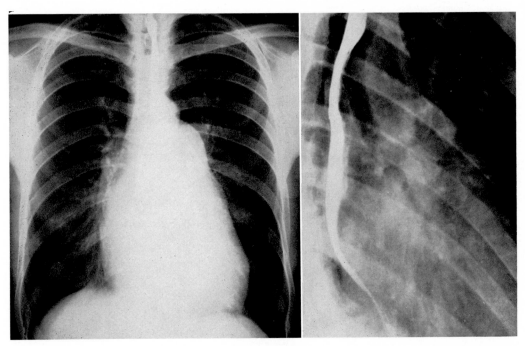

FIGURE 199

Roentgenograms of mitral stenosis. (*Left*) Postero-anterior view shows evidence of enlargement of left atrium, right ventricle, main pulmonary artery. Pulmonary vasculature increased. Lymphatics often congested, as shown by enlarged septae seen at the bases (Kerley lines). (*Right*) Anterior oblique view shows esophagus displaced posteriorly by enlarged left atrium.

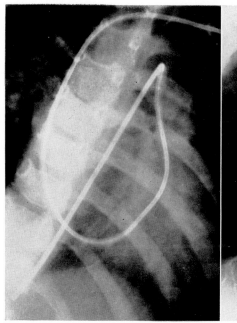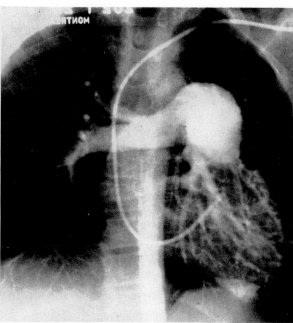

FIGURE 200

(*Left*) Angiogram of left intra-atrial mass shows lacunar shadow in opacified left atrium which may be due to (1) thrombotic or (2) tumor mass. (*Right*) Anterior oblique roentgenogram of cor triatriatum shows absence of posterior displacement of esophagus at left atrial level, but postero-anterior roentgenogram shows typical roentgenographic signs of mitral stenosis.

Errors in Diagnosis. When the semiology of mitral stenosis is complete, the diagnosis presents no difficulty. However, when some factors are lacking, other diagnoses must be considered, such as:

1. Essential pulmonary hypertension, which is rare and unlikely to be confused with mitral stenosis because (*a*) there is no left atrial enlargement, (*b*) auscultation at the apex is negative, and (*c*) pulmonary capillary pressure is normal despite a high pulmonary arterial pressure.

2. Intra-atrial mass. This diagnosis may be difficult, particularly when there is coexistent mitral stenosis. If the presence of a mass in the atrium is clinically suspected because of repeated syncope and uncontrollable arrthymia, angiocardiography must be done (see above).

3. Cor triatriatum. All diagnostic elements of mitral stenosis may be present, except (*a*) auscultatory signs at the apex, (*b*) absence of left atrial enlargement and (*c*) a long history of a heart condition dating back to early childhood.

4. Mitral stenosis with insufficiency. When mitral stenosis is complicated by the presence of mitral insufficiency, it is essential to determine which is the predominant lesion. The presence of mitral insufficiency is suggested by an apical systolic murmur, which, however, is present in 40 per cent of all cases of proved tight mitral stenosis. The presence of an apical systolic murmur in itself is not proof of the presence of a predominant mitral insufficiency unless it is associated with clear-cut electrocardiographic and roentgenographic evidence of left ventricular enlargement.

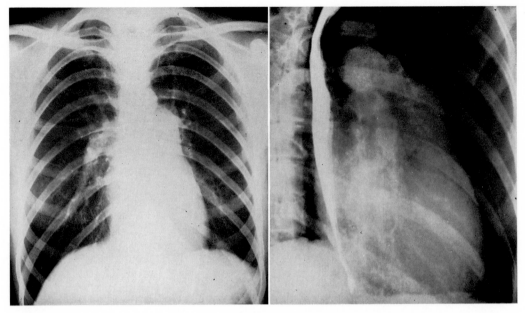

FIGURE 201

Pure pulmonary hypertension roentgenograms. (*Left*) Postero-anterior view shows enlarged pulmonary arteries; no evidence of venous and lymphatic engorgement (Kerley lines and hilar haziness are absent). Translucency of peripheral lung fields is increased due to the hypertensive changes in pulmonary arterial bed. (*Right*) Right anterior oblique view shows no signs of enlargement of left atrium, but prominent conus and right ventricle.

FIG. 202. (*Illustration on following page*)

Objective: To free fixed mitral leaflets along their commissures and separate fused chordae tendinae and papillary muscles when subvalvular stenosis is present. Approach is through the left atrium via the left or the right thoracic cavities. In the right-sided approach, the left atrium is entered through the interatrial septum. In the left-sided approach, the index finger enters the left atrium through its auricular appendage.

Errors:

1. Placing the purse-string too high on appendage.

2. Failure to enlarge opening. A tight opening in atrial appendage or atrial wall favors tears.

3. Not to place safety cotton sutures through the wall of the left atrium in line of possible tear when appendage is small.

4. Not to blow out atrium when thrombus is suspected.

5. Cutting of leaflets, chordae tendinae, papillary muscles and even circumflex artery.

6. To proceed through large atrial thrombus. Best to use extracorporeal circulation.

7. Insufficient opening of commissures.

8. Failure to detect and correct subvalvular stenosis.

9. Not to explore pulmonary veins.

10. Not to examine other heart chambers and the great vessels for the presence of thrills, and not to take intracardiac pressures when indicated.

11. To attempt to remove intra-atrial tumor or ventricular tumor without the aid of extracorporeal circulation.

12. Not to correct tricuspid stenosis when present.

OPERATIVE TREATMENT FOR MITRAL STENOSIS

1. indirect:(b)transaortic:

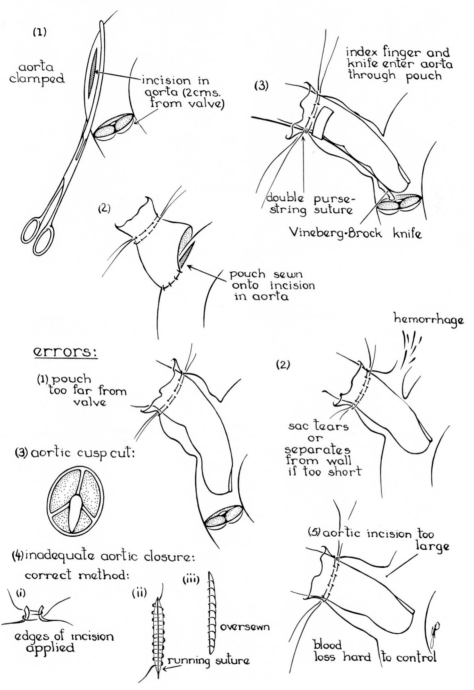

FIG. 202. Mitral Commissurotomy.

ACQUIRED AORTIC STENOSIS

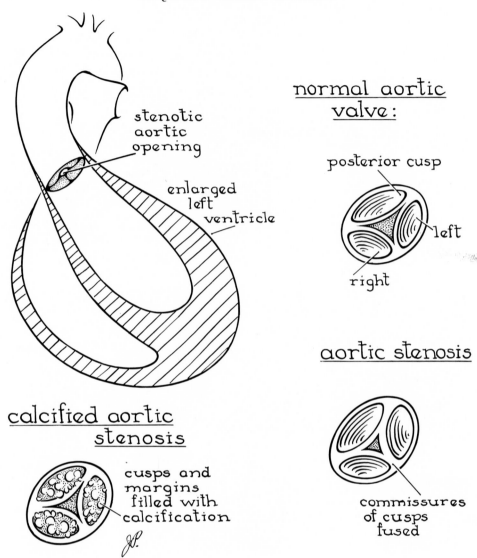

stenotic
aortic
opening

enlarged
left
ventricle

normal aortic valve:

posterior cusp

left

right

aortic stenosis

commissures
of cusps
fused

calcified aortic stenosis

cusps and
margins
filled with
calcification

FIGURE 203

History: A tight aortic stenosis is incompatible with a normal life span. Sudden death is a frequent result of this disease. In the early period of the disease, symptoms such as asthenia, palpitations and exertional dyspnea occur. Later, anginal pain and syncope on effort appear. In some cases death can occur without any symptoms.

Diagnosis: A systolic thrill is palpable over the second right intercostal space, where a very harsh systolic murmur, radiating to the neck, is heard. It may also be heard in the third left interspace. The second aortic sound is diminished or absent. At the left border of the sternum there is sometimes a faint diastolic murmur. The systemic arterial pressure is usually low.

FIG. 204. ECG shows left ventricular hypertrophy with systolic overload.

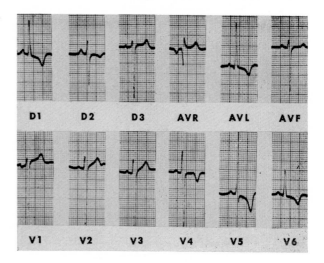

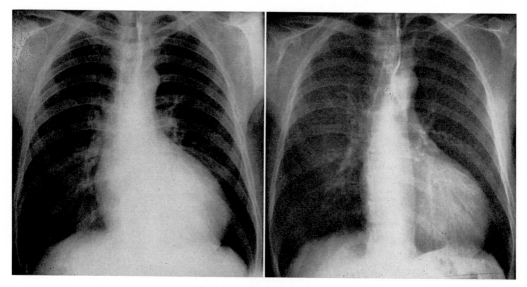

FIG. 205. Roentgenograms.

(*Left*) Postero-anterior view shows left ventricular enlargement. Calcification of the aortic valve is often present and may be extensive. (See right anterior oblique penetrated roentgenogram.) (*Right*) Right anterior oblique view (5° to 15°) will show aortic valve calcification on penetrated film with short-time exposure.

Left-Heart Catheterization: This is indicated in order to evaluate the tightness of the lesion and to make a differential diagnosis between the acquired and the subvalvular congenital lesions. Percutaneous left ventricular pressure readings recorded simultaneously with arterial pressure readings yield information with regard to the pressure gradient across the aortic valve and allow calculation of the ventricular output when dye-dilution curves are studied.

Errors in Diagnosis:

(1) Aortic systolic murmur of arteriosclerotic origin without true stenosis of the valve.

(2) Failure to estimate tightness of aortic stenosis and, in particular, the degree of associated aortic insufficiency.

(3) Failure to recognize other lesions, such as organic mitral insufficiency.

operative treatment

I indirect:(a)transventricular:

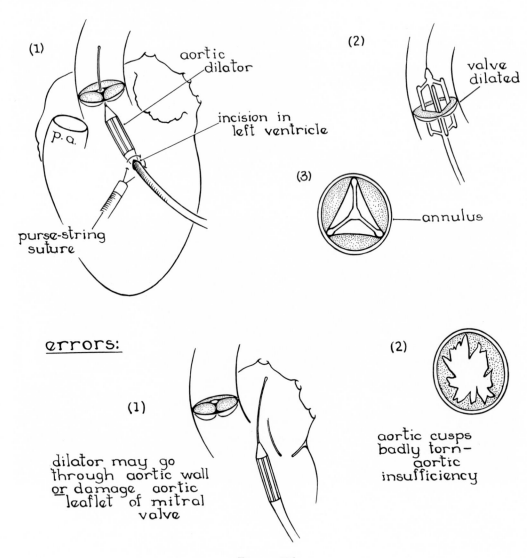

(1)

aortic
dilator

incision in
left ventricle

P. a.

purse-string
suture

(2)

valve
dilated

(3)

annulus

errors:

(1)

dilator may go
through aortic wall
or damage aortic
leaflet of mitral
valve

(2)

aortic cusps
badly torn—
aortic
insufficiency

FIGURE 206

Objective: To relieve stenosis and restore cusp function.

I. INDIRECT APPROACH

A. *Transventricular:* Dilator is passed through an opening in the left ventricular wall and is threaded through the stenotic aortic opening, where the valve is forcibly opened by expanding the blades of the dilator.

Errors:

1. Dilator is pushed through the aortic leaflet of the mitral valve or the wall of the aorta instead of through the stenotic aortic valve opening.

2. Fragmentation of the valve cusps may occur during dilatation, resulting in serious aortic insufficiency.

3. Improperly placed purse-string suture may

(*Continued on facing page*)

FIG. 206 (*Continued*)

result in uncontrollable hemorrhage from the left ventricle.

B. *Transaortic:* A sac is sewed on the aorta 2 cm. from the aortic valve, through which the index finger with a saw knife is passed into the aorta toward the stenotic valve. The commissures may thus be opened.

Errors:

1. The clamp occludes too much of the aortic lumen.

2. Too large an opening in the aorta permits bleeding between the sac and finger. The opening should be a little larger than the index finger.

3. A weak sac may tear. It must be (a) strong enough not to tear, (b) impermeable to blood and (c) long enough for operator's finger. Controlling purse-string sutures may break and permit leakage.

4. Aortic cusp may be cut instead of commissures, resulting in aortic insufficiency.

5. Leakage may occur from the aortic incision after closure. This can be prevented by the placing of interrupted mattress apposition sutures and continuous over-and-over sutures.

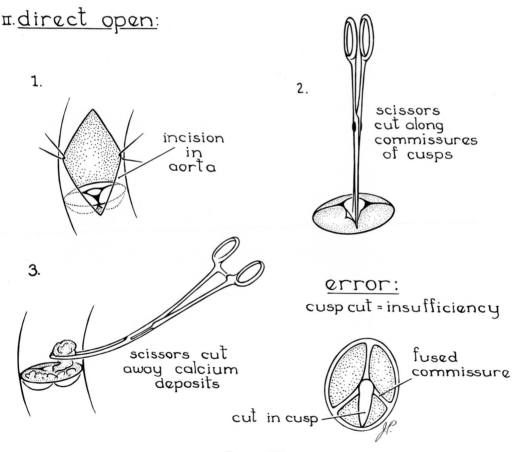

II. direct open:

1.

incision in aorta

2.

scissors cut along commissures of cusps

3.

scissors cut away calcium deposits

error:

cusp cut = insufficiency

fused commissure

cut in cusp

FIGURE 207

DIRECT APPROACH (Hypothermia or extracorporeal circulation): Commissurotomy may be done, with removal of calcium plaques under direct vision in a dry field through an opening in the anterior aortic wall.

Errors:

(1) Cutting of aortic cusp.

(2) If cusps are very still, an anatomically perfect commissurotomy may lead to left ventricular failure due to aortic insufficiency.

MITRAL STENOSIS AND ASSOCIATED STENOTIC VALVULAR LESIONS

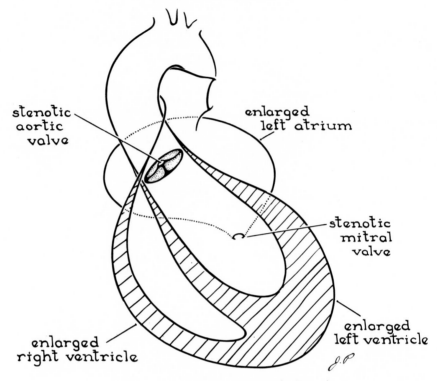

FIG. 208. Mitral Stenosis and Aortic Stenosis.

History: Mitral stenosis is often associated with aortic stenosis. The resulting heart condition is better tolerated than is aortic stenosis alone when the latter is tight. Anginal pain due to aortic stenosis may complicate the symptomatology of mitral stenosis.

Diagnosis: A harsh systolic murmur, radiation into the neck, is heard at the second right interspace. The second aortic sound is diminished, and the characteristic sounds of mitral stenosis can be heard.

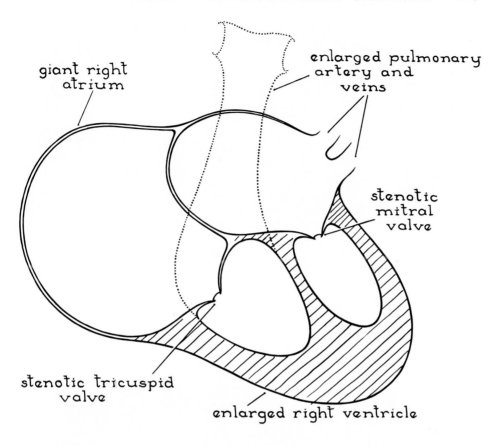

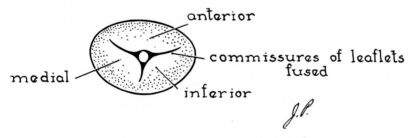

FIG. 209. Mitral Stenosis and Tricuspid Stenosis.

History: Mitral stenosis is rarely associated with a tight tricuspid stenosis. At first the tolerance of both lesions is the same as in mitral stenosis alone. Later, the combined lesions are poorly tolerated, and the prognosis is poor.

Diagnosis: The clinical picture of mitral stenosis is supplemented by (1) a presystolic pulsation of the jugular veins, (2) pulsating hepatomegaly and (3) enlargement of the right atrium.

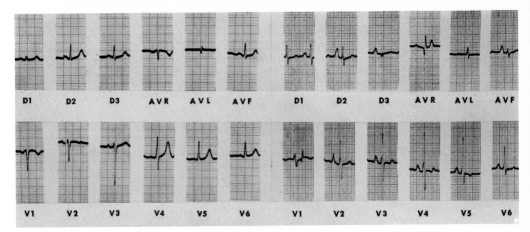

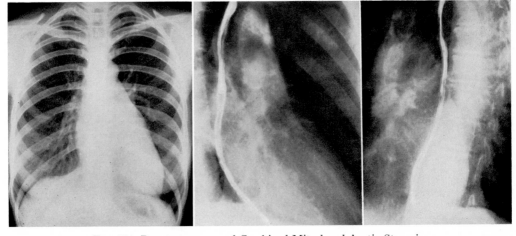

FIG. 210. ECG. (*Left*) Sometimes shows only left atrial enlargement. Left ventricular hypertrophy may be seen alone or combined with right ventricular hypertrophy.

(*Right*) In addition to the characteristic pattern of mitral stenosis, there is evidence of enlargement of the right atrium.

FIG. 211. Roentgenograms of Combined Mitral and Aortic Stenosis.

(*Left*) Postero-anterior view shows a prominent auricular appendage and an elongated left ventricular arch. The congestive lung vascularity is less pronounced than it is in pure mitral stenosis.

(*Center*) Right anterior oblique view shows an enlarged left atrium and left ventricle. The esophageal curve is less acute and is prolonged.

(*Right*) Left anterior oblique view shows enlarged left and right ventricles.

Catheterization: Right Heart. Hemodynamic studies must be done before considering surgery. Right-heart catheterization permits evaluation of the mitral lesion. Study of the brachial pulse shows a delayed anacrotic notch, indicating aortic stenosis. In some cases left-heart catheterization is needed. *Left Heart*. Through this method the degree of aortic stenosis is estimated by measuring the left ventricular output and the pressure gradient between the left ventricle and the aorta.

Errors in Diagnosis: Failure to evaluate properly (a) the degree of associated aortic stenosis and (b) the amount of possible aortic regurgitation.

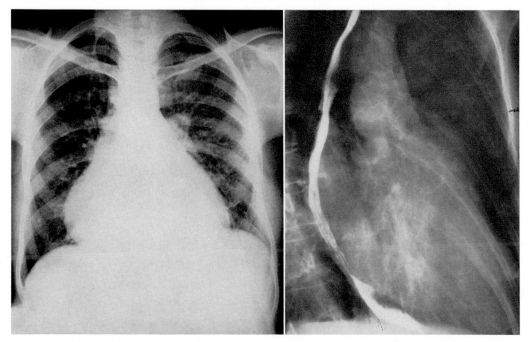

FIG. 212. Roentgenograms of Combined Mitral Stenosis and Tricuspid Stenosis.

(*Left*) Postero-anterior view shows enlarged right atrium. (*Right*) Right anterior oblique view shows enlarged left atrium, prominent right ventricle and pulmonary conus.

Catherization: Right Heart. A high systolic and diastolic pressure is present in the right atrium; this is associated with a diastolic pressure gradient between atrium and right ventricle.

Errors in Diagnosis:

(1) Right heart failure.

(2) Tumor mass in the right atrium.

operative treatment

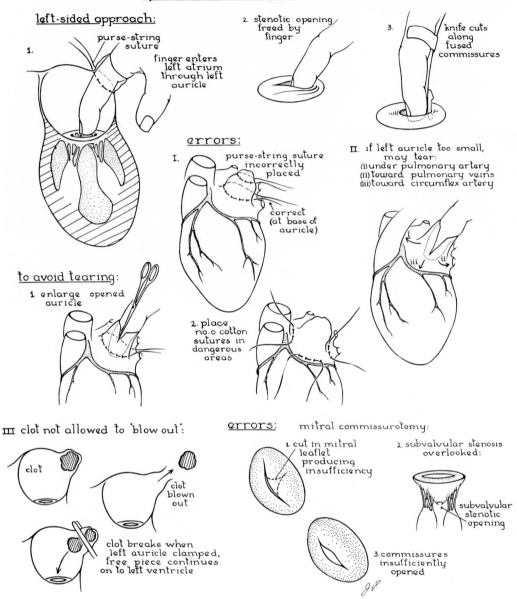

__left-sided approach:__

1. purse-string suture
finger enters left atrium through left auricle

2. stenotic opening freed by finger

3. knife cuts along fused commissures

__errors:__

I. purse-string suture incorrectly placed
correct (at base of auricle)

II. if left auricle too small, may tear:
(i) under pulmonary artery
(ii) toward pulmonary veins
(iii) toward circumflex artery

__to avoid tearing:__

1. enlarge opened auricle

2. place no. 0 cotton sutures in dangerous areas

III clot not allowed to 'blow out':

clot

clot blown out

clot breaks when left auricle clamped, free piece continues on to left ventricle

__errors:__   mitral commissurotomy:

1. cut in mitral leaflet producing insufficiency

2. subvalvular stenosis overlooked:
subvalvular stenotic opening

3. commissures insufficiently opened

FIGURE 213

right-sided approach for aortic and mitral commissurotomy:

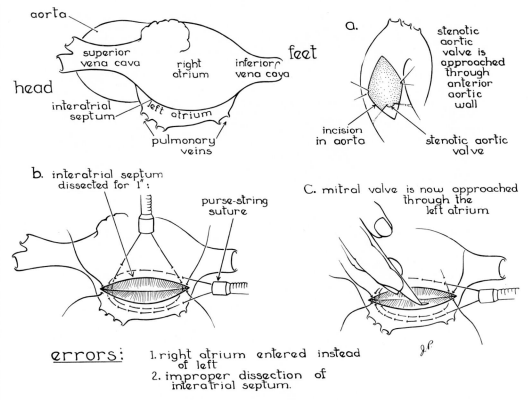

errors: 1. right atrium entered instead of left
2. improper dissection of interatrial septum.

FIGURE 214

Objective: To relieve aortic and mitral stenosis simultaneously. (For technics, see Aortic and Mitral Commissurotomy.)

Errors:

(1) Sternal splitting mid-line incision is an unsatisfactory exposure for mitral commissurotomy.

(2) Failure to open the aortic valve first.

MITRAL INSUFFICIENCY

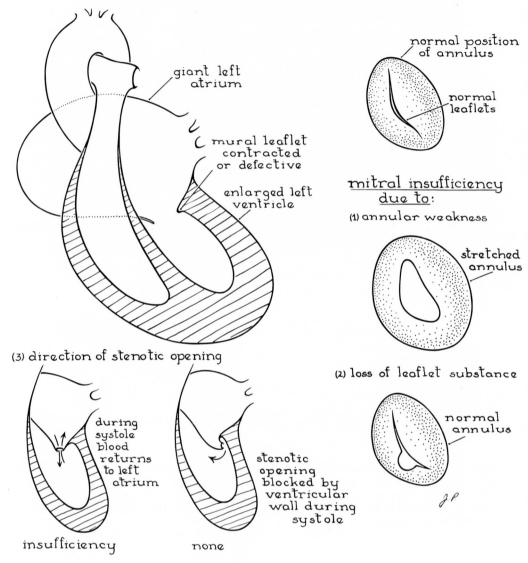

giant left atrium

mural leaflet contracted or defective

enlarged left ventricle

normal position of annulus

normal leaflets

mitral insufficiency due to:

(1) annular weakness

stretched annulus

(3) direction of stenotic opening

(2) loss of leaflet substance

during systole blood returns to left atrium

stenotic opening blocked by ventricular wall during systole

normal annulus

insufficiency

FIGURE 215

History: Mitral insufficiency is generally well tolerated except when there is extensive regurgitation. In such cases cardiac compensation becomes rapidly exhausted, and early signs of cardiac failure appear. Exertional dyspnea, palpitations and, later, symptoms and signs of left heart failure are present.

Diagnosis: There is often a systolic thrill at the apex, where a harsh systolic murmur radiating to the axilla is usually present. The first sound is obscured by this systolic murmur. The second pulmonary sound is sometimes accentuated.

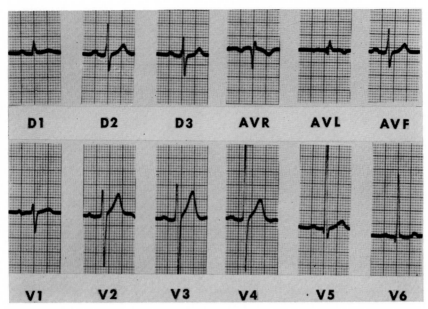

FIG. 216. *ECG* shows left ventricular hypertrophy, with diastolic overload and left atrial enlargement.

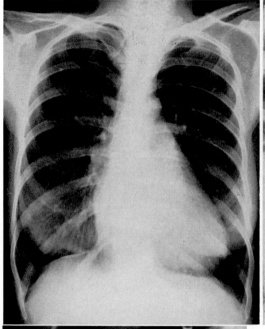

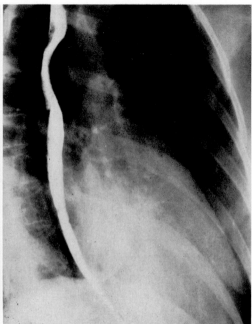

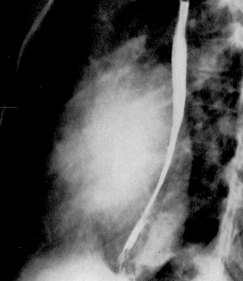

Fig. 217. Roentgenograms.

(*Top, left*) Postero-anterior view shows left ventricular and left atrial enlargement. (*Top, right*) Right anterior oblique view shows enlargement of left ventricle and left atrium. The latter displaces the esophagus in such a manner that it forms a shallow long curve. (*Bottom*) Left anterior oblique view shows enlargement of the left ventricle.

Errors in Diagnosis:

(1) Functional mitral insufficiency which may be secondary to essential hypertension

(2) Arteriosclerotic heart disease in which there is a systolic murmur at the apex

(3) In any severe anemic condition

(4) Nonspecific myocarditis

operative treatment

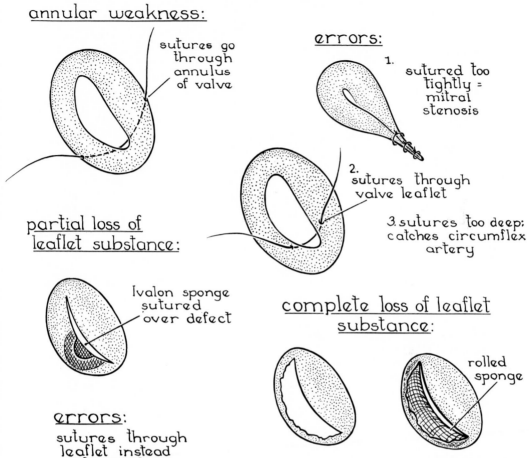

annular weakness:

sutures go through annulus of valve

errors:

1. sutured too tightly = mitral stenosis

2. sutures through valve leaflet

3. sutures too deep: catches circumflex artery

partial loss of leaflet substance:

Ivalon sponge sutured over defect

complete loss of leaflet substance:

rolled sponge

errors:

sutures through leaflet instead of annulus

FIGURE 218

Mitral insufficiency due to:

1. *Annular weakness.* Closed cross polar plication procedure of Nichols.

    Errors: (1) Failure to place suture through annulus.

             (2) Inability to reinforce closure.

Open with extracorporeal circulation.

    Errors: (1) Cerebral and coronary air embolism occurs if the left atrium is completely emptied, or if air remains trapped under aortic leaflet.

             (2) Failure to place sufficient sutures through annulus.

2. *Loss of leaflet substance.* Can be repaired only by open method. Dangers are the same as above. Valve substance loss should be covered by a piece of Ivalon sponge sutured into position.

3. *Mitral stenosis.* Improvement and often disappearance of mitral insufficiency occur following mitral commissurotomy. In such cases it is an error not to perform commissurotomy because of fear of increasing mitral insufficiency.

CORONARY ARTERY HEART DISEASE

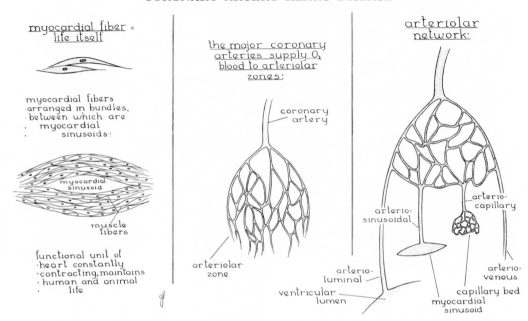

FIGURE 219

History: In coronary artery heart disease there is a pathologic change in the coronary arterial tree, causing a narrowing of the arterial lumina. As a result of this narrowing, myocardial anoxia occurs. Anginal pain, which is the characteristic feature of the disease, is a clinical manifestation of myocardial ischemia. The disease is a progressive one, of unknown etiology. Myocardial infarction is a frequent complication which may cause sudden death from ventricular fibrillation or may shorten life due to heart failure.

Diagnosis: The symptomatology is character-ized by anginal pain which occurs during or after exercise and may be the result of exertional dyspnea. The pain is severe, constricting in character and is usually localized to the retrosternal region, radiating to the left shoulder and the arm, sometimes to the neck and the jaw and rarely to the right arm or the back. The pain is relieved immediately when exercise is stopped or emotional disturbances are removed. When anginal pain persists in spite of cessation of the causative factors and nitroglycerin, the presence of myocardiai infarction must be considered.

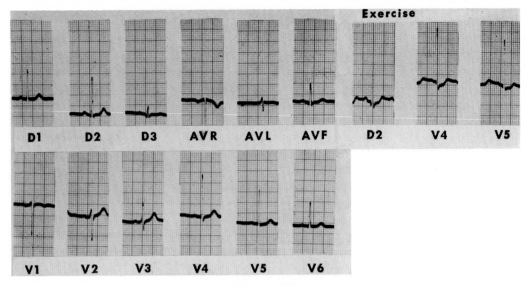

FIGURE 220

ECG: In many cases the ECG at rest is within normal limits. The exercise tolerance test or hypoxia tests may produce some significant modifications of the S-T segments of the T wave which point to myocardial ischemia. These tests must be used with caution and always after clinical evaluation of the patient. The extent of the test should be adapted to each patient and be medically supervised. The ECG is diagnostic of myocardial infarction, showing the electrical signs of myocardial necrosis. When the lesion is intramural, the ECG may fail to reveal its presence.

ROENTGENOGRAMS

Fluoroscopy: The heart may be normal in contour and size, but in coronary artery disease of long standing it is usually diffusely enlarged, especially if infarctions have occurred. The heart is generally hypodynamic, particularly at the apex, where poor ventricular contractions may be noted.

In atherosclerotic coronary heart disease, aortic parietal lines of calcification are noted, especially along the descending arch. Sometimes coronary artery calcification may be seen in the larger branches.

Angiocardiography: It is now possible with selective angiocardiography to visualize the caliber and the irregularities of the lumina of the major coronary arteries.

Errors in Diagnosis: (1) The following conditions may produce anginal pain due to myocardial ischemia without coronary atherosclerosis: (a) severe aortic stenosis and (b) severe anemia due to rapid blood loss.

(2) The causes which may simulate true anginal pain without any evidence of myocardial damage are: (a) cervicodorsal arthrosis, (b) biliary tract disease, (c) diaphragmatic herniation; upper gastric intestinal lesions, as well as pancreatic lesions and (d) spontaneous pneumothorax.

Dissecting Aneurysm of the Aorta. In these cases pain is persistent and simulates myocardial infarction. However, the ECG does not show the classic signs of myocardial infarction.

coronary artery insufficiency

Beck I operation for myocardial revascularization:

(a) partial ligation coronary sinus:

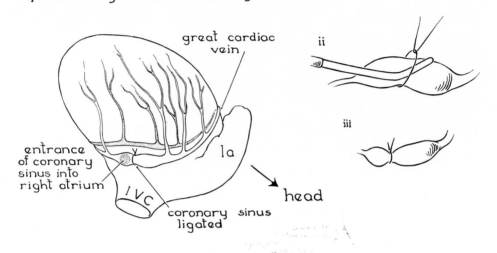

great cardiac
vein

entrance
of coronary
sinus into
right atrium

IVC

coronary   sinus
ligated

head

ii

iii

la

errors:

1. coronary sinus torn:
needle goes through
sinus

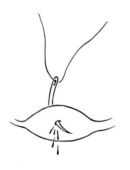

2. circumflex artery
occluded:

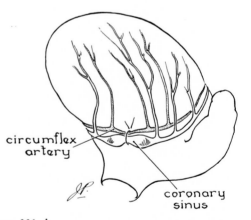

circumflex
artery

coronary
sinus

FIGURE 221 A

*Operations for Revascularization of the Heart
in Coronary Artery Heart Disease*

Objective: To relieve or prevent the effects of myocardial ischemia caused by narrowed or blocked coronary arteries, namely, (a) anginal pain; (b) acute or chronic myocardial fiber loss, with eventual left ventricular failure and death. There are two main ways in which this may be brought about. These are:

1. *Beck I Operation:* Beck is the proponent of better distribution throughout the myocardium of existing supplies of oxygenated blood. This is accomplished by partial ligation of the coronary sinus and the application of surface abrasives, such as asbestos powder, both of which stimulate

(*Continued on facing page*)

(b) pericardium and epicardium scraped:

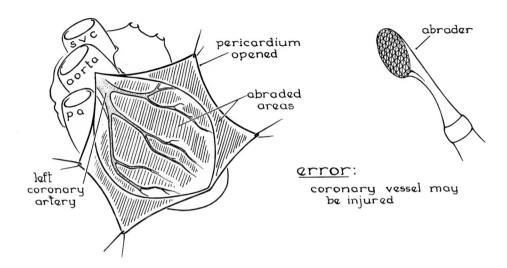

(c) pericardio-cardiopexy:

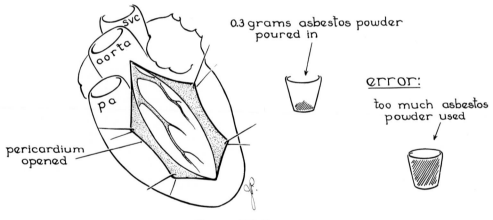

FIGURE 221 B

the opening of intercoronary arterioles or collaterals;

2. *Vineberg Internal Mammary Artery Implantation Operation*—By implanting the internal mammary artery into the left ventricular myocardium, Vineberg introduces systemic arterial blood to the heart muscle beyond the points of coronary artery occlusion.

Beck I Operation. The coronary sinus is partially ligated over a 3-mm. probe as close to its entrance into the right atrium as possible. The epicardium and the serous layer of the fibrous pericardium are roughened by a scraper. Asbestos powder is sprinkled over the myocardium, and the pericardial fat pads are sutured to the heart muscle.

Errors:

1. Ligation of the circumflex artery at the time of coronary sinus ligation.

2. Tear of coronary sinus.

3. Scraping of the epicardium over the coronary vessels which may be damaged.

4. The use of too much asbestos powder—not more than 0.3 Gm. should be used.

FIGURE 222 (*Illustration on facing page*)

Vineberg Internal Mammary Artery Implantation Operation. The left internal mammary artery is detached from the chest wall from the 6th interspace to the subclavian artery by double ligation and cutting all the intercostal vessels. The distal end of the internal mammary artery is doubly ligated and transected between ligatures. A tunnel is made in the left ventricular myocardium into which the internal mammary artery is pulled after first opening side holes in the part of the vessel to be buried in the myocardial tunnel. The artery is fixed in this position by one cotton suture tied around it as it emerges from the tunnel.

Errors:

1. Damage to the artery while freeing it from the chest wall by grasping it with forceps or having to catch torn intercostal vessels too close to the artery wall.

2. If the direction of the tunnel is not in line with the point of attachment of the internal mammary to the subclavian artery or the chest wall, there will be angulation.

3. If the artery is pulled into the tunnel without side holes open and bleeding satisfactorily, the vessel will thrombose.

4. If the fixation suture placed in the myocardium distal to the end of the tunnel is not deep enough, it may pull out and thus permit the artery to pull out of the tunnel.

5. If the artery after placement in the tunnel is on too much stretch, thrombosis will result.

6. Closure of the pericardium may nip the artery if insufficient room is left.

internal mammary artery implantation

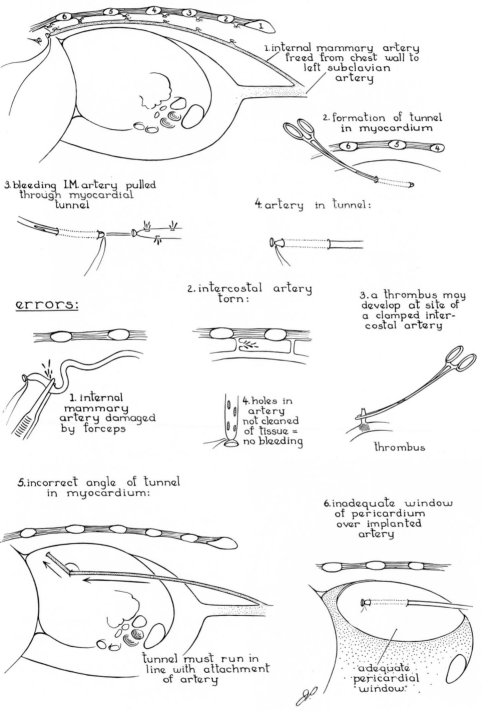

1. internal mammary artery freed from chest wall to left subclavian artery

2. formation of tunnel in myocardium

3. bleeding I.M. artery pulled through myocardial tunnel

4. artery in tunnel:

errors:

1. internal mammary artery damaged by forceps

2. intercostal artery torn:

3. a thrombus may develop at site of a clamped inter-costal artery

4. holes in artery not cleaned of tissue = no bleeding

thrombus

5. incorrect angle of tunnel in myocardium:

tunnel must run in line with attachment of artery

6. inadequate window of pericardium over implanted artery

adequate pericardial window

FIGURE 222 (*Caption on facing page*)

VENTRICULAR ANEURYSM

History: It is usually a complication of a previous myocardial infarction. It may be the result of trauma or abscess which occurs secondary to ulcerative endocarditis. There are no definitive symptoms, but anginal pain, with or without ventricular failure, occurs.

Diagnosis: Occasionally, the aneurysmal pouch may be felt pulsating in an interspace apart from the apical thrust.

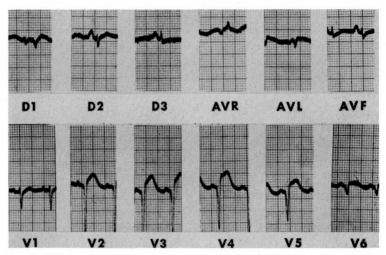

D1   D2   D3   AVR   AVL   AVF

V1   V2   V3   V4   V5   V6

FIG. 223. *ECG.* There are signs of previous infarction with persistence of some anomalies, such as elevation of the S-T segment.

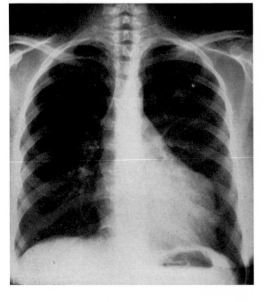

FIG. 224. Roentgenogram.

Postero-anterior view shows left ventricle with a localized bulge along the left ventricular contour of the heart. Calcifications are sometimes seen in the wall of the ventricular aneurysm.

Fluoroscopy: A small ventricular aneurysm may be detected at fluoroscopy as a localized area of paradoxical contraction. Under the fluoroscope a larger anuerysm shows a pronounced bulge of the left ventricular wall which does not contract during systole.

Errors in Diagnosis:

(1) Pericardial cyst

(2) Heart tumors

(3) Pericarditis with or without localized effusion

(4) Large pericardial or epicardial fat pads

(5) Right anterior ventricular aneurysm which is difficult to visualize

All the above errors may be avoided by visualization of the heart chambers through angiocardiography.

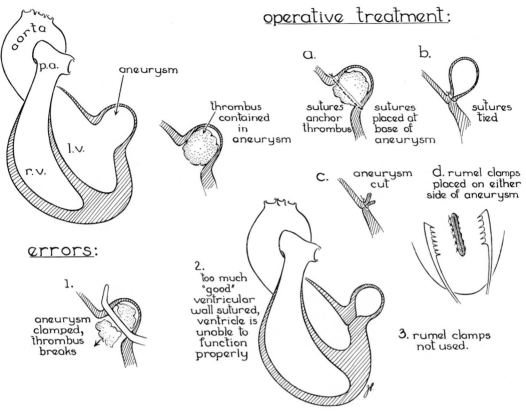

operative treatment:

aorta
p.a.
l.v.
r.v.
aneurysm

thrombus contained in aneurysm

a. sutures anchor thrombus   sutures placed at base of aneurysm

b. sutures tied

c. aneurysm cut

d. rumel clamps placed on either side of aneurysm

errors:

1. aneurysm clamped, thrombus breaks

2. too much "good" ventricular wall sutured, ventricle is unable to function properly

3. rumel clamps not used.

FIGURE 225

Objective: To resect the aneurysmal dilatation without dislodging intraluminal thrombi and without diminishing the size of the left ventricular cavity. Various technics for resection of left ventricular aneurysm have been described. One of the safer procedures seems to be that of placing interrupted mattress sutures through the base of the bulge in order to fix any intercavitary thrombus. Care must be taken to cut away only the aneurysmal sac.

Errors:

(1) Clamping of the aneurysm before occlusion of its base or blowing out of clot may dislodge thrombus.

(2) A too extensive resection diminished left ventricular cavity.

MAX THOREK, M.D.

14   The Abdomen in General

In a book designed for the use of trained and experienced medical men, it does not seem that it should be necessary to mention—let alone to stress—the imperative need for thorough knowledge and training before the undertaking of any form of surgery. Yet, all too often, one hears of cases—or witnesses their dire after-effects—in which some so-called surgeon has cut into the abdomen of an unsuspecting patient, with little practical knowledge of what he might reasonably expect to find there or to accomplish by his ill-advised efforts. It is for this reason alone that I have made bold to repeat and re-emphasize certain points which will be but truisms to those readers who deserve the honored title of Abdominal Surgeon.

No one who undertakes to open a human abdomen should ever do so unless and until he knows himself to be thoroughly grounded and experienced in anatomy, both normal and abnormal, and in differential diagnosis. Also, he himself should have made a complete physical examination of the patient and have evaluated all the findings, even those which may appear, superficially, to have little bearing on the current complaint. Even exploratory laparotomy should not be done unless there is clear evidence of an abdominal lesion; mere suspicion of such lesion is not enough. Incorrect diagnosis and failure to correlate symptoms combine to form one of the most prolific sources of surgical error. The "snap" diagnosis is usually the weapon of the over-enthusiastic and the underexperienced. The old adage "Make haste slowly" was never more appropriate than in the field of abdominal surgery.

PREOPERATIVE PRECAUTIONS

General Considerations

A small amount of pabulum in the digestive tract is desirable, as it is conducive to normal peristalsis following surgery. Strong purgatives which produce dehydration are to be avoided, especially before a celiotomy. Unless contraindicated by a history of recent hematemesis or evidence of perforation, the stomach should be aspirated, either immediately before the patient is sent to the operating room or even at the end of the procedure, but while he is still under the anesthetic.

The bladder should always have been emptied, either spontaneously or by catheter, immediately before any abdominal operation. Infections of the urinary tract may be avoided by adequate care both before and after surgery. The operating room must be kept warm and the patient well covered, especially his extremities, except, of course, the operative field itself. On no account allow the patient to wait about in chilly or drafty passages, since the effect is bad on both his body and his morale.

If a patient is extremely nervous or apprehensive, additional sedatives, beyond those normally given preoperatively, may be administered. Pentobarbital sodium or Pentothal sodium given intravenously are to be preferred for this purpose. If the patient has chanced to receive an overdose of a sedative, or has shown excessive reaction to a normal dose, avoid respiratory depression from nitrous oxide-oxygen anesthesia by adding a small amount of ether. Preoperative sedation for small children requires special precautions (see pp. 9, 33-34 and 381).

The nurse who prepares the patient for the operation should avoid scrubbing the site to the point of producing erythema. Care must also be taken to remove all residue of the cleansing agent from the navel. After cleaning, she should drop half-strength tincture of iodine or a saturated solution of picric acid in alcohol into the navel and seal with collodion, as previously suggested (Fig. 226).

FIG. 226. Swabbing the umbilical pit with iodine and sealing it with collodion.

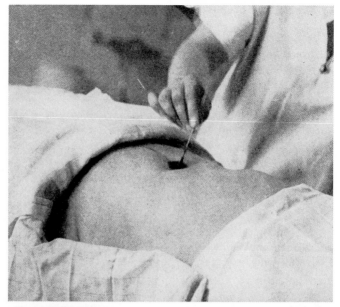

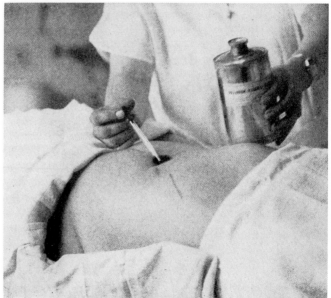

WATER AND SALT BALANCE

It is well for a surgeon to establish some set rule on his services by which all his patients are to be given routine quantities of fluids and salt unless some specific contraindication exists. This is particularly important if the patient be dehydrated and should be scrupulously observed both preoperatively and postoperatively. Keeping the patient warm throughout the operative period helps in this respect. Also, have his bed warmed before he is returned to it, but *under no circumstances* should any heating device be left in bed with him (particularly hot-water bottles).

Intestinal Obstruction. This condition calls for special consideration in the matter of regulation of fluids. Large quantities of saline can be dangerous; bear in mind the average daily intake required by a normal, well adult. It is well to remember also that excessive intake of saline should be avoided in the patient with *decreased renal function.*

Edema. Edema due to cardiac decompensation and congestive failure may be controlled both preoperatively and postoperatively with digitalis and derivatives of caffeine. Five hundred cc. of 20 per cent glucose with 10 cc. of aminophylline often improves cardiac function in such cases. If the edema is due to hypoproteinemia, it may be treated with a high-protein, salt-free diet, together with fluid intake of 1,000 to 1,500 cc. per day. High dosages of vitamins, especially B and C, should also be given.

Acidosis. After general anesthesia in *children,* acidosis is frequent. Glucose and saline per rectum should be given routinely, especially following emergency procedures.

POOR-RISK PATIENTS

Postoperative Pneumonia. Although the so-called poor-risk patient is naturally most liable to postoperative pulmonary complications, any person with a history of kidney, liver or lung malady, as well as the diabetic, the arthritic and the alcoholic, should receive special preventive attention, since all such conditions predispose strongly to postoperative pneumonia. The necessary precautions in this area have been covered elsewhere (see pp. 17-18, 31, 35, 43).

Cardiac Disease. Patients with severe angina pectoris or syphilitic aortitis, also those with a recent coronary thrombosis, should not be subjected to surgery except in desperate cases. In deciding the degree of operative risk for others with adverse heart conditions, bear in mind the following hazards: (1) exhaustion of cardiac reserve; (2) sudden myocardial ischemia; (3) gross derangement or cessation of ventricular function; (4) peripheral circulatory collapse and (5) massive pulmonary embolism.

During the preoperative period, those patients should be brought to the best possible condition by bed rest and the use of digitalis and diuretics. When faster effects are wanted, as in cases of auricular fibrillation, intravenous strophanthin in daily doses of 0.3 mg. may be used. For auricular flutter, quinidine, 4 gr. every 4 hours, may be given alone or with digitalis—or this may be combined with $\frac{1}{40}$ or $\frac{1}{30}$ gr. strychnine sulfate 2 or 3 times daily.

Choice of Anesthesia. *Spinal anesthesia* is not recommended for cardiac patients because it greatly lowers blood pressure. In the elderly, *ether* is contraindicated in the presence of bronchitic or pulmonary disturbances. Parenthetically, it should be stated that, wherever possible, surgery should be delayed until *any* respiratory condition, even a "common cold," has been cleared up. This applies to *all* patients, not simply to the "poor risks."

An adequate supply of *oxygen* should be kept at hand in the operating room. Be prepared to administer fluids, solution of acacia or blood intravenously in case of a drop in blood pressure during the procedure from shock, hemorrhage or loss of fluid.

Shock. In those desperate situations where one must operate on a patient in shock, blood plasma and serum, as well as physiologic saline, must always be given. Combat weakness of the heart with subcutaneous injections of camphor and caffeine. If the shock be due to hemorrhage, transfusion is always indicated.

Diabetes. Be sure that the diabetic condition is completely controlled before operating. The patient should have shown normal levels of blood sugar and sugar-free urine for several days prior to surgery. On the day of operation, keep the insulin dosage below the point of possible reaction. Avoid anesthetic materials that may cause postoperative nausea or vomiting, or have a toxic effect on the liver, or cause an abnormal rise in blood sugar.

Obesity. Figure 227 shows an extreme example of a condition to give pause to any abdominal surgeon. A moderate amount of fat is insurance of good reaction to surgery; however, the present-day desire for extreme thinness, especially among fashionable women, can lead to lowered resistance. On the other hand, a person who is markedly overweight, like the woman in this illustration, is even more prone to be a poor surgical risk. The obese are particularly liable to postoperative pneumonia; with this in mind, choose a position on the operating table that will interfere with respiration as little as possible.

If time permits, such hyperadiposity should be treated separately. A "fat apron" like that shown may be relieved by plastic surgery. Special attention should be given to diet, exercise and such other measures as will reduce weight and improve cardiovascular efficiency. Attempt to obtain the patient's co-operation by every possible means, since little may be accomplished without it. Under such conditions, it seems to me to be perfectly legitimate to play upon both his fear and his vanity, if need be, to obtain the desired ends!

PERITONEOSCOPY

This procedure has been in practical use for little more than 20 years, following the introduction of Ruddock's instrument. It is of some value under certain conditions, for instance, (1) where other diagnostic methods have failed or have been inconclusive; (2) for the injection of radiopaque materials into the gallbladder; (3) as an aid in the diagnosis of malignancy, particularly where biopsy is to be done; (4) as an aid in gynecologic diagnosis, including ectopic pregnancy; and (5) very cautiously, in some acute conditions, but only when laparotomy is to follow immediately.

CONTRAINDICATIONS

Peritoneoscopy is definitely contraindicated in cases of marked cachexia and weakness, abdominal wounds and injuries, in the presence of heavily developed muscles, extensive intra-abdominal adhesions or multiple operative scars, in severe cardiac or pulmonary disease, acute inflammation or active bleeding from the gastro-intestinal tract.

ADVANTAGES

Where indicated, this procedure has the advantage of requiring only brief hospitalization—often less than one day—and of causing little pain or distress in most instances. Mortality is extremely low, less than 0.5 per cent. However, it is subject to certain complications, among them (1) hematoma in the abdominal wall, (2) subcutaneous emphysema, (3) subsequent hernia through the site of the peritoneoscopy, and (4) probably most serious and startling, perforation of a viscus.

LIMITATIONS

This technic has a considerable number of limitations. Frequently the viewer must be satisfied with very little information, as the eye-

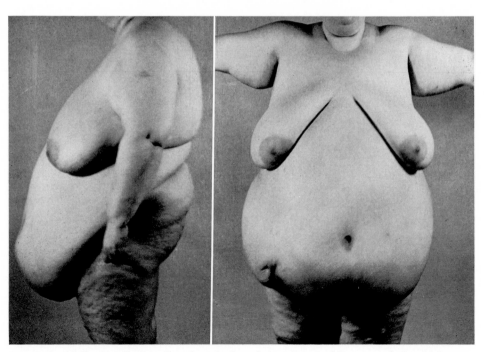

FIG. 227. Abdominal hyperadiposity. Such a deformity as this can and should be corrected by surgery, provided there are no systemic contraindications.

piece is apt to fog, the lighting gives abnormal brilliance to the surfaces, and retroperitoneal masses may be diagnosed only by deduction. Unless lesions give telltale external manifestations, peritoneoscopy may not be enlightening. Intrinsic stomach or duodenal lesions, including ulcers, are better sought for by gastroscopy or roentgenography.

The actual *technic* of peritoneoscopy may be found described in other texts, thus is not pertinent here. Suffice it to say that success and freedom from untoward sequelae depend largely on strict observance of detail and complete asepsis.

SAFEGUARDS DURING OPERATION

The precautions which every surgeon must take during the actual course of an operation fall into certain definite categories. The first of these, a thorough knowledge of anatomy, has already been mentioned.

ANATOMY

The surgeon should familiarize himself completely with the anatomic and surgical landmarks of the area, especially the normal surface anatomy—the position and relations of the viscera and the nervous and the circulatory supply (Figs. 228, 229 and 230).

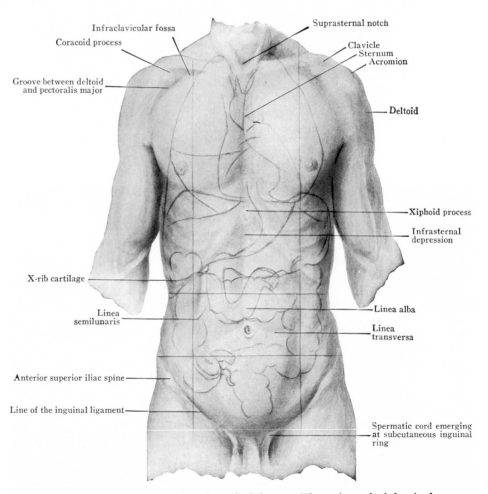

FIG. 228. Anterior surface of trunk and abdomen. Thoracic and abdominal organs are outlined. Bony landmarks are somewhat exaggerated. (Piersol: Human Anatomy, Philadelphia, Lippincott)

Fig. *229.* Abdominal organs in situ. (Davis: Applied Anatomy, Philadelphia, Lippincott)

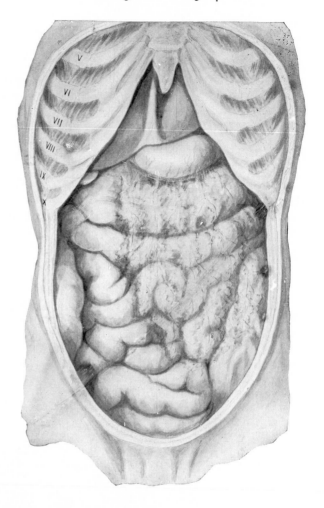

Here, as in so many other medical fields, one is impressed by the safeguards which Nature herself has provided for our assistance. The abdominal cavity, by virtue of various separating structures, is divided into compartments, vertically, horizontally and laterally, in such a way as to wall off and hold in check, almost completely, infectious or inflammatory processes when the normal resistance of the individual's system is intact. For this reason, it is imperative that the surgeon who opens the abdomen should, as far as possible, respect those subdivisions and confine his maneuvers to the immediate area concerned. To do so is to make use of the remarkable resorbtive powers of the peritoneum, which is capable of taking up almost unbelievable amounts of infective residue after a main source of sup-

puration, such as a gangrenous appendix or a perforated ulcer, has been removed.

Protection and walling off of healthy areas is obviously essential. However, in this same connection it should be added here that, although thorough inspection of the adjacent structures is extremely desirable, unnecessary rummaging is strongly to be decried. Respect —but do not misinterpret—Murphy's dictum to "get in and get out of the abdomen quickly."

Mechanical Safeguards

Protect the viscera with warm compresses during operation. Use only the type of *laparotomy sponges* having metal rings or something similar attached to avoid their being lost in the abdomen. Wherever possible, *clamps* should be applied only to tissues that are to be removed; otherwise they tend to produce thrombosis, with danger of subsequent embolism. *Gauze* is believed by some to cause postoperative tympanites, but there appears to be little real ground for such a belief. A decade or so ago, some surgeons recommended pouring ether into the abdomen; I have found this to be not only useless but also positively dangerous.

PHYSICAL PRECAUTIONS

These include such matters as co-operation among members of the operating-room team, position of the patient on the table, amounts of tissue to be removed and exact anatomic replacement of abdominal viscera (Fig. 231). Care in dealing with adhesions and in distinguishing between these and the peritoneum also come under this heading, as does the general matter of asepsis.

Co-operation of Operating-Room Team. It is of the utmost importance that the surgeon have as his aides only those who are as com-

pletely versed in his methods, technics and mechanical requirements as he is himself. He and they should be able to work together with the utmost smoothness, each doing his part promptly, accurately and without being told.

Position of Patient. A number of complications may arise from simple lack of care in placing or keeping the patient on the operating table. Prolonged Trendelenburg position may lead to torsion of the transverse colon, volvulus of the small intestine and dragging on the sigmoid flexure, especially in the obese. Also, acute dilatation of the heart may result, owing to heightened pressure of blood from the vena cava. If the patient is old and weak, he should be returned to level at least every 10 minutes.

So simple a matter as placing the patient's hands under his buttocks—a common practice—or allowing his feet to be overextended by the weight of blankets or by an assistant leaning on them can easily cause painful reactions during the first postoperative hours or days. These may seem to be small items, yet they can all add up to the difference between

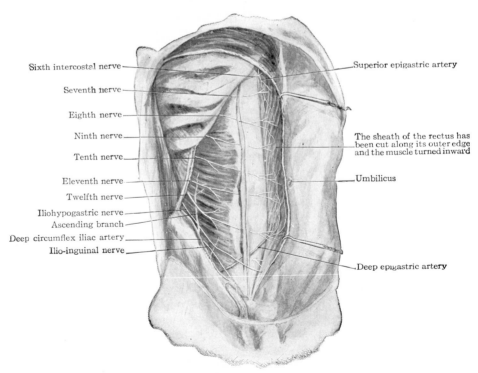

FIG. 230. Nerves and blood vessels of anterior abdominal wall. (Davis: Applied Anatomy, Philadelphia, Lippincott)

Fig. 231. Right and wrong methods of repositioning abdominal viscera after operation. (*Top*) Efforts here will be futile, and much trauma may result. (*Bottom*) When abdominal wall is lifted, as shown, viscera will fall back into place of themselves.

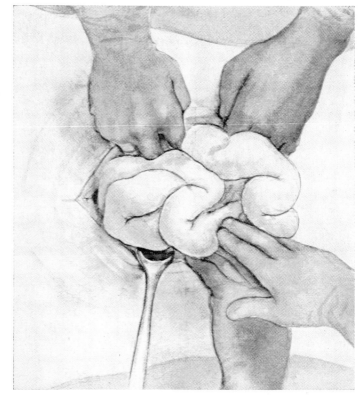

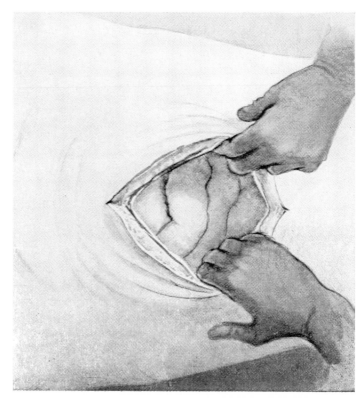

a good procedure and a middling-to-poor one.

Protection of Skin. Some surgeons consider it essential to protect the skin around the site with sterile towels, secured by Doyen or other clamps. Others do without, assuring us that they get equally good results. In either case, it is clearly a matter of practicing good asepsis at all times and in every detail.

Protection of Peritoneum. The peritoneum should be protected from exposure to infection by every available means. For all that it is extremely resistant, as already stated, such precautions are still essential, particularly in that infection within the abdominal cavity may well set up suppuration in the operative wound itself, whose tissues—muscle and fascia—are far more susceptible.

Hemorrhage. Bleeding must be arrested before the peritoneum is incised. Large vessels should be ligated, smaller ones clamped.

Underlying Structures. In the hands of the inexperienced, underlying structures are frequently damaged while the peritoneum is being opened. The following method will avoid this. The peritoneum having been exposed, it is picked up in dissecting forceps, elevated and given a little shake to disengage clinging organs beneath. A hemostat is then applied to the pinched-up fold, the forceps removed and the fold again shaken by the hemostat. The forceps again pick up the elevated peritoneum, while the hemostat, still attached, is handed to an assistant. Holding the scalpel nearly horizontal, the surgeon then incises the peritoneum.

Adhesions. When there have been one or more previous surgical invasions of the abdomen, adhesions can sometimes be mistaken for peritoneum. The intestines may be strongly adherent to the abdominal wall and could be incised accidentally. Chronic inflammatory conditions with their inevitable dense adhesions can produce similar misguiding conditions. The mistake is understandable; to fail to recognize and immediately correct it, when made, is inexecusable! Careless tearing of adhesions may also be a source of injury to the attached organs. Therefore, they should always be handled gently; it is often wiser to leave divided adhesive bands attached to the viscera rather than to jeopardize their continuity by careless manipulations.

Amount of Tissue To Be Removed. Naturally, this depends on the organ being treated. Patients have lived for years after nearly complete removal of either the stomach or the large intestine. However, with more than a minimal portion of the small intestine removed, chances of survival are slim indeed. These examples serve further to illustrate the absolute necessity for the surgeon to be completely familiar with both the physiology and the anatomy of the structures concerned.

Replacement of Organs. Replacement of each abdominal organ in its exact physiologic position is imperative (see Fig. 231). Also, be sure to replace the omentum accurately; this must never be neglected before closing the peritoneum.

CHOICE OF INCISION

I have experimented with most of the types of incisions recommended for use in abdominal surgery and have reached the conclusion that the less complicated they are the better they are. Longitudinal incisions are simplest, safest and least objectionable (Fig. 232).

For a definitely indicated, interval appendectomy, Battle and Kammerer's pararectus incision is best. Where possible pelvic lesions may have obscured the diagnosis, the use of a longitudinal transrectus approach is preferable. The paramedian incision is useful for general exploration. For specific exploration of the biliary passages, resort may be had to either the longitudinal pararectus or the transrectus incision, or the transverse. To reach the pylorus or the duodenum, use the longitudinal, xiphoid-to-umbilicus paramedian incision. For stomach and general intestinal procedures, longitudinal incisions may be planned so as to attain the best possible exposure. I personally never resort to the McBurney gridiron incision. Further, I reserve the Pfannenstiel incision for those cases in which, for esthetic reasons, it is definitely indicated.

In general, let it be said that the aim and desire of every conscientious surgeon should be to inflict as little damage on the tissues as possible. The simpler the incision—the more tissue it spares—the less is the chance of postoperative complications, especially hernia.

One precaution should be kept particularly

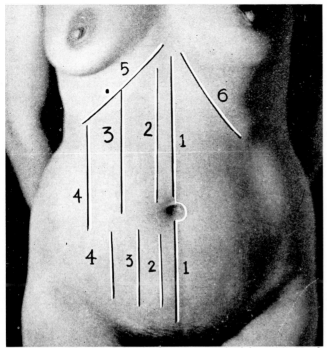

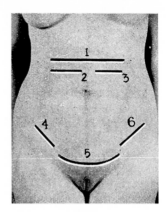

Fig. 232. Most used abdominal incisions.

(*Left*) Commonly used longitudinal incisions in approaching the abdominal viscera: (1) midline incision, (2) paramedian incision, (3) transrectus incision, (4) upper abdominal pararectus incision and lower abdominal pararectus incision, (5) Kocher's incision for exposure of the liver and biliary passages, (6) Fenger's incision.

(*Right*) Commonly used transverse and oblique incisions: (1) bilateral transverse incision, (2) right transverse incision, (3) left transverse incision, (4) gridiron incision for the exposure of the appendix, (5) Pfannenstiel incision, (6) left gridiron incision.

(*Bottom*) Extension of right rectus incision (Kammerer) for exposure of gallbladder. B'-B extension is parallel with nerves. (F. W. Bancroft.)

(Thorek, M.: Modern Surgical Technic, eds. 1 and 2, Philadelphia, Lippincott)

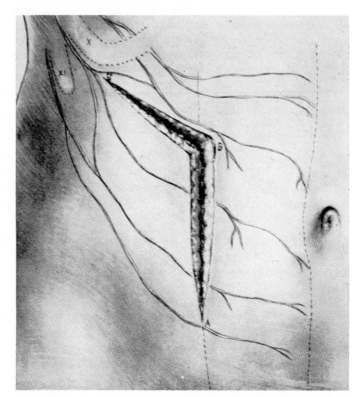

in mind. If, for any reason, it is desired to extend the incision upward beyond the apex of the ensiform process, there is always danger of broaching the pleural cavity, with its possible attendant complications, pneumothorax and cutaneous emphysema.

As previously mentioned, although it is wise to confine any exploratory operation as far as possible to the actual abdominal compartment where trouble is suspected, it is wise to try to get at least a general idea of the status of the entire area. To illustrate: A case was reported some years back of a woman who had a large diaphragmatic hernia that had gone undiscovered for some 15 years in spite of 3 operations at the hands of a skilled surgeon. Had he taken the precaution simply to pass his hand across the diaphragm and into the esophageal hiatus, he could have saved this patient years of distress and 2 of those 3 operations!

Obese Patients. These patients require many extra and special precautions all along the line. Routine methods and materials may not be suitable. Procedures, instruments, etc., should be chosen in the light of the surgeon's own wisdom and experience. Similarly, surgical landmarks are apt to disappear in heavy layers of fat. Fatty tissues are extremely friable, their blood vessels very easily lacerated. Capillary hemorrhage during operation can be very troublesome, increasing operating time and the risk of shock. Larger incisions as well as larger or longer instruments are needed. All the usual precautions against cardiac failure, wound infection, reopening of the wound and hernia must be redoubled with obese patients. They should be observed until healing of the wound is complete.

Wound Closure

In my opinion, many surgeons take the closing of the operative wound much too lightly. All too often they complete it hastily or, worse yet, leave it entirely to an assistant. Truly, wound closure and the method chosen are *as much a part* of the operative procedure as any of the earlier steps. A burst abdomen, resulting from a combination of careless or improper closure, or some unavoidable attacks of coughing or vomiting, may cause unpleasant consequences and some complications.

Many factors affect the choice of technic and of suture materials. For example, catgut sutures may be digested by ferments, as in acute pancreatitis; in the obese, tissues may be slow to heal. These things should be foreseen, especially in the presence of general debility. The intern or the inexperienced surgical assistant should be constantly on the alert.

Various considerations in this connection were discussed in some detail in Chapter 1. However, certain additional points should be made here.

Standard methods of closure, where thoughtfully chosen, will be effective, provided that approximation of each stratum is carried out carefully. A sound, smoothly healed scar will be obtained when (1) the incision has been clean and even; (2) muscle edges have not been frayed or torn; (3) wound edges have been protected from discharges and from mechanical damage; (4) perfect asepsis has been maintained throughout the procedure; and (5) sutures have been accurately placed in each layer to give adequate approximation and support without tension.

Again referring to the *obese patient*, it is well occasionally to place a small catheter along the whole length of the operative wound during the procedure, leaving this in place for 48 hours to draw off accumulated serum, which otherwise may become contaminated and produce infection. Some form of drainage is generally indicated because of the thin, oily exudate from fatty tissues which is likely to be profuse. Dead spaces and interstices between sutures must be sedulously avoided in closing the wound. Traumatizing fatty tissue with forceps not only results in slower healing but also may induce fat embolism. In addition, fat entering the circulation, as through an improperly ligated vessel, is another likely source of embolism. This may end when the fat reaches the lungs, causing complications, or the fatty droplets may be disseminated throughout the entire system, especially the brain, resulting in delirium, coma and death.

Figure 233 illustrates vividly what may occur if these general rules are ignored. Here we have a keloid resulting from improper closure. If such a disfigurement were to occur on a portion of the body which is normally

Fig. 233. Keloid formation on abdominal scar. (Negress). Such unsightly results may follow carelessness in closure of operative wounds.

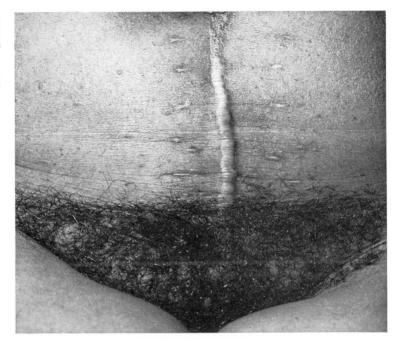

exposed, much embarrassment to the patient could result—and never forget that, in these days of ever-increasing public nakedness in warm weather, this matter of exposure may, besides being an annoyance to the patient, result in criticism of the surgeon.

When suturing the rectus muscle, it is a good plan to allow slight overlapping of the edges of its fascia. This produces a stronger scar and protects against hernia or eventration. In this last connection, I feel prompted to state my opinion that this accident is far more common than is generally admitted. This will be referred to again.

In certain cases, where some extra strain might be anticipated, tension sutures embracing all layers are a sound safeguard. Never cut catgut sutures short, as swelling of the tissues has a tendency to cause knots to loosen. Leave ends at least 1 cm. long. For cosmetic reasons, especially on women, intradermal sutures or Michel's clips are often advisable (Fig. 234).

DRAINAGE

Drainage of the peritoneal cavity may not allow the escape of more than a negligible amount of the fluid present, except in cases of definitely localized suppurative processes or when the whole cavity is filled with pus under pressure. While it is true that, in many instances, the presence of drains and the pressure that they exert undoubtedly prolong convalescence and may even cause phlegmons and fistulae, it is better, in certain cases, to combat these, where necessary, than to risk the patient's life by chancing the omission of drainage where it might be needed. On the other hand, statistics appear to show that the incidence of hernia increases quite directly, particularly in suppurating wounds, with the increase in the number of days that drainage is maintained.

When a drain is used in the abdomen it may not be advisable to place the drain through the original wound. Rather, in such cases, it may be well to insert the tube through a distant stab wound, anchoring it to the skin with a stitch passed through one side (rather than the center) of the tube or by a sterile safety pin to prevent its being lost. Suprapubic drainage—the preferred method for draining the pelvis and the peritoneal cavity—is required on occasion after the abdomen has already been opened.

Summary. The peritoneum is capable of dealing with considerable amounts of purulent material. Therefore, the direct indications for drainage should be (1) the presence in the peritoneal cavity of large quantities of free infective material; (2) oozing surfaces where complete hemostasis has not been possible; (3) in the obese; and (4) in the presence of an actual abscess (see also p. 594).

SUTURE MATERIALS

Considerable experimental work on materials and knots for fascial sutures has been done by Madsen.[7] He found that two of the newest materials, monofilament Nylon and Perlon, though permanently strong, had considerable tendency to slip and come untied. He found that plain catgut weakened too quickly. Chromatized peroxide catgut was reliable up to an average of 10 days, but different commercial makes varied noticeably; apparently the chromium content was the deciding factor. He concluded that silk (to which I would add cotton, as well) in the

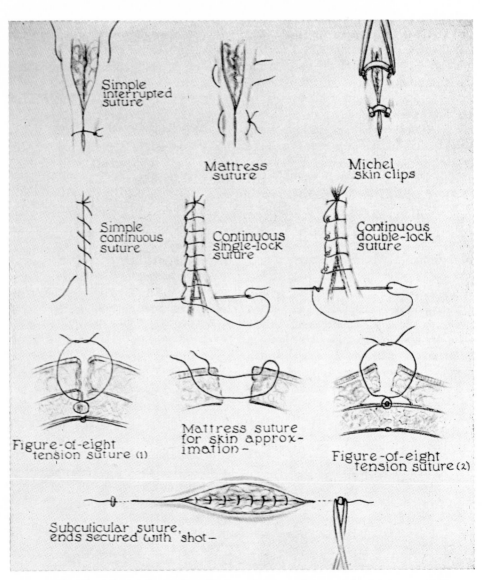

FIG. 234. Good methods of suturing where surface scarring must be kept at a minimum.

finer gauges was the most satisfactory all-round material. With regard to tying methods, he felt that in most places a triple knot was better than a "reefer," but that this depended somewhat on the nature of the suture material being used.

Since the Second World War, additional work, that is interesting if nothing else, has been reported in Europe on new suture materials. Perlon has been used in Germany, and one Polish writer even reports the use of nutria tendon as a suture material.

Woodruff[9] recommends stainless steel wire. He agrees with Madsen that the finer gauges do not seem to have any increased tendency to "cut out" as some have thought (Fig. 235).

One final word of caution—though it has been said before in these pages, it will bear repeating—before closing the abdominal wound, be *absolutely sure* that *nothing* has been left behind—a sponge, packing, rubber tubing (Fig. 236), a small instrument, *anything* that does not belong there—that later may cause mental, physical or legal complications. Accidents of this type happen often enough and are sufficiently dangerous that no amount of caution is too great!

GENERAL POSTOPERATIVE SAFEGUARDS

Nursing Care

Many of the precautions already cited apply after operation as well as before. They come under the general heading of good nursing care. A *special nurse* during the immediate postoperative hours, whether these be spent in a recovery room or in the patient's own bed, should be routine. However, in the case of the abdominal patient, the undivided attention of a special nurse should be maintained

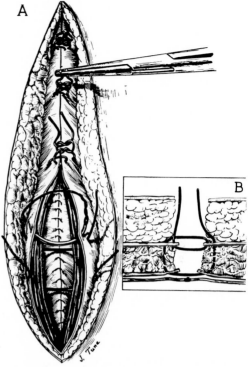

Fig. 235. Stainless steel wire, even in the finer gauges, when used as a suture material, holds well and does not "cut out." (A) The peritoneum has been closed with a running suture of chronic catgut. (B) Cross section showing wire inserted and ready for tying. (Woodruff, R.: Am. Surgeon 20:282)

for up to 36 or even 48 hours if at all possible. It should be her responsibility to see that he is kept warm, both by warming his bed before he comes from surgery and during the first 2 days following. However, hot-water bottles or warming pads should *never* be left in bed with him; use warmed blankets in-

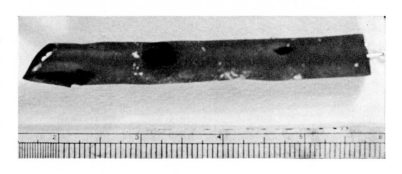

Fig. 236. Piece of rubber tubing found in inguinal region 9 years after operation for hip joint affection, performed elsewhere. (Author's service) (See also Chap. 1, p. 22 et seq.)

stead to avoid any possibility of having him burned or scalded while unconscious or helpless. *Venoclysis* requires continuous attention. Fluid should be kept at a constant temperature and rate of flow—an additional indication for continual supervision.

Bowel Movements. How soon after abdominal surgery and how often bowel movements should occur cause some differences of opinion. There seems to be little cause for real worry for 48 hours—certainly no purge should be used unless 4 or even 5 days pass without any evacuation. Enemas of olive oil or glycerine or glycerine suppositories may be used from the third day, if these seem to be indicated. Or, an aperient may be given on the third day, or earlier, if there is distention or vomiting, provided that there has been no suturing of the intestines.

Urination. Watch urination carefully. Retention is frequent following operations on the genitalia and the lower bowel. Never neglect daily emptying of the bladder. Much damage, even death from uremia, may result from failure to observe this apparently simple dictum. If turpentine has been used (a practice now largely outmoded) to relieve gaseous distention, watch the kidneys; suppression of urine may follow.

Diet. As a rule, diet is not a problem during the first 24 hours. *Water* is usually all that the patient will tolerate; in the opinion of many surgeons, fluid intake should be limited to avoid vomiting and distention. In my own experience, there is little foundation for this belief. Except in cases of actual stomach surgery, it seems needless to deprive the patient of reasonable amounts of water as his thirst demands. Solid food is not generally advisable until there has been a good bowel movement, and a full, general diet should be withheld for about a week.

Pain. If not caused by some definite complication, pain may be relieved during the first 48 hours by one or more injections of morphine or Demerol. Functional intestinal colic is relieved by pressure; however, if inflammation is known to be present, avoid pressure, as it will only aggravate the condition.

Rectal drop infusion (Murphy drip) may cause gas pains and nausea. It should be used only where definitely indicated. Venoclysis is preferable.

Distention. When uncomplicated, distention often yields to Prostigmin, administered hypodermically. The prophylactic use of eserine and strychnine, formerly well considered, is now thought to predispose to such postoperative complications as emesis, delayed voluntary urination and abdominal distention; therefore, these drugs should be avoided.

POSTOPERATIVE AMBULATION

Though used sporadically for more than 50 years, "early ambulation" could, even as recently as the end of World War II, raise a storm in any discussion group. Today, however, in many places, it has come to be almost routine, though, in my opinion, conservatism in its use is still advisable.

When a patient has no complicating, concurrent preoperative or postoperative malady, and has well withstood the operation itself, he may be allowed to exercise as much and as soon—both in bed and out of it—as his inclinations, coupled with the nature, the location and the extent of the surgery he has undergone, will permit. This is not to say that the human dynamo, inherently resentful of all physical restrictions, should be allowed to go leaping about the hospital corridors with the smell of the anesthetic still on his breath! It *is* to say that there is much evidence that early mobilization lessens nausea, promotes appetite, increases peristalsis and encourages bowel movements, diminishes the tendency to pulmonary complications, prevents wasting of muscles and greatly improves morale.

Blodgett[1] defines "early" ambulation as walking within 3 days of surgery. He believes that it should be used routinely except in cases involving the peritoneum. He stresses two points not generally noted. First, that time spent merely sitting in a chair is of little value; "ambulation" should be actual walking about. Second, that women patients should do their walking in shoes with heels of the height to which they are accustomed, *not* in flat slippers. He also notes, as have others, that the incidence of complications, such as hernia, shock, thrombosis, etc., is not increased much by the practice. Leithauser[6] states that he insists on actual ambulation on the very day of operation. This seems to me to be rather extreme. He further insists that "abuse" of the practice consists in "too little and too late" and suggests that contradictions in the literature result from greatly varying standards and interpretations rather than from really untoward results.

MINOR COMPLICATIONS

Although anything which interferes with steady recovery after surgery should rightly be considered seriously undesirable, the following items do fall into the class of "troublesome" rather than "dangerous" sequelae.

Hiccup. This may or may not be serious, but is more apt to be benign in nature, especially when unaccompanied by manifestations of developing peritonitis (see below). A case in point was that of a patient of mine, operated on originally for right, indirect, inguinal hernia. After the hernial sac was opened, an intestinal forceps was applied to the cecum and the ileocecal segment brought into view, revealing a chronically inflamed and adherent appendix, which was removed. For the next 48 hours, the patient suffered from persistent singultus with vomiting. Though temperature, pulse, bowel and bladder functions were normal, and recovery otherwise was uneventful, the patient was troubled and depressed, as is often true under such conditions. Obviously, the cause here was trauma to the bowel, the result of permitting the forceps to remain too long attached.

Persistent hiccup is a distressing complication, most often following upper abdominal operations, though by no means rare even in those who have undergone renal surgery. It upsets the victim and other patients within hearing and distracts the attendants. Morphine sometimes controls it, more often not. The best treatment seems to be inhalation of carbon dioxide. In severe cases, injecting the phrenic nerve with alcohol may occasionally be advisable, with crushing of the phrenic nerve as a last resort.

Necrosis of the Skin. This may follow careless administration of hypodermoclysis. It may even result from injections of saline alone.

Stitch Abscess. Extreme care must be exercised with stitch abscess to avoid even the smallest pressure, which may force infectious material into the peritoneal cavity, with possibly fatal results.

Wound Infection. Though it should seldom occur if proper asepsis has been observed during operation, wound infection is sometimes unavoidable. The surgeon who claims never to have had such an occurrence is scarcely being truthful. However, its incidence may be minimized by observing, in addition to scrupulous asepsis, avoidance of trauma to adjacent tissues, complete hemostasis and meticulous postoperative care.

Obstruction. Obstruction or, to be more exact, a condition simulating obstruction, may be due to omental torsion following handling of the viscera and faulty replacement (see p. 339). However, if the evidence of obstruction should be severe or persistent, this complication certainly should not be considered "minor" and is dealt with elsewhere (see p. 352).

DRAINAGE

The subject of drainage has already been touched upon in connection with wound closure (see p. 342). Certain points call for further discussion here.

METHODS

There is no ideal way to drain the abdomen. If tampons are to be used, give preference to plain sterile gauze; iodoform packs sometimes produce a reaction. Soft rubber appears to be a better material for tube drains than glass, as the latter may cause pressure necrosis. In the opinion of some, gauze drains appear to be fundamentally wrong, as they soak up blood and pus, which then coagulate and prevent further drainage. In our own work, we use rubber drains, cigarette drains and gauze packs, also the Mikulicz pack, in accordance with the requirements of the individual case.

REMOVAL OF DRAINS

As already indicated, removal of drains should be effected as soon as practical. There are several reasons for this. Adhesions may render drains ineffective within a short time, or they may become adherent to loops of small bowel and do serious damage when removal is attempted. Also, if retained for a relatively long period, drains may cause intestinal obstruction or fecal fistula from pressure necrosis.

SEQUELAE

Those postoperative complications which cause the most concern are:

1. Peritonitis
2. Postoperative evisceration and hernia in the line of incision
3. Postoperative ileus
4. Postoperative adhesions
5. Pulmonary affections, including thrombosis and embolism
6. Acute dilatation of the stomach
7. Postoperative diarrhea
8. Secondary hemorrhage and shock

Peritonitis

This may be circumscribed, e.g., abscess of the cul-de-sac of Douglas following appendectomy, or diffuse. Diagnosis can easily be confusing, as the early signs may be indistinguishable from the usual postoperative reactions. However, if the pulse steadily increases and pain fails to subside, if the bowels do not respond to stimulants, and distention and tympanites appear, peritonitis should be suspected. Add to these, persistent vomiting beyond 48 hours after the operation, particularly when accompanied by loss of bowel sounds, and abdominal rigidity, and the diagnosis becomes practically certain.

Etiology. Causes fall into the following three main groups.

1. OPERATIVE PROCEDURES. These include carelessness in preoperative preparation; insufficient sterilization of dressings, instruments, etc.; insufficient care regarding asepsis on the part of all members of the operating team*; excessive manipulation; peritoneal irritation from improper use of chemicals such as iodoform, iodine, etc., in the abdominal cavity; carelessness of any kind, such as ill-advised use of clamps causing devitalization and pressure necrosis. Peritonitis arising from

* A classic case in point is that of a series of operations followed by infection, in which the source was finally traced to a member of the operating team who was suffering from a nasopharyngeal infection which yielded a pure culture of streptococci of the hemolytic type. As soon as this man was removed from the team, the tragedies ceased!

any of these causes is inexcusable in this day and age.

2. FOCI OF INFECTION. The abdominal cavity may become contaminated through the opening, during operation, of some focus of infection, related or not to the current complaint for which the surgery is being performed.

3. SUTURE FAILURE. Occasionally, in spite of every safeguard (or so the surgeon believes), peritonitis will ensue because one or more sutures fail to hold. This may be the surgeon's fault, as, for example, when a knot slips because it was tied improperly, or the ends were cut too short; or it may result from failure of the suture material itself.

Treatment. As has already been pointed out, the ability of the peritoneum to deal with the residue of infections is remarkable. For this reason it is often unwise to reoperate, even in obvious cases of septic peritonitis, unless symptoms become actually alarming. Such operations are very often unsuccessful. However, if reoperation does seem to be indicated, to remove the cause of the infection and to evacuate exudate, surgical manipulations during the quest for the source of the trouble should be kept to a minimum. Excessive handling tends to promote shock and intoxication from exposure and cooling of the organs. In any such procedure, all the rules previously cited regarding preliminary and procedural precautions apply in double measure in view of the obvious fact that the patient is almost always in poorer condition than at the time of the original intervention.

Drainage. In the presence of suppuration or obvious progressive infection, drainage is nearly always indicated. Even when infection is limited to the pelvis (pelviperitonitis), I am convinced that it is wise to drain the area thoroughly, though I am fully aware that there are surgeons of unquestioned ability who disagree with me on this point. There is no disagreement on the value of the antibiotics and chemotherapy in such cases.

Parturition or Abortion. When general peritonitis follows parturition or abortion, the consensus favors immediate surgery, even if the patient appears to be acutely ill. Two drainage tubes should be passed into the pelvis, one in front of the uterus, the other into the pouch of Douglas. Until the infection has subsided, the patient should be kept in bed and on a restricted dietary regimen. Particular attention should be given to supervision of urination and the use of the bedpan. The patient should be instructed and helped to draw the feet well up, with the soles flat on the bed, to bring the thighs to a right angle with the abdomen.

Position of Patient. Parenthetically, it should be stated that the use of Fowler's position, formerly practically universal in the presence of abdominal infection, has lost its former popularity. Some surgeons have come to feel that a level position, either on the back or even face downward, serves as well or better. It is certainly more comfortable for the patient. The important item here is the character of the nursing care; it is imperative that the patient's position be changed frequently, at least once an hour, to prevent phlebitis and other circulatory and/or respiratory complications. This cannot be stressed too strongly.

Obstruction. Some years ago, I had under my care a young woman who came into the hospital with acute gangrenous appendicitis. An appendectomy was performed and drainage instituted, followed by satisfactory progress for 5 days. On the sixth day, however, she developed an intestinal obstruction with symptoms of rapid, progressive peritonitis. I decided to perform an *enterostomy*. Her reaction was prompt, and convalescence thereafter was uninterrupted, with ultimate complete recovery. This case is cited as an *exception to a rule*. At the time I performed this enterostomy, the patient's condition appeared to be beyond help; the choice of procedure was in the nature of a last resort, for such an operation in cases of advanced peritonitis is usually a failure. This experience is reported to show that all rules occasionally have to be broken.

Farquharson[3] states that enterostomy is much less frequently employed since the efficacy of gastroduodenal suction drainage has been recognized. However, he finds enterostomy of value in cases of gross distention of an *isolated segment* of the small intestine but adds that it is actually no more than an adjunct to other measures for relief of obstruction, providing a sort of "safety valve" for

the flaccid loop until its tone has been restored. He states specifically that he has abandoned the use of enterostomy for *generalized* distention, as in paralytic ileus.

Specific Organisms. Cases of peritonitis due to specific organisms call for differing methods of treatment. In *pneumococcal* peritonitis, the peritoneal cavity should be drained. In primary *streptococcal* peritonitis —fortunately a rare, though usually fatal, condition—suprapubic drainage, continuous intravenous infusion and administration of antibiotics form the only treatment. So-called *acute tuberculous* peritonitis—more likely, an acute exacerbation of a pre-existing chronic infection—usually comes to operation only on account of an incorrect diagnosis.

Each case of peritonitis is actually a law unto itself and calls for the closest attention and scrutiny. Some patients do well simply on supportive treatment. Others, as previously suggested, may require enterostomy, as in one case of *gonococcic* peritonitis, in which the patient was losing ground rapidly under all forms of treatment, yet recovered fully following a "last resort" enterostomy.*

POSTOPERATIVE EVISCERATION AND HERNIA

Evisceration. This complication has been referred to briefly elsewhere in these pages. Here it will be dealt with in more detail. The latest figures on this subject show some improvement over those cited in earlier editions of this work, but there is nothing in such statistics to indicate any need for lessening any of the precautions recommended earlier for preventing these accidents.

Farquharson notes—and I agree—that burst abdomen is most likely to occur in debilitated subjects and in conditions of wound infection, with persistent cough, vomiting and distention as contributing causes. He also states, as has been observed earlier (see below), that disruption is most likely to occur a week or 10 days after operation. "As a rule," he adds, "it develops suddenly . . . the patient complains that 'something has given way,' and the surgeon is summoned hastily because one or more coils of intestine are seen to have prolapsed onto the abdominal wall."[3] There may or may not be any warning

* Dr. Philip Thorek's case.

signs beforehand. An important warning may be the appearance of a serosanguineous transudate on the dressings, in which case an inexperienced resident may wrongly conclude that he is dealing with an infection and, more often than not, proceed to remove some of the sutures. *This should not be done* if no actual prolapse of bowel or omentum is found. *Leave all sutures in place.*

Many years ago, Dr. Baldwin of Columbus, Ohio, called attention to the fact that evisceration is frequently due to too early removal of sutures. He cited a large series of cases in which possible evisceration was avoided by leaving all sutures in place for a fortnight or longer.

When protrusion actually is manifest, immediate operative repair is imperative. While the operating room is being readied, first-aid treatment consists of covering the parts with sterile towels wrung out of warm saline solution, these in turn being covered with sheets of absorbent cotton and a firm binder. The patient must be warned to avoid coughing if at all possible.

When the patient reaches the operating room, the protruding abdominal contents are wrapped in fresh packs wrung from warm saline. After the skin has been toweled off, the viscera are gently washed with saline, dusted with sulfonamide powder and returned to the abdominal cavity, where they are retained by the introduction of a moist pack into the wound. Repair of the incision is carried out by through-and-through sutures, traversing all layers of the wall from skin to peritoneum about an inch from the edge. Mattress sutures will give the most secure closure and are best tied over small swabs so that they will not cut out. To avoid trapping any loops of bowel in the closure, the retaining pack should be left in position until just before the last stitch is tied. Additional sutures may be placed to secure the aponeurosis and the skin, but these should not be tightened excessively. Throughout the entire procedure, every precaution mentioned in connection with primary surgery must be observed with even greater care.

Some years ago, in a large series of laparotomies at Michael Reese Hospital, Chicago, an incidence of 0.43 per cent of eviscerations was observed, occurring twice as often in females as in males. It was especially frequent following hysterectomy. Mortality stood at 37.5 per cent. These incidents generally took place between the sixth and the ninth postoperative days, and no surgical reason was assigned in the report. Elsewhere it has been stated that the length of time before removal of sutures seems to have some bearing. As stated above, serosanguineous discharge from *clean* operative wounds should *not* be allowed to prompt early removal of sutures. First, be *sure* that you are actually dealing with infection!

Postoperative Hernia. This is one of the most unfortunate and embarrassing sequelae of abdominal surgery. The causes, some mentioned previously, include:

1. Prolonged drainage
2. Wound infection
3. Defective sutures or suturing methods
4. Vomiting, cough, meteorism or adhesion of bowel to abdominal wall
5. Poorly chosen incisional site
6. Hematoma of abdominal wall

Most of these items have been dealt with elsewhere in this chapter. However, it may not be amiss to add emphasis here on some particularly pertinent points. For instance, it has been asserted on good authority that with through-and-through sutures 50 per cent of herniae have been observed, while two-layer suture reduced this figure to 16.5 per cent and three-layer to 5.5 per cent. In my own experience, it would appear that these percentages are too high; nevertheless, they merit thought.

Choice of incision can be an important factor. Lahey[5] recommended that in making an incision the knife should go between the recti muscles and that, when closing, all small blood clots, which favor infection, should be removed by washing each layer with saline before suturing. I would add that perfect hemostasis and exact approximation should give good results. The lower midline incision is by far the most potent cause of strangulated incisional herniae; strangulation of other incisional herniae is comparatively rare. In such cases, the sac almost always contains small intestine, and—probably because the intestine has become entangled in adhesions—the symptoms of obstruction may be masked. Such patients seem to tolerate the resulting toxemia to a remarkable extent, even while gangrene proceeds. Therefore, one should not be misled by the lack of indisputable signs of obstruction, as a conservative course will often spell disaster. *Operate at once!*

SUTURES. The importance of sutures and suturing methods also merits additional attention. Smooth wound healing, resulting from good anatomic reconstruction, is the best preventative of postoperative hernia; this has been stated before. The fibers of the aponeurosis (the tendinous structure of the lateral abdominal muscles), when cut across, do not heal readily. The suture material used must not be quickly absorbable. Chromic catgut seems to be best suited for this situation, although for some time I, personally, have been using cotton sutures instead. Some surgeons favor kangaroo tendon. The edges of the aponeurosis should overlap, as edge-to-edge approximation often does not suffice to withstand lateral muscle tension, especially when the patient coughs or strains. In suturing the aponeurosis, taking in too much tissue favors necrosis. Also, every interstice or "dead space" left in the wound is the possible site for a *locus minoris resistentiae* and invites hernia. Factors predisposing to wound infection, apart from gross soiling (for which there can never be any possible excuse) are:

1. Small hematomas due to incomplete hemostasis
2. Inclusion of too large segments of tissue within sutures
3. Failure to exclude skin from the wound edges
4. Excessive length of incision
5. Irregular or jagged incision

With regard to the matter of length of incision, I might also say that though a short incision is more favorable to the production of a smooth, strong scar, the surgeon should not allow himself to be intimidated into resorting to incisions too small to permit a thorough, unhampered procedure and complete visualization.

SCAR HERNIAS. These may appear as early as 4 or 5 days after operation or, in rare instances, as late as 20 years. About one third of all such manifestations appear within 6 months, another 20 per cent within a year.

If an abdominal wound heals poorly, it is usually wise to perform a secondary prophylactic operation as soon as the patient is in fit condition to endure it. In experienced hands, excision of the scar and reconstruction of the abdominal wall are usually relatively simple. The same course is to be recommended where a small, asymptomatic hernia is already present, since this is apt to increase in size and be more difficult to deal with later on. I have seen a scar hernia such as this in which the abdominal viscera were separated from the outside world only by skin and a little fatty tissue. Under such conditions, any unusual strain could cause trouble. Further, the owner of such a scar—either immediately liable to hernia or already herniated—is often the victim of neuroses—and small wonder, in view of the handicaps, physical and usually economic as well, to which he has fallen heir.

When a hernia results from a poor incision that has not permitted proper union of the structures, or where there is a large defect, it may become necessary to resort to some procedure such as fascial transplant, pedicled muscle flaps, transposition, and the like. However, in this type of case, recurrence is always a possibility.

Cokkinis[2] reports reasonably good results even in cases of enormous (10 or 12 *inches*) gaps in the abdominal wall following surgery through the use of tantalum gauze mesh as a reinforcing material. He also mentions Fortisan fabric as being valuable for the same purpose but is careful to state that, so far, its use has been only experimental. In this connection, he points out that our long-established ideas regarding the failure of infections to heal in the presence of any sort of foreign body in the wound appear to need revision insofar as such inert materials as these are concerned.

Hernias affecting only the inner layers of the abdominal wall may sometimes follow infectious processes. In such instances, partial evisceration may occur, and loops of the intestine become incarcerated in the incompletely broached wall. This is especially likely to coincide with persistent vomiting during the second postoperative week.

BINDERS. One final point should be made. When a wound is unusual in any way, such as length, liability to infection, prolonged presence of drains, etc., a good abdominal binder not only protects the wound itself but is also an added support against pressure on the sutures. It is especially indicated with very long vertical incisions.

POSTOPERATIVE ILEUS

Paresis of the bowel may complicate the picture in peritonitis. Needless to say, the proverbial "ounce of prevention" is most valuable here. If all the procedural precautions already listed are strictly adhered to, the incidence of intestinal paresis will be greatly reduced. Nature is likely to make an attempt to immobilize the bowel by suspending peristalsis, in an effort to overcome the plastic peritonitis which inevitably follows, to some extent, every abdominal intervention. Gaseous distention may take place, depending on the bacterial activity. Impeded heart action, respiratory embarrassment and general discomfort make up the clinical picture. There will be obstipation, but little, if any, rise in temperature. In severe cases, the abdomen becomes like a kettledrum, in which condition the patient may die if not promptly relieved.

My own practice is to leave the patient alone as much as possible during the first 48 hours after surgery, even in the face of some evidence of bowel paresis. A glycerine enema may be administered if this seems to be indicated, and Prostigmin is given hypodermically every few hours.

It is most unwise to make a diagnosis of progressive peritonitis simply from tympanites associated with simple paresis. Many patients have been subjected to unnecessary secondary surgery because of such erroneous assumptions. The standard methods of stimulating peristalsis should be resorted to first. In uncomplicated cases, these usually will give prompt relief. If they do not, then one may safely assume that one is dealing with something more dangerous—specifically, some form of ileus, as well as peritonitis.

In watching over any abdominal patient who is having a stormy postoperative course, the possibility of ileus should always be kept clearly in mind, especially following appendectomy. Distention and symptoms of obstruction commencing within the first 3 days after operation may be due to paralytic ileus. This type of obstruction may be distinguished from true mechanical obstruction by its timing, since the mechanical form seldom appears before the sixth to tenth day.

Treatment. Confine treatment to conservative measures for a brief time only. When the diagnosis of organic obstruction is definite, the earlier surgical intervention is instituted the better. Prompt action often spells the difference between life and death.

POSTOPERATIVE ADHESIONS

The word "adhesions" has come to have a sinister significance in the minds of the laity and, unfortunately, in the minds of some members of the medical profession as well. Actually, postoperative adhesions may have their uses and should be considered, at least, with guarded respect. Naturally, it is better to secure healing without the formation of adhesions because of the likelihood of various untoward consequences of their presence, particularly obstruction. Exact peritonealization of every part of the abdominal viscera where the overlying serosa has been broached (i.e., all parts show a serosal defect, especially sutured areas) appears to be the most effective way of preventing adhesions. Handle all parts and structures gently. Avoid irritation from whatever source, whether rough wiping with gauze pads, use of excessively hot compresses, introduction of strong disinfectant solutions, or even of oils and emollients. Foreign fluids of *any* kind are more likely to cause rather than prevent (as some have claimed) the formation of adhesions.

Unskillful suturing of abdominal wounds, picking up underlying structures, is very likely to cause adhesions or even peritonitis. Do not break up indiscriminately adhesions found already formed at the time of laparotomy. Others, more extensive and permanent, are likely to form in their place. Also, bear in mind that, to a certain extent, adhesions tend to retrogress spontaneously once their work of walling off and isolating infection has been completed.

PULMONARY COMPLICATIONS

Pneumonia. The chief sequela under the heading of pulmonary complications is postoperative pneumonia. Every possible precaution should be taken to prevent it. Preoperative emptying of the stomach reduces risk of *aspiration* pneumonia. Patients with a tendency to bronchitis should not be anesthetized via the respiratory passages, if it can be avoided. In cases involving high pulmonary risk, spinal anesthesia appears to have definite advantages, especially in males in whom alcoholism and abuse of tobacco may be influential factors. The anesthetic should not be allowed to reach a level high enough to produce intercostal paralysis. Use of the Trendelenburg position both during and after operation tends to prevent hypoventilation and atelectasis. However, judgment is required in this, as pointed out on page 338.

Patients with *bronchiectasis* or *pulmonary tuberculosis* are especially liable to postoperative pneumonia. Sputum should be examined and, usually, bronchoscopy aspiration resorted to where indicated. Postural drainage best controls the symptoms. Administration of iodides is often advisable. Iodides in appropriate dosage are also of value for *asthmatic* patients, who should also be kept in dust-free or air-conditioned rooms.

For persons with any form of pre-existing pulmonary affection, postoperative treatment consists in preventing dissemination or aspiration of infectious material and, as previously stated, avoiding hypoventilation and resultant atelectasis. These tendencies may be reduced by limiting the use of opiates, encouraging expectoration (in patients with productive cough), proper use of the indicated chemotherapeutic and antibiotic agents and administration of intermittent inhalation of a mixture of carbon dioxide and oxygen. Routine use of carbon dioxide toward the end of anesthesia is sometimes advised in order to prompt the patient to breathe deeply and expand his lungs. This internal "bath" has only the drawback of increasing liability to anesthetic gas explosion (see Chap. 2).

If pneumonia does develop (statistics give an incidence of about 4%), treatment should not differ from that for pneumonia appearing under any other circumstances. However, one thought should be kept in mind: In what is probably a high proportion of cases of postoperative pneumonia or pleurisy developing suddenly between the fifth and tenth days after operation, there may actually have developed a small pulmonary embolism.

Pulmonary Embolism. There is the definite danger in pulmonary embolism of a larger embolus developing later. As long ago as 1922, deQuervain stated that following operations on the stomach, three quarters of the so-called true operative deaths were due to lung complications of this sort. There is no reason to believe that this is much changed even now.

VENOUS STASIS. Venous stasis (a preliminary to embolism) may be caused by rough handling of the viscera, infection or injury to blood vessels in the operative area. It has been variously ascribed to circulatory changes in the vessels near the operative wound, to general vascular and cardiac changes resulting from narcosis and to a weakened condition of the patient himself. It most frequently complicates operations in the lower abdominal regions. It usually becomes manifest about 2 weeks after gynecologic operations and is more frequent in patients who have been "pulled down" by previous hemorrhages.

The tragedy of fatal pulmonary embolism in patients who seemed to have been started toward early recovery is frequent enough to impel the conscientious surgeon to take every precaution to prevent it. Limitation of use of Fowler's position, deep breathing (respiratory gymnastics) and leg exercises, early ambulation (where not definitely contraindicated), use of sodium citrate, Dicumarol, heparin, etc., to lower coagulability of the blood and prophylactic massage beginning the day after operation, all appear to aid in the prevention of embolism.

Thrombosis. This is most apt to appear in the lower part of the left leg any time from 2 to 40 days or more after operation. Once established, the treatment must change from preventive (see above) to that aimed at forestalling the consequences. The patient must be kept in bed with the affected limb at rest, preferably slightly elevated. If in an accessible position, it may be desirable to remove the blood clot surgically. Above all, *never* allow massage of a thrombosed vessel! The same rule applies to *phlebitis* of the femoral vein, which may appear about 2 weeks postoperatively.

To recapitulate, prevent embolism and its attendant complications; forestall the clotting that causes thrombi by keeping always in mind the following safeguards:

1. Always handle all tissues with the greatest gentleness.

2. Avoid infection.

3. Avoid trauma.

4. Bear in mind the venous anatomy of abdomen and pelvis.

5. See that the patient is encouraged to change his position in bed and take suitable exercise frequently during his convalescence.

ACUTE DILATATION OF THE STOMACH

It was once thought that this condition arose from air swallowed during the operation. Now it is believed to be due to delayed shock, though this is by no means certain; the actual cause still remains obscure. It is less frequent following gastric surgery than after other types of operation, but it may follow no operation at all! Since it *is* a rarity, it is not surprising that the diagnosis may be missed until too late.

Early *symptoms* include (1) obliteration of the normal, slight concavity beneath the costal margin (in obese patients this may not be evident); (2) rising pulse; (3) subjective discomfort, even without actual pain; (4) scanty urine; (5) occasionally, persistent hiccup. In the later stages, vomiting becomes increasingly frequent and violent; the patient drools uncontrollably, while his mouth, inside and out, becomes eroded and painful from the corrosive action of the stomach contents. The hypochondrium will be bulging, tense and drumlike. With these signs, death will inevitably ensue if the condition is not promptly relieved.

Treatment. Provide continuous aspiration of the stomach by tube, discontinue all food by mouth (though the patient may be allowed to swallow water as he wishes), continue intravenous saline to replenish fluid, and administer eserine 1/200 gr. every 4 hours for 3 doses. The tube should be left in place for 36 hours or longer—even if the aspirated fluid is clear—at least 24 hours after symptoms have subsided.

POSTOPERATIVE DIARRHEA

This condition is a true enteritis; if profuse, it is often fatal. Like dilatation of the stomach, it is not confined to abdominal operations. It is probably caused by changes in the motility and the chemistry of the intestinal tract. It seems to appear in some 6 per cent of abdominal operations, usually after a week or so of apparently uneventful convalescence. If the stools are slimy, bloody or puslike in character, the prognosis is poor, especially if the diarrhea appears sooner than a week after operation.

Treatment. Treat this the same as any septic diarrhea.

POSTOPERATIVE HEMORRHAGE AND SHOCK

These two conditions are distinct but may sometimes be almost indistinguishable. As differential diagnosis is of the utmost importance, the examiner must be thoroughly familiar with the cardinal signs.

Hemorrhage. In general, postoperative hemorrhage results from errors in technic or undiagnosed and untreated blood conditions. These have been indicated earlier. Sutures and ligatures improperly secured and extensive injury to the capillaries play a leading role. Chief precautions include care in ligation, use of sufficient pressure on all oozing surfaces (Oxycel, etc.) plus secure hemostasis. Allow adequate length for suture knot ends.

Where *blood transfusion* is indicated, the dangers and the difficulties of the usual methods must not be ignored, especially under emergency conditions, where one may be forced to work with inadequate equipment. Under such circumstances, intraperitoneal infusion of citrated blood may be worth a trial, since the technic is relatively simple and generally familiar. However, a careful watch must be kept for 48 hours for possible reaction, which occurs in an appreciable proportion of cases. Chief symptoms of such reaction are dyspnea, muscular pain, fever, occasionally hemolysis, jaundice and, rarely, even death.

Abdominal distention is an important sign of serious trouble following any surgery. However, in the presence of other symptoms, it is never safe to assume that the trouble is not serious simply because distention happens to be missing. In the differential diagnosis of intra-abdominal hemorrhage and postoperative shock a number of other guideposts are reliable. If standard treatment for shock is followed by prompt improvement in the patient's condition, hemorrhage may tentatively be ruled out, but the surgeon must still remain alert for delayed indications that bleeding actually continues. Is the patient restless? Is he cold and clammy? Is there shifting dullness in the abdominal area? Do dressings or drains show fresh bloodstains? Is the blood pressure falling? Is the patient anemic? Is the pulse accelerated and thready? An affirmative answer to *any* of these questions calls for immediate action. As a further check, also ask if these symptoms are stationary or progressive. If they are caused by shock, they tend to remain stationary or even to regress. In hemorrhage, they are progressive.

Once the diagnosis of hemorrhage has been made, or even if there is still some doubt, it is often better to reoperate than to risk having the patient bleed to death. This should be the rule whether the patient has been under surgery or is suspected of ruptured extra-uterine pregnancy, gastric or bowel perforation or some other "spontaneous" source of hemorrhage.

Shock. The ideal treatment for shock—as well as for dehydration from vomiting, oliguria and many forms of toxemia—is a slow continuous flow of saline supplied intravenously. However, as pointed out by Kirwin:[4]

An important thing to remember in shock is that many a person has been "killed by kindness." Close, trained observation is essential; but all the various ways of bedeviling a sick man, by unnecessary hospital routine measures, should be scrupulously avoided. More patients have been brought out of shock by intelligent neglect, after proper stimulative treatment has been given, than by elaborate routines which continually annoy the shocked patient.

OTHER POSTOPERATIVE COMPLICATIONS

EMPHYSEMA

Postoperative emphysema will seldom be encountered if good technic is followed during operation. Press all air out of the abdomen before final wound closure and see that each layer is leakproof. *Essential emphysema* predisposes to postoperative pneumonia; the degree of danger in this condition is measured by a preoperative determination of vital capacity. If this has been less than 60 or 70 per cent of normal, the patient falls into the "poor-risk" class. Respiratory reserve may be estimated by having the patient hold his breath as long as he reasonably can. If he is able to do so for only 20 or 30 seconds, reserve should be considered as restricted.

Surgical emphysema is usually a complication of rib fracture, though occasionally of other conditions. Minor degrees of surgical emphysema require no treatment; absorption takes place within a few days. If the involved area is considerable, and especially when it shows signs of spreading, do not hesitate to open the subcutis under local anesthesia and let out the air. In my opinion, this simple and effective procedure should be resorted to much earlier and more often than is the prevailing practice.

ASCITES

In abdominal ascites, paracentesis is the treatment of choice. See that the bladder is empty. Make the puncture precisely in the midline to avoid not only injury to the large blood vessels but also penetration of the viscera by the trocar. Evacuate the fluid slowly.

HEMATOMA OF THE ABDOMINAL WALL

This may follow injury to the deep epigastric vessels (see Fig. 230) or some of their branches and will delay healing and predispose to scar hernia as well as to threatening hemorrhage. Further, careless handling of these vessels can cause thrombosis and embolism. Very occasionally, also, one might be confronted with the problems involved in diagnosis of spontaneous hematoma in the rectus abdominis muscle. This is a rare condition and seldom recognized preoperatively.[8] It may arise from some definite cause, such as trauma or strain, but may also appear, under certain conditions of debility or disease, from no discoverable immediate source. Chief symptoms are paroxysms of pain, which are increased by bending forward or flexing the thigh on the affected side. There are no visible bulges or peristaltic waves, but on attempting palpation, tenderness is so marked that the patient will be unable to endure it. In a case of mine, a preoperative diagnosis of twisted ovarian cyst was made, but operation revealed an extensive hematoma in the lower right quadrant of the rectus abdominis muscle.

TETANUS

Following surgery, tetanus occurs, I believe, somewhat more often than its rare mention in the literature might lead one to believe. It is understandable that no one, even for the sake of helping others to avoid similar tragedies, is overanxious to spread forth in print the helpless remorse that follows such a calamity. *Catgut* carrying the germs may be responsible for many of those cases appearing after clean, correct surgical technic. It is certainly well worth while for every medical student and every surgeon to keep in mind the possibility of such a disaster, especially in abdominal work where the Kitasato organism may be latently present, awaiting only the chance to cause a flare-up when afforded the opportunity through surgical disturbance.

PAROTITIS

Parotitis following surgery is now infrequent. It appears usually about 5 or 6 days postoperatively, with pain and swelling in the region of the parotid gland. Rarely, it will proceed to the stage of abscess formation.

If suppuration follows, prognosis is bad. Oral hygiene throughout the hospital stay and keeping the oral mucosa moist are the best preventives. If infective parotitis threatens, no effort should be spared to cleanse the mouth and prevent reinfection of the duct. When treating an established case, do not wait for signs of fluctuation, for the pus may lie deep beneath the parotid fascia. If symptoms continue for several days, with increasing swelling or an increase in temperature, incision must be carried out, and antibiotics should be administered.

MESENTERIC THROMBOSIS

Though rare, this possibility may be guarded against by gentle manipulation and careful replacement of the viscera at operation. If it develops, reoperation is indicated.

FECAL FISTULA

This is an unpleasant sequel. It may be verified by the passage of flatus with the discharge. If this sign is not definitely present, one may be dealing merely with foul, fecal-smelling pus being discharged from the wound.

RETENTION OF URINE

This is relatively common after operations for such conditions as strangulated hernia, as well as following the use of spinal anesthesia. This, incidentally, is one of the reasons, even if not the most important, why spinal anesthesia is being used less and less frequently by many of the leading surgeons of today, particularly in the fields of abdominal and urologic surgery. When a distended abdomen is found, see that a catheter is passed, if necessary, and that the bladder is emptied *first*, before considering any other possible causes for such apparent distention.

REFERENCES

1. Blodgett, J. B.: Early ambulation following surgical procedures, Bull. New York Acad. Med. 25:176, 1949.
2. Cokkinis, A. J., and Bromwich, A. F.: Tantalum repair of very large incisional hernia: healing after secondary repair, Brit. J. Surg. 41:623, 1954.
3. Farquharson, E. L.: Textbook of Operative Surgery, Edinburgh, Livingstone, 1954.
4. Kirwin, T. J., and Lowsley, O. S.: Clinical Urology, ed. 3, Baltimore, Williams & Wilkins, 1956.
5. Lahey, F. H.: The management of some complications following abdominal operations, J.A.M.A. 89:1735, 1927.
6. Leithauser, D. J., et al.: Prevention of embolic complications from venous thrombosis, J.A.M.A. 147:300, 1951.
7. Madsen, E. T.: An experimental and clinical evaluation of suture materials, Surg., Gynec. & Obst. 97:439, 1953.
8. Thorek, Max.: Hematoma of the rectus abdominis muscle, J. Internat. Coll. Surgeons 16:355, 1951.
9. Woodruff, R.: Management of surgical incisions of abdomen, Am. Surgeon 20:282, 1954.

PHILIP THOREK, M.D.

15   The Esophagus

The diseases to which the esophagus is subject are numerous and bizarre. For most of them, only surgery can provide relief. Therefore, the clinician should be alert to the many pitfalls which present themselves in diseases involving this organ. It is indeed embarrassing to misinterpret cardiospsam as coronary disease, to overlook a hiatus hernia as the cause of an "idiopathic" secondary anemia or to consider the cyanosis of a newborn infant as due to a tetralogy of Fallot rather than a tracheo-esophageal fistula. As we learn more about the esophagus, these errors are becoming less frequent.

CARDIOSPASM

Cardiospasm is characterized by dilatation, hypertrophy and tortuosity of the esophagus (Fig. 237). Theories as to the cause of cardio-spasm are numerous and nebulous; they will not be discussed here. However, it is sufficient to say that there is no known pathologic origin of the condition. It is twice as common in women as in men, and in a large proportion of cases, a history of emotional strain or psychic trauma can be elicited. Cardiospasm is the cause of 20 per cent of all cases of dysphagia.

The outstanding symptoms are dysphagia, regurgitation and retrosternal pain. Complete esophageal obstruction of varying duration, even to a point where the patient cannot swallow his own saliva, has been observed. Difficulty in swallowing is associated first with liquids and then with solids. The retrosternal pain varies from mild to severe, and prolonged use of morphine for relief may result in addiction to the drug.

Kramer and Ingelfinger have described the methacholine (Mecholyl) chloride test as an aid to the diagnosis of cardiospasm. When this parasympathomimetic drug is injected into normal persons, there is only a slight increase in tone and magnitude of esophageal contractions. However, in patients with cardiospasm,

FUSIFORM ──────▶ FLASK STAGE ──────▶ SIGMOID STAGE

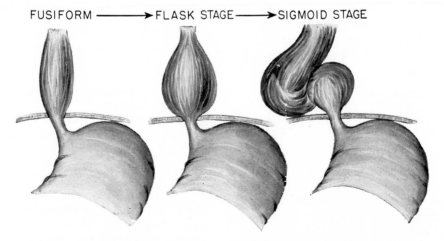

FIG. 237. Achalasia of the esophagus (cardiospasm). The idiopathic dilatation of the esophagus commences as a simple fusiform dilatation. If uncorrected it proceeds to a flask-shaped type. The sigmoid type reveals the far-advanced phase of this condition. (Thorek, P.: Diseases of the Esophagus, Philadelphia, Lippincott)

marked esophageal spasm and contractions follow administration of the drug. Roentgenograms and esophagoscopy confirm the diagnosis. It is well to remember that in cardiospasm the esophagus is markedly dilated; in carcinoma, dilation is moderate; in strictures, there is only mild dilatation.

Complications which may be associated with the condition are bronchitis, bronchiectasis and pulmonary abscess, all of which may be caused by aspirated matter regurgitated from the esophagus.

Medical management includes the use of psychotherapy, antispasmodics and dilatation. Many surgical procedures have been devised, including cardiomyotomy, resection and anastomosis.

ESOPHAGEAL SPASM AND TENSE ESOPHAGUS

Esophageal spasm and tense esophagus are frequently overlooked or misdiagnosed. The condition is a functional derangement of the esophagus that is a somatic expression of psychic disturbances and is manifested primarily by an increase in muscular tonus in the absence of any demonstrable local organic disease. A frequent error is to confuse it with cardiospasm. *Tonus* is the muscular tension present in the noncontracting state or during diastole. *Esophageal muscular tonus* produces pressure in the lumen; hence, this pressure varies according to the state of relaxation, and esophageal pain may be produced by an increase of muscle tonus. In some persons, transit time can be temporarily slowed by emotional tension.

Errors in the Diagnosis of Tense Esophagus

States of diastole involve different levels and have a wide range of severity. The condition termed *globus hystericus* is probably a mild increase in tonus in the upper esophagus. Patients with this condition should not be dismissed as neurotics, for they can be successfully and sympathetically treated. Tension states involving the middle and the lower parts of the esophagus are associated with frequent belching, "heaviness" and dull pain; a frequent error is to mistake these same symptoms for signs of gallbladder derangement or gastrointestinal diseases. In severe forms of this condition, there is usually excruciating substernal pain accompanied by dyspnea, pallor, sweating and syncope. If these manifestations are erroneously associated with coronary disease, the patient may become an unnecessary "cardiac cripple." It has been proposed that the term *tense esophagus* be applied to increased esophageal diastole and that the term *esophageal spasm* be reserved for the more acute and severe attacks suffered by patients with a tense esophagus.

Every case of tense esophagus must be investigated thoroughly before a purely functional etiology is accepted. Errors made in overlooking cases of this type impress us with the truism: *When the treatment does not work, do not condemn the therapy but suspect the diagnosis.* General treatment for tense esophagus is the same as treatment of functional derangements elsewhere in the body. In severe or refractory cases, medical therapy and bougienage almost always give rapid and dramatic relief.

ESOPHAGEAL DIVERTICULA

Diverticula of the esophagus can be classified in two ways: (1) by location or (2) by structure. There are three possible locations for an esophageal diverticulum: in the *upper* (pharyngo-esophageal), the *middle* (thoracic) or the *lower* (epiphrenic) esophagus (Fig. 238).

With regard to structure, if a section of mucous membrane herniates through the muscle layer, it is called a *pulsion diverticulum*, but if all layers of the esophageal wall are pulled to form a pouch, it is known as a *traction diverticulum*. The so-called traction type is usually located in the region of the bifurcation of the trachea where chronically inflamed tracheobronchial lymph nodes will be found. These diverticula rarely produce symptoms since they usually have a wide ostium forming a neck. More important than classification is recognition of the pathologic physiology, which explains the signs and symptoms. Weakness of the muscular wall is believed to be a prerequisite for a pulsion diverticulum. No symptoms are manifested so long as the opening into the diverticulum is large.

As food slowly packs into the pouch, it increases in size and drops downward. This process continues until the weighted diverticulum brings pressure to bear on the esophageal wall, causing obstruction. It should be noted that in such a fully developed diverticulum, food has easier access to the pouch than to the normal esophageal lumen. Dysphagia is the chief symptom, while diverticulitis, perforation and mediastinitis are common complications. Roentgenograms and esophagoscopy confirm the diagnosis and prevent errors which might be made if one depended on physical examination alone.

Avoiding Surgical Errors

In this day of chemotherapy, improved surgical technic, modern anesthesia and proper postoperative care, *the 1-stage diverticulectomy* is preferred to the 2-stage operation. However, diverticulopexy also has its place. In this procedure, the diverticulum is dissected free and is stitched upward to the surrounding structures. It is a safeguard for the poor-risk patient who has manifested esophageal symptoms. After the operation, food no longer has access to a hanging diverticulum, and thus the symptoms are alleviated.

ESOPHAGEAL VARICES (PORTAL HYPERTENSION)

A ruptured esophageal varix results from increased pressure in the portal system (either intrahepatic or extrahepatic). It almost always occurs at the lower end of the esophagus. The usual cause of intrahepatic block is cirrhosis of the liver, and so long as cirrhosis remains a common disease, esophageal varices will continue to be a threat to life. Extrahepatic block may be caused by phlebitis, thrombosis, fibrous stenosis or cavernomatous transformation of the portal vein. It may be congenital or acquired. Differential diagnosis of gastroduodenal ulcer and an esophageal varix often challenges the physician's diagnostic ability, hence errors are frequent. The cirrhotic habitus (the man with no hair on his chest) and the presence of gynecomastia and telangiectasis are often signs of liver abnormality. Banti's syndrome is characterized by splenomegaly, anemia, esophageal varices, ascites and leukopenia. If the block is due to an intrahepatic lesion, the findings of liver-function tests will be abnormal, whereas if

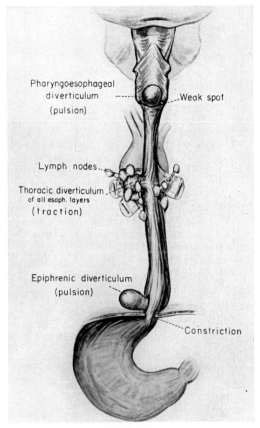

Fig. 238. Esophageal diverticula. The three types of diverticula are depicted. Their anatomic relations are clearly shown from behind. (Thorek, P.: Diseases of the Esophagus, Philadelphia, Lippincott)

the portal block is extrahepatic, results of the tests will usually be negative. If the disease is in a quiescent stage, it might be safe to take an esophagram, which would reveal pathognomonic "beaded" appearance near the cardia.

Safeguards Against Recurrence

Since hemorrhage from a ruptured esophageal varix may be rapidly fatal, definite measures must be taken to prevent recurrence. Some of the therapeutic procedures advocated are injection of the varix with sclerosing agents, tamponade through the esophagoscope, ligation of the coronary vein, esophagogastric resection to remove the "diseased" area and the various forms of portacaval shunts. This last group of procedures has become popular in the past few years, and various types of anastomoses intended to shunt the blood from the portal to the caval system have been attempted. More recently, splenic and hepatic artery ligations have been advocated.

ESOPHAGEAL HIATUS HERNIA

An *esophageal hiatus hernia* is that type of diaphragmatic hernia in which the upper part of the stomach herniates through the esophageal hiatus (Fig. 239). Three types of esophageal hiatal hernias have been described: the *para-esophageal type,* in which the stomach herniates through the hiatus and lies parallel with an esophagus of normal length; the *sliding type,* in which the stomach is herniated through the hiatus but has pushed an esophagus of normal length upward, rendering it tortuous; and the *hiatal hernia* with a congenitally short esophagus, in which the upper part of the stomach is herniated through the hiatus because the esophagus has never attained its normal length. The last type can be diagnosed by the appearance of gastric mucosa at an unusually high level. Hiatal hernias may be a coincidental finding in a routine gastro-intestinal roentgenogram. Such hernias rarely, if ever, produce any symptoms. Although many advocate no treatment, the danger of strangulation with resulting putrid empyema and rapid death is always present. On the other hand, many patients with hiatal hernias complain of epigastric distress, bloating, belching, anorexia, loss of weight and retrosternal pain. Such cases have been erroneously diagnosed as gallbladder disease, peptic ulcer, gastritis or coronary disease. These errors can be avoided if esophageal hiatus hernia is kept in mind, particularly if roentgenograms are taken with the patient in the Trendelenburg position, which would readily demonstrate an otherwise missed herniation.

Surgical Procedures

Left phrenic nerve avulsion should always be considered, since it may relieve pressure and symptoms by relaxing the left side of the diaphragm. Surgical repair of a para-esophageal or sliding type of hernia is simple, since all that is necessary is a reduction of the herniated stomach and a tightening of the esophageal hiatus. Hernia with a congenitally short esophagus is the most difficult to treat successfully.

CONGENITAL DEFECTS

Recently much has been learned about congenital atresias and tracheo-esophageal fistulas, so that they now can be properly classified and treated. Various combinations of these anomalies are possible. The most common defect is that in which the proximal end of the esophagus terminates as a blind pouch, while the distal end joins the trachea to form

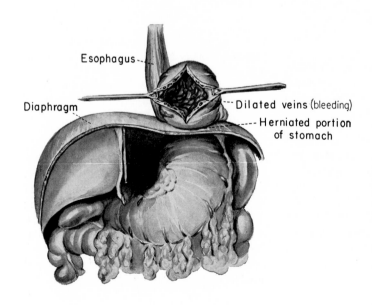

Esophagus

Diaphragm

Dilated veins (bleeding)

Herniated portion of stomach

Fig. 239. Secondary anemia caused by esophageal hiatal and diaphragmatic hernias. The distended veins in the constricted supradiaphragmatic portion of the stomach may bleed slowly or rapidly. (Thorek, P.: Diseases of the Esophagus, Philadelphia, Lippincott)

a tracheo-esophageal fistula. Such a defect may be suspected if a newborn infant has a symptom complex of coughing, choking and cyanosis, especially with an abnormal amount of drooling and/or rhinorrhea. These cases should be considered as emergencies, for the child may die of aspiration pneumonia. The roentgenologist can determine the type and the site of such lesions by merely noting the presence or absence of gas in the stomach and the bowel and by injecting a small amount of iodized oil (Lipiodol) through a nasal catheter into the proximal esophagus. *Barium injections should never be used.* If these few pertinent facts are kept in mind, the error of considering every "blue baby" as having a tetralogy of Fallot will be avoided, and immediate and proper therapy may be instituted. Treatment of congenital esophageal defects is by surgery, and with modern methods a high percentage of cures can be expected.

CARCINOMA OF THE ESOPHAGUS

A defeatist attitude no longer can be assumed with regard to carcinoma of the esophagus. What was considered a hopeless and inoperable condition only a decade ago is now regarded as being worthy of every surgical effort. *Early diagnosis* is of paramount importance in increasing the survival rate in esophageal carcinoma. It may be said that any change in the swallowing habit that *persists* is a symptom of carcinoma of the esophagus until proved otherwise. If this dictum were followed and such symptoms further investigated by means of esophagoscopy and roentgenographic study, many errors in the diagnosis of esophageal neoplasms would be avoided and early recognition and treatment would be instituted.

Dysphagia is usually the first symptom, and the patient will change his eating habits progressively from steak to hamburger, to soft foods and finally to liquids. There may be periods during which the patient believes the difficulty has passed. Although a tumor may involve a great portion of the circumference of the esophagus, symptoms may be minimal because of the distensibility of the remaining normal esophageal muscle. Pain and regurgitation are later manifestations. Esophagoscopy with biopsy is the only method by which a positive diagnosis can be made. The preferred treatment is surgical; irradiation therapy is only of palliative value.

16   The Stomach

GENERAL REMARKS

What was said in the chapter on surgery in general relating to operations on the abdominal organs applies also to surgery of the stomach. The need for a thorough knowledge of the specialized anatomy of the region is equally as imperative (Fig. 240). Also important is to be certain of the diagnosis and recognizing the definite indications for surgical intervention. X-ray findings are valuable only as corroborative evidence. Alone, they are not necessarily conclusive. Neither are chemical tests invariably decisive.

DIFFERENTIAL DIAGNOSIS

When confronted with a combination of symptoms which at first glance seem to incriminate the stomach alone, the surgeon must bear in mind that any one or a combination of morbid changes elsewhere in the body frequently produce symptoms referable to the gastric region. Some of these are (1) appendicitis, (2) biliary disease, (3) cardiovascular disease, (4) renal disease, (5) syphilis, (6) carcinoma, (7) genito-urinary disease and (8) metabolic and pulmonary disturbances. In one reported case, a patient treated for suspected duodenal ulcer was revealed, at autopsy, to have been suffering from a malignancy of the vertebral column!

Even such apparently conclusive symptoms as hematemesis and epigastric tenderness combined with chronic indigestion *may* arise not from gastric disease alone but from such other conditions as kidney stones, allergy or even certain neuroses. Perhaps in no other part of the body is the incautious surgeon so apt to make the unpardonable error of operating in response to purely subjective, neurotic or psychoneurotic symptoms with no background of physical cause. Let me repeat, it is essential to make *sure,* before deciding to operate, that definite *anatomic* lesions actually do exist.

Close co-operation between internist and surgeon will pay dividends when caring for a patient with symptoms referable to the stomach. Even if the stomach actually has been opened and the surgeon believes that he has found nothing to cause the symptoms complained of, it is well for him to remember that an ulcer may be overlooked, quite as surely as a diagnosis of ulcer may be made when none actually exists.

Again, when no suspicion of ulcer has been entertained, indurations and cicatricial contractions may be found. Always palpate the accessible lymph nodes of the stomach (Fig. 241); if they are enlarged, this alone is sufficient indication of the existence of some pathologic condition. On the other hand, it is not just to say "cancer" without sufficient corroboration (microscopic, etc.). Such a "cancer" could also be syphilitic or tuberculous in origin.

The possibility of *acute dilatation of the stomach* should be kept in mind when dealing with what appears to be perforation of a gastric ulcer. Perforated ulcers may not be located at the "classic" site; occasionally they are found on the posterior wall of the stomach. In one of my cases, a perforated duodenal ulcer simulated acute appendicitis. Also, in the presence of hematemesis, such possibilities as cirrhosis of the liver, blood dyscrasias or gumma should be excluded. Because of such vagaries, the surgeon must think of *every* possibility, even the most remote, before fixing on a definite diagnosis. Even then, after surgery actually has been undertaken, he should still be prepared to meet and cope with whatever situation he may find, no matter how unexpected (Fig. 242).

HEMORRHAGE

One exception to the cautious approach advocated above is in the case of definite evidence of continued arterial bleeding. Under such circumstances, even brief delay may cost the patient his life. Yet, surgical intervention may not prevent tragedy, for the surgeon may fail to find the bleeding point, or the patient may be unable to withstand the procedure in addition to his existing troubles.

CARCINOMA

When ulcer of the stomach or gastric carcinoma is suspected, the stool is usually examined for occult blood. However, it must be remembered that even if blood is found, this may indicate nothing worse than a red meat diet! Even more chance of error lies in the decision as to whether or not a carcinoma is still in an operable stage, as well as to whether such a growth actually does exist. All enlarged nodes are not necessarily cancerous; simple lymphadenopathy may be present as a result of some inflammatory condition.

Even the decision regarding operability is subject to some division of opinion. Charles H. Brown of the Cleveland Clinic[2] states categorically that many patients who earlier would have been considered to be beyond the aid of surgery can now undergo resection and survive for 5 years or more. Even when the lesion has extended to the esophagus or other neighboring organs, surgery, in the present view, is not necessarily contraindicated. He believes further, that x-ray examination is of doubtful value in estimating operability. Frankness with the patient regarding the whole question is of the utmost importance, since those who

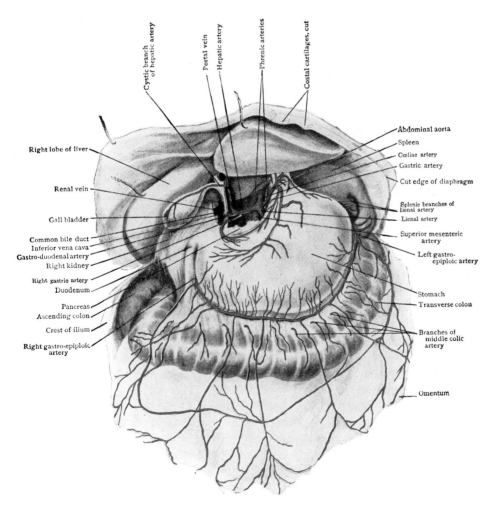

FIG. 240. Blood supply to the stomach. (After Piersol)

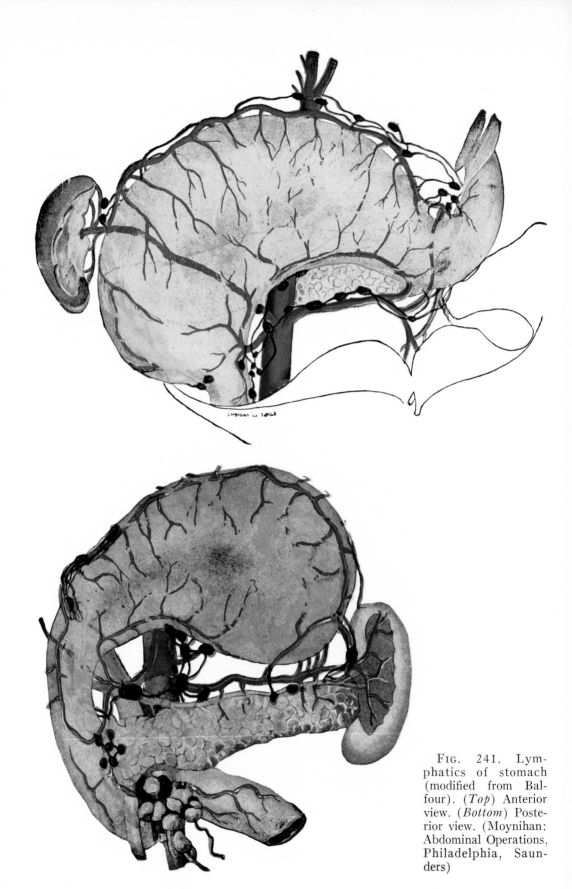

FIG. 241. Lymphatics of stomach (modified from Balfour). (*Top*) Anterior view. (*Bottom*) Posterior view. (Moynihan: Abdominal Operations, Philadelphia, Saunders)

are not told the truth may turn to faith heal-
ers and quacks to avoid the radical operations
which alone have any real chance of saving
their lives.

PREOPERATIVE PREPARATIONS

To assure as much success as possible,
every effort should be made to bring the patient to the best attainable general condition.
The mouth, the teeth and the throat should
receive any necessary corrective treatment,
e.g., diseased tonsils, infected teeth, etc.
The entire upper digestive tract should be
reasonably clean to safeguard against postoperative infection.

Here, as in other surgery, certain points
must be observed if success is to be attained.
These include (1) careful and complete history taking, (2) judicious selection of patients,
(3) proper choice of operative procedure and
(4) adequate surgical skill and experience.
The final results of the surgeon's efforts also
depend largely on meticulous preoperative and
postoperative care, as well as the handling of
any unforeseen complications.

DIAGNOSTIC PRECAUTIONS

When gastric ulcer is suspected, caution
must be exercised in the use of a stomach
tube. It could produce hemorrhage or hasten
an impending perforation. This is particularly
true in the presence of severe melena or in
cases with a history of recent hematemesis.
Care should also be taken with regard to
"test meals" and other diagnostic measures
which could put added strain on an already
weakened stomach wall. A classic case in point
is that of a patient who died within a few
hours after being fed a barium meal for an
x-ray study, the mere weight of the barium
apparently having been enough to cause perforation of an ulcer and release of the stomach contents into the peritoneal cavity.

Not, strictly speaking, a point of preoperative care, but falling into that general category,
is the matter of *inspecting the stomach* when
any procedure necessitates exposure of that
organ. Examine it thoroughly from cardia to
pylorus, making sure that each area is sur-
veyed accurately.

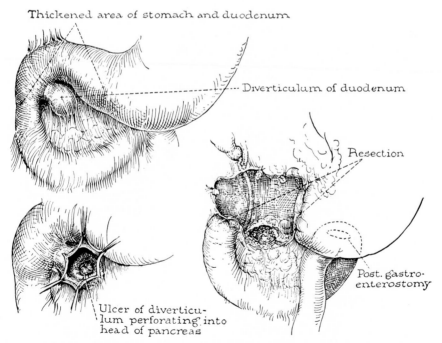

FIG. 242. Operation to remove ulcer in diverticulum of duodenum perforating into head of pancreas. Ability to deal with the unexpected marks the
competent gastric surgeon.

POSTOPERATIVE CARE

Regardless of whether the procedure has gone smoothly or has involved complications, any patient who has been subjected to a gastric operation requires the closest supervision by the surgeon. Meticulous attention to detail contributes to ultimate success.

Vomiting

If more than minimal, vomiting should be dealt with according to circumstances. This is discussed elsewhere in this chapter.

Feeding

Food by mouth is customarily forbidden at least during the first 72 hours following operation since suction is usually resorted to for that period. After this time, feeding may begin gradually, testing the tolerance of the stomach at each step. It should never be taxed with large amounts of food, since after any surgical intervention on the digestive tract, the innervation and peristaltic functions of the organ or organs involved have been impaired. Only gradual increases, supplemented, if necessary, by parenteral feeding, should be permitted.[4]

Diet

After the patient leaves the hospital, he should still be governed by strict dietary rules, and full explanation of the risks involved in disregarding these instructions should be stressed. A successful operation does not consist merely in discharging the patient in good condition. It includes continuance of his treatment until all danger may reasonably be assumed to have passed.

Hematemesis, Adhesions and Damage to Adjacent Structures

Special postoperative precautions of importance in interventions on the stomach include care with respect to (1) hematemesis, (2) formation of adhesions and (3) damage to adjacent structures.

Hematemesis. Sometimes hematemesis may prove to be unavoidable, as when it results from blood dyscrasias, metabolic aberrations and the like. However, if it is the result of imperfect placement of sutures, the responsibility lies right at the surgeon's door, for this is as inexcusable as it is avoidable.

Adhesions and Scar Tissue. These are quite often serious complications in dealing with "cured" duodenal ulcers which have been treated by medical methods such as alkalinization or lavage. Scar formations, in time, can and do produce pyloric obstruction or duodenal stricture. About one-third of such patients later require surgery.

Injury to Ducts. Injury to the pancreatic and the common bile ducts often complicates resection of a duodenal ulcer in the vicinity of the pancreas. If these cannot be dissected without harm, they should first be protected. A new implantation of the common bile duct may be made if it seems to be indicated. Injury to the common bile duct is usually recognized by the appearance of bile, but damage to the pancreatic duct is not detected so easily.

GASTRIC AND DUODENAL ULCERS

In order to avoid confusion, let me first define the terms used here in referring to various types of so-called stomach ulcers. Differential diagnosis and proper classification are essential because, though differing ulcers have many symptoms in common, treatment must vary according to the type of ulcer. Chronic *gastric* ulcer becomes malignant in about 20 per cent of cases, while malignant transformation of *duodenal* ulcer is a rarity.

Simple ulcer is the term applied to one which presents a chronic and regularly recurrent typical clinical picture, i.e., pain relieved by food or alkalies or by vomiting. A *penetrating ulcer* is one which has involved some adjacent organ, such as the pancreas. A *perforating ulcer* is one which is progressing toward perforation but has not as yet penetrated the serosa. These last two types are characterized by a subjective history of pain which increases in intensity, is continuous and is not relieved by vomiting or the ingestion of food or alkalies.

A *perforated ulcer* produces sudden, dramatic and painfully acute symptoms. The picture is too familiar to need further description. However, two points should be mentioned. One is that the term "ruptured" ulcer should not be used in this connection; "rupture" refers strictly to the results of trauma. The other point has to do with the so-called *forme fruste* ulcer, in which a minute perforation occurs which promptly reseals itself, allowing minimal leakage and soiling, and which does not produce the characteristic symptom picture. Such patients may arrive at the hospital under their own power.

Perforated peptic ulcer has two identifying signs: (1) the "silent abdomen," which occurs more promptly here than with any other condition; and (2) the "spontaneous pneumo-peritoneum," i.e., air under the diaphragm demonstrable by roentgenogram and found in 70 to 80 per cent of all cases of perforated ulcer (Fig. 243). This sign may be missed, however, if the patient is prone or supine during examination. He should be sitting up or lying on his left side, so that the "air bubble" will show up between the liver and the diaphragm.

One further point bears repetition. Perfo-rated ulcer is *very rarely* seen in females—so rarely, indeed, that it is a reasonably safe assumption, when the characteristic symptoms appear in a female, that one is dealing with a *perforating carcinoma* instead. In over 40 years of hospital service and private practice, I have seen only 1 case of true perforated gastric ulcer in a female. One of my col-leagues has seen but 4 in more than 30 years' experience.

PROGNOSIS

When perforation has occurred, the *sooner the patient is operated on, the better the prog-nosis*. Many of these patients go into shock within an hour; if this occurs, it is better to delay operation for a reasonable time until they respond to treatment for shock. In this situation I always operate within 24 hours, if at all possible, after which conservative meas-ures (Levine tube siphonage, drainage, trans-fusion) are administered. These patients must be watched for development of subphrenic and perigastric abscesses.

I cannot agree with those who, when per-foration has occurred, recommend resection of the ulcer or a gastroenterostomy, or even a

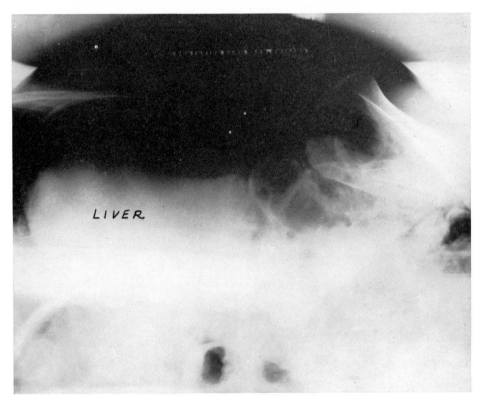

FIG. 243. Perforated peptic ulcer. Note enormous air space between liver and right lateral chest wall. (Patient in left lateral decubitus.)

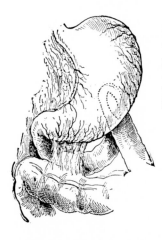

FIG. 244. Posterior gastroenterostomy completed. (Davis: Applied Anatomy, Philadelphia, Lippincott)

routine gastric resection. As a standard procedure, we do nothing more than suture the perforation and place an omental pad over it.

GASTROENTEROSTOMY

Some years ago this procedure was held to be practically a "sure cure" for duodenal ulcer. More recent opinion concludes that its greatest usefulness is in stenotic conditions of the stomach and the duodenum. It is most often done for pyloric obstruction. Because the results in these cases were excellent, it was illogically assumed that it should be the treatment of choice for *all* gastric ulcers. However, it soon became apparent that the end-results, in cases of chronic ulcer near the cardia or upon the midsection of the stomach, were apt to be less satisfactory in the long run, even though the patients usually did experience some immediate relief. For ulcers elsewhere than at the pylorus, especially if small, excision by knife or cautery seems to give better results than gastroenterostomy. Small ulcers on the lesser curvature may be excised with no resultant deformity. If the ulcer is large, excision may be combined with gastroenterostomy (Fig. 244).

Some years ago, Sir Hugh Devine stated:

The surgeon should make himself intimately acquainted with the physiologic conditions . . . [and] study carefully the pathology of the lesion as seen by X-rays. This knowledge is necessary so that the technic . . . can be individualized. The information required is as follows: (1) the shape and size of the patient's stomach; (2) the presence of even mild degrees of pyloric stenosis—a complication which is not infrequently associated

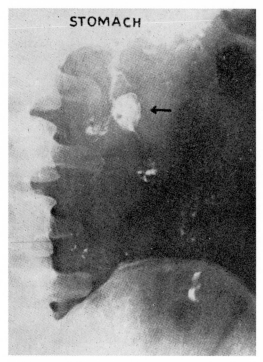

FIG. 245. Postoperative peptic (jejunal) ulcer.

with chronic peptic ulcer . . . (3) the situation and degree of chronicity of the ulcer; (4) the degree of gastric acidity; (5) the possibility of any malignant degeneration.

He further points out that two decisions may be predicated on these findings: (1) whether gastroenterostomy may be done without giving rise to undesirable by-effects, and (2) whether the stomach in question will be amenable to cure by this procedure; some ulcers are of too long standing and so located that results may be unfavorable.

With this information, he adds, the surgeon may then decide where to place the stoma, how large to make it and whether or not the formation of a jejunal ulcer may result (Fig. 245). All these decisions are predicated on the gastric muscle tone, the age of the patient and the acidity of the gastric juice.

Parenthetically, I might add that, in some of these cases, *pyloroplasty* (see Fig. 251) does not disturb the structures of the stomach itself but permits resection of an ulcer-bearing area and eliminates the possibility of pylorospasm by cutting the pyloric sphincter (Fig.

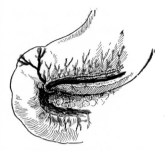

FIG. 246. Veins at pyloric sphincter.

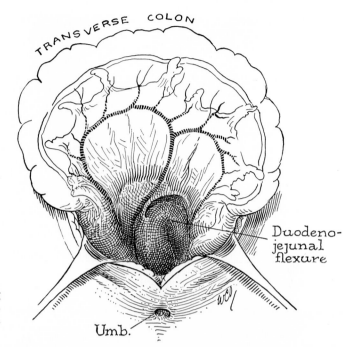

FIG. 247. Diagram showing proper method of locating duodenojejunal flexure during gastrojejunostomy.

246). This technic has been used only to a very limited extent for some years but recently has returned to greater favor as an adjunct to *vagotomy*.

Certain technical errors may occur in the performance of a gastroenterostomy. The stomach may accidentally be sutured to some portion of the bowel other than the jejunum, such as the lower end of the ileum or even the colon. (This seems unlikely, but cases of this type of error actually have been reported.) A fairly common mistake is suturing the jejunum to the stomach in such a way that it can become kinked at the anastomosis (Fig. 247). Owing to steady improvements in technic, such errors are less frequent than formerly, yet no surgeon can feel fully assured that complications will not occur. They can happen even with the best procedure and the most elaborate precautions. Here again, skill and experience are the indispensable ingredients for favorable results (Fig. 248).

As far back as 1942, Rudolf Nissen offered some valuable suggestions and described many technical details in the treatment of complicated ulcers in the duodenum. In brief, his method consists of mobilizing the anterior wall of the duodenum so as to give access to the

ulcers situated on the posterior wall, which constitute by far the larger number of "nonresectable" lesions.

The pancreatic or the common bile ducts may be injured if the ulcer has invaded the region of the papilla. While these may be repaired, additional risk is involved. When the ulcer is small, the anterior wall of the duodenum should be opened directly below the pylorus and the posterior wall incised from within, taking care to prevent escape of duodenal contents. If the ulcer is large, the opening should be made from without. Incise the dorsal wall of the crater of the ulcer and proceed to dissect through the wall. The ulcer itself should not be incised; large blood vessels at its base, if seen, should be ligated.

The operation is a delicate one, and special caution should be exercised in suturing after this procedure. In the first line of sutures, include the anterior duodenal wall and the opposite margin of the crater; in the second (invaginating) suture, the anterior duodenal wall and its distal margin; in the third, the peritoneal coat of the pancreas (usually thickened, because of chronic inflammation) should be pulled over the anterior duodenal wall and united with the omentum. Before placing this

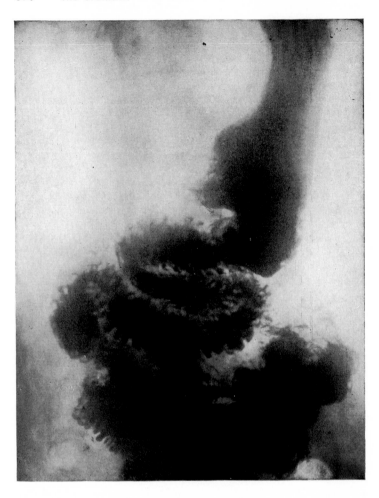

FIG. 248. Well-function-
ing gastroenterostomy.

final suture, be sure to determine the exact location of the superior pancreaticoduodenalis artery so as to avoid injury to it. Sutured in this manner, drainage from the floor of the ulcer is impossible. In theory, an open accessory pancreatic duct (if one exists) could evacuate into the space between the first and second rows of sutures, causing them to disintegrate. Finsterer thought that this had happened in one fatal case of his; since this report, Nissen has allowed an outlet into the duodenum, and his operative mortality has been 3.5 per cent.

POSTOPERATIVE COMPLICATIONS

Complications which may follow gastro-enterostomy include:

1. Hemorrhage
2. Regurgitant vomiting ("vicious circle")
3. Obstructive conditions
4. Internal hernia
5. Retrograde intussusception
6. Separation of the viscera
7. Adhesions about the anastomosis
8. Postoperative peptic (jejunal) ulcer (Fig. 249)
9. Thoracic complications
10. Subphrenic abscess
11. "Dumping syndrome"

Hemorrhage. Bleeding may follow improper suturing of the stomach or the jejunum. A continuous suture, embracing all layers, should be used and drawn up firmly but not too tightly. The mucosal edge should be turned outward so that any bleeding points may be seen easily and secured at once.

Hemorrhage may also result from ulceration of the jejunum, due to obstruction at the anastomosis or to imperfect neutralization of the gastric juice by the pancreatic and duodenal secretions. Sepsis and the use of non-absorbable suture materials have sometimes

Fig. 249. Gastrojejunal ulcer (at arrow), following gastrojejunostomy.

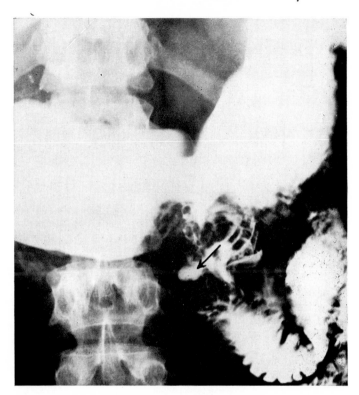

also been incriminated. A slight showing of bright blood in vomited material may be due to oozing along the suture line. This can usually be controlled by injections of morphine and icebags applied to the epigastrium. Severe hematemesis calls for immediate reoperation to locate the source of the bleeding.

Regurgitant Vomiting. Vomiting of the regurgitant or "vicious circle" variety is probably due to some obstruction at the stoma in the efferent loop opening and to disturbances of peristalsis. It may also result from a true mechanical ileus, the immediate cause probably being the twisting of one of the loops involved in the gastroenterostomy or the incarceration of a loop of small intestine in an opening in the transverse mesocolon (in posterior gastroenterostomy).

In this connection, some authorities believe that all ileus, following such procedures, is both mechanical and paralytic in nature and should be treated accordingly.

In the early days of gastroenterostomy, vomiting was observed in a number of cases and sometimes proved to be fatal. Today, when hypoproteinemia and hypochloridemia are better understood and controlled, trouble

from this particular complication is no longer formidable.

Obstruction. The classic treatment for postoperative obstruction, according to Aird,[1] is still saline drip infusion plus gastro-intestinal suction drainage. However, he points out that the Miller-Abbott tube cannot pass the pylorus against the pressure from below when the obstruction is mechanical in nature; nevertheless, it does help, indirectly, to relieve such pressure. On the other hand, when the obstruction is paralytic, the tube passes readily through the pylorus. He further states that no drugs should be given to restore peristalsis if water and salt balance are maintained and protein needs fulfilled.

If the gastroenterostomy fails to function and the patient's condition is poor, reoperation, though indicated, could be fatal. In such a case, a jejunostomy may save the patient's life, as it can even be perfomed under local anesthesia. The best location for such a jejunostomy is a few centimeters from the plica duodenojejunalis.

Hernia. Internal herniae of all types can usually be avoided by suturing the edges of any opening in the transverse mesocolon to the stomach or to the jejunum and by seeing that no loop of intestine comes between the duodenojejunal flexure and the anastomosis.

Retrograde Intussusception. This may occur 4 or 5 days after operation. The etiology is obscure. Symptoms are sudden griping pains in the epigastrium with hematemesis. Here, immediate reoperation is imperative.[10]

Separation of the Viscera. This is infrequent when proper care has been used in suturing. Because thick catgut is too heavy for the thin walls of the intestine, and because, at times, fine gut may be absorbed too rapidly, I have come to use cotton, with gratifying results. I still use tanned catgut for suturing the stoma, but, for safety, I prefer cotton for reinforcing the stoma sutures and for serosa-serosa appositions.

"Dumping Syndrome." The so-called dumping stomach usually results from lack of care regarding the size of the anastomotic opening. It should not be any wider than the jejunum at the point of the anastomosis, otherwise too rapid evacuation of the stomach will result.

Length and Disposition of the Jejunal Loop

Much has been said and written regarding the importance of the length and the disposition of the jejunal loop in gastroenterostomy operations. When the loop is to be relatively long, it is considered best that it be arranged in an isoperistaltic position. With a very short loop, on the first portion of the jejunum, an antiperistaltic arrangement is preferable. After experimenting with both, I have found the results to be about the same in either case. More important, apparently, is the length of the loop. A short loop (no more than 8 cm.) or no loop at all is considered by many to be the better choice when performing the von Hacker posterior gastroenterostomy. However, I have found the no-loop method to yield less satisfactory results than use of a loop measuring about 1½ inches from the beginning of the jejunum to the proposed jejunal stoma. In anterior gastrojejunostomy (to which I now resort in the majority of cases), the loop should be of sufficient length to make possible the construction of a jejunojejunostomy. However, here as elsewhere, moderation and common sense must be the guiding principles.

Location of Incision

In order to ensure good function of the neo-pylorus, an oblique or, better yet, a vertical stomach incision appears to be the best choice. Even quite recalcitrant gastric material is efficiently discharged into the efferent tract, and with this type of opening, there is the least chance of setting up the "vicious circle." Experiments appear to show that, so far as drainage is concerned, the anastomosis tends to function best if placed at the incisura angularis, particularly in a stomach of normal size. Locating the orifice as near as possible to the greater curvature also helps to ensure adequate emptying.

The *size* of the opening is also important. It must not exceed that of the jejunal loop, lest evacuation be too rapid, producing the condition commonly called "dumping stomach" (see above).

Strangulation of the small bowel, in posterior gastroenterostomy, may be avoided by suturing the opening in the transverse mesocolon to the peritoneum of either the stomach or the jejunum. Do this after the anastomosis has been completed.

Much might be said regarding *choice of operation*, but it is my feeling that the Stanischeff method (Fig. 250) is the simplest and most effective and has the added virtue of eliminating the disadvantages of those methods which utilize a posterior anastomosis.

A word about postoperative *diet* is appropriate here. Those who have undergone a good gastroenterostomy and "recovered completely" are all too prone to become indiscreet in the matter of food. They feel that they have been on starvation rations long enough! However, they should be made to understand clearly that such indulgence can lead to unhappy complications. The surgeon is doing less than his full duty if he fails to supervise their diet for several months, pointing out to them that both mechanical and chemical changes have been made which require considerable adjustment, mentally as well as physically.

Some specialists feed their gastroenterostomized patients on bland foods almost from the first day, feeling that if the anastomosis has been properly done, the risk that the sutures will give way is negligible. This is a

Fig. 250. Stanischeff's oblique anterior gastroenterostomy. (Thorek, Max: Modern Surgical Technic, Philadelphia, Lippincott)

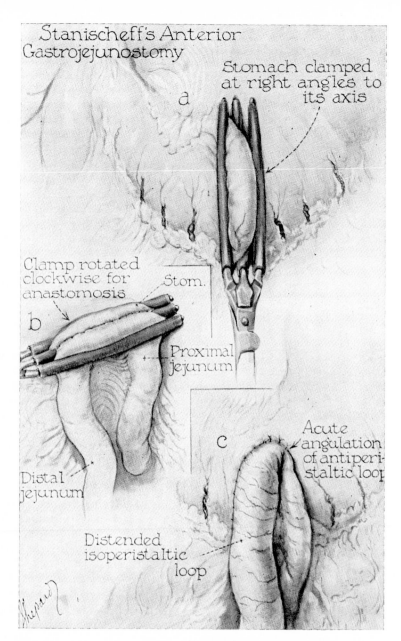

Stanischeff's Anterior Gastrojejunostomy

a — Stomach clamped at right angles to its axis

b — Clamp rotated clockwise for anastomosis — Stom.

Proximal jejunum

c

Acute angulation of antiperistaltic loop

Distal jejunum

Distended isoperistaltic loop

Fig. 250. Stanischeff's oblique anterior gastroenterostomy. (Thorek, Max: Modern Surgical Technic, Philadelphia, Lippincott)

reasonable conclusion, as the patient whose sutures are not milktight and watertight will not live long enough to enjoy much food of any kind. However, I prefer to begin feeding these patients very gradually, with nothing solid for at least a week.

RESECTION FOR ULCER

INDICATIONS

It is my belief that resection of the upper part of the duodenum and the pyloric end of the stomach is the operation of choice in the treatment of peptic ulcer, in spite of the excellent results that, on occasion, may be obtained in cases of obstruction through a good gastroenterostomy. However, there can be situations where, even though resection seems to be indicated, it had better not be undertaken. The decision should depend on the degree of technical experience and the type of assistants and physical equipment available. Where some or all of these conditions are doubtful, the patient's interests may be better served by performing a gastroenterostomy rather than a resection.

Two important points must never be overlooked: (1) the surgeon must not overestimate his own ability, and (2) he must not be too optimistic about the general condition of the patient at the time of operation. His personal skill must be more than equal to the situation, and so must the general physiologic condition of the patient. It must be remembered also that many patients suffering from *duodenal ulcer* may recover under medical management alone. In such cases, there is usually time to operate later on, if need be. In *gastric ulcer*, the opposite is likely to hold—procrastination may be dangerous. Medical care should be given a fair trial, but if a medical regimen fails, operate promptly.

Where controlling conditions *are* favorable, resection is indicated in certain deeply excavated *duodenal* ulcers with considerable hemorrhage, as well as in extensive *gastric* ulcer. Where there are several ulcers, as found in 8 to 25 per cent of cases, excision is usually contraindicated.

EXTENT OF RESECTION

When resection is undertaken, the aim is to remove the ulcerated area *and* to prevent recurrence. Figures show that if enough of the body of the stomach is removed to reduce the acidity by 50 per cent, recurrence will probably be prevented.

Short-circuiting operations of various types only partially control excessive gastric acidity. Therefore, the best procedure seems to be removal of that part of the stomach having the least amount of acid-secreting tissue, namely, the pyloric end, adding only such amount of the body and the fundus as necessary to reduce substantially—but not to eliminate completely—the number of acid-forming cells. This also makes possible, without untoward results, the removal of ulcers which have bled repeatedly, or have closed after perforation, become adherent to adjacent structures or are located at a stoma or in the contiguous areas of the jejunum.

SAFEGUARDS DURING OPERATION

Here, as elsewhere, the primary requisite for success is adequate practical experience derived from experimental work on animals and through assisting other more competent and experienced surgeons. The acquisition of experience through work on animals should also be the rule when a new procedure is to be undertaken. However, it is better to gain a high degree of skill in a single procedure and stick with it than to accept every new idea before it has been proved by the test of time.

The Billroth II operation is safer than the Billroth I (Fig. 251). However, certain precautions apply. During the preliminary steps, care must be taken, when ligating the right gastroepiploic artery, not to injure the middle colic artery. Such injury would probably result in gangrene of the transverse colon. When working on the duodenum, the various possible positions of ducts emptying into it should be kept in mind. I once inadvertently divided an aberrant pancreatic duct, with fatal results. If the common bile duct should be divided accidentally, endeavor to repair it either by end-to-end anastomosis or by implanting it into that portion of the duodenum which will be left intact.

Above all, it is imperative to have a clear view of the whole operative area and never to cut blindly. Aim for perfect hemostasis. Special care is essential when closing the open end of the duodenum; if in doubt, add one or more extra rows of sutures. Leakage often results in fatal peritonitis.

Hemorrhage and some other complications are usually more frequent and severe after *gastric resection* than after *gastroenterostomy*. In resection for *duodenal ulcer*, hemorrhage from the numerous small vessels located near the head of the pancreas is often troublesome. Therefore, complete hemostasis must be the surgeon's first concern.

Gastric Lavage. Large amounts of gastric and duodenal secretions may be lost through use of a nasal gastric tube during or after stomach surgery. Replacement of fluids and electrolytes is essential.

SINGLE-STAGE VS. MULTISTAGE PROCEDURES

While it may be advantageous to complete a complicated procedure during a single session, nevertheless, if the patient's condition is poor, such a major undertaking may cost him his life. Better to perform 2 or even 3 operations at suitable intervals than to have the patient die as a result of too much surgery in one stage.

In some cases of gastric resection, it may be best to perform a gastrojejunal anastomosis, followed later—when safe—by removal of the involved segment of the stomach.

POSTOPERATIVE COMPLICATIONS

Gastric *retention* may be treated by aspiration or, if persistent, by jejunostomy. Even severe *pulmonary conditions* will usually yield to chemotherapy, which should not be discontinued too soon. *Pulmonary embolism* should be treated with sedatives, and oxygen should be administered promptly. *Urinary infections* also are usually amenable to chemotherapy.

Delayed Hemorrhage. Early postoperative hemorrhage is usually attributable to blood which accumulated in the stomach during the operation, or, if profuse, it may be an indica-tion of technical error, such as loosening of ligatures or an ulcer overlooked during the operation.

Hemorrhage appearing later is more difficult to explain. It may be due to intragastric or extragastric factors. Causes within the operative field may be (1) multiple ulcers at different levels of the gastroduodenal tract; (2) an ulcer missed during the operation; (3) peptic ulcer developing after the operation; (4) poor evacuation of the gastric stump, causing venous stasis; (5) gastritis; or (6) duodenojejunitis. Extragastric causes may include (1) uremia; (2) blood dyscrasias; (3) hypertension; (4) intoxication; (5) concurrent infectious disease; (6) cirrhosis; (7) splenomegaly; (8) liver insufficiency; (9) cholecystitis; (10) pancreatitis; (11) diverticulosis; or (12) esophagitis.

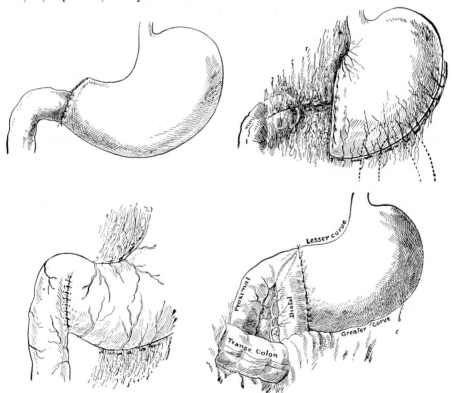

FIG. 251. Representative types of gastric resections. (*Top, left*) Billroth I operation. (*Top, right*) Billroth II operation. (*Bottom, left*) Finney pyloroplasty. (*Bottom, right*) Reichel-Polya procedure.

TREATMENT. Hemorrhage of this type is usually diffuse, without erosion of blood vessels, and does not immediately threaten life. Therefore, medical treatment is indicated until inflammatory processes have subsided. Prophylaxis should include elimination of focal infections, if present, and institution of supportive treatment. After the bleeding has been arrested, choice of surgical treatment depends on the etiologic factors involved. Adhesions should be separated, any eventration corrected and necessary changes or improvements in the anastomosis made. Gastroduodenitis will improve under a regimen of rest with suitable diet and medication.

PYLORIC EXCLUSION

Under some conditions (e.g., excessive crippling by adhesions) it is not wise to resect the first portion of the duodenum, even in cases of long-standing callous duodenal ulcer associated with hyperacidity. These are the cases which do not yield to medical treatment. For these, pyloric exclusion has long been recommended. This procedure includes removal of the pyloric mucous membrane up to the outlet of the stomach, with closure of the pyloric stump, followed by subtotal gastrectomy. This ensures adequate reduction of acidity and should be coupled with an anterior type of anastomosis.

GASTRIC RESECTION

This type of procedure has three objectives: (1) removal of the ulcer and the affected areas around it; (2) permitting alkaline reflux into what remains of the stomach; and (3) removal of part or all of the acid-secreting glands. Gastrectomy at a high level promises the best results and should be undertaken in cases where the risks involved may reasonably be assumed. Some surgeons recommend even so radical a step as *total* gastrectomy for some of these patients, but very recently there has been a trend away from such extreme measures.

INDICATIONS

In the past few years better medical management has served to reduce the number of peptic ulcers coming to operation to about 1 in 10. The other 9 can be expected to progress satisfactorily without surgery. Surgery is definitely indicated when perforation, obstruction or hemorrhage occur, when other symptoms persist under nonsurgical treatment or when there is a possibility of some malignant change in a gastric ulcer. Surgery should also be undertaken when pain persists in spite of a thorough trial of medical management. The threshold for pain varies with individuals; it is governed by the patient's mental reactions and consequent disability. The obligation of the internist is, first, to institute the best possible medical regimen, and, second, if this is less than successful, to discuss frankly with the patient the pros and cons of surgery in his particular case.

Massive Hemorrhage. This is an indication for surgery when (1) the patient is over 50 and has a definite history of peptic ulcer; (2) the condition has not responded to medical treatment; (3) there is no response to transfusion; and (4) there is evidence of continuing or frequently recurring bleeding. Under these conditions, the best plan is to attack the bleeding point directly, performing either a pylorectomy or a transfixion of the base of the ulcer.

Perforation. In dealing with a *perforation*, it should be remembered that this incident, of itself, often has a tendency to promote healing of the ulcer. Delayed surgical intervention in the form of supplementary gastroenterostomy is only a further affront to what the system has already suffered and may simply increase the chance of failure by helping to spread infection in the peritoneal cavity. Recurrence, hemorrhage and stenosis seldom follow a primary perforation. Besides, gastroenterostomy alone does not necessarily relieve symptoms or prevent recurrence. Evaluation of the clinical course is essential.

Careful scrutiny of the literature tends to indicate that *closure alone is the best procedure. In addition, it should be borne in mind that promptness is far more important to success than the type of procedure used.*

PROGNOSIS

The prognosis depends on several factors, of which promptness of intervention is the most decisive. The location of the perforated ulcer is also of some significance, perforated *gastric* ulcer showing a somewhat higher mortality

Fig. 252. Congenital pyloric stenosis.

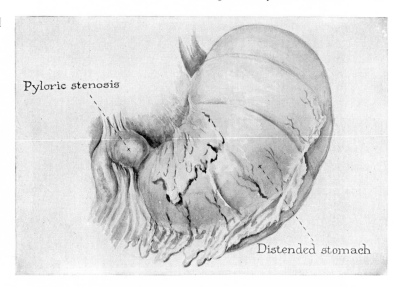

Pyloric stenosis

Distended stomach

rate than perforated *duodenal* ulcer. Finsterer, in a large series, found that 23.8 per cent of deaths from ulcers in these areas involved perforation; about 15 per cent of all deaths were due to hemorrhage. More recent statistics show some improvement over these averages.

Recurrence. For long-range success in these cases, it is important that the patient who has been operated on for a perforated ulcer be kept under medical supervision for an extended period. Symptoms of recurrence should be given prompt attention, yet these may not be recognized as dangerous by the patient himself if left to his own devices.

Safeguards

As soon as it becomes evident that perforation has occurred, operative intervention is urgently indicated. It is far better to open the abdomen and find no perforation than to procrastinate and lose the patient.

A perforation should be *completely* closed and covered with a tag of omentum sutured in place over the site of the perforation.

Atypical Sites. Perforations may occur in regions other than those one would normally expect. Some years ago, I operated on a young man in whom an ulcer was found in a duodenal diverticulum, with penetration into the pancreas (see Fig. 242). Since such diverticuli are usually asymptomatic, it seems reasonable that they might give no indications suggestive of

ulceration until penetration or perforation has taken place.

Penetrating Gastric Ulcer. When the patient is in generally poor condition and a large penetrating ulcer has been diagnosed high on the lesser curvature near the cardia, *gastrojejunostomy* is the procedure of choice. This will usually yield even better results if combined with excision of the ulcer whenever possible.

Wedge Resection. This may be done safely *only* when the ulcer is small and movable. It should never be attempted in large ulcers, inaccessibly located ulcers or in those which have become fixed to some adjacent structure.

Gastrojejunocolic Fistula. This complication calls for extreme care in preoperative medical management. When such precautions are observed, statistics show a sharp decrease in mortality following a 1-stage corrective operation (i.e., dissociation of jejunum from stomach, resection of affected loop of jejunum, end-to-end or side-to-side anastomosis of jejunum and closure of opening in stomach).

CONGENITAL PYLORIC STENOSIS

A condition more likely to be noticed first by the family physician rather than by the specialist is congenital pyloric stenosis in infants (Fig. 252). In order to be successful, treatment of this condition must be prompt and simple, with early diagnosis and a rapid method of surgical correction.

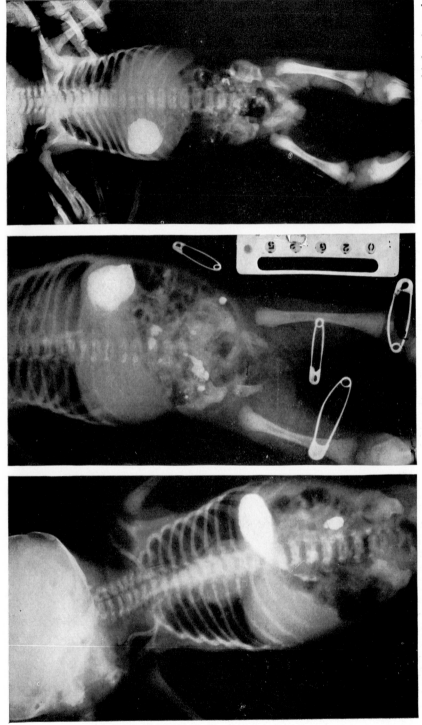

Fig. 253. Case of congenital pyloric stenosis. (*Left*) Fifteen minutes after ingestion of opaque meal. (*Center*) Three hours after ingestion of meal (almost complete retention of meal). (*Right*) Six hours after ingestion of meal (two thirds of meal still retained).

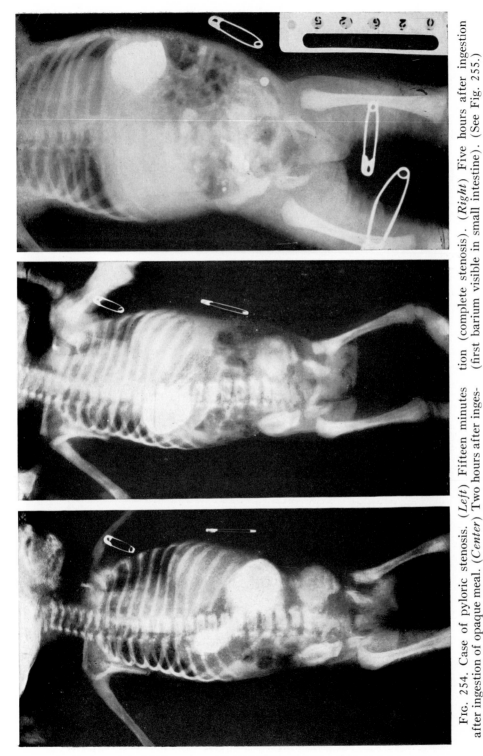

FIG. 254. Case of pyloric stenosis. (*Left*) Fifteen minutes after ingestion of opaque meal. (*Center*) Two hours after inges- tion (complete stenosis). (*Right*) Five hours after ingestion (first barium visible in small intestine). (See Fig. 255.)

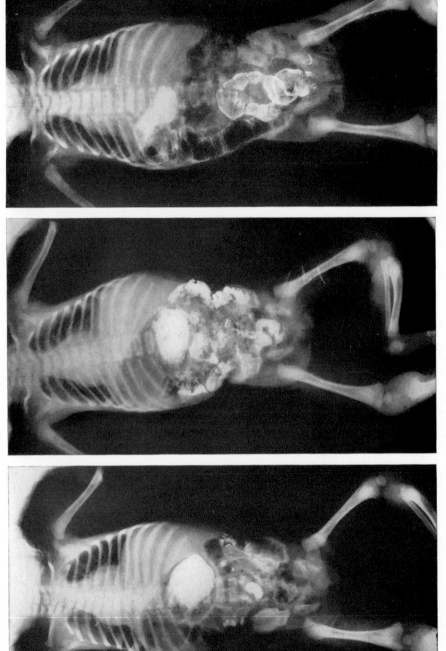

FIG. 255. Same case as Figure 254. (*Left*) Seven hours after ingestion (about two thirds of meal still retained in stomach). (*Center*) Same patient, fourth postoperative day (30 minutes after ingestion of opaque meal). (*Right*) One hour after ingestion of meal (stomach two thirds empty).

ETIOLOGY

The origin of this condition is still moot. It has been variously ascribed to hypertrophy of the pylorus, to congenital malformation, to an inflammatory hyperplasia and to simple pyloric spasm. Strauss believed that it begins prenatally and is brought about by rhythmic contractions of the pylorus due to some abnormal stimulation, in other words, that it is actually only an advanced stage of pylorospasm. There is also some evidence that it may be hereditary. An interesting study made in England and published recently involved 50 follow-ups on patients who had been subjected to surgical correction of pyloric stenosis in early infancy and who now had children of their own. There was a definitely higher incidence of the condition among this new generation than in the population as a whole. The general figure is about 1 in each 400 male births.

DIAGNOSIS

Many experts believe that the presence of a palpable *tumor* in the pyloric area is pathognomonic, being found in all but a very small proportion of proved cases. On the other hand, some say that no tumor is demonstrated at operation in the very instances where it has been most prominent preoperatively, all of which goes to bear out Strauss's contention that pyloric stenosis and pylorospasm are but varying stages of the same condition.

X-ray Examination. The most useful adjunct to the diagnosis of this condition is x-ray examination (Fig. 253), though some believe that the clinical findings alone are all that are needed to decide whether medical methods offer a good chance of success or whether surgery is indicated. The best single index appears to be whether and how much weight is being lost by the infant. The operative mortality among infants who have lost 20 per cent or more of their optimum weight is as much as *6 times greater* than in those who have lost less. Whether a given case will be amenable to medical management or demands surgery may also be judged by the proportion of a bismuth-milk meal passing the pylorus in a given time—say, 4 hours (Figs. 254 and 255).

TREATMENT

Requirements for treatment are relatively

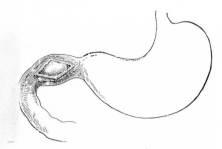

FIG. 256. The Ramstedt operation.

simple. A young infant has little resistance to trauma and shock, yet will soon starve to death if stenosis at the pylorus is not relieved. *Ergo,* the *sine qua non* is a method that will cure the spasm permanently by the fastest effective procedure. If we accept Strauss's view of the etiology of this condition, medical treatment will usually be ruled out. The need for a quick, simple procedure also eliminates such formidable operations as gastroenterostomy and pylorotomy or other pyloroplastic methods. There remains the Ramstedt modification of the operation first performed nearly half a century ago by Fredet, now known as the Fredet-Ramstedt procedure (Fig. 256).

This technic has become so standardized that it need not be described in detail here. However, I would like to call attention to my own modification of the classic operation, which is clearly shown in Figure 257. My method involves not merely the splitting of the pyloric muscularis but also the excision of a wedge lengthwise leaving the serosa and the mucosa untouched and the gap unsutured. In my experience, this has given a somewhat better result and takes little or no more time than the standard technic.

PRECAUTIONS

Because of the frailness of these tiny patients, special care must be taken to keep bleeding at a minimum. Any considerable loss of blood is far more dangerous than for an adult. With regard to anesthesia, it has been found that infants stand ether even better than adults. Add to this the need for having the patient relaxed and quiet, and it will be obvious why local anesthesia should not be used.

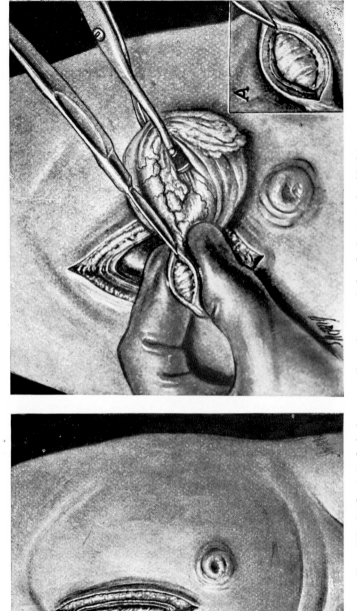

Fig. 257. Author's technic for correction of congenital pyloric stenosis. (*Left*) Incision. (*Right*) Exsection of muscularis (insert shows same in detail).

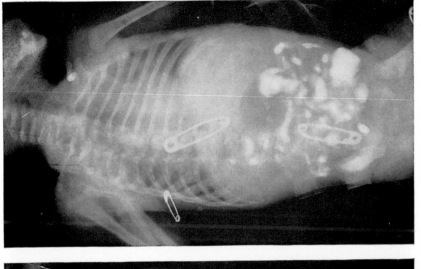

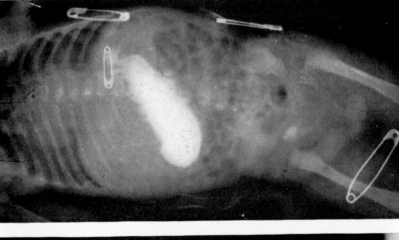

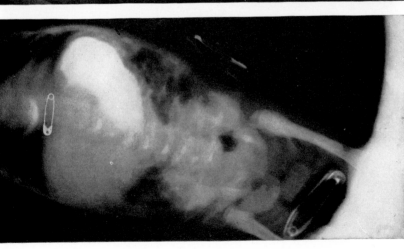

Fig. 258. Roentgenograms taken on third postoperative day.
(*Left*) Immediately after ingestion of opaque meal. (*Center*)
One hour after ingestion (beginning peristalsis). (*Right*) Three
hours after ingestion (stomach completely emptied, normal
peristalsis).

Little attention seems to have been paid in the literature (with the exception cited on page 381 to long-range studies of the results of this operation. In those results that have been published, gastric motility was found to be normal and the end-results good in every case. My own case histories bear this out (Fig. 258).

CARDIOSPASM

The condition most usually known as cardiospasm (i.e., a spasmodic contraction of the cardia) is also designated by a number of other terms, each referring more or less directly to the opinion of some expert or group of experts as to its etiology and exact nature. Plummer thought the name "cardiospasm" confusing, as it apparently has not been established conclusively that spasm of the cardia actually does cause dilatation of the esophagus directly above it.

ETIOLOGY

Some disturbance of the neuromuscular mechanism of the esophagus seems to be the exciting cause of this condition, since there exists no anatomic sphincter at the entrance to the stomach. Because many of these patients are not seen until the condition has reached a terminal stage, it seems somewhat futile to say so, but the best real hope of cure lies in prevention, and with the internist rather than the endoscopist or the surgeon. Eggers suggested that the inflammatory and nutritional causes behind the exciting disturbances, especially a vitamin B_1 deficiency, might be etiologic factors in this connection.

DIAGNOSIS

Esophagoscopy is of considerable value, but for purposes of differentiation between cardiospasm, benign stenosis and carcinoma, the best method is to pass a sound over a previously swallowed silk thread. In the presence of cardiospasm, only slight elastic resistance will be met rather than the definite evidence of stricture present with the other conditions cited.

TREATMENT

Numerous operations for the relief of this condition have been devised. The methods of procedure are divided into (1) conservative and (2) radical. Conservative treatment consists chiefly of gradual dilatations. Radical methods include a variety of surgical operations.

DIET

Long-continued supervision of diet is usually needed. Some patients find that soft foods and bland liquids cause the least trouble. Others incline to an opposite view. In general, in working out a practical regimen, the following suggestions will prove to be helpful: (1) eat slowly; (2) take smaller meals at more frequent intervals; (3) give preference to warm food; (4) use carefully chosen, mild sedatives and antispasmodics. Temporary relief is often obtained by the passage of a tube or a bougie.

DILATATION

Since the methods suggested above tend to treat only the symptoms, eventually most of these patients will come to the endoscopist or the general surgeon. A number of methods of effecting permanent dilatation of the constricted area have been tried. Passing successively larger sounds of sizes ranging from No. 41 F. to No. 60 F. may be effective, or additional stretching with a Russell hydrostatic dilator may be needed. Another method involves a start with a No. 28 F. mercury-filled bougie, one half hour after administration of $1\frac{1}{2}$ gr. Nembutal, and spraying the patient's throat with 2 per cent cocaine. This treatment is followed at intervals of 1 week by the passage of No. 30 and No. 34 bougies, each left in place for up to 5 minutes. These, in turn, may be followed by a Mosher bag pumped up to 4 pounds. However, it must be remembered that some individuals have much genuine difficulty in swallowing the bag; *one should be patient with these!*

Some technicians perform these maneuvers under fluoroscopic guidance. Others prefer to depend on measurements.

VOLVULUS OF THE STOMACH

When faced with an obscure abdominal condition that defies the usual diagnostic methods, volvulus of the stomach should come to mind. This may simulate a number of other more common conditions, notably

FIG. 259. Acute vol-
vulus of stomach (au-
thor's case). Not diag-
nosed preoperatively;
twisted stomach simu-
lated ovarian cyst with
twisted pedicle.

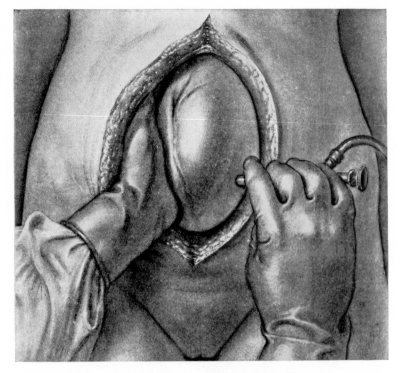

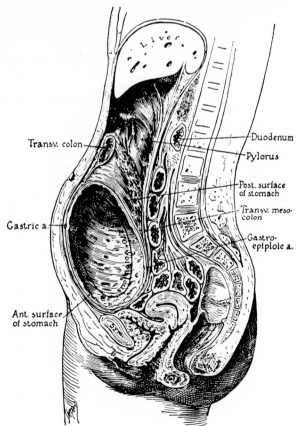

FIG. 260. Same case as Figure 259;
diagram showing degree of torsion
(270°) of stomach; note relative positions of pylorus and cardia.

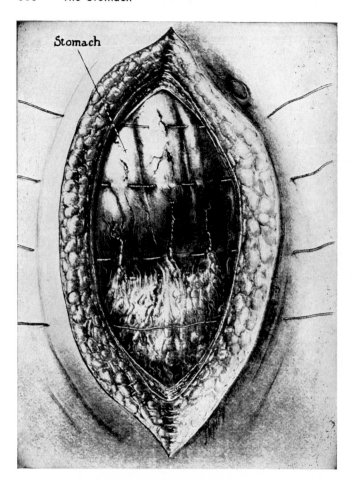

Stomach

FIG. 261. Same case as Figure 259; gastropexy after detorsion. This was followed by complete recovery.

ovarian cyst with twisted pedicle and acute intestinal obstruction. In a case of my own, reported in 1924, in an elderly woman, the stomach was so much twisted, enlarged and displaced that it was mistaken, even during the early part of the operation, for an enormous, twisted ovarian cyst (Fig. 259). Following detorsion and gastropexy, the patient recovered (Figs. 260 and 261). In a similarly exaggerated case, reported in *Science* in 1938, there were 4 inches of stretched and twisted esophagus within the abdomen, and the stomach had become a much distended closed loop. This patient died.

Jenkinson,[3] in discussing the rarity of this condition, cites Gohar's report in 1940 of 75 cases, plus some 25 that have appeared since then in British and American literature, and states that he believes many of these were not true incidents of volvulus as that condi-

tion is defined. His own patient was treated by surgical reduction and gastroenterostomy, which was followed by recurrence but with less severe symptoms. He feels, in retrospect, that gastropexy would have yielded better results.

Weiss[11] has reported what he believed to be a unique case. A newborn infant showed typical symptoms of obstruction, which proved to be due to a congenital torsion of the stomach, caused by bands running from the greater curvature to the gastrohepatic ligament. Weiss did not call this volvulus, although the conditions found were similar and the results the same. All adjacent structures were normal, and dividing the bands gave complete relief.

OCCURRENCE AND TYPES

Volvulus may be *total* or *partial,* the distinction being whether or not the stomach has rotated a full 180° about the cardiopyloric axis. Rotation almost always occurs in an isoperistaltic direction, i.e., from back to front (Fig. 262). In the rare instance where it is antiperistaltic, it is likely to be only partial. According to its evolution, volvulus may be acute or chronic, idiopathic or complex. It is designated as *idiopathic* when there is volvulus alone without apparent coexisting pathologic conditions within the stomach. When associated with ulcer, hernia or other complication, it is more apt to be *partial* only. In practice, all forms may be classified into two main types: (1) total idiopathic and (2) partial subacute or complex.

MECHANISM

Strictly speaking, no volvulus of the stomach can be total, for its attachments by the phrenogastric ligament, the cardia and the pericardial peritoneum do not give way except under extraordinary stress. The pylorus is not so fixed and may allow complete rotation of the organ from below upward. Torsion rarely exceeds 180°. The axis of movement is the

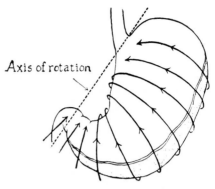

FIG. 262. Volvulus of stomach; diagram showing axis of rotation.

smaller curvature. As rotation progresses, the pylorus moves toward the cardia, causing the lesser curve to become, first a deep V, then a mere sulcus (Fig. 263). In rare cases, the pylorus and the cardia meet, and the organ then twists about them as on a single pivot.

PATHOLOGY

Volvulus is usually only partial, the cardiac

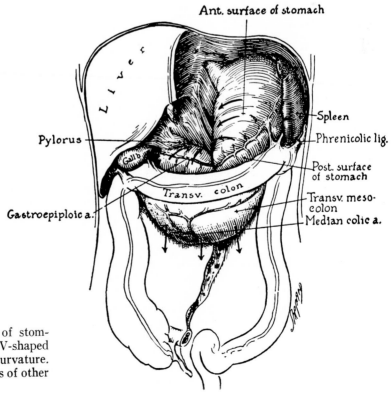

FIG. 263. Volvulus of stomach; diagram shows V-shaped infolding of lesser curvature. (Note relative positions of other viscera.)

end of the stomach remaining in place while the pyloric part rotates. The organ then appears to be in two sections, one upward to the left and vertical, the other lower and horizontal.

In the rare situation of total idiopathic volvulus, when the abdomen is opened, the posterior wall of the stomach will be found presenting, covered by the mesocolon (unless this has already ruptured). Often the organ is hugely distended due to occlusion of the orifices, while adjacent structures are displaced and distorted. The transverse colon may have assumed a position approaching the vertical. Occasionally, the displaced stomach may even herniate through the diaphragm. Also, in the case of a partial volvulus, hernia may take place through some opening in the peritoneum.

Functional Effects. These are definite and self-perpetuating. The esophagus is stretched downward. The obliteration of the stomach orifices not only hinders evacuation but also, due to the characteristic mediogastric "kink" at the junction of the vessels of the lesser curvature, there is a tendency for the formation of isolated cardiac and pyloric sacs.

Dilatation. On the other hand, dilatation has, up to a point, a tendency to reduce the volvulus spontaneously. It is only when this balance is upset and the stomach becomes incarcerated between the anterior wall of the abdomen and the diaphragm that spontaneous reduction is no longer possible.

Evacuation. In volvulus, evacuation of the stomach contents may be hindered not only by external pressure and stricture but also by intrinsic kinks and flexures. Both of these factors increase in importance as the rotation progresses.

Symptoms

In total idiopathic volvulus the symptoms form a characteristic picture. The onset is sudden, the development rapid and the end-result, if unrelieved, quickly fatal. The main symptom triad is (1) acute meteorism, (2) impossibility of passing a stomach tube and (3) signs of ileus. To these might be added (4) a sensation of torsion in the gastric region, (5) a sensation of traction near the heart and (6) displacement of the spleen. When other causes have been ruled out, these signs are valuable aids to the diagnosis of this condition.

It is also true that such symptoms as those more usually associated with intestinal obstruction, i.e., distention, dilatation and congestion, may suggest total idiopathic volvulus.

In partial volvulus, the symptoms are less striking and may be preceded by some digestive disturbance. Occlusion is only partial, and remission of symptoms is frequent.

Differential Diagnosis

Various other conditions first must be ruled out, even if one is definitely thinking of volvulus. The situation is so rare that few physicians ever see it at all. For this reason, as well as others, it has been confounded with most of the more common abdominal lesions—intestinal ileus, pancreatitis, perforative peritonitis. The sudden, extreme meteorism of volvulus will serve to distinguish it from other stomach conditions, as will the presence of a large, tympanitic tumor in the gastric region and a change in the fluid level when the patient shifts his position.

Treatment

In this condition treatment must be surgical. Correct appraisal of the situation, whether before surgery or after the abdomen has been opened, is essential to saving the patient's life. When volvulus is recognized promptly, complete relief may be secured by evacuation of the stomach contents, followed by detorsion and fixation of the organ.

The condition of the patient at the time of surgery, together with any coexisting lesions, must determine the operative steps to be taken. The volvulus can properly be considered as being fully corrected only when the ramifications of the coronary arteries of the stomach have been restored to their normal anatomic positions. Subsequent, complementary procedures may be a gastropexy to fix the organ in good position or, if there is associated stenosis, a gastroenterostomy or a jejunostomy. Here, as in so many other situations, the simpler the procedure, the better.

Prognosis

Where correct diagnosis and prompt treatment have followed the development of volvulus, even in the total form, the prognosis appears to be relatively favorable. In cases of partial volvulus, the percentage of recoveries is very high.

FOREIGN BODIES IN THE STOMACH

Foreign bodies in the stomach present several chances for errors in diagnosis. These arise both from the nature of the objects themselves and from the character and the intentions of the patient. Children swallow all sorts of things, some of which, such as glass marbles, are only slightly radiopaque. The insane compound the trouble by attempts at concealment. So also, on occasion, do "professional" swallowers (Figs. 264 and 265). Add to all this the wonderful powers of the stomach to accept a wide variety of foreign objects and substances and still to continue to function at near normal levels over varying periods of time, and it will be seen that chances for mistaken diagnoses are numerous indeed!

Trichobezoars and Phytobezoars

In addition to the numerous foreign objects introduced, concretions that form within the stomach present further problems. Persimmon seeds, in geographic areas where this fruit is plentiful, may undergo certain chemical changes which cause them to build up into phytobezoars sometimes of astonishing size (Fig. 266). The largest on record weighed 6½ pounds! Persian cats have no monopoly on hairballs (trichobezoars); children[6] and

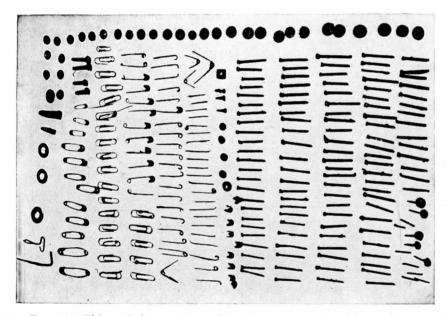

Fig. 264. This varied assortment of hardware was removed from the stomach of a single "professional swallower" at one operation (one eighth actual size). (See Fig. 265.)

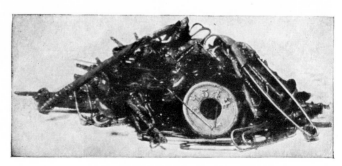

Fig. 265. Same case as in Figure 264. Objects clustered to give an idea of the amount of space they took up in the patient's stomach. Note ordinary paper clip, lower right, for scale.

the mentally deranged occasionally also fill their stomachs with hair (Fig. 267), sometimes to an extent that produces severe symptoms of malnutrition with all its attendant sequelae.

SYMPTOMS

The symptoms are similar to those of acute gastritis: pain, emesis, diarrhea, foul breath, offensive stools and, eventually, emaciation.

DIAGNOSIS

Great care in history taking and accurate use and evaluation of x-ray examination are the chief elements on which diagnosis rests (Fig. 268). Questioning should include not only the patient himself—or his parents, in the case of a young child—but also anyone else who may be familiar with his personal habits, especially if he is known or suspected to be mentally unbalanced.

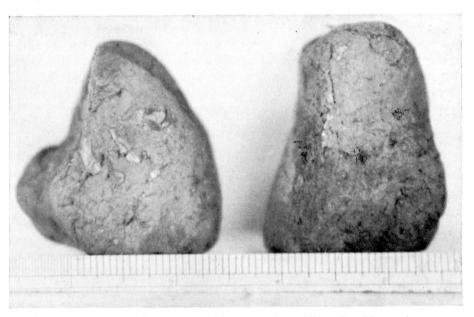

FIG. 266. Phytobezoars found in stomach. (Philip Thorek's case)

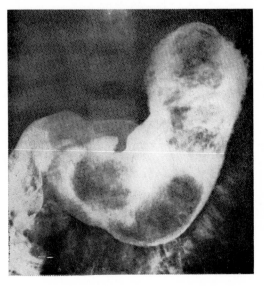

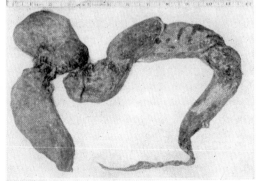

FIG. 267. Trichobezoar (hairball) reported from England. (*Left*) Five hours after a barium meal. (*Right*) The mass removed at the operation. (Morris, H.: Brit. J. Radiol. 25:672)

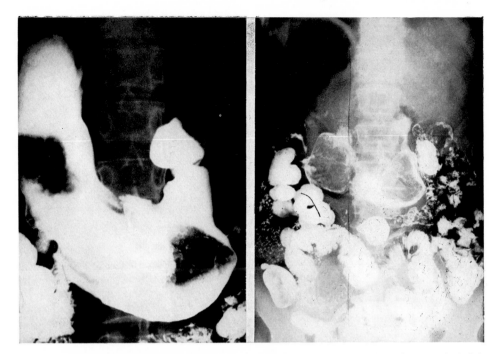

FIG. 268. Phytobezoars in stomach. (*Left*) Bezoars diagnosed as carcinoma. (*Right*) Outline of bezoars easily seen in empty stomach.

Several special procedures in the use of roentgenography for the location of foreign bodies have been developed recently. One of these[7] is deceptively simple but appears to give excellent results, namely, the use of a carbonated soft drink as a contrast medium. As described, this procedure has several advantages. It will reveal such translucent materials as glass and china, by the filling of the stomach with gas, and will be taken readily by those, especially children, who may refuse barium and the like. To be effective, the drink must be given *very cold*, so that the dissolved gas will be released slowly enough in the stomach to avoid eruction. The amount should be limited to 1 ounce for an adult and to no more than a couple of "swallows" for a small child. More will dilate the stomach so much that the value of the test is lost. Also, it is of little use if the patient has recently eaten a heavy meal.

The soft-drink method is especially useful where the presence of a foreign body has already been demonstrated by conventional x-ray methods but its location is uncertain,

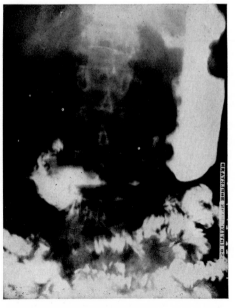

FIG. 269. Showing case in which carcinoma has attacked both cardiac and pyloric ends of stomach.

i.e., whether it is still in the stomach or has moved farther along the digestive canal.

CARCINOMA OF THE STOMACH

ETIOLOGY

Like all other neoplasms, those originating in the stomach are still largely of unknown origin. However, some facts are known, and the accusing finger points definitely in certain directions.

DIAGNOSIS

Templeton[9] makes a number of points that are sometimes missed regarding the differential diagnosis of stomach cancers. He stresses particularly that the primary function of the radiologist is to discover the presence of the lesion (Fig. 269); other, surer methods may then be employed in differential diagnosis. He observed that a "hindsight review" of a series of proved gastric cancers shows some identifiable signs in early roentgenograms on which the findings had been reported as "normal" less than 1 year previously. Character and growth of the tumor cannot be blamed for such errors. Divided attention (e.g., looking at an ulcer) seems to be a likelier cause. This might best be overcome by combining a spot-filming technic with fluoroscopy. Experience and excellence of technic are more valuable than improved mechanical aids, and it is no disgrace to admit to the patient that clear indications were not obtained in the first examination—if such be the case—and that repeated studies are necessary.

Here, as elsewhere, early recognition is of prime importance. Since fully one third of all malignancies are located in the gastric region, and in view of the frequently great difficulty in diagnosing this particular type of growth, the surgeon is confronted with a complex of questions, upon the correct answers to which rest all chances of success. First, it must be definitely determined whether the symptoms are caused by malignancy or by some benign lesion; also, if benign at the moment, whether or not the lesion may later become malignant. What and how many diagnostic procedures are called for to give accurate information in the particular case at hand? How far should medical methods be carried before resorting to surgery? If surgery is indicated, what procedure is to be used? These are but a few of the points that must be decided.

If one seeks inspiration from the current literature, he is confronted with an embarrassment of riches. Unlike many commonly encountered medical problems, which by their very frequency discourage further publication, stomach carcinoma continues to call forth a veritable stream of written observations and opinions, leading the reader to the inevitable conclusion that none of the methods proposed is entirely satisfactory or successful.

DIFFERENTIAL DIAGNOSIS

The first step in differential diagnosis is to determine whether one is confronted with an ulcer or a carcinoma (see also p. 394). If a tentative diagnosis of ulcer is made, then it must be decided whether there is a possibility of cancer developing later, or even of carcinoma actually being in the process of developing, superimposed upon the ulcer. Of primary significance here, in evaluating the roentgenograms, is the evolution of the characteristic "niche" while the patient is under active treatment. Other criteria are (1) localization, (2) size (of minor importance in the early stages), (3) form of the "niche," (4) irregularities of the contour and the surface of the "niche" and (5) condition of adjacent tissues.

Nearly 20 years ago, Gutmann described 3 forms of gastric carcinoma that could be differentiated roentgenographically: (1) the *infiltrating* form, of which the chief sign is rigidity of the stomach wall, which may assume a variety of forms and, at first, may cause functional "pseudo-defects"; (2) the *vegetating* form, of which the principal sign is a filling defect; and (3) the *ulcerating* form, mentioned above. Next to history taking and the finding of blood in the stool, the x-ray study is still our most valuable diagnostic aid. Though more conclusive in the later stages of the disease, even in its incipience—as described above—it still forms our most reliable guide. By the time a carcinoma begins to give any clinical symptoms, it can also be demonstrated radiologically to the trained and observant eye. However, it is most unwise to expect roentgenograms *alone* to be conclusive; without corroborative evidence from other diagnostic procedures, entirely wrong conclusions may be drawn, and operation undertaken where it is unnecessary, or the reverse!

A special x-ray technic is that known as the "relief method." In principle, this depends on administering an opaque medium in small quantities, thereby permitting only the spaces between the rugae to be filled and, at the same time, applying compression by some means (Fig. 270). Thus we are enabled to study the behavior of the mucous folds with respect to their secretion, movement, consistency, coordination and continuity, as is not possible with full intake of an opaque meal. A much more detailed picture of conditions is thus obtained.

Newest of the weapons at our command are those chemical and microscopic tests introduced within the past few years—the outgrowth of work done under the stress of World War II and part of the benefits derived from it—which give promise of becoming the best and most conclusive yet devised. However, it is too soon to take them at face value. We can only wait on the outcome of continuing experiment and observation, and hope and pray that we are actually on the threshold, so long sought for, of the discovery of the *cause* of cancer, followed, as it must be, by development of positive methods of cure.

Gastroscopy. In experienced hands, gastroscopy may be used, especially in early diagnosis, without danger and with only slight discomfort for the patient. In spite of its drawbacks (e.g., inability to observe certain areas or likelihood of failing to recognize small, early lesions), it is a valuable adjunct to x-ray examination, particularly where roentgenographic interpretation is doubtful or inconclusive. In differential diagnosis between a callous ulcer and a carcinoma, gastroscopy may even be superior to direct examination of a resected specimen precisely because it is performed on living tissues rather than on those the appearance of which has changed because of the cessation of the blood supply. It is also superior in some instances to roentgenography in distinguishing among different gross pathologic types of tumors, making it possible to select those of varying degrees of malignancy and operability. However, in this connection, it must be borne in mind that the

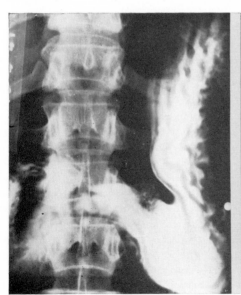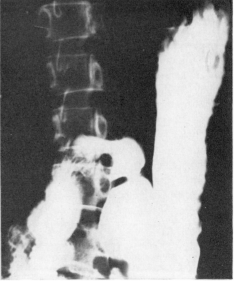

FIG. 270. Roentgenogram of normal stomach. (*Left*) Immediately after one swallow of opaque meal; relief of rugal folds easily seen; course and width of folds give useful information in differential diagnosis of gastritis, peptic ulcer and carcinoma. (*Right*) After full opaque meal, both curvatures are outlined, but no further information on condition of mucous membrane is given.

appearance, the evolution and the frequency of gastric lesions vary according to the site of the growths.

Gastrophotography. Like gastroscopy, gastrophotography is most valuable as an aid to interpretation of x-ray findings. Though by no means conclusive, due to wide possible margins for error, it does furnish useful additional observations, plus a permanent record for later evaluation and study. Like gastroscopy, it is subject to failure when the growth is close to the cardia or is hidden by a peristaltic wave. Conversely, in a photograph, a noncancerous gastric lesion may be mistaken for malignancy.

To summarize, x-ray examination, supplemented by other methods as indicated in each individual case, gives us our best present means of discovering gastric cancer. However, we are still handicapped by the fact that these particular lesions in their early stages give few characteristic signs and may easily be mistaken for ulcers and other nonmalignant conditions. Even exploratory laparotomy may fail to reveal an incipient carcinoma, especially when an ulcer is already present. Knowing this, *it is wise to consider as malignant any suspicious gastric lesion which shows persistently suggestive roentgenographic and clinical symptoms.*

PRECANCEROUS CONDITIONS

For many years there has been wide divergence of opinion as to the relation between ulcer and mucous polyp on the one hand and malignancy on the other. Some experts are of the opinion that any ulcer should be treated as though it might become malignant; they advise resection as a preventive and claim that they could save 90 per cent of their patients by so doing. Others take an exactly opposite view, claiming that no more than 5 per cent of patients with benign ulcer will ever develop gastric carcinoma. The truth probably lies somewhere between, as is so often the case with widely divergent beliefs. Certainly the presence of an ulcer is no guarantee against carcinoma.

It is more important that the general practitioner, who is not likely to be in a position to recognize gastric cancer in its early stages, should be strongly urged to send any patient over 35 who shows persistent gastric symptoms (beyond 2 or 3 weeks' duration) to an expert diagnostician for all indicated examinations. Likewise, the patient with any of those conditions which our present knowledge indicates may predispose to cancer should be given prophylactic treatment to allay gastritis or other chronic or inflammatory lesions—no matter how trivial they may appear—thereby reducing the number of those likely to develop carcinoma. Even changes in diet and dietary habits may lessen the chances of developing cancer. Gastric irritation may result from consumption of such common foods as rye bread and spices, from eating things too hot and, obviously, from excessive use of alcohol and cigarettes or chewing tobacco.

Early Diagnostic Criteria. Where no tumor is palpable, early diagnostic criteria are thought to include:

1. Achylia gastrica of short duration, with appearance of blood in the washings from the fasting stomach

2. In patients with a long history of peptic ulcer and hyperchlorhydria, a combination of pain, low HCl in gastric contents and the presence of occult blood and Oppler-Boas bacilli

3. In patients with no gallbladder lesion, cardiospasm of brief duration.

PROGNOSIS

Klass[5] points out that, of late years, one seemingly contradictory fact has become clear: the longer the history of cancerous symptoms, the better, relatively speaking, the prognosis. In other words, slow-growing lesions constitute a less immediate threat to life and permit of more hopeful treatment than those whose rapid development is usually associated with wide involvement of adjacent organs, as well as extensive and often distant metastases.

With the improved diagnostic methods and more radical operations that have been developed within the past decade, we are now able to give somewhat more hope to victims of gastric cancer. We have learned that even a palpable tumor does not always indicate that the lesion is inoperable. We have found that resection can be done at a higher level than was dared even 10 years ago. Yet, with all these improvements, we are still faced with a

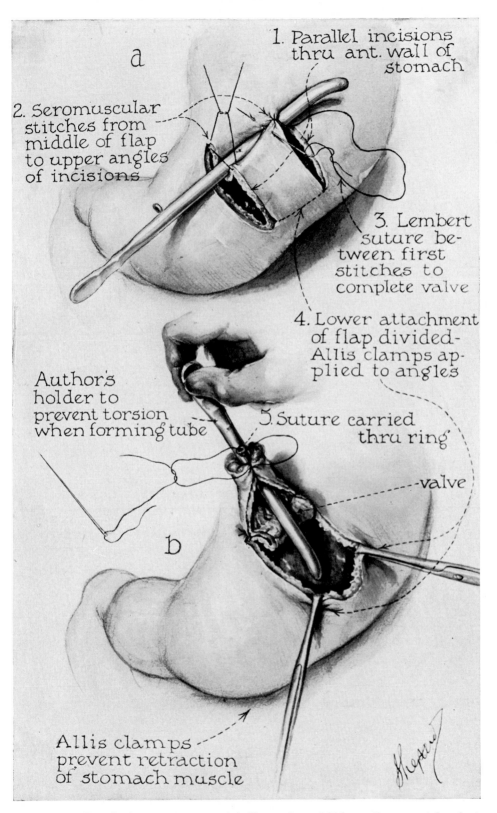

a

1. Parallel incisions thru ant. wall of stomach

2. Seromuscular stitches from middle of flap to upper angles of incisions

3. Lembert suture between first stitches to complete valve

4. Lower attachment of flap divided— Allis clamps applied to angles

Author's holder to prevent torsion when forming tube

5. Suture carried thru ring

valve

b

Allis clamps prevent retraction of stomach muscle

Fig. 271. Tubovalvular gastrostomy. (a) Formation of Dépage-Janeway tube, first stage. (b) Same, second stage.

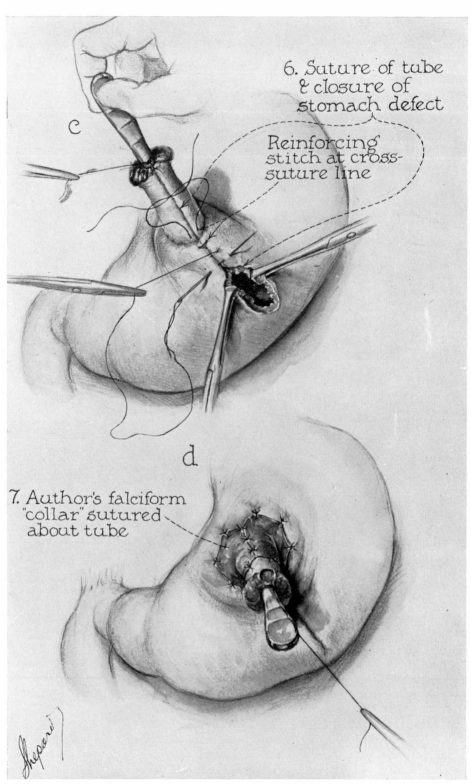

6. Suture of tube & closure of stomach defect

Reinforcing stitch at cross-suture line

c

d

7. Author's falciform "collar" sutured about tube

Fig. 271 (*Cont.*). (c) Dépage-Janeway tube completed; closing stomach wall. (d) Reinforcing a vulnerable point (author's method).

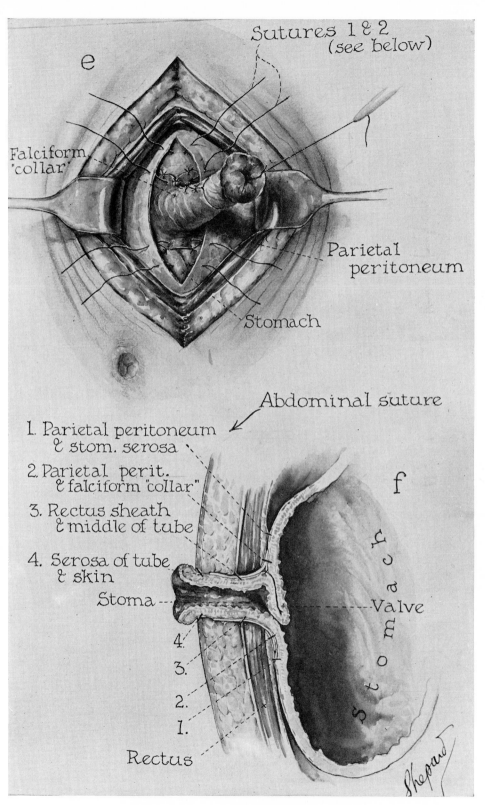

e

Sutures 1 & 2
(see below)

Falciform
"collar"

Parietal
peritoneum

Stomach

Abdominal suture

1. Parietal peritoneum
   & stom. serosa

2. Parietal perit.
   & falciform "collar"

3. Rectus sheath
   & middle of tube

4. Serosa of tube
   & skin

Stoma

f

Stomach

Valve

4.

3.

2.

1.

Rectus

FIG. 271 (*Cont.*). (e) Method of implanting newly formed tube into abdominal wall, with suture to superimposed structures.

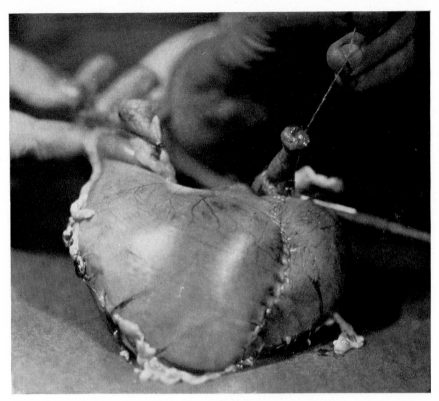

FIG. 272. Tubovalvular gastrostomy (experimental specimen); note tube made from anterior stomach wall.

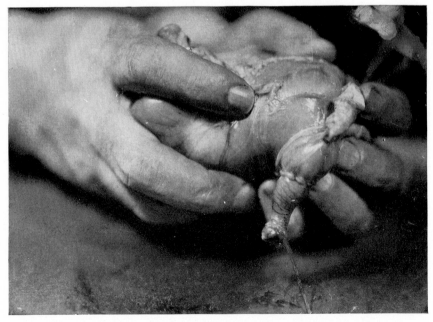

FIG. 273. Same case as Figure 272. Even when filled with water and subjected to marked manual compression, there is no escape of fluid, proving water tightness.

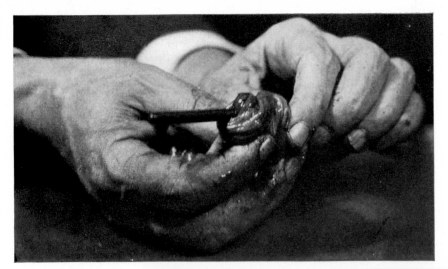

FIG. 274. (*Top*) Same case as Figures 272 and 273, showing construction of valve. Catheter passes through opening.

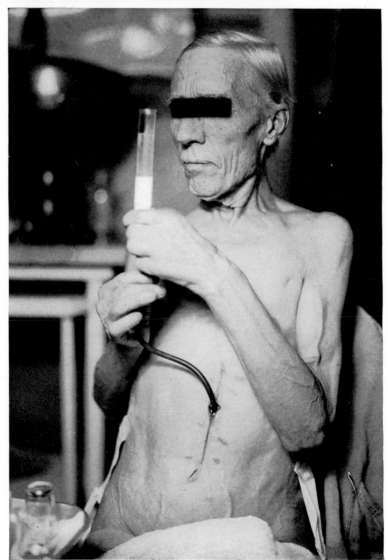

FIG. 275. (*Right*) Tubovalvular gastrostomy in use. This patient suffered from obstructive carcinoma of the esophagus. Gastrostomy was put into use 4 days after it was made.

discouragingly small percentage of 5-year survivals. In spite of all the efforts that have been made to educate the public, all too many cancer patients are still being seen for the first time too late to permit of anything more than palliative treatment and the prolonging of life by a tragic few months at most. This is particularly true in the field of gastric surgery, for reasons indicated in the preceding paragraphs.

In discussing the future with the gastric cancer patient and his family, it should be made quite clear that (1) unless he undergoes surgery, the surgeon will not be responsible for the consequences; (2) gastroenterostomy will prolong his life for a limited time; and (3) gastrectomy, radical though it appears to the layman, and for all its inescapable limitations and drawbacks, is still his best hope, giving promise of additional years of fairly comfortable, even useful life.

Surgical Treatment

Partial Gastrectomy. We now know that gastrectomy gives greater life expectancy in cases of gastric cancer than any of the formerly preferred palliative "short-circuiting" procedures. It stands to reason that radical removal of the growth should improve the patient's general condition and may even lead to complete recovery in some instances. Wider resections are being done today than ever before, with satisfactory results, and in the hands of a skilled surgeon, these may be submitted to with reasonable confidence. Simon[8] suggests performing a supplementary enteroanastomosis as a routine following gastric resection, claiming that this eliminates possible stagnation in the duodenal stump.

For satisfactory results, even the most skilled and experienced surgeon must keep certain points clearly in mind when performing operations of this type. Ligation of the left gastric artery is difficult and, in careless hands, dangerous; ligatures are apt to slip, and the resulting hemorrhage can be extremely hard to control. When incising the omentum close to the liver, extreme care should be exercised to avoid injury to the common bile duct. Also, be very sure to identify and avoid the middle colic artery; if it is ligated accidentally, gangrene of the transverse colon may result. *Never undertake any of these procedures without a complete and detailed knowledge of the anatomy of the area, especially its blood supply.*

Gastrostomy. Where limited experience on the part of the surgeon or some other consideration forbids resort to gastrectomy for the relief of gastric carcinoma, the much older procedure of gastrostomy may be undertaken. This has been practiced in various modifications since before the days of asepsis, but real success has come only in recent years with the introduction of the tubovalvular technic (of disputed origin) (Figs. 271-274): even now it is subject to some complications and, at best, is only palliative. Further, since the tubovalvular gastrostomy requires a higher degree of skill and experience than simpler methods of gastrostomy, in the hands of those not so skilled, the latter will better serve the interests of the patient.

Indications for gastrostomy are (1) for feeding the patient when there is some constriction or obstruction of the esophagus (Fig. 275), and (2) for such therapeutic purposes as dilatation of the cardia.

REFERENCES

1. Aird, I.: Management of acute intestinal obstruction *in* Techniques in British Surgery, p. 308, Philadelphia, Saunders, 1950.
2. Brown, C. H., Kane, C. F., and Harrington, V. A.: Changes in surgery for carcinoma, Cleveland Clin. Quart. **20**:276, 1953.
3. Jenkinson, D. L., and Bate, L. C.: Volvulus of the stomach; report of a case, Am. J. Roentgenol. **69**:54, 1953.
4. Johnson, A. H., McCorkle, H. J., and Harper, H. A.: Problem of nutrition following total gastrectomy, Gastroenterology **28**:360, 1955.
5. Klass, A. A.: Carcinoma of the stomach; the case for total gastrectomy, Canad. M.A.J. **68**:350, 1953.
6. Morris, H.: Unusual trichobezoar; case report, Brit. J. Radiol. **25**:672, 1952.
7. Roberts, W. E.: Carbonated soft drinks in roentgen diagnosis of foreign bodies in the stomach, Am. J. Roentgenol. **71**:239, 1954.
8. Simon, M. M.: Enteroenterostomy; a useful

but neglected procedure in gastric resection, J. Internat. Coll. Surgeons **24**:28, 1955.

9. Templeton, F. E.: Errors in diagnosis of gastric carcinoma, Gastroenterology **28**:378, 1955.

10. Thorek, M.: Modern Surgical Technic, ed. 2, Philadelphia, Lippincott, 1949.

11. Wiess, F., and Dwyer, J. C.: Torsion of the stomach in the newborn; report of a case, J. Internat. Coll. Surgeons **23**:89, 1952.

17   The Intestines

GENERAL CONSIDERATIONS

ANATOMY

A thorough knowledge of anatomy is, quite obviously, the first requisite for any surgeon; possibly it is more important to the abdominal surgeon than to any other. This specialist must be completely familiar with, first, the normal anatomy of the intestinal tract, especially the vascular and the nervous elements (including the intricacies of their branches and connections), and, second, with all the usual anatomic anomalies (Figs. 276 and 277). Time spent intermittently reviewing a standard textbook of anatomy is never wasted; no matter how busy the surgeon may be, he will find that he can sometimes forget even the truisms that he learned in medical school!

OPERATIVE PRECAUTIONS

Filled loops of bowel may present an operative hazard; if at all possible, the intestinal contents should be evacuated before any surgical procedure. When this is not possible, the portion to be worked on should be emptied by gentle digital manipulation.

Distention. The difficulties of any operation on the intestines are greatly increased by distention. Various methods of deflating the bowel are familiar.

When returning the loops to the abdominal cavity, avoid all rough handling; cover with gauze strips, as described on page 351 (Chap. 14, Abdomen in General).

Exteriorization. The loop of bowel to be operated on should first be drawn out of the wound and isolated. This avoids the danger of spilling the contents and contaminating the peritoneal cavity.

Clamps. Avoid tight clamping of the bowel; undue pressure may cause mucosal ulceration. When a clamp must be used, a flexible type is least dangerous, even when the bowel is distended.

Sutures. The chief danger directly connected with suturing the bowel is peritoneal infection due to leakage. This may follow faulty or inadequate closure, with resultant opening of the suture line. Leakage is more apt to occur following end-to-end anastomosis than after lateral joinings, especially if there has been some error in suturing technic.

When suturing a damaged portion of the bowel, be sure to place all sutures in healthy tissue capable of resisting intrinsic pressure and infection.

An intestinal anastomosis demands perfect technic; any fault may cost the patient his life. One should be scrupulous in approximating the apposing structures in placing of sutures and in hemostasis. All blood vessels of any size must be carefully ligated.

Micro-organisms find a favorable medium in cut and sutured surfaces, especially if stagnant blood is present. As suturing progresses, keep a constant watch for bleeding points. From the point of view of infection, a circular suture is more dangerous in the large bowel than in the small intestine, due to the more septic contents. Lateral anastomosis in either site is a procedure gaining in favor, especially when the parts to be joined are of different caliber. Where a lateral joining is to be used, the incision in the bowel should be from 2 to 2½ inches long to allow for possible contraction in healing. Each cut end should then be closed with reinforced circular sutures, after inverting it into its lumen. Patients requiring intestinal resection and anastomosis frequently are extremely ill and in poor condition. They would be unable to withstand the long operation that is necessary when doing the ideally exact suturing called for by fine technic. Speed may outweigh all other considerations. To meet such a demand, a number of methods have been devised for obtaining mechanical continuity of the intestine, as well as for support of the structures during suture.

Some of these have been in use for a great many years (the Murphy button or some similar device). Their advantages include ease and speed of application, minimum manipulation of parts, being watertight and gastight, etc. Dangers inherent to their use are pressure necrosis, obstruction, extravasation following slough and failure to be eliminated promptly.

However, the surgeon's own experience is better than any set rule. He should use those methods and materials that have proved to be most satisfactory in his own hands, even though they may seem unconventional by usual standards. For example, I have found

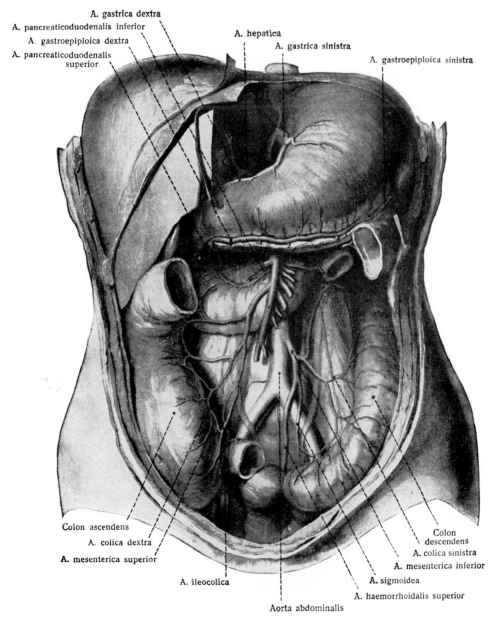

FIG. 276. Arteries of the abdominal viscera, superficial layer, front view. (After Spalteholz)

cotton, in suitable sizes, to be the most generally dependable suture material. Others rely on Nylon, stainless steel or other material; experience is the best guide. The same is true of methods.

The *mesentery,* where breached, must be carefully closed to avoid the possibility of a loop of bowel slipping through the opening and becoming strangulated. Most important is meticulous care for its connection with the intestine; detachment of the mesentery may cut off nutrition of the bowel, causing necrosis.

Similarly, *peritonealization* of all sutured surfaces must be carried out painstakingly. This applies especially to the site from which any segment of intestine has been removed.

The *ureters* must be carefully guarded from injury when doing resection in the vicinity of the cecum, the ascending and the descending colon and on both sides in abdominoperineal resection. One should be especially careful to identify these structures before cutting or ligating *any* tissues in the area.

DRAINAGE

Modern practice leans to the belief that drains can be effective for only a few hours postoperatively at most. In my own practice, I do not use drainage as routinely as I once did; however, I still believe that in cases where it is definitely indicated, it should by no means be skimped or omitted. Also, drains of whatever type should not be removed too early but should be shortened daily to prevent damage from the development of adhesions. Final removal should be done gradually and with the utmost gentleness.

ANTIBIOTICS AND CHEMOTHERAPY

Since the appearance of the fourth edition of this text, medicine and surgery have almost literally been turned upside down by the in-

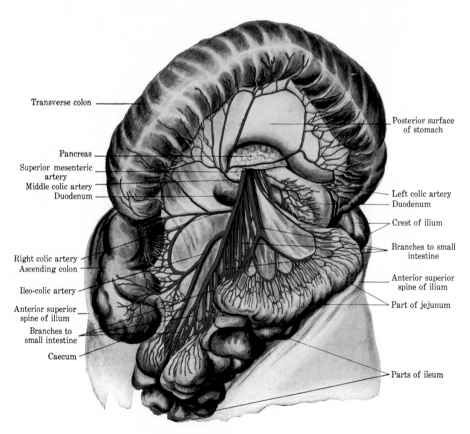

FIG. 277. Superior mesenteric artery and its branches; transverse colon and stomach have been turned upward. (After Piersol)

troduction and the development of the "wonder drugs."[?] The laity as well as the medical profession are constantly dazzled by the crescendo of claims for the ever-increasing efficacy of these medicaments. Truly, they *have* done wonders; there is hardly a corner of the realm of healing that has not felt their impact. Yet, for this very reason, I feel that we *must* "make haste slowly." Unjustified and untested claims have been made for many of them, and, as pointed out by Till,[24] "the subject is complicated by the frequent production of new preparations which are extolled before the proper clinical use of the last has been evaluated." He also cautions that intraperitoneal sulfonamides sometimes are not well absorbed by inflamed tissues, that they are inactive in the presence of pus, that the less soluble forms may cake, thereby acting as foreign bodies and promoting adhesions, and that, occasionally, they may actually introduce concurrent infection if they themselves have not been well sterilized.

However, in spite of their drawbacks, if properly used, these drugs can reduce dramatically the mortality from postoperative as well as primary infection in the abdominal cavity. In one series, a reduction in mortality of general peritonitis and peritoneal contamination was reported from 55.5 per cent to 8.3 per cent!

With the advent of the antibiotics, the limelight swung somewhat away from the sulfa drugs. *B. coli,* the most commonly present organism in general peritonitis, can destroy penicillin, but, in the massive doses usually used, it can still act as a bacteriostat for this bacillus. Streptomycin has a wider bacterial spectrum and is likely to prove to be more effective. The value of terramycin, Achromycin and neomysin are lauded presently.

INTESTINAL OBSTRUCTION

ETIOLOGY

No complication that the surgeon is called on to cope with is more dangerous and few are more frequent than intestinal obstruction. The sources of this condition are well known (see section on Ileus). However, some points will bear further elucidation here.

Broadly speaking, obstructions may be classified as follows:

1. Organic or mechanical
2. Functional or spastic
3. Reflex

Organic Obstruction. If there is a history of previous abdominal surgery, organic obstruction may be suspected. In such case, it may result from adhesions, volvulus or intestinal kinks, or it may result from an intussusception or the strangulation of a hernia (internal, external or diaphragmatic) or cholelithiasis.

Functional Obstruction. This will yield to administration of atropine (see section on Ileus). X-ray studies are valuable, especially in chronic cases. Rodney Smith[22] believes that "the so-called paralytic ileus of general peritonitis is seldom truly paralytic, for the obstruction is organic, at least in part; multiple sites of adhesion, edema, and kinking providing a mechanical element." He also states that a "true paralytic ileus without peritonitis is rare, but may be neurogenic in origin, caused by multiple fractures or any severe trauma, for instance, or by painful renal conditions or . . . certain toxic states, such as pneumonia or uremia."

Reflex Obstructions. These may result from renal colic, tabes or hysteria. In obscure cases, these possibilities must not be forgotten.

Maingot[11] uses a somewhat different classification from that cited above. He divides obstructions, first, into two main types, i.e., mechanical and paralytic, then, from the standpoint of causative factors, as (1) mechanical, (2) nervous and (3) vascular. He quotes Wangensteen (1949) to the effect that "a satisfactory classification for both clinician and pathologist can be made only by correlating in the more common types of obstruction, the factors of causation and pathological appearances." He also observes that obstruction of the small bowel is *5 times as common* as that of the large bowel and notes that "postoperative adhesions have now ousted strangulated hernia as the chief cause of small-gut obstructions."

DIAGNOSIS

Prompt and accurate diagnosis is of the utmost importance. The earlier the situation is fully appraised, the better the patient's chances for recovery.

Abdominal auscultation yields much infor-

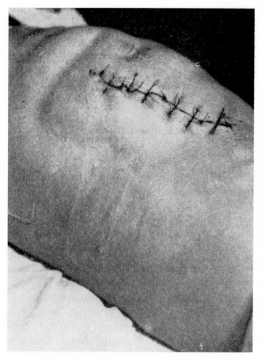

FIG. 278. Intestinal obstruction. Note distended intestinal coils.

mation to the trained ear. This can be especially valuable in *differential diagnosis*. Abdominal sounds fall into three distinct groups: (1) diminished, (2) augmented and (3) abnormal.

1. The "silent abdomen," indicating complete intestinal paralysis, results more or less promptly in perforated peptic ulcer, diffuse appendiceal peritonitis, penetrating wounds, acute pancreatitis and acute effusions of blood, bile or urine. Incomplete paralysis, producing a quiet but not completely "silent" condition, follows some forms of peritonitis (such as Neisserian infection), acute appendicitis without perforation, ruptured ectopic pregnancy, bleeding corpus hemorrhagicum or corpus luteum and hemorrhage (without peritonitis) from other causes.

2. Increased peristaltic sounds are heard in incomplete mechanical ileus, during spinal anesthesia and active catharsis, in intra-intestinal hemorrhage and in bleeding peptic ulcer. In ulcer, they can be a prime diagnostic aid in distinguishing between intra-intestinal and intraperitoneal bleeding.

3. The most important of the abnormal peristaltic sounds are "obstructive borborygmi." When these sounds are metallic and tinkling,

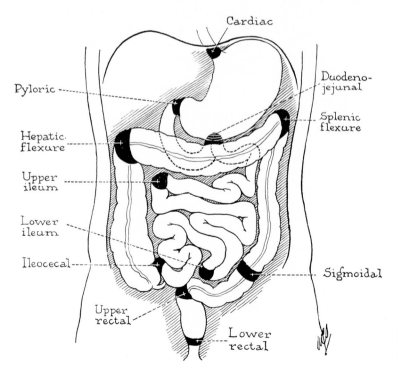

FIG. 279. Diagram showing most likely sites of intestinal obstruction.

Fig. 280. Flat plate, showing paralleling or "stepladder" appearance in small bowel obstruction. (See also Fig. 283.)

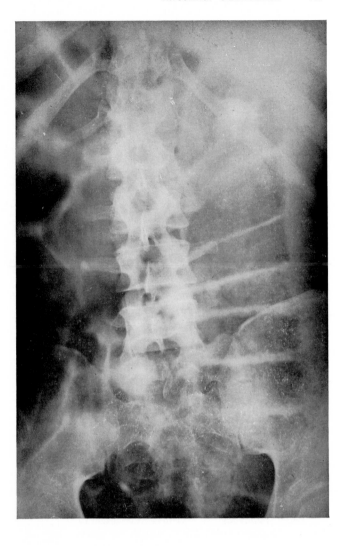

bubbling or loud and resonant in character, they are pathognomonic of incomplete mechanical ileus; they are heard thus in no other condition. They should be listened for both before and after attempting to reduce a hernia; if present beforehand, they gradually change to a normal tone following reduction. If reduction of the hernia does not relieve obstruction, the borborygmi remain. Other abdominal sounds include transmitted cardiac and respiratory sounds, splenic or liver friction rub, the splashing of pneumohydroperitoneum, *bruit d'airain,* the bruit of abdominal aneurysm and crepitation of subcutaneous emphysema.

Obstruction Syndrome. Intestinal obstruction is a symptom complex, not a disease per se. When confronted with the symptom triad, obstipation, vomiting and distention (Fig. 278), we should think at once of obstruction. Pain, its nature and location, can also be indicative. Colic—abdominal pain—can be significant during auscultation. Of all the known colics, only that which is synchronized with peristalsis originates in the intestines; this may be considered as pathognomonic of obstruction. We must then determine the site of the trouble, i.e., whether in the large or the small bowel, also whether complete or incomplete and if a strangulation exists. Upon these points rests the decision regarding therapeutic measures to be followed.

Locations. Some speak of "high" and "low" obstruction; to me these terms are confusing.

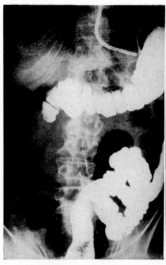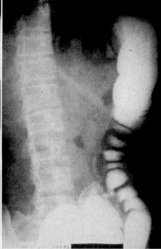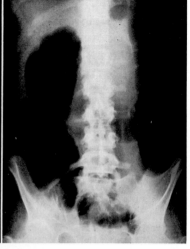

Fig. 281. Obstruction of large bowel. (*Left*) Typical appearance of obstruction at hepatic flexure. (*Center*) Obstruction at splenic flexure. (*Right*) Obstruction at hepatic flexure.

Large or *small bowel* obstruction seems to be clearer, and the differential diagnosis is all-important. Whether vomiting is early or late is significant. *Patients with small bowel obstruction vomit early and often; those with obstruction in the large bowel vomit little and late or not at all.* It has been correctly stated that the higher the obstruction, the greater the amount of vomiting.

"Fecal Vomiting." I consider this term to be a misnomer; "feculent" would be more correct. I believe that true fecal vomiting could occur only in the presence of a gastro-colic fistula or, as has unfortunately been known to happen, where some monumental error has been made during a gastro-intestinal anastomosis (e.g., performing a gastrocolostomy or a gastrosigmoidostomy instead of a gastrojejunostomy). Vomitus in intestinal obstruction is often brown in color and has a feculent odor, but this is due to the action of *B. coli* or other micro-organisms on the small bowel contents, not to the presence of actual fecal material. If intestinal obstruction is accompanied by feculent vomiting, the stomach should be thoroughly washed out before administering an anesthetic.

SITES OF OBSTRUCTION

Figure 279 shows the usual locations of obstruction throughout the entire length of the digestive tract. Obstructions affecting the stomach have already been discussed in Chapter 16.

Duodenal obstruction occurs only rarely, usually as the result of a congenital anomaly, and is often confused preoperatively with some other condition such as Hirschsprung's disease. Obstruction at the *duodenojejunal junction* will be accompanied by distention over the epigastrium, vomiting of bile and possibly evidence of interrupted mesenteric circulation. Obstruction elsewhere in the *upper ileum* will be similarly manifested; this is usually due to congenital bands, adhesions, internal hernia, intussusception or neoplasm. In the *lower ileum*, distention is more marked, the vomitus is somewhat feculent, and the patient becomes dehydrated. Roentgenograms show a characteristic "stepladder" pattern (Fig. 280). Obstruction associated with *Meckel's diverticulum* is rarer than the anomaly itself; it will be indicated by symptoms centered in the lower right abdominal quadrant. Following an appendectomy or some intervention on the

FIG. 282. Carcinoma of sigmoid causing obstruction. Note markedly dilated and haustrated horseshoe-shaped colon proximal to site of obstruction.

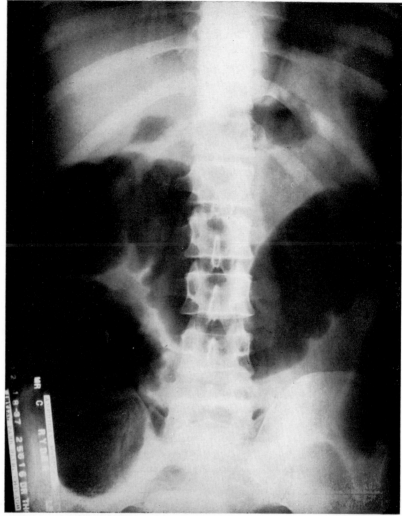

female genital tract, obstruction may appear at the *ileocecal valve*. It may also appear here due to a tuberculous tumor. Symptoms will point to the right iliac fossa, particularly in the early stages of the condition. Carcinoma at this point will give few clinical signs.

In obstruction at the *hepatic flexure* of the large intestine, the history is important. Chief symptoms are a palpable mass, distention of the cecum and the ascending colon and late vomiting. X-ray study after intake of opaque material will indicate an obstruction (Fig. 281). If the obstruction is incomplete, stools may be normally formed. Where carcinoma is suspected, the patient's age and a thorough study of the roentgenograms are of utmost importance. When the obstruction is at the

splenic flexure, distention will be localized in this area, but the tympanites will be more or less general. Again, stools may be formed if obstruction is incomplete. At this point, the trouble is usually caused by carcinoma, rarely by any other condition. At the *sigmoid flexure* (Fig. 282), obstruction causes distention backing toward the cecum; there will be little peristalsis. A barium enema will clarify the diagnosis. If obstruction is incomplete, varying bowel action (alternate constipation and diarrhea) may be present. Again, carcinoma is the most likely cause.

In the *upper rectum*, obstruction produces tympanites, irregular bowel action, loss of body weight, bloody or ribbon-shaped stools and mucus. The cause may be carcinoma,

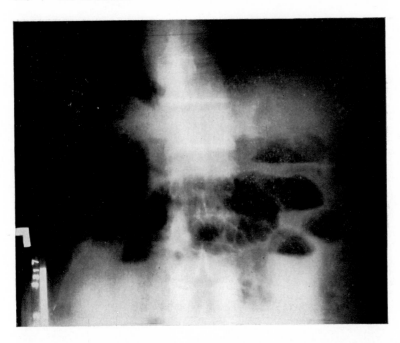

Fig. 283. Small bowel obstruction with fluid levels and distention.

syphilis or other tumors. The results of high proctoscopy, barium enema, Wasserman tests and bimanual examination will usually establish the diagnosis. In the *lower rectum,* there is a possibility of fecal impaction (ask if the patient has been taking bismuth). Proctoscopy

and roentgenograms will suggest a connection, if any, with causes farther up in the digestive tract.

Roentgenography. Use of scout films has become routine in all cases where the nature or even the existence of an occlusion is at all

TABLE 2. DIFFERENTIAL DIAGNOSIS BETWEEN SIMPLE AND STRANGULATED BOWEL OBSTRUCTION[3]

	STRANGULATED	SIMPLE
Pain	Sudden onset and fulminating; severe, cramplike; may be continuous	Onset gradual; less severe; tends to disappear during periods of inactive peristalsis
Vomiting	Occurs at onset of pain; severe, continuous, sustained and may have little relation to peristaltic pain	Begins at considerable interval after onset of pain; tends to be simultaneous with peristaltic action
Shocklike manifestations	May appear early at onset; persistent with progressive severity	Appear late in course of obstruction; tend to be less severe
Response to conservative therapy	Poor	Usually good
Peritoneal fluid	Invariably bloody	Clear
Scout roentgenogram	Isolated loop may be present	Isolated loop rarely present
Mass	May be present	Rarely present
Tenderness	May be marked	Usually not marked
Abdominal spasm	Frequently present and marked	Usually absent
Rectal examination	Bloody rectal discharge may be present	Blood rarely present
Blood studies	Dehydration and hemoconcentration do not respond to therapy; white cell count may be elevated	Dehydration and hemoconcentration respond to therapy

FIG. 284. Proper method of examining for suspected bowel tumor. Note position of thighs to ensure relaxation of abdominal muscles.

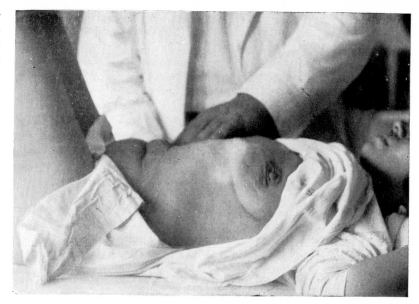

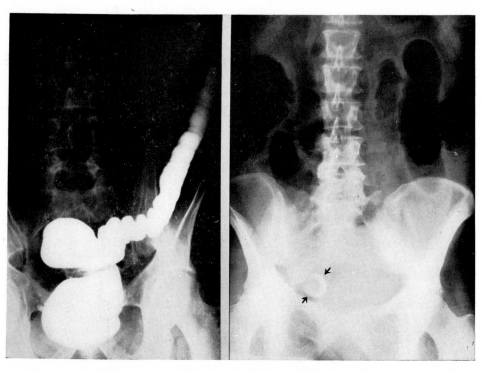

FIG. 285. Two cases of obstruction. (*Left*) Large bowel obstruction due to carcinoma at splenic flexure. (*Right*) Small bowel obstruction caused by impacted gallstone (arrows). Note fine cross striations of jejunum ("herringbone" appearance due to Kirkring's folds).

questionable. Gas and fluid accumulate above the obstruction; when the patient is upright, these cause a series of "fluid levels" (Fig. 283). When he lies supine, the amount and the distribution of gas in the intestinal loops becomes apparent. The pattern and the amount of distention of the involved loop or loops confirm a doubtful diagnosis and indicate or suggest the location of the trouble.

Differential Diagnosis

The most important point to keep in mind regarding obstruction is that the cases in which there is the gravest and most immediate danger to life are those involving interference with the blood supply. Nothing is more vital than to distinguish between *simple* occlusion and that involving *strangulation*. Table 2 will provide some assistance in distinguishing between the two.

Indications for the *location* of the obstruction have already been given, as suggested by the amount and the character of vomiting, the extent and the location of distention, the character of pain, the presence or the absence of shock symptoms and the location of a palpable mass, if any (Fig. 284). Diagnosing the *cause* of the obstruction is the third and final step (Fig. 285). Before operation this is often difficult or even impossible and, in any event, may be of little more than academic interest. However, sometimes it can be deduced from such factors as the age of the patient, his long-range history (particularly for previous ab-

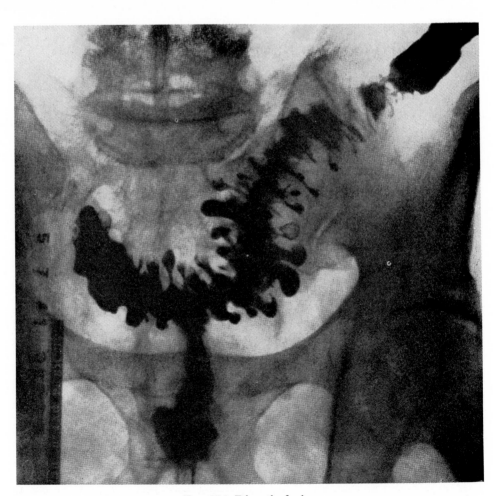

Fig. 286. Diverticulosis.

dominal surgery) and such signs as recent loss of weight or dehydration. Maingot groups these signs as follows:

1. *Congenital Causes.* Imperforate anus or rectum; infantile pyloric stenosis; congenital duodenal atresia or stenosis; congenital atresia or stenosis of the small intestine and the colon; intestinal obstruction of the newborn resulting from meconium ileus; acute obstruction due to malro-

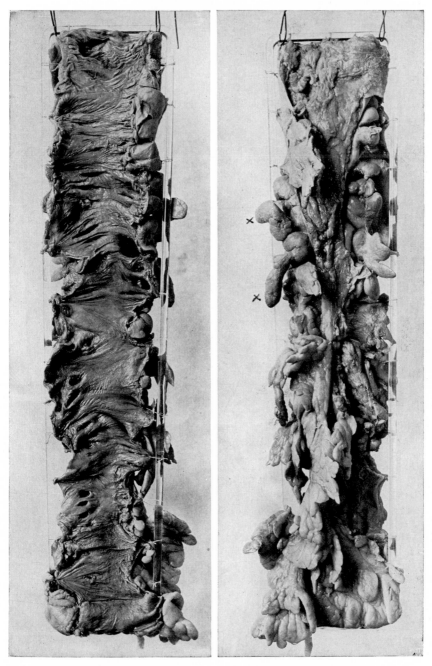

FIG. 287. Diverticulosis of large bowel. Note appendixlike diverticula at x-x that have undergone inflammatory changes. (deQuervain)

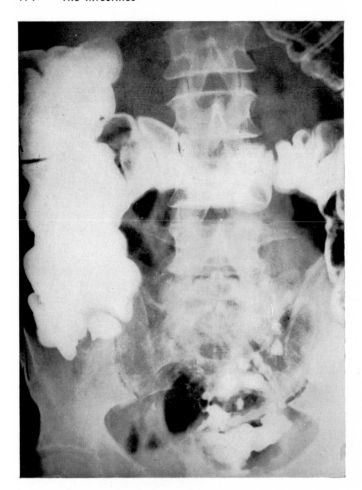

FIG. 288. Obstruction at rectosigmoid junction caused by carcinoma of prostate with diverticulosis.

tation of the intestines, annular pancreas, foreign bodies and duplication of elements of the alimentary tract.

2. *In Early Life.* Intussusception, Meckel's diverticulum, strangulated hernia, adhesions or bands—congenital or acquired.

3. *In Late Life.* Cancer of the intestine, strangulated hernia, fecal impaction, diverticulitis, volvulus, gallstones, adhesions or bands.

4. *With Previous History of Operation or Inflammation.* Adhesions or bands near appendix or gallbladder, in the pelvis or under an abdominal scar; paralytic ileus.

5. *Cases with Special Symptoms or Signs.* Strangulated hernia, intussusception, carcinoma of the colon, gallstone ileus, volvulus and mesenteric embolism and thrombosis.

Diverticulosis. Statistics show that nearly 1 person in 10 over the age of 40 has diverticula of the colon. The incidence of diverticulosis (Fig. 286), the precursor of diverticulitis, is not easy to establish, nor is it confined to those in the older age group. Often a congenital diverticulum causes no trouble for its owner and is discovered accidentally or not at all. Acquired diverticula may ulcerate, perforate or contribute to the development of fistulae (Fig. 287). There appears to be no conclusive proof that they predispose to the formation of neoplasms, but the fact that they do appear in patients of the "cancer age group" makes it inevitable that the two conditions should sometimes appear concurrently (Fig. 288).

A suggestive history includes recurrent attacks of lower abdominal pain and tenderness, together with constipation, general malaise and sometimes a rise in temperature. Use of a barium enema and sigmoidoscopy usually will serve to distinguish, in cases where there is doubt, between diverticulitis and carci-

Fig. 289. Duodenal diverticulum, immediately after ingestion of barium.

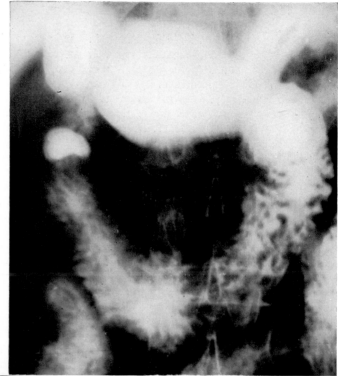

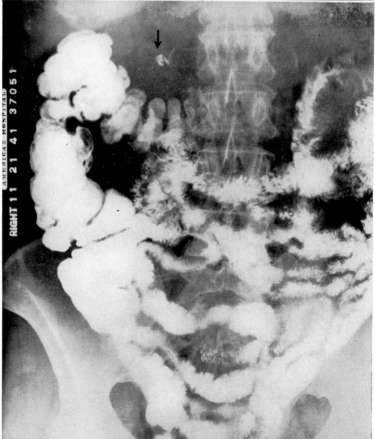

Fig. 290. Duodenal diverticulum. Same patient as in Figure 288, 8 hours later. Note barium residue in diverticulum (arrow).

noma. The presence of a large fixed mass in the region of the sigmoid, in an otherwise well person, usually eliminates the possibility of a malignancy. However, where all signs appear to point to benignancy, early indications of a neoplasm could be missed; keep this in mind. If there is blood in the stool, it is safer to consider the case as suspected carcinoma until proved otherwise. Where it is impossible to make a definitive diagnosis between the two conditions, as occurs in a small proportion of patients, surgery should be instituted and the affected area removed, even though it is usually possible to cure a true diverticulitis (Figs. 289 and 290) by conservative, non-surgical means.

Roentgenography is extremely helpful in the diagnosis of diverticulitis. By use of the barium enema, the diverticulum can usually be demonstrated, together with an area of spasm, "saw-toothing" and a narrowed sigmoid, unlike the "filling defect" of carcinoma. At times, at operation, it is almost impossible to ascertain definitely whether one is dealing with an inflammatory process or malignancy until microscopic evidence is at hand.

Foreign Bodies. Occasionally, foreign bodies may cause obstruction. These may be things swallowed (see Foreign Bodies in the Stomach, p. 389), as well as wandering biliary calculi or even objects getting in from the outside as a result of trauma. If an impacted gallstone causes intestinal obstruction (see Fig. 285), it may be enough simply to remove it, but such stones at times reach the intestine through a suppurating fistula from the gall-bladder. The lining of the bowel in the vicinity of the impaction should be examined very carefully, as it is likely to have been severely damaged. Under such conditions, it is better to resect the damaged portion of the bowel; this is also true under any condition where the bowel wall has been seriously injured in connection with an obstruction. When it is necessary to remove a foreign body by enterostomy, the intestinal incision should be made lengthwise and sutured transversely in order to avoid subsequent stenosis.

Volvulus. This may be the cause of some obscure cases of obstruction. The only cure is immediate surgical intervention. However, de-torsion alone (Fig. 291) is not enough. The *causes* of the volvulus must be sought for and removed if cure is to be permanent (see

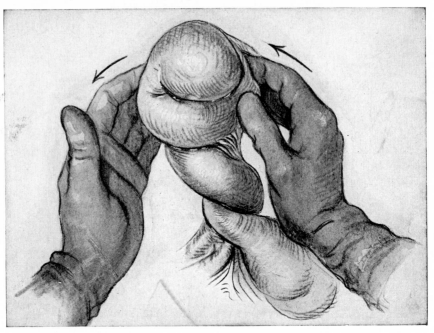

FIG. 291. Shows proper method of reducing intestinal volvulus.

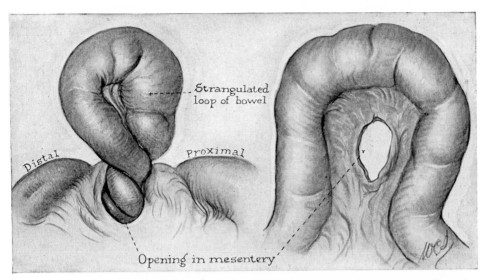

FIG. 292. (*Left*) Shows how opening in mesentery may permit loop of bowel to slip through and become strangulated. (*Right*) Loop reduced, detorsion accomplished, and opening in mesentery ready for closure.

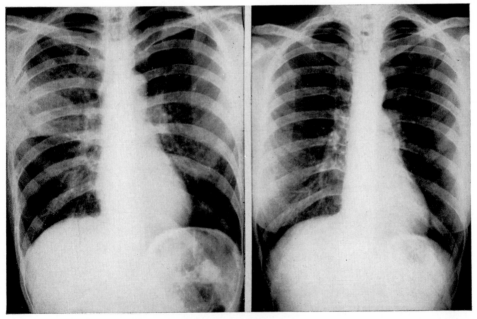

FIG. 293. Paralytic ileus in lobar pneumonia. (*Left*) On admission this patient showed marked abdominal distention and other signs of partial obstruction. Roentgenogram shows marked meteorism in both large and small bowel, gas-filled jejunal loop with typical "herringbone" pattern below left dome of diaphragm, pneumonic infiltration of right, middle lobe (not diagnosed clinically). (*Right*) Same patient, 1 week later. After chemotherapy, pneumonic infiltration cleared, meteorism disappeared, and the left diaphragmatic region is normal.

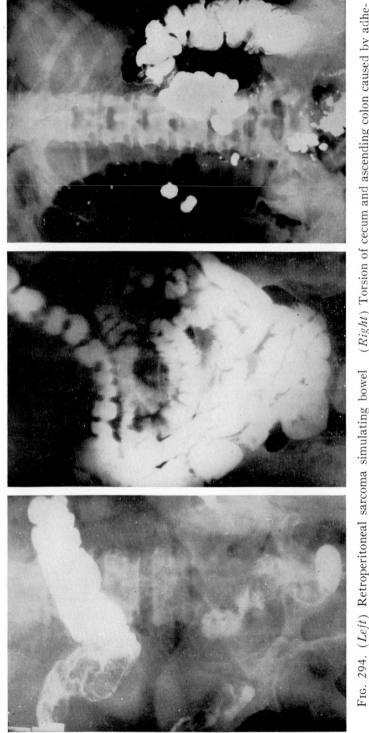

FIG. 294. (*Left*) Retroperitoneal sarcoma simulating bowel lesion; note apparent filling defect. (*Center*) Patent ileocecal valve; barium enema filled greater portion of small bowel. (*Right*) Torsion of cecum and ascending colon caused by adhesions. Preoperative diagnosis (roentgenographic) was carcinoma; clinical diagnosis was hysteria.

Volvulus of the Stomach, p. 384). Figure 292 illustrates a common cause of this condition. Here, the opening in the mesentery is the obvious reason; this should be repaired. Needless to say, to leave such an opening during any operative procedure is to invite trouble in the future.

Strangulated Hernia. When the etiology of the obstruction is doubtful, another possibility is strangulated hernia. Careful history taking, when done in the light of a thorough knowledge of the diagnostic criteria and of the possible sites of occlusion, together with the individualizing signs of each, should serve to differentiate this source of blockage from other possibilities. Operative treatment of this condition is dealt with elsewhere in these pages (see Chap. 20, Hernia).

Additional Factors. Some additional pointers regarding diagnosis in various forms and locations of obstruction include the following.

HERNIAL RINGS. When obstruction is evident, a thorough examination of the hernial rings should never be omitted. The most frequent error is to mistake a small femoral hernia in a fat woman or a congenital inguinal hernia for the site of an intestinal obstruction. The origin of the pain should be carefully studied as to location and radiation. If its onset was sudden, it usually signifies either strangulation, acute invagination or torsion.

DISTENTION AND METEORISM. These are important signs in obstruction (Fig. 293). If the blockage is caused by strangulation or torsion, the affected bowel segment will become distended with gas. If this condition can be studied early enough, it sometimes gives a useful clue to the location of the trouble. Meteorism may be visible from the outside. If it is centrally located, the occlusion involves the small intestine; if it is in the right iliac region, it is beyond the cecum; if it is on both sides, an occlusion or atony in the whole course of the large bowel is indicated. The affected bowel segment may be palpable. A distended loop without peristaltic movements will have an elastic or sometimes a hard, resistant feel to the palpating hand. Regrettably, this valuable sign is soon masked by widespread meteorism.

Confusion in the diagnosis of obstruction may arise from the fact that some of the symptoms may be those of peritonitis, while others are those of occlusion due to intestinal infarction, thrombosis of the mesenteric vessels, internal herniae or acute pancreatitis. Under these conditions, both peristalsis and meteorism may be completely absent. Here, exploratory laparotomy may be the only means of ascertaining the true state of affairs.

LEUKOCYTOSIS. An increased white blood cell count will be found in inflammatory states, whereas in obstruction the count will be normal.

RETROPERITONEAL TUMORS. Occasionally a roentgenogram will show what appears to be a definite abnormality of the bowel, which, nevertheless, turns out to be of extraperitoneal origin (e.g., a retroperitoneal new growth).

HYSTERIA. Very occasionally, symptoms of occlusion may be actually due to some mental disturbance, but the diagnostician would be well-advised to be very slow in ascribing purely subjective symptoms to neurotic causes. More than one case has been reported where supposedly imaginary woes have turned out to be the result of quite definite physical causes, such as adhesions, etc. (Figs. 294 and 295).

PROGNOSIS

Happily, in recent years there has been a definite decrease in deaths from obstruction. Much of this decrease comes, indirectly, from improved understanding of the nature of the body's reaction to the effects of occlusion. A clear comprehension of what Maingot calls the "lethal effects" of a group of "vicious circles" that follow development of any of the various forms of obstruction will help to reduce the number of these deaths still further. He lists these vicious circles as:

1. Irreversible ileus
2. Kinking of distended loops
3. Shock syndrome
4. Reflex spread of distention
5. Compression of the thorax
6. Impairment of caval, portal and peripheral venous flow

To this list I would add, along a slightly different line of thought, two factors tending to lower the death rate: (1) earlier diagnosis, especially of postoperative occlusions, and (2) prompt elimination of toxins. Toxins developing in the intestine following obstruction are highly poisonous. Further, it is now known that dehydration and loss of the vital blood chlorides are important causes of death from obstruction. Forewarned, we know what to do to counteract these losses. Intravenous blood and saline, together with inhalation of 95 per cent oxygen (this last is especially valuable in children), and administration of vitamin C (orally or parenterally, as indicated by circumstances) with appropriate antibiotics serve to restore body chemistry and metabolism to normal as rapidly as possible.

To recapitulate, lowered mortality figures and better end-results will follow observance of the following:

1. Rapid and accurate diagnosis

2. Prompt surgical intervention where indicated

3. Discrimination in the use of accessory measures, methods, medications and appliances both before and after operation (e.g., intubation)

4. Recognition of the significance of pain in all its forms.

MANAGEMENT

In handling all types of obstruction, it is helpful to remember the 5 "S's" of treatment: (1) suction, (2) saline, (3) sanguine (blood), (4) surgery and (5) sulfas (chemotherapy).*

* Dr. Philip Thorek.

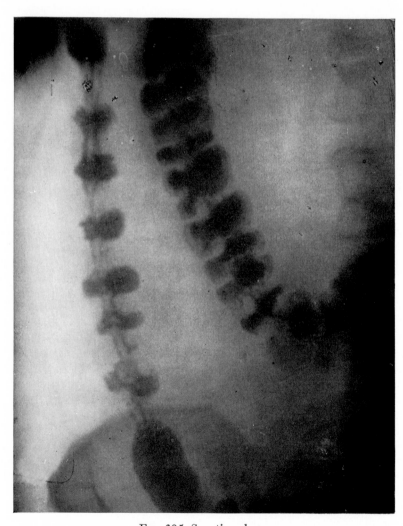

FIG. 295. Spastic colon.

Suction. Since its introduction in 1934, the use of the Miller-Abbott drainage tube has become almost the invariable method of choice in cases of small bowel distention. In my own hands, this device has yielded quite satisfactory results. However, to quote Maingot again:

All too frequently, the tube obstinately refuses to be guided through the pylorus in just those cases in which intestinal suction drainage is most desirable. Again, the mere presence of the double-lumen tube in the stomach appears to throw the pyloric sphincter into an obstinate and whimsical spasm, and when this muscle eventually relents and relaxes, the onrushing stream of pent-up intestinal fluids hurls the balloon aimlessly about in the capacious gastric cavity. At times, the tube will kink back on itself and lie coiled in the stomach and even tie itself into a knot! No one has, as yet, devised the ideal tube for intestinal intubation. A stubborn persistence in attempts to pass a Miller-Abbott tube through a recalcitrant pyloric canal and the over-zealous employment of intestinal suction drainage are responsible for a number of deaths in cases of mechanical acute intestinal obstruction.

It is certainly true that in large bowel obstruction suction is not only useless but also may waste precious time. In some forms of small bowel obstruction, however, suction may not only aid in the treatment but also, by itself, may bring about a cure. In this category belong those obstructions which are associated with peritonitis (such as postoperative appendiceal or gonorrheal), where a limited portion of the terminal ileum is kinked in the inflamed area. Suction with a Wangensteen or the much longer Miller-Abbott tube (which is designed to reach to the ileocecal valve and is even reported to have come out of the anal orifice) may cause the loops to "unkink." However, the results are not always so striking. It should be pointed out that the removal of *swallowed air* can be as useful as the removal of liquid material.

Saline. When suction is instituted, it must never be forgotten that important chloride ions are being lost to the system because of the removal of gastric hydrochloric acid. These must be replaced. It has been well said, "As soon as the tube goes in the nose, a needle should go into a vein." The value of this combination has been adequately demonstrated in animal experimentation. However, the mistake should not be made of believing that the administration of saline is, of itself, a *treatment* for obstruction; it is merely a necessary *part* of such treatment, in that it prevents hypochloridemia.

Sanguine. Transfused blood has become one of our most valuable weapons in many surgical fields, nowhere more than in the treatment of obstruction. With the setting up in more and more places of blood and plasma "banks," and our ever-increasing knowledge of the entire subject of blood transfusion, it cannot but follow that with each passing year many more lives will be saved by this means.

Surgery. The type of lesion naturally determines the surgical procedure to be followed.

Acute Large Bowel Obstruction. This usually calls for only a "ventilating" operation, since it seems unwise to attack, for example, a carcinoma in the presence of distention. The entire left side of the abdomen should be left alone for the time being, the immediate intervention being limited to a simple cecostomy.

Small Bowel Obstruction. As already suggested, small bowel obstruction may be relieved by suction and saline in preparation for whatever surgery may be indicated for the future. On the other hand, if the obstruction shows definite signs of being caused by a strangulated hernia, surgery cannot wait. When tenderness localizes at a specific point, it usually indicates the onset of gangrene.

Sulfa. The use of antibiotics and chemotherapy is now so routine that little need be said about it here. Each new type that is introduced, as Till pointed out (p. 405), is likely to be acclaimed as a "cure all" but actually will prove to add only *something more* to our armamentarium. With any of them, a careful watch must be kept for signs of toxemia.

Choice of Operation

When decompression and detoxication fail to relieve an obstructed bowel, the surgeon must decide between the advisability of doing (1) a simple resection or (2) enterostomy with drainage. In any event, the technic must be chosen with regard to individual requirements.

Simple Resection. Where indicated, simple resection must include all of the damaged portion of bowel. In some instances, where the patient's condition is good, resection may be combined with anastomosis and drainage at a distant point.

Primary Colostomy or Ileostomy. On the other hand, with the obstruction left to be removed at a later time, primary colostomy or ileostomy will sometimes give better end-results. The deciding factor is to obtain detoxication first; radical procedures can wait.

Enterostomy. When tubal decompression fails, enterostomy is the most effective procedure, in that it permits emptying the obstructed bowel segments, detoxicates and promotes re-establishment of peristalsis; always bear in mind that its use must be predicated on the patient's condition. Remember also that drainage may not show any results during the first few postoperative hours.

In any procedure for the relief of obstruction, bear in mind the likelihood of aspiration of vomitus and its often fatal consequences. Preoperative lavage should be routine with these patients.

PRECAUTIONS

Regurgitant Vomiting. During operation, regurgitant vomiting may be prevented by shutting off the upper jejunum with a pair of intestinal clamps, but all the precautions previously cited must be kept in mind concerning the use of this device.

Anesthesia. Make use of the best anesthetist, anesthetic materials and methods available. Spinal block is often recommended, but the possibility of untoward sequelae (e.g., sterility in the male) must be given due consideration.

Operative Precautions. Injury to dangerously distended loops of bowel must be avoided by every available means. In obscure cases, use a median incision and be extra cautious to avoid damage to the distended loops beneath. Even though some surgeons routinely exteriorize excessively distended bowel segments, it has been my own practice to do so only when that seems to be absolutely necessary.

If the bowel contents must be evacuated through an intestinal incision, peritoneal soiling should be avoided. If the patient's condition is poor, and the surgeon's skill not of the highest order, the best interests of all concerned will probably be served by doing a simple decompression or colostomy rather than by attempting a more radical procedure.

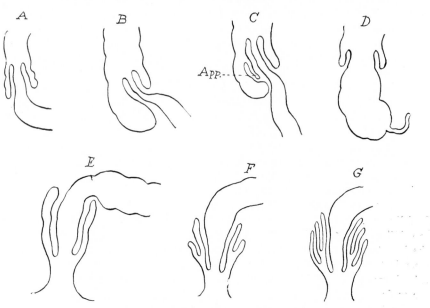

FIG. 296. Simplified diagram showing types of intussusception. (A) Ileo-ileal. (B) Ileocolic. (C) Cecocolic. (D) Colic. (E) Rectocolic. (F) Double. (G) Triple.

Postoperative Occlusions. To summarize, let me again call attention to the fact that obstruction follows surgery for other conditions. In particular, paralytic ileus of the small bowel will occur after gynecologic interventions during the first few days after the operation. A successful outcome depends on immediate and accurate diagnosis with prompt and proper treatment.

The possibility of mesenteric thrombosis, internal herniae, volvulus, obstructive adhesions or obstruction by foreign bodies must all be considered in making a diagnosis. In infants, think of acute intestinal invagination; in older children, the subacute variety should come to mind. Occlusion of Meckel's diverticulum, volvulus of the pelvic portion of the colon and obstruction by polyps or neoplasms are more frequent in persons in the later age groups, particularly males.

INTUSSUSCEPTION

Every precaution should be taken to avoid

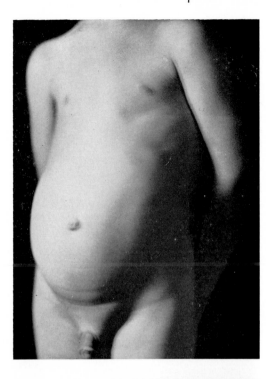
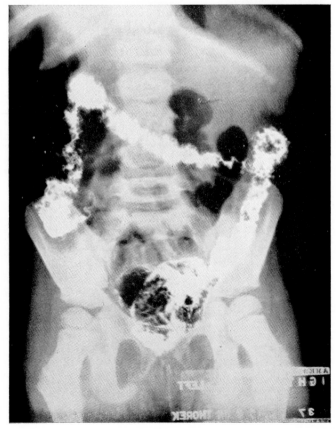

FIG. 297. (*Top*) Congenital obstruction of duodenum, diagnosed preoperatively as Hirschsprung's disease. (See also Figs. 299 and 300.) (*Right*) Duodenal obstruction causing enormous distention of stomach and clinical manifestations leading to diagnosis of Hirschsprung's disease. Gastrojejunostomy followed by good recovery. (See also Fig. 300.)

errors in diagnosis when dealing with the possibility of intussusception either in children or in adults (Fig. 296). There is definite risk in "waiting to see" whether the condition will resolve of itself. Simple methods of treatment are sometimes successful, but if there is any indication of persistence of trouble, surgical measures should be resorted to promptly. Short-circuiting operations should be avoided. They seldom succeed in anything except delaying an inevitable resection. Reduction performed in time may save the patient's life. The following should be borne in mind:

1. An invagination may be overlooked or its symptoms misinterpreted. This happens oftenest in early infancy, when symptoms may be mild and transient. If the patient demonstrates pain, vomiting and diarrhea without any other apparent cause, and is otherwise well, always think of the possibility of in-

vagination. The same should come to mind if there is obstinate constipation and distention; here, rectal examination occasionally may clinch the diagnosis. Also, a palpable tumor will be present in about half the cases. These signs, together with blood in the stool, should always be looked for and evaluated properly.

2. In adults, tumor is often difficult to find, and, if found, because it is apt to be inflammatory in nature, the condition may be mistaken for appendicitis or diverticulitis. Invagination will be characterized by incomplete obstruction and alternating constipation and diarrhea. In the elderly such signs are particularly likely to be mistaken for intestinal or vascular spasms or a gradually stenosing tumor. Here x-ray examination may be of special assistance.

3. When the condition is chronic, it may

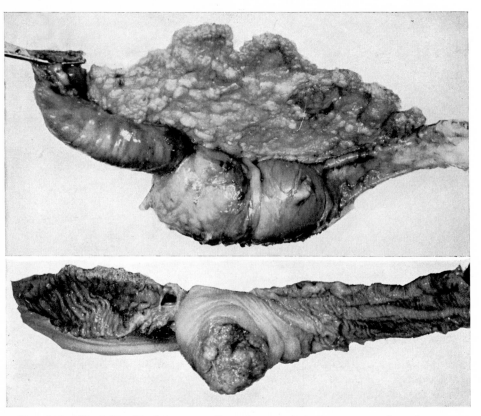

Fig. 298. (*Top*) Double intussusception of cecum into transverse colon, due to carcinoma. Note enlarged lymph nodes. Very poor prognosis, but, following microscopic examination, all specimens proved to be inflammatory, and the patient made a good immediate recovery. (*Bottom*) Same patient. Polypoid carcinoma of cecum protruding into ascending colon; note edematous mucous membrane.

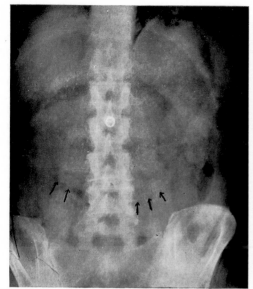

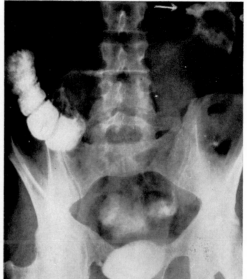

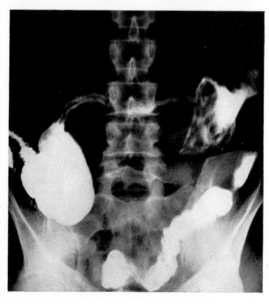

FIG. 299. Intussusception of cecum into transverse colon due to carcinoma. (*Top, left*) Curved line marked by arrows, resembling border of tumor mass, represents inner contour of markedly distended transverse colon (the intussuscipiens). (*Top, right*) Arrow marks cap-shaped tumor mass which pulls narrow band of ileum into transverse colon. Note outlines of enlarged transverse colon. (*Lower, right*) Same as preceding.

not be recognized. Children thus afflicted become emaciated and may be thought to suffer from Hirschsprung's disease (Fig. 297) or intestinal tuberculosis. Here, too, operation may be delayed unjustifiably. Cases illustrative of this point have been reported in both children and adults. One man of 50 had multiple intussusceptions due to melanotic sarcoma. An infant of 11 months showed an obviously long-standing intussusception and signs indicating that there had been another sinister episode which had reduced itself spontaneously by means of retroperistalsis. In a man of 30, who was operated on for obstruction, it was revealed that the telescoping was due to a pedunculated tumor which had dragged the affected segment of bowel into its abnormal position (Figs. 298 and 299).

4. Even when a correct diagnosis has been made, valuable time may be lost in trying to reduce the invagination by conservative means.

In such instances the prognosis rapidly grows worse; devagination succeeds only in early cases; late resection has a high rate of mortality. Therefore, operation should be undertaken as early as possible.

During devagination, the invaginated portion of the bowel should not be pulled on; rather, a "milking" action should be undertaken to push it out, and all attempts to disengage it should be abandoned if they do not succeed easily (Fig. 300). If the patient's condition is poor, immediate treatment should be the formation of an artificial anus above the site of the invagination; devagination or resection should then be delayed until the patient's condition has improved.

PRECAUTIONS IN REDUCTION

In addition to being careful not to pull on the invaginated segment of bowel, it is vital to make sure, after the invagination has been reduced, that the involved segments are fully viable. Make sure of unimpaired circulation, especially in the invaginated portion. Circulation is not so apt to be interfered with in the enveloping portion. Never put back into the abdomen any part of the intestine that shows any signs of circulatory damage; if in doubt, always resect!

I am convinced of the value of exploratory laparotomy in all cases where the diagnosis is doubtful. While it is true that every reasonable effort should be made to arrive at a correct diagnosis before operation, it does not follow that operation should be postponed because of doubt. It is a gross surgical error to delay intervention when an exploratory celiotomy is urgently indicated by the clearly observable signs.

MESENTERIC OCCLUSION

ETIOLOGY

Two distinct types of conditions are generally included under this heading. The first is mesenteric infarction from thrombosis or embolism; the second is one which Grégoire, many years ago, aptly described as "intestinal apoplexy," resulting from what was then known as "anaphylactoid shock." Any of these conditions may simulate intestinal obstruction and, indeed, actually produce obstruction of a sort. The prognosis is grave, and the condition ends fatally in a large proportion of cases; figures reported by different workers run from 58 to 92 per cent mortality.

DIFFERENTIAL DIAGNOSIS

Thrombosis may originate from any focus of infection, especially in the portal area, sometimes spreading from the portal or splenic veins. Splenic anemia, with or without splenectomy, sometimes produces fatal thrombosis. Complete intestinal obstruction generally results; however, the condition seldom is diagnosed correctly, sometimes being missed even after the abdomen has been opened.

Laden[10] believes that thrombosis is more common than embolism. If the occlusion is *venous*, there will be hemorrhagic infarction and, later, typical signs of shock. Little dilatation takes place above the involved segment, as there is no real obstruction, the condition being one of a nonfunctioning intestinal loop rather than a true blockage. He states that spontaneous recovery is a "surgical curiosity."

When the occlusion is *arterial*, there will be pain, cramps, vomiting, diarrhea, gradually

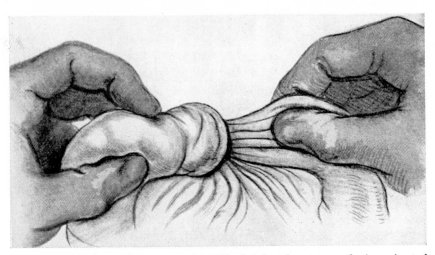

FIG. 300. Reducing an intussusception. The left hand expresses the invaginated portion, while the right exerts gentle traction.

developing mild distention and possibly hematemesis or blood in the stool. Shock appears early. Peritonitis develops later on. In possibly 10 per cent of cases, a vague, "doughy" mass may be palpable. In patients past the age of 50, this condition should be suspected when sudden, left-sided pain develops, with little rigidity and mild distention, and, later, a "silent abdomen." Resection of the affected segment is the only chance for these patients. The use of coagulants and antibiotics, advised by some, should be reserved for those who refuse operation and for postoperative treatment. It is further believed by Laden that this

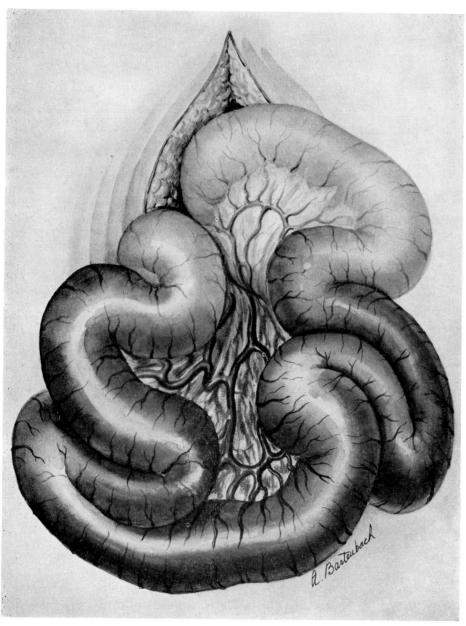

FIG. 301. Mesenteric occlusion. An almost classic example of "infarction" of allergic origin. This patient recovered under conservative treatment.

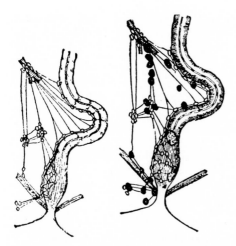

Fig. 302. Lymph supply of lower bowel.
(After Davis)

condition is more common than is generally supposed.

Different workers have reported varying degrees of success with resection for this condition. Some years ago (before the days of chemotherapy), one series showed a mortality of 32.6 per cent. Laden reports a resection on a man of 70, from whom he removed 4 feet of gangrenous bowel, and who was alive and well 4 years later.

Rosenman and Gropper[17] call attention to the fact that while the effects of massive infarction are well known, it is not so generally recognized that more limited involvement may have long-range effects that are nearly, if not quite, as serious. From an elaborate study they conclude that fibrosis and stricture may develop long after the original occlusion, with results as lethal as those of more acute processes.

As previously indicated (p. 426), a second and rather more puzzling form of infarction appears to derive from allergic reactions. In recent years our understanding of such systemic behavior has increased vastly, and, in the light of such knowledge, we are now somewhat better able to diagnose and to deal with these conditions, wherever in the body they may be found. My personal surgical experience over a half century convinces me that had I possessed the know-how that we have today, my procedure in many so-called infarction cases would, on numerous occasions, have

been quite different from the procedure I actually used.

Intestinal apoplexy caused by allergy may regress spontaneously under suitable therapy. Though we cannot always distinguish, even now, the clinical differences between true mechanical infarction and allergenic apoplexy, there are some guideposts to rely on, particularly the suggestive triad of sudden onset, drop in blood pressure and bloody stools. The aphorism of Grégoire, "Every form of medication capable of counteracting shock of intolerance and raising arterial tension is capable of remedying intestinal apoplexies without vascular lesions," still holds good, even though we now know far better how to bring about these ends than he did when he laid it down. Figure 301, though dating from 1938, could hardly be improved upon as being typical of the sort of condition which Grégoire had in mind. The case report which this accompanied showed, preoperatively, a nearly classic picture of acute appendicitis, yet laparotomy revealed the condition shown, and, acting in line with Grégoire's observations, adrenalin therapy was instituted, with ultimate complete recovery. Though the medications employed today might be different, the over-all treatment probably would be similar.

Symptoms

In all cases, shock and acute intestinal upheaval are the symptoms. Occasionally, very early operation may show the condition in its initial stage, before the occurrence of hemorrhage into the involved tissues. Contrary to the usually observed (in mechanical infarction) dark color of the affected segments of bowel, the color is bright red, and the appearance of the intestine is sausagelike, resembling the edema of Quincke. Hemorrhagic manifestations are absent in the ileum but are already present in the mesentery, as demonstrated by scarlet patches and a few ecchymotic plaques. When operation is not performed so early, preoperative roentgenograms may show either the typical picture of occlusion or localized changes only.

Digestive complaints, which frequently are reported previous to the onset of acute clinical manifestations, may be considered as being sensitizing factors. Pulmonary shock has been reported following an attack of intes-

FIG. 303. Blood supply of lower bowel.

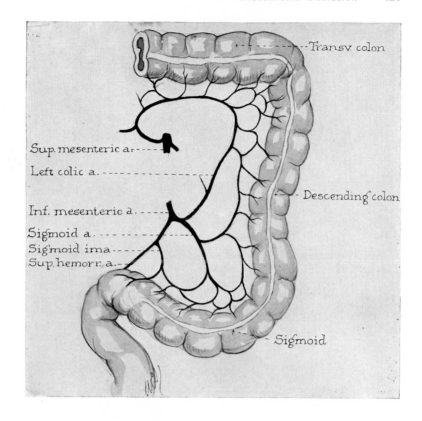

Transv. colon

Sup. mesenteric a.

Left colic a.

Descending colon

Inf. mesenteric a.

Sigmoid a.

Sigmoid ima

Sup. hemorr. a.

Sigmoid

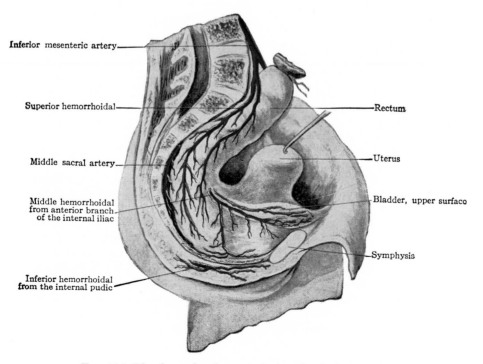

Inferior mesenteric artery

Superior hemorrhoidal

Middle sacral artery

Middle hemorrhoidal from anterior branch of the internal iliac

Inferior hemorrhoidal from the internal pudic

Rectum

Uterus

Bladder, upper surface

Symphysis

FIG. 304. Blood supply of rectum in female. (After Davis)

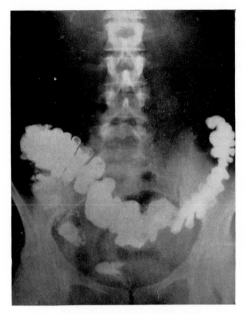

FIG. 305. Ptosis of bowel.

tinal apoplexy and might be considered as simply being an additional evidence of sensitivity. However, if it fails to respond to the treatment for allergy, it is more likely to be due to postoperative embolism, thereby again linking the two forms of occlusions.

TREATMENT

Treatment should include both medication for allergy and, imperatively, laparotomy. Since operative intervention is also urgently indicated for mechanical occlusion, the various steps involved may be guided by the surgeon's own judgment and experience, still further proof, if such be needed, of my oft-repeated injunctions to know beyond all doubt the basic principles involved.

SURGERY OF THE COLON

GENERAL CONSIDERATIONS

Operations on the colon (Figs. 302, 303 and 304) may be divided into two general classifications: those performed for the removal of malignant neoplasms and those for treatment of various benign conditions (Fig. 305). The surgical treatment of malignant tumors in the cecum and the ascending colon is accepted and time-honored; as this is dealt with else-

where in these pages, only a few words are needed here. Anastonosis between the transverse colon and the ileum, followed after 2 or 3 weeks by removal of the entire right colon is, in my opinion, a dangerous procedure, as it may result in leakage and peritonitis. Lahey advised a modified Mikulicz plan of excision which largely eliminates these dangers, although at the cost of considerable temporary discomfort to the patient. In using this procedure, be sure that the spur is made long enough. Otherwise, when the patient returns for the second stage of the operation, the septum may be so shortened, due to swelling and cicatrization, that further cutting will be necessary. Also, do not attempt to re-establish bowel continuity before the lapse of at least 2 months. Earlier, edema will not have subsided in the wound, and the peritoneum will not have become firmly attached to the implanted intestinal loop.

INFLAMMATORY LESIONS

The Distal Colon. In one series of patients suffering from chronic ulcerative colitis, Lahey found that more than 40 per cent did not respond to medical methods. Surgery should be resorted to when (1) the condition does not yield readily to medical therapy; (2) the patient is incapacitated for more than one quarter of the time; (3) subacute perforation or abscess is present; (4) there are fistulae or sinuses; (5) in the presence of massive hemorrhage, polyposis or obstruction. It might also be noted that major operations on the intestinal tract frequently are followed by enteritis, especially a type of colitis resembling dysentery. Operative procedures of value in treating these conditions include ileostomy, partial colectomy and complete colectomy.

PRECAUTIONARY CONSIDERATIONS. In dealing with benign conditions in the distal colon, time and invalidism are not usually factors that need be considered. The distal colon may be defunctioned for a year or more, if necessary, when it is desirable to obtain the germ-free, quiescent operative field which will give the most hopeful outlook for long-range results. Several advantages may be secured by such defunctioning well in advance of operation, including absence of septic feces, collapsed and retracted colonic walls and low bacterial content, resolution of inflammation, disappear-

FIG. 306. Steps in temporary colostomy.

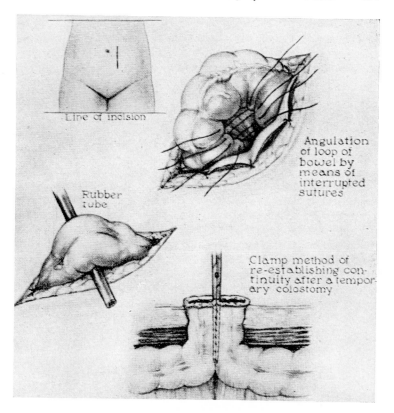

Line of incision

Angulation of loop of bowel by means of interrupted sutures

Rubber tube

Clamp method of re-establishing continuity after a temporary colostomy

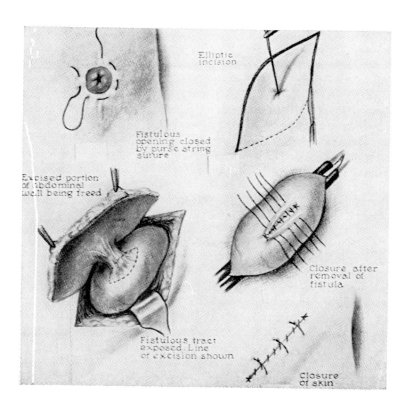

Elliptic incision

Fistulous opening closed by purse string suture

Excised portion of abdominal wall being freed

Closure after removal of fistula

Fistulous tract exposed. Line of excision shown

Closure of skin

FIG. 307. Intraperitoneal closure of colostomy.

ance of adhesions which may have bound the inflammatory tumor or other lesion to neighboring organs, and, frequently, the possibility of removal of previously inoperable tumors, as well as avoidance of removal of bowel which was formerly inflamed but otherwise healthy. This method has stood the test of time, enabling the successful performance of quite drastic procedures on aged or otherwise poor-risk patients and working even better on those in less precarious states.

The ends to be sought in preparing for the removal of benign growths by production of a temporary artificial anus are that it should (1) disconnect completely, (2) be more or less continent, (3) be capable of being easily closed when no longer needed and (4) be situated well away from the area later to be resected. These ends may be secured by a 3-stage procedure in which (1) a disconnecting anus is done and the entire area explored (Fig. 306), (2) the tumor or other lesion is resected, and (3) normal function is restored (Fig. 307). The details of the classic method are to be found in any standard surgical text and are not germane here; comment only is called for. This technic produces, during the first-stage operation, an anus fulfilling all the cited requirements and permitting of the long period of dysfunction which best serves the desired ends.

In this connection, however, it should be noted that where the treatment is planned for cure of malignancy, the defunctioning period cannot be extended to more than 3 weeks or a month, in contrast with the year or more that is practical and often desirable in some of the nonmalignant lesions. Yet, precisely because of this difference, the inflammatory conditions often yield far more dramatic results under such treatment than would be possible otherwise.

CLOSING THE ARTIFICIAL ANUS. In operations for eliminating the colostomy, thoroughly wash and irrigate the wound with copious amounts of soap and water (both before the operation is started and again when dissection is complete) followed by normal saline. Avoid strong antiseptics; depend on alcohol alone. Dissect back far enough extraperitoneally to permit closure in layers. Limit the number of sutures and knots. Use interrupted sutures of silk or cotton.

COLOSTOMY

Preoperative Considerations. When determining the advisability of producing a permanent colostomy, several considerations are of almost equal import. The first, naturally, is whether or not the patient's life would be jeopardized by something less radical than complete removal of the anorectal apparatus. This involves the second consideration, absolute certainty of diagnosis; has every available diagnostic aid been called into play, and do all the results point to the same conclusion? Unless the surgeon has had broad experience in this field, he would be well-advised to seek consultation with others more experienced than himself, because here, almost more than in any other field of medicine or surgery, the mental, emotional and economic, as well as the purely physical, future of the patient is involved. In practice, it may safely be said that one should *never* condemn the patient to spend the rest of his life with an abdominal anus until it is completely certain that the rectal disease is malignant in nature and incurable by any lesser procedure.

The third consideration is the method of attack to be employed. Whether the approach should be perineal, perineo-abdominal, abdominal or sacral depends on many factors that can be weighed only in the light of the surgeon's skill and experience. Each method has its advocates; at least a theoretic familiarity with all of them is a basic requirement.

Comment. Some aspects of the question of colostomy seem not to have been covered as thoroughly as might be in other texts, though the periodical literature offers much helpful advice. Dubois[6] says that a "colostomy is as uncertain as New England weather." What we consider as "normal home life" is actually pretty irregular and may lead to mechanical complications for the owner of a colostomy. He may be helped to deal with these difficulties by careful guidance in selecting his diet. He should be advised to avoid all rough or gas-forming foods such as cabbage. Also to be avoided, at least during the first few months, are raw fruits and vegetables, cocktail party foods and overeating of any kind. The French have a saying to the effect that a gourmand is never constipated—which, to a certain extent, is exactly what the owner of a colostomy must always strive to be.

In talking with the patient, never try to gloss over his problems but, at the same time, be as encouraging as possible with regard to his ability to live a normal life, physically, socially, even sexually. Emphasize these last, not only to the patient himself but also to his family. Teaching him to live with his colostomy takes time and patience but is an essential part of the surgeon's responsibility. Even before the dressings are removed, his lessons should begin. Let the patient become acquainted with the new apparatus and instruct him in its routine care and use. In connection with this last item, let me emphasize the importance of using the simplest devices possible (Fig. 308).

One of the most inspiring things I have encountered in this connection is an article by Secar,[21] herself the owner of a colostomy, in which she shows how successfully one may adjust to the complications and the problems involved and attain a life so completely normal that literally "no one knows" she has a colostomy, except those she had told in her continuing campaign to convey her own outlook to others in the same situation.

Marino et al[12] also offer some suggestions regarding the teaching of the patient. They

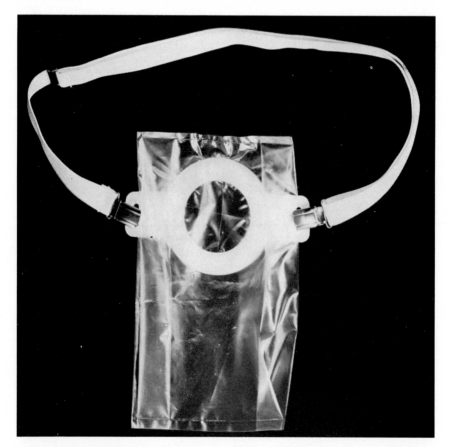

FIG. 308. A simple and effective permanent colostomy apparatus. This postoperative aid permits the use of a disposable pouch which is made in a number of sizes. The pouches are made of flexible material and adjust themselves closely to the shape and the contour of the abdomen. It is held in place by an adjustable band. The disposable feature following each use allows for cleanliness and the avoidance of dermatitis. (Marsan's Single Service Saf-T Pouch for colostomy patients, Colostomy Appliance Lab., Chicago, Ill.)

suggest telling him that the colostomy will shrink as time goes on and also emphasize that dietary indiscretions and emotional upsets will have the same effect on his digestion that they always had, except that the mechanical results may be far more unpleasant. Demonstrate to the patient that gentle manipulation of the colostomy opening is painless, even before healing is complete, and especially discourage him from demanding help in caring for it any longer than is absolutely necessary. Failure to observe this point will simply prolong his hospital stay and delay his return to society.

Marino also makes some useful suggestions regarding medication. For persistent looseness of bowels, give bismuth subcarbonate, 15 to 60 grains, with paregoric, 1 dram, t.i.d., before meals, or tincture of opium, 5 to 20 drops, t.i.d., before meals. If looseness still persists, rule out achylia gastrica; use dilute HCl, 20 to 60 drops, with 1 enseal pancreatin, t.i.d., before meals. Paregoric should be used only as a temporary measure. Habituation must be guarded against. Castor oil should be taken occasionally. When normal control has been established, close the enterostomy. Use a simple binder. Some patients like to use cellulose tape to fasten the dressing to the skin. More often they prefer the simpler open systems of control. Cellucotton dressings are inexpensive, disposable and odorless. Kaolin also reduces odor, as well as helping to solidify the fecal material. Marino also recommends enteric-coated capsules of activated carbon 90 per cent, plus phenylsalicylate 10 per cent. He adds that limiting intake of fish and eggs will reduce odor.

For a high stoma where liquid feces are unavoidable, Fox[7] recommends a new 5-piece device made chiefly of foam rubber and plastic which does away with many of the unpleasant problems produced by earlier, more cumbersome methods. This has the advantage of being nonirritating to the skin, since it uses no adhesive cement, of allowing earlier ambulation, of being easily cared for and inexpensive to buy and to maintain and, in general, contributing greatly to improved morale.

Operative Safeguards. In connection with the actual surgical production of the colostomy, a number of precautions should be taken. The fascia should be closed more loosely than the peritoneum; stricture may result from too tight suture of the anterior fascia to the skin. The entire blood supply of the distal portion of the colostomy may traverse an appendix epiploica. Extreme care should be exercised to avoid sacrificing the circulation of the terminal end of the bowel. The colostomy should be anchored to the parietal peritoneum and to the fascia to avoid having loops of bowel retract and possibly cause obstruction.

ANORECTAL SURGERY

GENERAL CONSIDERATIONS

Catharsis. The use of drastic purges prior to anorectal surgery is to be condemned because (1) the whole intestinal tract may be emptied so completely that it may be several days before the patient is again able to defecate and (2) an irritation may be set up which will cause a desire to defecate to remain for several hours, resulting in discomfort to the patient and soiling of the operative wound.

Anesthesia. It is axiomatic that there is no such thing as an ideal anesthetic material for any surgical procedure. In anorectal surgery, as anywhere else in the body, the best we can do is to arrive at some sort of compromise which will give us the optimum results.

The technics and the precautions in the use of various types of anesthesia have been covered in Chapter 2. Here, it is only necessary to say that certain types, while eminently suitable elsewhere, should be used with caution in the anorectal area. Sadove[19] favors certain of the new regional anesthetic agents, such as lidocaine, because (1) they act rapidly, giving more of a true anesthesia than mere analgesia, (2) they have a definite "spreading factor," (3) they cause only slight local irritation, and (4) they give approximately twice the duration of an equivalent strength of procaine. Sadove also speaks well of the relatively new "saddle-block" technic but cautions that it should be used with extreme care where there has been heavy premedication or if the individual is weak or a poor risk from any other cause. In spite of this, he feels that this method is relatively safe in experienced hands and has only one real disadvantage, that of postoperative headache in from 6 to 14 per cent of patients. He warns further, with regard to spinal anesthesia, that it is not a technic to be used lightly, i.e., the anesthetic equipment should be carefully checked ahead of time and asepsis maintained at an even higher level than is considered necessary for surgical instruments. Also, the patient so anesthetized should be watched closely; the level of anesthesia, the blood pressure, the pulse and the respiration should be checked every 5 minutes.

Further, Sadove says, "The ability to inject into the spinal canal does not constitute a knowledge of spinal anesthesia"! Also, keep at hand at all times oxygen, apparatus for administering artificial respiration and means for supporting blood pressure. This applies not only to spinal but also to all types of anesthesia. In short, equipment must be available for adequately combating the potential hazards of any and every anesthetic technic.

On the other hand, Schneider[20] feels that perianal infiltration is probably the safest, especially in elderly or debilitated persons. In a series of 357 patients, he used this method with satisfactory results in all types of anorectal procedures, both major and minor. Principal contraindications are the presence of active suppurative conditions and, possibly in some instances, the presence of severe hypertension, though the use of Cobefrin in place of Adrenalin may serve to minimize the hypertensive effects.

Postoperative Care. A number of important points regarding general care of the anorectal surgical patient should be mentioned. Fear of the first postoperative bowel movement can produce what is known as "fear constipation," even when a long-acting anesthetic has been used. Many persons are preconditioned to this fear by loose talk from the uninformed. This type of constipation is definitely harmful in that long-held stool becomes bulky and dry and, when finally passed, may damage the wound.

Mineral oil should be given on the night prior to the time when the first bowel movement is desired. However, too much oil will leak from the bowel and may cause pruritus. Moreover, mineral oil alone appears to slow the healing process. On the other hand, preparations including psyllium have a directly beneficial action because they exert an internal soothing effect, reducing the frequency of narrowing by stricture or stenosis in a manner that is better, easier and much more frequent than any form of digital manipulation could possibly be.

HEMORRHOIDS

Incidence. Hemorrhoids most frequently appear in persons in the second half of life and in pregnant women. In older persons, they are often of very long standing and frequently have been "treated" by a variety of inefficient or even dangerous home remedies. In the gravid female, they may appear for the first time and, with proper care, will disappear after parturition, recurring, if at all, only during some subsequent pregnancy. In the younger age groups, hemorrhoids are rare but not unknown. One case of verified acute, bleeding hemorrhoids has been reported in a little girl of 4, another in a boy just learning to walk. Both of these young patients were cured by routine surgery. In each case, a history of persistent constipation from birth was undoubtedly the predisposing factor, as is often the case with older patients. I mention these instances to show that it is unwise to discount the possibility of this condition when the signs point to it simply because the patient happens to be very young.

Preoperative Preparation. This is of especial importance before a hemorrhoidectomy. It is inconvenient, to say the least, to have an evacuation of the patient's bowels occur in the midst of surgery. Thorough preparation will help to avoid this accident, as will the introduction of a gauze pack high up in the rectum before beginning to operate. *Do not neglect to remove the pack at the end of operation.*

Operative Methods. There is no one "best" procedure; the choice rests with the individual surgeon. The best operation is the one with which the individual surgeon is most familiar. That procedure should be chosen which will promise the best long-range results in each individual case, i.e., the one which will remove the offending veins without causing subsequent stricture, cause no damage to surrounding tissues and not endanger the integrity of sphincteric control. Also, avoid leaving "anal tags"; these, while of no real

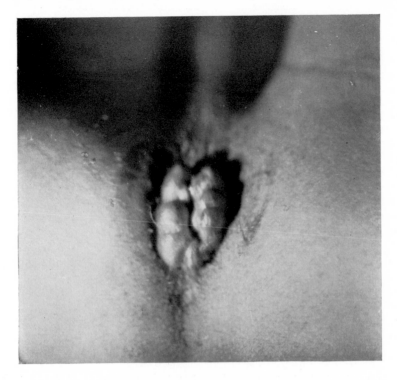

FIG. 309. This patient was operated on for external hemorrhoids and discharged as cured. A week later, the condition depicted here was revealed when the patient was asked to strain. *Always examine for internal hemorrhoids.*

importance, give the patient the impression that he still has hemorrhoids left by a careless surgeon, when he "has paid his good money" to get rid of them.

Injection. The injection of various sclerosing solutions is a method of treatment used by some. Personally, I am not favorably disposed toward it. Failures are frequent; disastrous results have followed injections. As a rule, permanent success is assured by adequate surgery.

Operative Precautions. ANESTHESIA. Either caudal or "saddle-block" anesthesia is most frequently favored at present. Be sure that the anesthetist is thoroughly competent and experienced, as untoward results can follow poor technic here as surely as after more serious operations. The same is true of the actual performance of whatever operative procedure has been chosen. In this connection is possibly the best place to repeat my firm belief that "there is no such thing as minor surgery—there are only minor surgeons."

Postoperative Complications. BOWEL MOVEMENTS. Do not be in too much haste to have the patient's bowels move after the operation. If there is no evacuation for a minimum of 3 days, the patient who has been properly prepared will not suffer systemically, and there will be much less pain and discomfort.

PAIN. Postoperatively, pain is often the most pressing problem. Long-acting local anesthetics are of help here. So also is preoperative mental preparation of the patient (see p. 5). If he can be helped to understand that spasm, pain and mental and physical tension form a "vicious circle," and that up-to-date methods will eliminate much of the anticipated suffering, he can often do a great deal in his own behalf during the first postoperative days. For intense pain, small doses of sedatives are indicated.

HEMORRHAGE. *Primary* hemorrhage usually comes from some small, oozing point that the surgeon had thought could be controlled by pressure or which was overlooked in an enfolding edge of mucous membrane. *Secondary* hemorrhage may result from straining, the slipping of a ligature or the separation of necrotic tissue during defecation. Under normal conditions, separation should occur between the eighth and twelfth days; if it occurs sooner, it may indicate local sepsis. Internal bleeding may remain unrecognized, owing to spasmodic contraction of the anal sphincters. Also, all bleeding from the rectum is not of hemorrhoidal origin. When in doubt, resort to thorough proctoscopic examination to eliminate the possibility of overlooking ulceration, fissure in ano, carcinoma (see p. 443) or other more serious conditions that otherwise might escape notice. Also, do not be satisfied that you have found all the trouble when external hemorrhoids have been eliminated. Careless or superficial diagnostic methods may miss internal hemorrhoids completely (Fig. 309).

OTHER POSTOPERATIVE COMPLICATIONS. If there is undue pain, or if fever develops, investigate; remove the sutures if necessary. Use every precaution, both preoperatively and postoperatively to avoid infection. Watch especially for *stitch abscess* and for abscesses following infection of *hematomata. Edema* of the skin sometimes follows when the operation has involved the mucocutaneous border, particularly if skin tags have been left. This condition can be very painful and a source of spasm of the anal sphincter that may delay healing. *Retention of urine* may occur not infrequently following hemorrhoidectomy; this is due to the intimate connections of the nerves of the contiguous structures.

FISTULA IN ANO

Of late, much more attention has been

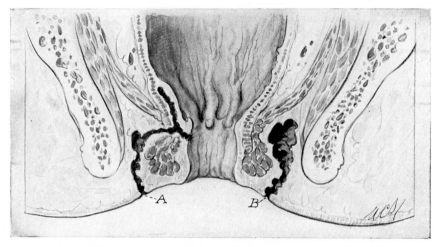

FIG. 310. Fistula in ano. (A) Complete fistula, with submucosal branch. (B) External, incomplete fistula. (After Drueck)

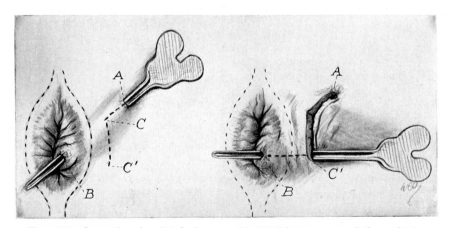

FIG. 311. Operation for fistula in ano. (*Left*) Director passed through sinus at A emerges at B. Skin incision exposes external sphincter at C, continuing along outer border to C'. (*Right*) Director moved to lie at right angles to muscle; incision continued onto internal orifice. (After Drueck)

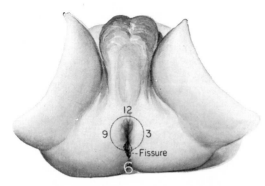

FIG. 312. Fissure in ano located at the 6 o'clock position (patient in lithotomy position). (Thorek, Philip: Surgical Diagnosis, Philadelphia, Lippincott)

given to the problem of fistulae in the anus than heretofore (Figs. 310 and 311). Several new methods were introduced to be used for surgical correction. Pain and fear of pain are among the most troublesome problems in most anorectal surgery.

Bell[1] and Ross[18] speak of the importance (long understood but still sometimes disregarded) of cutting the sphincters, where necessary, *at right angles to their long fibers.* If these fibers are cut obliquely, partial or complete incontinence may follow. The actual surgical procedures involved may be found detailed in standard surgical texts; however, certain precautions may need further emphasis. Be sure to open up fistulous tracts *completely.* In yielding to the occasional temptation to keep the wound small, remember that doing so may simply court further trouble at a later time. Operations for this condition fail often enough, for a variety of reasons beyond the control of the surgeon; there is certainly no need to *invite* complications by failure to expose *all* existing tracts if in any way possible.

Coughlin,[5] in a recent paper, sets up an excellent classification of these lesions, grouping them according to their origin and pointing to the specific surgical approach indicated for each. He also mentions the importance of keeping granulation tissue under control by curetting and of preventing all bridging or shelving. The drainage exit must be kept open, even if reincision is needed. He recommends use of a potassium permanganate solution in about a 1:8,000 strength as an irrigation after bowel actions.

Special care must be used in dealing with elderly patients and with those of limited mentality. Poor, slow healing can limit the success of the corrective procedure, while ignorance and superstition may prompt tampering that can undo even the most meticulous surgery.

Also, keep in mind that many such cases are tuberculous in origin. The lungs of every patient who consults the surgeon for this condition should be examined thoroughly. In discussing the treatment with the patient, he should be made to understand the possibility of failure and of the chance that further surgery may be needed later. To do so is to protect the patient from disappointment and the surgeon from legal complications in the occasional instance where treatment is unsuccessful.

FISSURE IN ANO AND ULCER

Fissure in ano is defined as a *painful linear ulcer* at the anal margin. The important word is "painful." As already indicated, so many nerves are concentrated at the anus that even the most trifling abrasion or interruption of the continuity of the anal mucosa is exquisitely painful, while the septic nature of the bowel ejections frequently cause infection of even the smallest crack, still further irritating the nerve tendrils of the anal tissue. Every bowel movement increases the anguish, until— if left untreated—sleep will be banished and the victim may be subjected to much suffering. In other parts of the body, a lesion so minor would cause little disturbance and certainly would never be considered for surgical treatment. But even the modern "wonder drugs" have failed to deal adequately with this condition, because each time the anal sphincter is stretched, the "crack" splits wide open, so that healing from below cannot take place without surgical assistance (Fig. 312).

Diagnosis. In this condition, diagnosis is easy, in fact, practically self-evident. However, there is considerable chance for error in selecting the proper method of treatment.

Anesthesia. General considerations on anesthesia for any procedure in the anal region have been given at the beginning of this section (p. 434). Anal fissures are usually seen in the elderly, many of whom have also been suffering for years from hemorrhoids or other painful conditions in the lower rectum and the anus. The surgeon and his anesthetist should do all in their power to allay the patient's fears and to reassure him as to the efficiency of the anesthetic to be used. One should not make the mistake of treating such a condition as unimportant; the anguish it can cause is out of all proportion to the dangers involved, making it, from the patient's point of view, a most painful affair.

Treatment. There are 3 ways of attacking this problem: (1) forcible dilatation, (2) incision and (3) a combination of the two, which is usually the best. *Forcible dilatation,* even under complete anesthesia, causes the patient at times such terror that it has largely been abandoned by modern proctologists. *Incision* should be done at the base of the ulcer, making the cut a little longer than the lesion itself. When the ulcer lies directly over the anterior or the posterior commissure, it is better to make a V-shaped cut at either one of these points. Better still, *curet* the entire floor of the ulcer (in addition to the cut) and, with curved scissors, trim away any overhanging edges. Search for *polyps,* which, when found, should be removed.

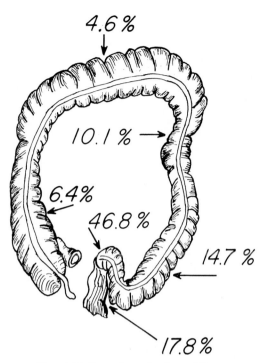

Fig. 313. Location of polyps. Diagram indicates the distribution of polyps found in 100 patients in this series. (Van Buskirk, W. C.: Ann. Surg. 141:234)

PROCTITIS

Inflammation in the anorectal region is usually a symptom rather than a clinical entity. The underlying cause should be determined and often will be found to be some inflammatory lesion in an adjacent area. If so, it would certainly be an error to treat the proctitis and neglect the real etiologic source, which may be in the pelvis or the prostate. Venereal infections or tuberculosis may be etiologic factors. In homosexual individuals, venereal disease is an especially likely source of trouble.

Proctoscopy. In examining this region with instruments, force should never be used. A diseased rectum may easily be perforated by the proctoscope. The result of such an accident may prove to be rapidly fatal unless surgical repair is instituted immediately.

RECTAL PROLAPSE

The standard operation for repair of prolapse of the rectum is that of Miles, devised in 1933. This operation is safe, technically simple and suitable for general application in cases of *complete* prolapse. However, special cases present special problems.

In *children,* eversion of the anal mucosa during defecation is physiologic; if it is repeated frequently, as in diarrhea or constipation, it may become exaggerated and the rectal mucosa start to protrude. Partial prolapse may also take place during attacks of childhood diseases or during any prolonged or wasting illness capable of reducing the supporting areolar tissue of the rectum and thus predisposing to the condition. Spontaneous cure is common.

In *adults,* partial prolapse is usually the result of confluent hemorrhoids or may appear as a sequel to Whitehead's operation or to repair of extensive anal fistulae. The only minor surgical procedure worth considering is Thiersch's operation;[24] in elderly patients, this is especially useful. In those better able to withstand major surgery, repair of the pelvic floor either from below or above, combined with obliteration of the pouch of Douglas, is the rational treatment. However, in the obese, middle-aged patient, the technical difficulties of such an operation are much increased. The difficulty confronting the surgeon is the choice and application of method to the wide range of patients who present themselves with this type of condition. Various methods of treatment are now available and are described in the texts on surgical technic. In desperate cases, in those patients who have already had one or more unsuccessful operations and are incontinent, a well-constructed colostomy may be the treatment of choice.

In those patients in whom radical surgery is contraindicated, the use of electrical stimulation of the sphincter may be tried.[15]

In my own experience, one other point stands out, namely, the importance of keeping in mind the fact that reduction of any prolapse of the anus must be accompanied by treatment of the sphincters. Sphincter exercises are of value here. Also, if cauterization is to be a part of the treatment, enough normal mucous membrane must be left between the cauterized areas to eliminate the possibility of stricture (see also below).

Complications. The possibility of stricture formation during the early postoperative period must not be forgotten. A finger should be passed on the seventh postoperative day and at weekly intervals thereafter until the suture line is completely healed (see also Hemorrhoids).

The bowels should be kept confined for at least 5 days, and on no account should an enema be given for fear of perforating the suture line. In females, the posterior vaginal wall may easily be damaged, resulting in formation of *rectovaginal fistula*. Should this occur, at times a temporary colostomy may be resorted to until repair has been completed. *Separation of the suture line* is not uncommon. *Secondary hemorrhage* may appear from 8 to 10 days after the operation.

Neoplasms

Polyps. Van Buskirk[25] states categorically that polypoid lesions are premalignant. Polypoid carcinoma is often associated with polyps elsewhere in the intestinal tract. In a series of 100 patients treated between 1946 and 1951, he reports that 78 per cent had lesions visible by sigmoidoscopy, while 11.5 per cent of the lesions were above the rectosigmoid junction. Thirty-five per cent had multiple polyps; 18 per cent of these could be detected digitally (Fig. 313). In 52 per cent, bleeding was a symptom, while 30 per cent were asympto-

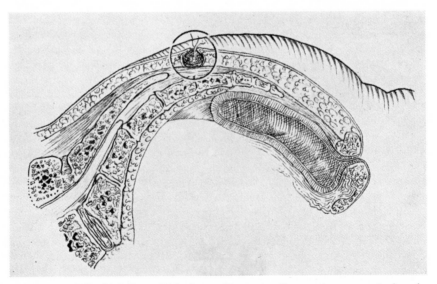

Fig. 314. Pilonidal Cyst. This figure illustrates the most common lesion, in which the pilonidal sinus opening connects with one or more subcutaneous cystic dilatations. The sinus opening may be single or multiple and is usually located in the region of the sacrococcygeal articulation. A small tuft of hair may project from the sinus opening, or is found in the cyst cavity during surgery. (Cantor, A. J.: Am. J. Proct. 3:321)

matic. "Rectal complaints" were not specific for polyps but were a general indication of serious trouble of some sort. The barium enema, while not always a reliable index, nevertheless is the best source of information available to us thus far, particularly when one resorts to a double contrast enema. Routine early eradication of polyps would notably reduce the incidence of rectal carcinoma. This should be done thoroughly. If the polyps are multiple, the whole affected segment of the colon should be removed. If the base of a polyp is cancerous, this is also an indication for removal of the whole affected segment of bowel. Also, prolonged follow-up for recurrence is important.

In removing a solitary rectal polyp, the pedicle should always be ligated first. Attempts to remove a polyp by curettage may be followed by hemorrhage. If this accident occurs, the sphincter should be dilated, the bleeding point secured immediately, and blood transfusions should follow.

As indicated previously, bleeding is an outstanding symptom of polyps in the sigmoid. Moderate obstruction may also be present. In addition to the barium enema, sigmoidoscopy and contrast air studies should establish the

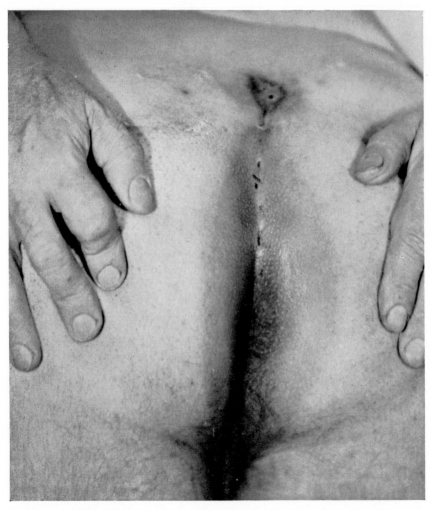

Fig. 315. Pilonidal cyst with 7 cutaneous openings. Several previous attempts at operative cure had failed; dissection en bloc was followed by prompt recovery.

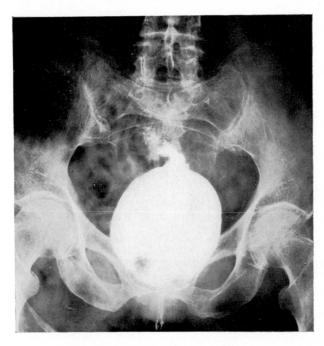

Fig. 316. Obstruction at sigmoid flexure caused by band of adhesions. Preoperative diagnosis was carcinoma. (See Fig. 281, *right*.)

diagnosis. Large polyps in this area should not be removed by fulguration through the sigmoidoscope because of the danger of hemorrhage or perforation and because of technical difficulties. Resort should be had to sigmoidostomy, with yearly follow-ups for at least 5 years by sigmoidoscopy and contrast enema to be alert for the possibility of malignancy.

PILONIDAL CYST

Fistula or Sinus? In dealing with conditions in what is generally called the perianal region, exact delimitations cannot be drawn. The best we can do is to include all those affections which are, can or may be directly connected with the anus or the rectum. Hill[8] of the Mayo Clinic gives an excellent résumé and classification of such lesions, with special emphasis on pilonidal disease but also including such related problems as comedo, sebaceous cyst, furunculosis, hidradenitis suppurativa, dermoid cyst of the sacrum or the coccyx, infection of Bartholin's glands in females and osteomyelitis. He draws a distinction between the "fistula" which connects with the lumen of the anus or the rectum and the "sinus" which, while located within the general confines of the perianal region, does not so connect. The treatment of all these conditions,

whether early or advanced, is usually surgical.

The cause of most nonfistulous sinuses in the perianal region is evident in the history, the physical examination, the pathologic findings or all three. Sometimes, however, the exact nature of the condition is not evident on microscopic examination because the infection has destroyed the tissues involved. On occasion, it may be necessary to study extensive sinuses radiologically after injection with radiopaque substances. For our purposes here, suffice it to say that, as in the case of fistula in ano, when the conditions call for surgical intervention, the chief precaution is to be sure that the entire tract is cleared out completely (Figs. 314 and 315).

CARCINOMA

In spite of all the good work that has been done by such organizations as the American Cancer Society toward making the public "cancer conscious" and familiar with the early signs of development of this disease, it is still practically axiomatic that patients with carcinoma of the lower bowel all too often consult us only when they are already beyond help! We know that when recognized early, surgery offers a fairly good prognosis; we can

FIG. 317. Spasm consequent to inflammation, causing filling defect simulating carcinoma of bowel.

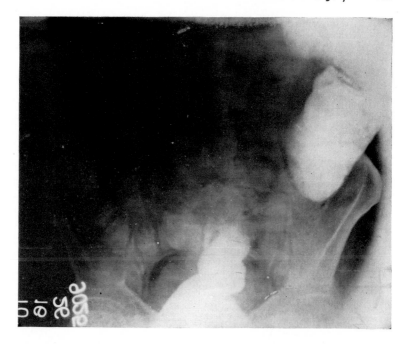

only hope that continuing and improving public education will bring these patients to us in ever-increasing numbers soon enough for success.

As suggested earlier in this section, if there is sudden development of hemorrhoids or other acute symptoms referable to the anorectal area, as well as of "sciatica" without an ascribable cause, the patient should be given a thorough proctologic examination with the thought of possible malignancy well in mind. Patients previously treated for hemorrhoids alone and inadequately examined furnish the greatest number of cases of inoperable carcinoma of the rectum!

Differential Diagnosis. In earlier editions of this work I said, "Never be cocksure about the diagnosis of rectal carcinoma" unless there has been definite corroborative microscopic evidence. *This bears repeating*. Several other diseases may simulate carcinoma of the bowel (Figs. 316 and 317). Inflammatory conditions may produce what appear radiographically to be typical "filling defects." Leukoplakia also can deceive even the wary, on occasion (Fig. 318). Further, endometriosis may be mistaken for carcinoma and resection done for a cancer which does not exist—truly a tragedy! Both proctoscopy and biopsy should always be used.

BIOPSY. An interesting new biopsy technic has been introduced recently and is aptly called "sponge biopsy." This involves using a sponge ½ inch square by ⅛ inch thick cut from Onkasponge No. 1 or Gelfoam No. 12, which is touched to the cleansed surface of the suspected lesion and then processed in the laboratory in the same manner as a block of tissue.

INDICATIONS. It has been well said that "every patient who has any type of bowel disturbance should be examined as a potential sufferer from carcinoma of the colon until proven otherwise" (Reynolds), though common sense dictates that this be modified to eliminate those in whom age, general health and the trivial nature of the complaint make this obviously inapplicable. (Even here one may be deceived. Witness a recent case of an elderly woman, apparently in good health, who suffered an attack of "indigestion" and died *5 days later* of an inoperable carcinoma of the lower bowel. The only prior finding was a loss of some 20 pounds during the preceding 6 months, for which no physician had been consulted.)

Familiar as the general signs of carcinoma of the bowel are—or should be—it can do no harm to list them once again:

Change of bowel habit

Alternating constipation and diarrhea

Sudden, apparently complete obstipation of several days' duration

Rectal bleeding

Hemorrhoids

A subjective sense of inadequate emptying of the bowel after stool

Urgency to defecate, but with inability to produce stool

Unexplained anemia

Obesity. For some reason, cancerous growths seem to spread more rapidly in persons who are markedly overweight. The obese patient also poses another problem; there is sometimes a temptation to attempt an end-to-end anastomosis deep in the pelvis for the sake of expediency. This is extremely trying and dangerous and may result in resecting a too short length of bowel and an inadequate amount of surrounding tissue for the particular situation. In such patients, abdominoperineal resection is a more thorough, more effective and less dangerous procedure.

Choice of Operation. Opinions vary widely as to the best method to be used for extirpation of the lower bowel. Quite possibly, here as elsewhere, there is no one "best" method (see also under Colostomy, p. 432). Some years ago, figures from certain European clinics appeared to indicate that mortality dropped from 31.4 per cent for a single-stage procedure to 5.9 per cent for a 2-stage operation. The introduction of chemotherapy and of additional types of operations in recent years undoubtedly has somewhat changed this picture. Perusal of the current periodical literature appears to indicate a trend away from the older, multiple-stage procedures to correspond to the more radical and extensive resections that are also gaining in favor.

Neal *et al*[16] have had good success, in a small series (unselected), with an extremely radical departure in the form of a 2-team technic which accomplishes somewhat the same ends as the more conventional 2-stage operations but completes all surgery at one time. They claim to have obtained better results with less postoperative shock, less chance of recurrence and, most important, *no mortality.* A large proportion of their patients, having carcinoma of the rectum, had multiple neoplastic lesions, often malignant, proximal to the primary growth. A left hemicolectomy permits wide en bloc removal of lymph-bearing tissue, avoids necrosis and left-gutter herniation and also allows wider removal of cancer-prone areas of the colon.

Various other technics, some of them "classic" (in the sense that they have proved to be satisfactory in many hands over long periods

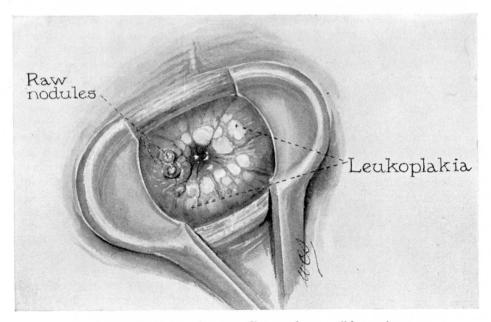

Fig. 318. Leukoplakia of rectum diagnosed as possible carcinoma.

of time) and some relatively new and radical, may be found described in any standard textbook of surgery. The chief point to remember here is that the procedure chosen should be the one which experience indicates will give the best results in the available hands and under the existing conditions.

Operability. Operability of a carcinoma of the rectum depends chiefly on (1) its regional fixation and (2) whether or not there is metastasis and, if so, its extent. When a tumor is fixed, operability is doubtful and failure or recurrence probable. Similarly, extensive metastases render such growths inoperable. A study of Figure 302 will serve to demonstrate the rich lymphatic supply of this area, indicating the complexity of the problem of metastasis. When the lesion is located high in the rectum, its operability often can be determined only by exploratory laparotomy. From observations on a series of 122 patients, ranging in age from 4 to 79, Judd and Burleigh[9] conclude that this type of lesion remains a problem of management and state that the "record is not brilliant." Local excision should be avoided except in very rare instances. They feel that the enthusiasm for treatment by radium and x-ray is unwarranted and has often led to loss of valuable time. Poor survival statistics for "early" radical operations are due, they believe, to the fact that actually most of these were performed *too late;* if they were truly done "very early," satisfactory results should usually follow. Theoretically, radical resection with bilateral dissection of the inguinal lymph nodes should give a good prognosis; in practice, there is too little verified evidence to bear this out. Some patients apparently have been cured without it, while, in their experience, none with proved inguinal involvement, has survived for 5 years.

Operative Precautions. The first step in operation for removal of a carcinoma of the rectum is establishment of a colostomy. This may be located in the suture line in a left rectus incision. Experience has shown that a midline colostomy may get in the patient's way, especially in younger persons who are still sexually active. Anchor the colostomy to the parietal peritoneum, as well as to the fascia, to avoid loops of bowel slipping in later and becoming obstructed.

It is desirable to remove all genital organs from females, unless urgently contraindicated by youth or some other consideration, since it makes the balance of the procedure simpler, and genital carcinoma is frequently associated with carcinoma in the colon or the rectum.

Berman[2] summarizes the precautions to be taken to avoid complications as follows:

A. Be certain of the preoperative diagnosis and rule out endometriosis.

B. Avoid postoperative intestinal obstruction (the most common complication) by:
   1. Proper placing of the colostomy and suturing of colon to peritoneum and fascia
   2. Meticulous peritonealization of pelvic diaphragm and at times converting a female type of pelvis to a male pattern

C. Dissection of rectum to levator ani

D. Complete visualization of both ureters

E. In the perineal part of the operation, the bowel must be pulled down with clamps rather than the hand inserted up in the pelvis.

Whenever possible, avoid opening the rectum, thus reducing the chance of contamination; if it be opened accidentally, close it again at once. Some surgeons recommend ligating the bowel on either side of the site of resection before beginning this part of the procedure to prevent possible forcing of cancerous material into healthy sections of the lumen. Every routine precaution against infection must be observed (e.g., exact and adequate suturing; use of suitable chemotherapy). Avoid interfering with the blood supply of the proximal segment of bowel; this can only be accomplished through a thorough prior familiarity with the anatomy of the circulation of the entire region. Be especially careful not to injure the genito-urinary system; catheters placed in the ureters help to locate and protect them during extirpation of the rectum. Be equally sure to avoid both injury to the sacral plexus and infection of the dural canal. Also, the strictest hemostasis should be observed. Drainage should always be instituted. As a further precaution, the whole colon should be examined before completing the procedure. About 4 per cent of patients will be found to have additional *primary* lesions elsewhere in the area; multiple primary malignancies of the same or a *different sort* may coexist. It should also be noted that metastasis to the liver does not necessarily render the lesion in-

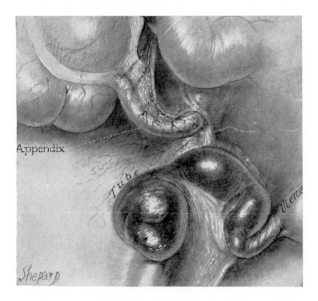

FIG. 319. Torsion of fallopian tube simulating appendicitis. Note thickening of surrounding structures.

operable, since removal of the primary growth has a tendency to retard development of metastases. Small localized metastases in the liver may be removed by partial hepatectomy.

ABDOMINAL EMERGENCIES

We come now to that linguistic abomination, the "acute abdomen," used by the indolent as a convenient dumping place for any and all abdominal affections that are in some way difficult to classify accurately. It is no more concise to speak of an "acute abdomen" than it would be to refer to a "chronic nose" or a "subacute great toe"! Nevertheless, there is a general group of acute conditions, of which the most important is appendicitis, which can and should be considered together for a number of reasons. This group includes, besides appendicitis, ruptured ectopic pregnancy, perforated gastric ulcer, twisted ovarian pedicle, torsion of the fallopian tube (Fig. 319), volvulus of the stomach, hemorrhages of pelvic origin, torsion of the omentum and certain renal and biliary conditions, as well as some other affections sufficiently rare to be disregarded unless all more likely situations have been eliminated. Some of these are considered in detail in other sections of this work; the rest will be discussed in the pages that follow.

Because several of the acute conditions occurring within the abdominal cavity have a disconcerting habit of simulating one another, it is necessary, in this discussion, to be somewhat repetitive in the various sections on differential diagnosis. The reader is asked to bear this in mind, especially when confronted with some symptom complex exhibiting these confusing similarities.

In avoiding catastrophe, two factors are of the utmost and equal importance: *time* and *intervention*, i.e., early diagnosis and, where indicated, prompt intervention. As we have already observed (p. 376), in *gastroduodenal perforations*, the hopefulness of the prognosis is in direct proportion to the promptness of surgical intervention. In this, they differ from some cases of *appendicitis*, where delay is permissible under certain conditions. Nevertheless, in appendicitis also, intervention at the earliest possible moment should be the rule.

A study of the frequency of different acute abdominal conditions discloses that appendicitis is still by far the most frequent, even though mortality figures for this affection, especially since the advent of the "wonder drugs," have fallen to a commendably low level. To avoid errors, certain points must be observed routinely, viz., careful and detailed history taking, proper evaluation of symptoms, good surgical technic and adequate preoperative and postoperative care. Differential diagnosis is also extremely important, because, as previously indicated, so many acute abdominal conditions may mimic one another. In order of frequency, these conditions may be listed as:

Acute appendicitis
Acute intestinal obstruction
Perforated gastric ulcer
Ruptured ectopic pregnancy
Acute pancreatitis
Mesenteric occlusion
Perforation of intestinal malignancy
Perforated diverticulum
Perforation of Meckel's diverticulum

DIAGNOSIS

Muscular Rigidity. This indicates irritation of the parietal peritoneum and the subserous tissues and is caused by a motor-sensory reflex, the result of infection. It is always indicative of peritonitis. *Palpation* should proceed methodically, should be superficial only and be performed with warm hands. Rigidity, if elicited, must be correlated with other existing signs. The *degree,* the *location* and the *extent* of resistance are all indicative. In cases of pelvic origin, such as retrocecal appendicitis, rigidity is less marked. In hemorrhagic pancreatitis, in intestinal obstruction and in hematogenous peritonitis of blood-borne infections it may or may not be present at all. Neither is it constant in typhoid perforation. In cases of gangrene of the appendix or of the gallbladder, as well as in ruptured extrauterine pregnancy, it is usually absent.

Pain. This is an important sign in all acute abdominal conditions. The onset, the source and the character of the pain are all of diagnostic significance. Bear in mind that pain does not always localize in the area that is actually affected.

In appendicitis the pain almost always begins in the epigastrium or in the umbilical region, localizing in the lower right quadrant only later on when the pathologic involvement of the appendix is already well established, indicating the need for immediate treatment. *Never give sedatives* until the diagnosis is firmly established!

Pain in the shoulder is frequently observed in perforation of gastroduodenal ulcer and in ruptured ectopic pregnancy; this last is also often accompanied by sudden, acute pain in the lower abdomen, sometimes particularly marked in the right iliac fossa, often radiating into the flank, the epigastrium and the hypo-

chondrium. In neglected cases, there may also be pain in the chest.

Distention. This is one of the most important signs in the diagnosis of acute intestinal ailments. However, if it is absent, especially following trauma, one should never conclude that operative intervention may be delayed. It is also an error, and one which may prove to be fatal, to think that distention, which is a reflex of irritation of the peritoneal structure, is the result of infection.

Hemorrhage. Progressive intra-abdominal hemorrhage is always indicated by acute anemia, but one *should not wait for this,* because it often apepars only when it is too late for successful intervention. Ruptured extrauterine pregnancy may cause serious intra-abdominal hemorrhage; however, in this particular condition, death seldom follows, as there may be spontaneous hemostasis. This should not be relied on, however, as bleeding may reappear days or even weeks later, with fatal results. The same is true of injuries to the spleen, the liver or the kidneys resulting from trauma. Because bleeding has ceased, the surgeon should not be lulled into unwariness; cases have been reported of severe secondary hemorrhage as much as a month after symptoms appeared to have subsided.

Other Signs. Giddiness, accelerated pulse rate (slight or extreme), increased respiration, nausea and vomiting and metrorrhagia are other signs particular to ruptured ectopic pregnancy which are of assistance in distinguishing it from appendicitis. The abdomen will usually be sensitive but not necessarily distended. A zone of dullness indicates profuse hemorrhage.

Errors in Diagnosis. Diagnostic errors among the conditions mentioned here may not be as serious as might appear at first, because the true condition, whether it be gastric or duodenal perforation, twisted ovarian pedicle, torsion of the fallopian tube or whatever, usually requires immediate laparotomy in any event; the error will be manifest when the abdomen has been opened and can be promptly corrected.

APPENDICITIS

GENERAL CONSIDERATIONS

Though much has been learned and enormous strides made in lowering the mortality

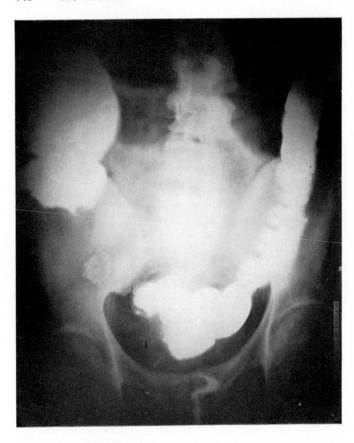

Fig. 320. Barium enema given this patient with suspected appendicitis caused perforation of appendix, followed by fatal peritonitis.

from acute appendicitis in the past 2 decades, so that percentagewise we appear to "have the situation well in hand," the actual figures are not so rosy. Some 65,000 persons still die each year in this country alone from this condition, *most of them needlessly!*

Mistakes and delays in diagnosis still stand at the head of the list of causes for this waste of human life; improper or inadequate treatment and ill-advised delay come close behind (Fig. 320). Too much or too protracted use of antibiotics and chemotherapy, which may mask some of the symptoms, can also be blamed for some fatalities and much morbidity. *If antibiotics fail to reduce symptoms promptly, they should be discontinued.* Also, the two following special areas merit thought.

1. In the elderly (in this connection, persons of 40 or over), symptoms may be masked by the general slowing up of all bodily functions. Conditions which will "come to a head" in a matter of hours in young persons may take days to arrive at the same state in older patients. Definitive signs, such as abdominal

rigidity, may be reduced or absent because of flaccid muscles or layers of fat. Systemic reactions to infectious or suppurative processes may be less marked and slower to develop. By the same token, resistance to such processes may also be reduced and the danger and the incidence of peritonitis proportionately increased. Pain may be less severe, and apparently unrelated symptoms such as headache, backache, malaise, hiccup and rectal bleeding may mislead the unwary. The existence of some concurrent disease may confuse the picture further. Boyce[4] cites an aphorism to the effect that it is "most unsafe to have an acute illness in a hospital while undergoing treatment for a nonacute disease" and quotes deTarnowsky's warning not to pay too much attention to a previous history of organic disease in older persons suspected of acute appendicitis. The list of cases of mistaken diagnosis in the elderly is "monumental"; the fact that the observed conditions often prompt a leisurely diagnostic routine indicates how mild the whole symptom complex may some-

Fig. 321. Polypoid tumor of ileum simulating appendicitis. (Actual size of tumor about one half that shown.)

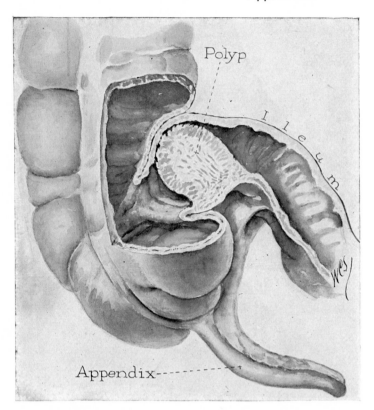

times be and helps to explain why there are *5 times* as many instances of wrong diagnosis in cases of appendicitis in the elderly as there are in the young. With these older patients, the single most useful diagnostic aid is to *remember the possibility* of this condition. It is well to remember that *prompt operation is more important* for them than for the young.

2. In cases of appendicitis in young children, the mistake is sometimes made of thinking that because the sick child sleeps fitfully, operation may safely be delayed. *Never think it!* He is simply sleeping from sheer exhaustion. Experience in one series of 118 cases showed that more than half had developed peritonitis by the time they came to operation, and this in spite of the fact that most were operated on within 24 hours of becoming ill!

Still another point is worth noting; lower abdominal pain, usually one of the most definitive signs, can itself sometimes lead one astray. In females, especially adolescents, the pain of developing appendicitis may be mistaken for menstrual "cramps" if it happens to coincide in time with the monthly "period" and if such cramps are a common experience with the particular individual.

DIFFERENTIAL DIAGNOSIS

In order to avoid the dangers of wrong diagnosis, the surgeon must be thoroughly conversant with every contingency that may arise and be prepared to meet it adequately. Though it may truly be said that there is no such thing as a "typical" case of appendicitis, the usual picture should be kept well in mind. As a rule, the onset is described by the patient as an "upset stomach" with abdominal pain, either general or localized in the umbilical area. This will be followed by anorexia and, usually, nausea and vomiting. In 12 to 24 hours or longer (see above), the pain will localize in the right lower abdominal quadrant. During this time, the blood picture (leukocytosis) also will become characteristic, though this sign alone should never be deemed conclusive; it is of value only when considered in connection with all other clinical manifestations.

Simulation of Other Conditions. The ability

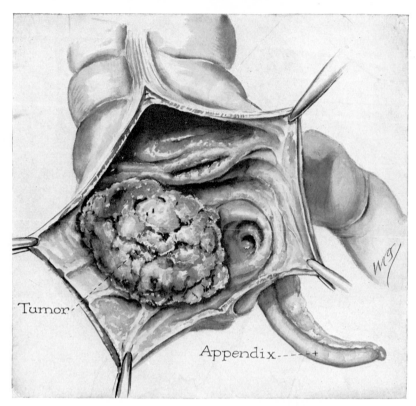

FIG. 322. Carcinoma of cecum simulating appendicitis.

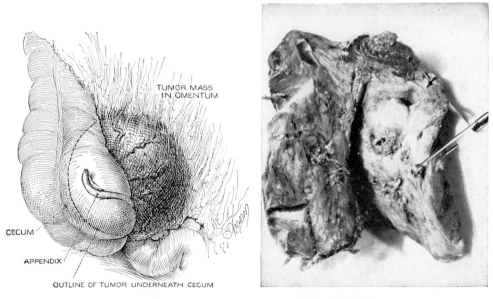

FIG. 323. Leiomyoma of greater omentum diagnosed preoperatively as appendicitis. (*Left*) Shows tumor in situ. (*Right*) Operative specimen opened down the middle.

FIG. 324. Ileocecal tuberculosis diagnosed as chronic appendicitis.

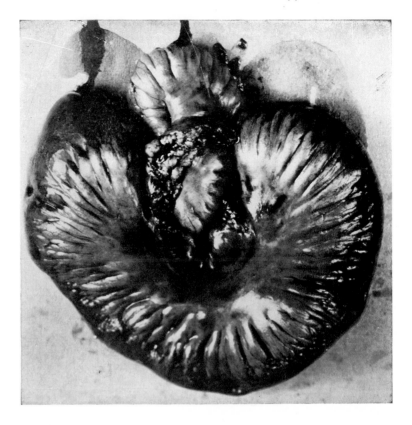

of the various acute abdominal conditions to simulate one another has already been pointed out (Figs. 321-324). Every surgeon of experience has seen instances of this. No one symptom, nor even any one limited group of symptoms, may safely be thought of as being pathognomonic of acute appendicitis or, for that matter, of any of the several other conditions as listed on p. 447. In *children*, errors of diagnosis are particularly likely to occur, being most frequent in girls between the ages of 4 and 10. In *pregnant women*, diagnosis also may be difficult; the gravid uterus may push the right colon upward and outward so that, under these circumstances, pain and tenderness never localize in the usual area. In this connection, it should be noted that (1) pregnancy or even tubal pregnancy does not necessarily contraindicate operation for acute appendicitis, and (2) when operating on a pregnant patient, the initial incision should be made not at some arbitrary "classic" location but rather *over the point of maximum tenderness*.

The prodromal stages of concurrent acute infection or contagious disease may confuse the picture still further, as may a pre-existing hernia. Mucocele of the appendix may simulate or complicate appendicitis.

Many erroneous diagnoses could be eliminated by more careful examinations, but a certain number of cases will continue to come to operation which do not reveal the condition preoperatively diagnosed. When the patient has shown the classic picture of acute appendicitis, yet the appendix appears normal at operation, it is advisable to explore the distal 2 feet of the ileum, not only for possible Meckel's diverticulum, but also for a regional ileitis (which is found most often in the distal portion of the ileum) (Fig. 325). Also, this is probably as good a place as any to mention an observation made recently by an English woman surgeon to the effect that "the small intestine is approximately 22 feet long, as any medical student can tell you because he read it in his anatomy texts," when as an actual matter of fact, the small intestine may be as short as 11 or 12 feet in a small woman to as long as 28 or 30 feet in a large man, a detail

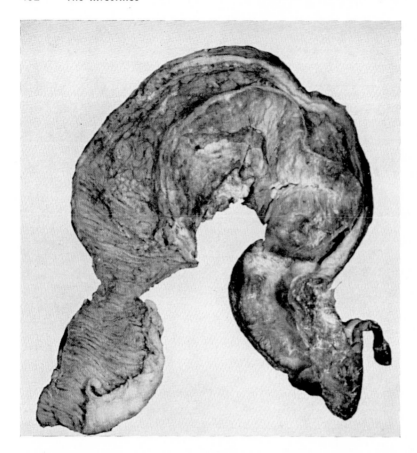

Fig. 325. Regional ileitis involving distal 18 cm. of ileum. Note sharp line of demarcation between involved and uninvolved areas. Intestinal wall much thickened and of firm consistency; superficial ulcers in mucosa.

which could spell the difference between life and death for the patient in some operative procedures!

SEMINAL VESICULITIS. When acute, seminal vesiculitis may also present symptoms confusingly similar to those of appendicitis. Detailed and accurate evaluation of the urologic and possible venereal history of any patient with doubtful symptoms is well worthwhile. Also, it is unwise to perform an appendectomy without first making a thorough rectal examination; fears of rupturing an abscess are practically groundless. If the seminal vesicles are involved, the spermatic cord will commonly be quite sensitive, even if not actually painful, and epididymitis of varying degree may be present. Pass the examining finger up along the median sulcus of the prostate until its upper border is reached, then out to the extreme end, where the seminal vesicle is most often found. A large thumblike, or even sausagelike, mass will indicate a diseased condition of the vesicle. If there is inflammation, there will

usually be much pain, swelling and exquisite tenderness. It has been estimated that chronic prostatitis and vesiculitis occur in some degree in nearly a third of all adult males, with only about two thirds of these showing a history of antecedent gonorrhea. Common causes of *nonspecific prostatitis* are infections of teeth, tonsils and nasal sinuses. A satisfactory procedure for determining the presence of these types of infection is to examine under the microscope the secretion obtained after massage of the prostate with the bladder empty. Failure to obtain any secretion is indicative of trouble, not of a lack of trouble, as is commonly believed. Such chronic infections frequently "light up" into an acute condition often suggestive of appendicitis.

Other conditions less frequently found but still to be considered in doubtful cases include lead colic, tabetic crisis, encephalitis lethargica, atheroma of the abdominal vessels, acidosis, spinal caries, disease of the right hip joint and pyelitis with other renal conditions arising in pregnancy. When symptoms are mild and haste is apparently not indicated, the patient should, nevertheless, be kept under close observation.

I still feel that the patient's own story may be more enlightening than even the most exhaustive laboratory and other tests. Actually, in my own experience, one sign that is more constant than any other is *anorexia,* though this is seldom stressed—in fact, is often not mentioned at all—in textbook discussions of the "classic picture" of appendicitis.

Fever. Never say, "This cannot be appendicitis because the fever is so low." It is not unusual, in the early stages, for the patient with appendicitis to have *no fever at all.* Because the acute inflammation begins on the mucous membrane side, there will be little or no elevation of temperature until the suppurative process reaches the serosa, when increasing fever indicates peritoneal involvement.

Location of Pain. "McBurney's point" is something that sticks more in the mind of the laity today. We prefer to ask the patient himself to show us "where it hurts the most," as he is not prejudiced by prior knowledge and will localize far more accurately than we are likely to do.

Rectal Examination. This must never be omitted, especially in children.

Location of Appendix. Regardless of what may have been stated in the medical-school texts, there is no "classic" location for the appendix, even when it is not diseased. The most dangerous type of appendicitis and, in our experience, the *most common* is that involving an appendix located *retrocecally.* Oftentimes, when so placed, it will produce no rectal tenderness and no muscular rigidity in the lower right quadrant. When the preoperative diagnosis has been definite and the offending organ does not immediately come into view, look for it first behind the cecum; 8 or 9 out of every 10 appendices will be found there.

Obstruction. To digress for a moment, let me remind the reader that appendicitis is, in the last analysis, a condition involving *obstruction* and, in many respects, should be treated as such. By the same token, it often accompanies or complicates obstruction from some other source, occurring in neighboring portions of the bowel. In the same way, inflammation in the appendix may be the causal factor behind obstruction in adjacent areas. Cases have been reported in which *carcinoma of the cecum* (which often gives no early signs) has produced directly or been accompanied by inflammation of the appendix. In fact, since more than half of all cases of appendicitis involve obstruction of the lumen of the appendix, the combination, according to Miller,[14] in theory should be more common than the reported cases appear to indicate. At operation, the appendix may have disappeared completely in the abscess. Three factors mitigate against the recognition of the presence of carcinoma of the cecum as an underlying process in acute appendicitis:

1. The neoplastic process may be mistaken for the induration of the cecal wall which is often present in acute appendicitis.

2. It is not considered good surgical judgment to explore extensively in the presence of an acute inflammatory process.

3. Our preconceived ideas about the age distribution of the two conditions may make us less likely to suspect their coexistence.

Trauma. Though not reported too often, there appear to be enough authenticated cases of traumatic appendicitis to make it advisable to keep this possibility in mind. Boys and young men, by virtue of their work and play habits, are especially likely victims of traumatic injuries in the lower abdomen, which can either light up a pre-existing chronic condition or, by violently forcing feces and gas into the lumen of the appendix, bring on distention and changes in the tissues, which, in turn, encourage the onset of infection and inflammation.

Torsion of the Omentum. Special mention might be made of this somewhat rare condition because it may be indistinguishable, preoperatively, from acute appendicitis, and its results, if uncorrected, can be equally lethal. However, exact differential diagnosis is often a matter of academic interest only, since the important point to be recognized is that *some* grave condition exists which calls for immediate surgical intervention. To delay in such circumstances over hairsplitting diagnostic procedures would be no help to the patient and no credit to the surgeon. Torsion of the omentum, as well as most of the other condi-

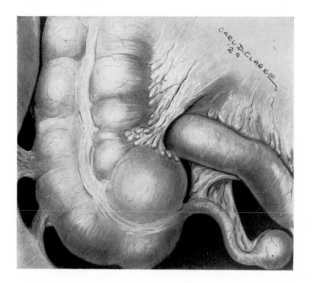

FIG. 326. Carcinoid tumor of appendix. (After Wilmoth)

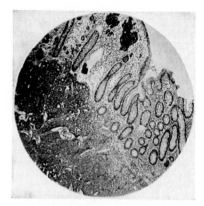

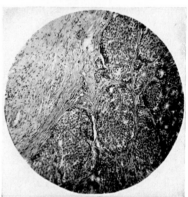

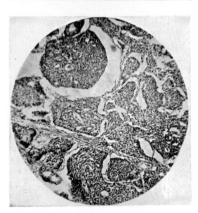

tions already mentioned as being potential sources of confusion, does call for immediate laparotomy; often correct preoperative diagnosis is little more than a fortunate guess.

Other Rare Conditions. Only mention need be made of other rare conditions simulating acute appendicitis. These include, among others, tumor of the ileum, malignant disease of the cecum, primary omental infarction and primary tumors in the greater omentum or elsewhere (Figs. 326 and 327).

OPERATIVE CONSIDERATIONS

The operative procedure of appendectomy is truly "classic," even though the condition it serves to correct is not. Again, it need only be said that the technic may be found in any standard surgical text. However, certain specific comments do appear to be in order. Massie and Vance,[13] in a recent paper, make one point which may be missed precisely by virtue of the "classic" nature of the treatment. In a series of 87 cases of perforated appendicitis occurring in the last 5 years, they used *drainage* routinely and had practically no complications. They believe that drainage should always be instituted, especially if the surgeon knows himself to have no more than average skill and experience. Opponents of routine drainage say that it is manifestly impossible to drain the whole peritoneal cavity. This is true, but it is also true that it *is* possible to cover the small but most vital area;

FIG. 327. (*Top*) Carcinoid tumor of appendix. Tumor cells chiefly in submucous layer, but invading mucosa. (*Center*) Typical arrangement of carcinoid cells in submucosa and muscularis of appendix. (*Bottom*) Typical carcinoid cells arranged in clumps. (After Wilmoth)

therefore, drainage is definitely indicated when the existing situation is in any way doubtful. Massie further states his firm conviction that improved postoperative care and the use of antibiotics are *not contraindications for applying the sound principles of surgery as first advanced by Yates in 1905*.

REFERENCES

1. Bell, R. H.: Management of common ano-rectal conditions with special emphasis on prevention of pain, Am. Surgeon 19:382, 1953.
2. Berman, H., and Mainella, F. S.: Complications and pitfalls of abdominoperineal resections, Am. J. Proc. 3:282, 1952.
3. Berry, R. E. L.: Diagnosis and treatment of acute intestinal obstruction, J.A.M.A. 148:347, 1952.
4. Boyce, F. F.: Special problems of acute appendicitis in middle and late life, A.M.A. Arch. Surg. 68:296, 1954.
5. Coughlin, B. D.: Anorectal fistulas; anatomic classification and principles of treatment, Am. J. Surg. 88:768, 1954.
6. Dubois, E. C.: Hints on the management of a colostomy, Am. J. Nursing, 55:71, 1955
7. Fox, J. D., and Bush, B. E.: A new ileostomy-colostomy device with disposable plastic bags and no cement, J.A.M.A. 156:1398, 1954.
8. Hill, J. R.: Infections and sinuses other than fistulas in the perianal region, Am. J. Surg. 88:829, 1954.
9. Judd, E. S., and Burleigh, E. deT., Jr.: Squamous-cell carcinoma of the anus; results of treatment, Surgery 37:220, 1955.
10. Laden, P.: Mesenteric vascular occlusion, J. Internat. Coll. Surgeons 22:598, 1954.
11. Maingot, R.: Abdominal Operations, ed. 3, New York, Appleton, 1955.
12. Marino, A. W. M., Caliendo, A. J., and Marino, M., Jr.: Modern management of colostomy, South. M. J. 47:1172, 1954.
13. Massie, J. R., and Vance, J.: Treatment of perforated appendix, Am. Surgeon 20:1194, 1954.
14. Miller, C., and Wooldridge, B. F.: Acute appendicitis with abscess formation as complication of carcinoma of the cecum, Am. J. Surg. 88:500, 1954.
15. Morel, J.-J.-Y.: Traitement du prolapsus rectal de l'adulte par l'électro-thérapie du sphincter anal, Thèse de Paris, 1953.
16. Neal, W. B., Jr., et al.: Abdominoperineal resection of the rectum by the 2-team technic, Ann. Surg. 137:325, 1953.
17. Rosenman, L. D., and Gropper, A. N.: Small intestinal stenosis caused by infarction; an unusual sequel of mesenteric artery embolism, Ann. Surg. 141:254, 1955.
18. Ross, S. T.: Treatment of anorectal fistulas, J. Internat. Coll. Surgeons 22:607, 1954.
19. Sadove, M. S., and Kowalski, L. F.: Anesthesia for anorectal surgery; a status evaluation, Am. J. Proc. 3:182, 1952.
20. Schneider, H. C.: Hyaluronidase with local anesthesia in anorectal surgery, Tr. Am. Proc. Soc. 53rd Session, pp. 703-706, 1954.
21. Secar, S. M.: New hope for colostomy patients, Nursing Outlook 2:642, 1954.
22. Smith, R.: Progress in Clinical Surgery, Boston, Little, 1954.
23. Thompson, H. R.: Rectum prolapse, Brit. Surg. Pract. 7:373, 1950.
24. Till, A. S.: Progress in Clinical Surgery, Boston, Little, 1954.
25. Van Buskirk, W. C.: Polyps of the large bowel, Am. Surg. 141:234, 1955.

18 The Liver and the Biliary Duct System

Part One: The Liver

The surgeon who operates on the liver and the biliary system must have a most thorough and complete knowledge of the anatomy and the physiology of the parts involved, under both normal and pathologic conditions. This is a branch of surgery in which errors are very likely to occur and certainly one in which every possible safeguard against accident and inefficiency is most necessary. Biliary surgery is no work for the tyro. It requires the highest type of skill—that which can be attained only by long experience.

Surgery of the liver has made great advances during the 20th century, especially in its second quarter. Liver-function tests and such diagnosic aids as cholangiography and needle puncture now give assistance to the surgeon in making his preoperative diagnosis, but they also impose upon him an added responsibility in preventing errors in their interpretation and require keener surgical judgment in the management of the conditions which they reveal.

ANATOMIC RELATIONS

These are shown in the schematic drawing, Figure 328. Keep in mind anomalies in the position of the liver (transposition). Movable livers (hepatoptosis) have been mistaken for neoplasms. In *liver enlargement from any*

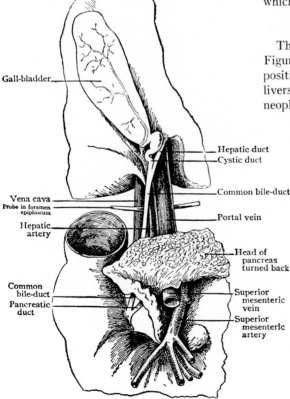

Gall-bladder

Hepatic duct
Cystic duct

Common bile-duct

Vena cava
Probe in foramen epiploicum
Portal vein

Hepatic artery

Head of pancreas turned back

Common bile-duct
Pancreatic duct

Superior mesenteric vein
Superior mesenteric artery

FIG. 328. Schematic drawing showing principal structures of the biliary system in their anatomic relationships. (After Piersol)

cause, careful percussion and roentgenography will aid in avoiding misinterpretation by establishing the height of the diaphragm resulting from upward displacement of the organ. In emphysema or pneumothorax, the upper as well as the lower limits are lowered; the same is true in empyema.

There are no tests which can demonstrate the exact functional capacity of the liver, because, of all the organs of the human body, the liver has the most diversified activities. Not only does it share in metabolic processes but it also promotes coagulation of the blood by producing fibrinogen and maintaining an adequate prothrombin level. It also removes toxins from the blood by conjugation, oxidation and the action of the endothelial system, to mention only a few of its most important functions. Bacteria entering the blood stream are regularly destroyed in the liver; in all types of surgery the liver acts as a detoxifying agent.

DANGERS ATTENDING THE USE OF LIVER-FUNCTION TESTS

Many tests have been devised to measure the liver's functional ability in certain of the activities in which it regularly participates. If its functional capacity could be measured accurately, the diagnosis of diseases which attack the biliary system would be greatly simplified, for the surgeon would then have a guide as to the ability of the affected organ to withstand the effects of surgical intervention, should such treatment be found advisable.

The limitations of any one test of liver function must be recognized and the value of the results of such tests estimated accordingly. *Within these limits,* certain tests of liver function are very useful diagnostic aids. It must be remembered that there is a tremendous reserve of liver tissue, which enables this organ to carry on normal function despite extensive damage. Functional insufficiency becomes detectable only after this reservoir is depleted. The demonstration of impaired liver function by laboratory tests usually indicates serious damage to this organ and sets out a danger signal to physician and surgeon alike. *Yet, the absence of laboratory evidence of impaired liver function is not a guarantee that the patient has a normal liver.* When surgery is contemplated in the presence of biliary tract disease, the only safeguard is to assume that considerable liver damage has taken place *despite normal function* as demonstrated by tests.

SURGERY OF THE LIVER

Before the 20th century surgery of the liver was practically unknown. It was in 1899 that W. W. Keen, then the first surgeon of his time, reported 3 cases of *partial* hepatic resection, with a review of 73 other cases which he had found in the literature. In contrast, the second edition of my *Modern Surgical Technic,* published in 1949, has 55 double-column pages devoted to hepatic surgery alone, giving an idea of the enormous progress made in this branch of operative technic in the past half century.

Yet, even today, if we open the usual classic surgical textbook, we will not find a great amount of space devoted to this subject, usually 3 chapters at most. One chapter usually will concern drainage of liver abscess or extirpation of hydatid cyst. Another will deal with what the French term "cuneiform resections," which are not often performed and then only in more or less fear and uncertainty on the part of the average general surgeon, with the by no means negligible risk of severe hemorrhage. These operations are carried out mostly for traumatic injuries close to the edge of the liver, where a wedge-shaped piece may be "carved out" without damage to any large blood vessels. A third type of procedure consists merely of tamponade for hemostasis in extensive injuries when immediate suture is not feasible.

Progress in the technic of administration of all types of anesthesia has reduced the amount of toxins that the liver is now obliged to take care of during any operative procedure. When it is itself undergoing surgery, this improvement is particularly advantageous. The surgeon now has sufficient time to do his work with deliberation if the patient's chest is kept open for any length of time. The generalized use of new incisions, based on the present concept that the liver is quite as much a thoracic as an abdominal organ, permits us to go about reaching it by more direct routes. French surgeons recommend the "thoraco-phreno-right laparotomy," passing by the eighth rib, which, they claim, gives complete

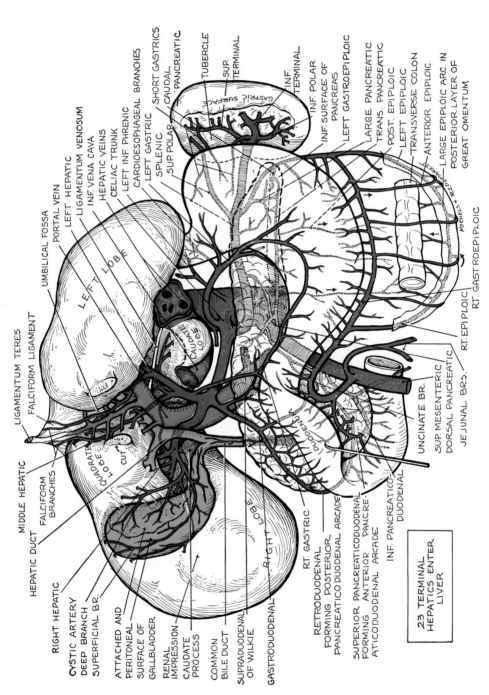

Fig. 329. Typical pattern of blood supply of the upper abdominal organs. (Michels, N. A.: Blood Supply and Anatomy of the Upper Abdominal Organs, Philadelphia, Lippincott)

Fig. 330. "Normal" arrangement of biliary ducts and gall-bladder and their blood supply. These arrangements account for about 82 per cent of cases; the remaining 18 per cent present an astonishing number of variations. (After E. Friend)

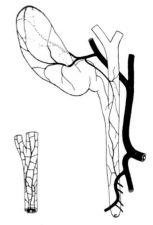

exposure of the entire surface of the liver, with the hepatic pedicle and the hilum as well as the inferior vena cava and the subhepatic veins.

STUMBLING BLOCKS TO SUCCESS IN HEPATIC SURGERY

The liver is a highly vascular organ. How to effect hemostasis has always been the problem the surgeon had to solve beforehand. Not until painstaking animal experimentation had demonstrated how liver hemorrhage could be controlled was there any sure prospect of success even under the most favorable conditions. With the anatomic facts supplied to us by such investigators as John E. Healey, Jr.,[4] of Philadelphia, who discussed the anatomic

aspects of radical hepatic surgery before the International College of Surgeons in 1953, surgery of the liver will be robbed of many of its terrors, and the chances of error will be greatly lessened.

HEPATIC CIRCULATION

Embryologically, the liver arises as an

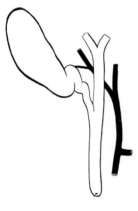

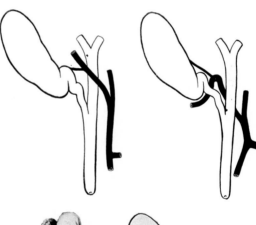

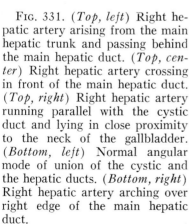

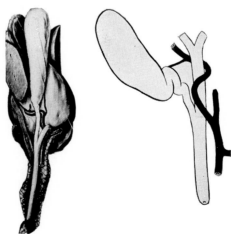

Fig. 331. (*Top, left*) Right hepatic artery arising from the main hepatic trunk and passing behind the main hepatic duct. (*Top, center*) Right hepatic artery crossing in front of the main hepatic duct. (*Top, right*) Right hepatic artery running parallel with the cystic duct and lying in close proximity to the neck of the gallbladder. (*Bottom, left*) Normal angular mode of union of the cystic and the hepatic ducts. (*Bottom, right*) Right hepatic artery arching over right edge of the main hepatic duct.

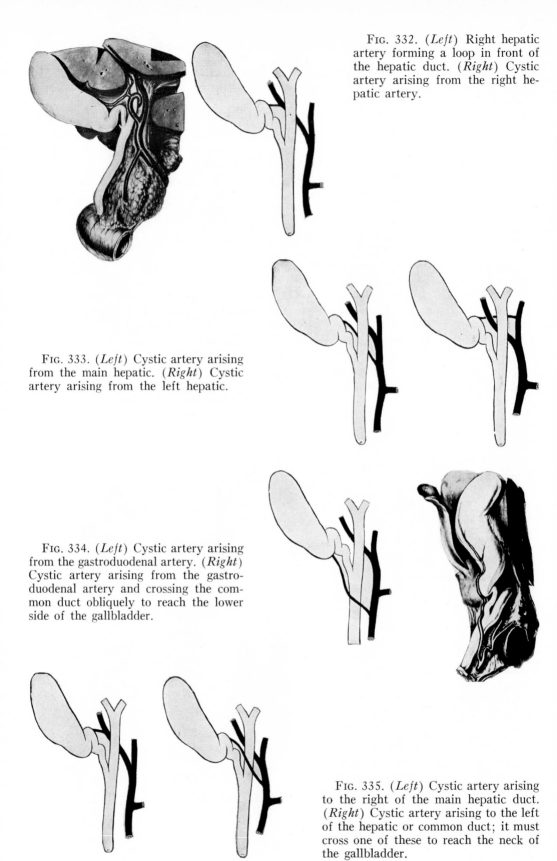

Fig. 332. (*Left*) Right hepatic artery forming a loop in front of the hepatic duct. (*Right*) Cystic artery arising from the right hepatic artery.

Fig. 333. (*Left*) Cystic artery arising from the main hepatic. (*Right*) Cystic artery arising from the left hepatic.

Fig. 334. (*Left*) Cystic artery arising from the gastroduodenal artery. (*Right*) Cystic artery arising from the gastroduodenal artery and crossing the common duct obliquely to reach the lower side of the gallbladder.

Fig. 335. (*Left*) Cystic artery arising to the right of the main hepatic duct. (*Right*) Cystic artery arising to the left of the hepatic or common duct; it must cross one of these to reach the neck of the gallbladder.

FIG. 336. (*Left*) Cystic artery arising on the left side of the main hepatic duct and crossing the latter to reach the neck of the gallbladder. (*Right*) Cystic artery arising behind the main hepatic duct.

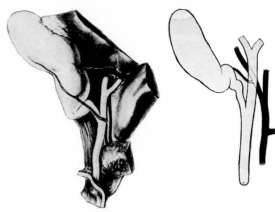

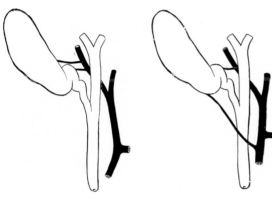

FIG. 337. (*Left*) Two cystic arteries arising from the right hepatic. (*Right*) One cystic artery arising from the right hepatic and the other from the gastro-duodenal artery.

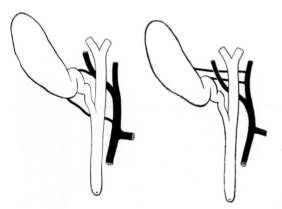

FIG. 338. (*Left*) Accessory cystic artery arising from the main hepatic. (*Right*) Two cystic arteries arising from the left hepatic.

FIG. 339. (*Left*) Pancreatico-duodenal artery crossing the common duct. (*Right*) Specimen showing pancreatico-duodenal artery crossing the common duct.

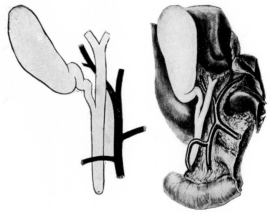

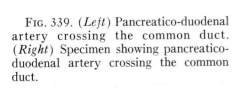

461

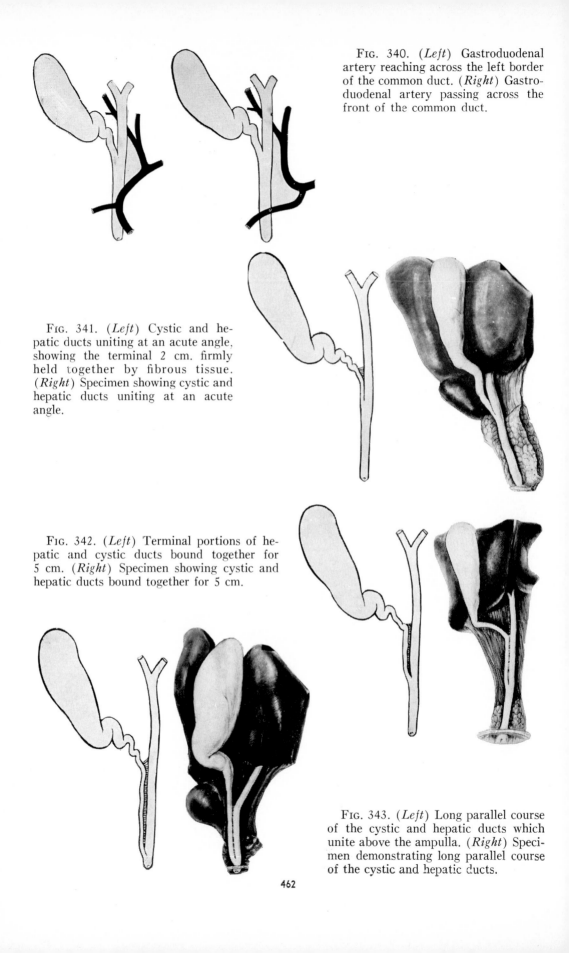

FIG. 340. (*Left*) Gastroduodenal artery reaching across the left border of the common duct. (*Right*) Gastroduodenal artery passing across the front of the common duct.

FIG. 341. (*Left*) Cystic and hepatic ducts uniting at an acute angle, showing the terminal 2 cm. firmly held together by fibrous tissue. (*Right*) Specimen showing cystic and hepatic ducts uniting at an acute angle.

FIG. 342. (*Left*) Terminal portions of hepatic and cystic ducts bound together for 5 cm. (*Right*) Specimen showing cystic and hepatic ducts bound together for 5 cm.

FIG. 343. (*Left*) Long parallel course of the cystic and hepatic ducts which unite above the ampulla. (*Right*) Specimen demonstrating long parallel course of the cystic and hepatic ducts.

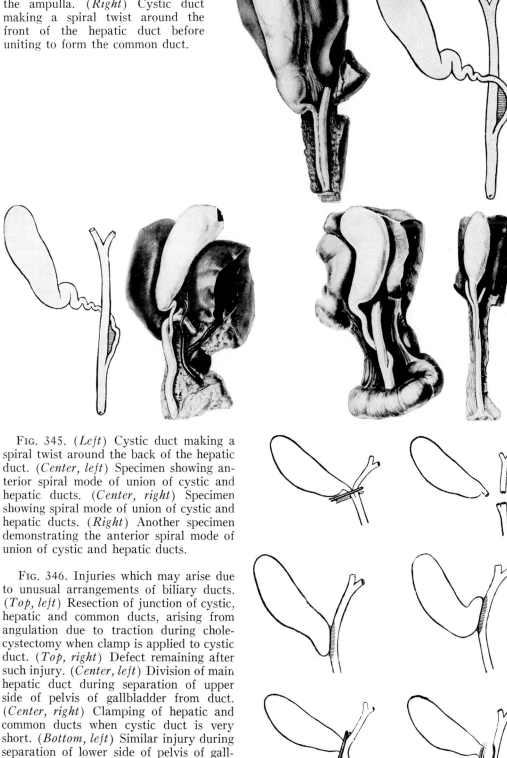

Fig. 344. (*Left*) Specimen demonstrating a long parallel course of the cystic and hepatic ducts uniting above the ampulla. (*Right*) Cystic duct making a spiral twist around the front of the hepatic duct before uniting to form the common duct.

Fig. 345. (*Left*) Cystic duct making a spiral twist around the back of the hepatic duct. (*Center, left*) Specimen showing anterior spiral mode of union of cystic and hepatic ducts. (*Center, right*) Specimen showing spiral mode of union of cystic and hepatic ducts. (*Right*) Another specimen demonstrating the anterior spiral mode of union of cystic and hepatic ducts.

Fig. 346. Injuries which may arise due to unusual arrangements of biliary ducts. (*Top, left*) Resection of junction of cystic, hepatic and common ducts, arising from angulation due to traction during cholecystectomy when clamp is applied to cystic duct. (*Top, right*) Defect remaining after such injury. (*Center, left*) Division of main hepatic duct during separation of upper side of pelvis of gallbladder from duct. (*Center, right*) Clamping of hepatic and common ducts when cystic duct is very short. (*Bottom, left*) Similar injury during separation of lower side of pelvis of gallbladder. (*Bottom, right*) Defect remaining after such injury.

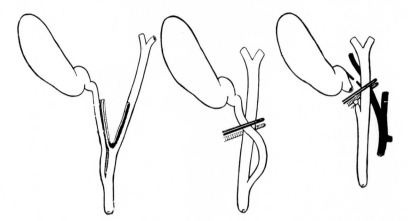

FIG. 347. (*Left*) Injury to hepatic duct when it runs parallel with cystic duct for a long way. (*Center*) Injury to hepatic duct when cystic duct winds around in front of it. (*Right*) Injury to hepatic duct during effort to catch bleeding cystic artery.

FIG. 348. (*Left*) Injury to common duct during effort to catch bleeding anomalous cystic artery arising from gastroduodenal artery. (*Right*) Hemorrhage from overlooked second cystic artery.

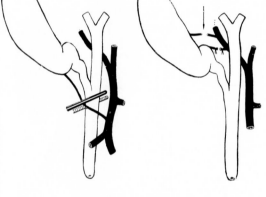

endodermal outpouching from the foregut, giving rise to a central tubular structure which becomes the biliary passages, with 2 sets of afferent blood vessels: the *hepatic artery* and its branches, which may be regarded as being primarily nutritive, and the *portal vein,* which is primarily functional (Fig. 329). The *hepatic veins* are a single set of efferent vessels. According to Healey, there is a segmental distribution of the bile ducts, the hepatic artery and the portal vein in the liver. This investigator has sought to establish a "prevailing pattern" of the branching of the bile ducts and the hepatic artery and of the hepatic venous system (Fig. 330).

There are, of course, many variations (Figs. 331-345) from this "norm," but with a knowledge of the intrahepatic branchings of the vascular and the biliary channels, especially their segmental and intersegmental arrangement, hepatic resection may be approached, he thinks, with a brighter outlook. A partial resection of the liver based on sound surgical anatomic principles is certainly the most logical approach, whether the aim be resection of an entire lobe, a segment or an area (Figs. 346-348).

It thus appears that the greatest *error* which can be made in surgery of the liver is to undertake any hepatic operation without the most complete comprehension of the vascular pattern of the entire gland. On the other hand, the best *safeguard* is complete comprehension.

HEPATOLOBECTOMY

Resection of the left (smaller) lobe of the liver has been done for a comparatively long time, as mentioned in the first page of this chapter. However, I find no mention of *right* hepatolobectomy before the cases of Quattlebaum[9] and of Pack and his associates[8] in 1953. These later surgeons were able to profit by the mistakes and the technical improvements of the pioneers, while they, in turn, have handed on to the next generation the results of practical experience which are now releasing the general surgeon from what one writer has called "the unwarranted foreboding of major hepatic surgery which has generally prevailed" heretofore. The careful anatomic approach which pulmonary surgeons long have deemed essential in their work is equally important when operating on the liver. Prior to any such procedure, a large portion of the blood supply to the projected operative field must be dissected out and carefully ligated before transection. With this safeguard, there will be no fearful bleeding such as often is encountered when these precautions are not taken. Such an approach does away with the need to use tourniquets, overlapping mattress sutures, cauteries or similar deterrants to bleeding.

After the right hepatic artery and the first branch of the portal vein are ligated, there will be very little bleeding during transection of the right lobe. The amount of postoperative bleeding and the accumulation of bile will be found to be relatively small in most cases, so that the employment of drains is seldom necessary. Lorimer recommends ligation of the vascular channels in the hilus in continuity rather than ligation and division.

Lobectomy, either right or left, is now regularly employed in extirpating tumors. The majority of liver neoplasms are metastatic, the primary growth frequently being located in some distant part of the body. Rarely will a tumor primary to the liver metastasize itself elsewhere. Such conditions greatly confuse diagnosis but do not lessen the importance of avoiding errors in hepatic surgery.

In 1944, a technic for complete *left* hepatic lobectomy was described for the first time, with a report of 3 cases and the statement that only 2 such procedures had been previously attempted. In the decade following, more and more reports on this particular procedure were published, but no one had had the temerity to attempt to resect the *right* lobe of the liver. However, in 1952, the French surgeons Lortat-Jacob and Robert published in *La Presse Médicale* the description of an operation by which the entire right lobe of the liver may be resected "with precision and strict adherence to the principles of good surgical technic." Since 1952, this operation has been performed a number of times, yet it remains confined to the hands of the most expert and experienced of abdominal surgeons. Though surrounded by all the safeguards known to up-to-date surgical practice, the chances of error remain very great.

Using the technic of Lortat-Jacob and Robert, surgeons at the Memorial Hospital, New York City, through an incision just to the right of the falciform ligament, removed the entire right lobe of the liver of a 61-year-old woman, together with the quadrate and most of the caudate lobe. Though they thought that all vessels had been properly ligated before division, "one sizable branch of the portal vein to the right lobe had been inadvertently overlooked . . . and was injured," so that brisk hemorrhage with moderate blood loss ensued until this vessel could be secured. Into the large dead space resulting from removal of the right lobe, the surgeons placed a Mikulicz pack, from which profuse biliary drainage issued until the fourth postoperative day when the flow gradually diminished. The pack was being removed piecemeal until the tenth postoperative day, when all of the remaining pack prolapsed out of the wound, leaving the large intra-abdominal dead space imperfectly drained, and a low-grade subphrenic abscess developed. A right thoracentesis removed 600 cc. of cloudy but sterile bile-stained fluid. Thereafter, the biliary drainage grew less, and the patient's septic course resolved by lysis. During the next 6 weeks, anorexia and nausea with progressive weakness and mental depression developed insiduously, until jaundice appeared 10 weeks after the lobectomy, at which time she was readmitted to the hospital. She had received multiple blood-bank transfusions prior to and during the operation on the right lobe. An interval of 2 months elapsed between the last blood transfusion and the appearance of jaundice. The symptoms enumerated are quite in keeping with a diagnosis of homologous serum hepatitis. The authors of this report comment: "That the patient survived the operation at all is indicative of the fact that the operative technic is sound." Resection of the entire right lobe of the liver was carried out successfully for metastatic leiomyosarcoma 7 years after surgical control of the primary tumor. Two months after resection the patient developed symptoms, signs and laboratory findings of homologous serum hepatitis. She remains living and well 1 year later, in spite of the fact that only 500 to 600 gm. of liver tissue in the *left* lobe were known to have been left at the time of the right hepatic lobectomy.

Total right hepatic lobectomy can be done only after it has been established that the remaining lobe is fully capable of functioning alone. Perhaps the chief error in such surgery would be failure to ascertain the precise condition and functional capacity of the unoperated side. Yet, even when this obvious precaution has been taken, there remain certain other contraindications which must be weighed carefully before proceeding to operate. Extension of a growth *primary to the right lobe* into the opposite lobe, even though the malignant cell growth is small and sharply localized, plainly indicates that the condition has advanced too far to make it worth while for the patient to undergo such an extensive intervention as complete lobectomy. Recurrence or further extension is practically inevitable, so the short postoperative period of freedom is out of proportion to the suffering undergone and the immediate risks involved. Tumor thrombi in the hepatic veins and the inferior vena cava, with consequent Chiari's syndrome, is sufficient criterion for inoperability. Moreover, there is always a possibility of independent primary cancers existing in the left lobe. Growths which have invaded the portal fissure and the hepatoduodenal ligament may cause insurmountable technical handicaps in the necessary surgical dissection of this region (Pack).

LEFT HEPATECTOMY

INDICATIONS

Aside from primary malignant disease of the left lobe, resection of that side of the liver may be advisable because of extensive malignant processes from other organs or metastasis from distant foci in other unrelated organs. Primary *benign* tumors are found occasionally. *Abscess* or *hydatid* or other *cysts* may also require resection or even entire removal of the left lobe of the liver.

The greatest chance of error here is in establishment of the diagnosis. It is seldom possible to tell whether or not a liver growth is primary or metastatic or benign or malignant before it is surgically exposed, and then it may be too late to adopt the best surgical procedure for the conditions found to exist. The use of liver-function tests may be of help, but in hepatic surgery, the surgeon has no such reliable physical and laboratory procedures as are, for example, at his disposal in renal surgery.

SAFEGUARDS IN SURGERY OF THE LEFT HEPATIC LOBE

The technical difficulties offered by operation on the left lobe of the liver are generally less than those encountered by the surgeon intervening upon the right lobe. The operative field must be adequately exposed and the lobe itself completely mobilized, bringing blood vessels and bile ducts into full view at the porta hepatis. To effect this, the lobe must be pulled well toward the right, which permits safe and satisfactory ligation of the vessels and the left hepatic bile duct, using an aneurysm needle by passing the ligatures and securing them before division. This is a special safeguard in any type of hepatic surgery. Most important is identifying and ligating the left hepatic vein. Guard against tearing the hepatic veins which open into the inferior vena cava. To do this is a serious error which may induce troublesome or even fatal hemorrhage. If ligation is properly carried out, there should be very little bleeding, and what small amount of hemorrhage does occur can be readily stopped by cauterization, as directed in my technic of electrocoagulation of the gallbladder (p. 487).

REPERITONEALIZATION OF THE RAW SURFACE OF THE RIGHT LOBE

Removal of the left lobe will leave a considerable raw surface exposed on the adjacent aspect of the right lobe. To cover this, the fold of peritoneum which remains after division of the longitudinal ligament is sutured to other peritoneal folds which the coronary ligament and the gastrohepatic omentum have formed. The hepatic artery, the common hepatic duct and the portal vein will likewise be enveloped in peritoneal folds, and these should be sutured in place as an additional safeguard.

SKIN GRAFTS AS HEMOSTATIC AGENTS IN LIVER SURGERY

At the Duke University School of Medicine, Frank Masters and co-workers carried on a series of animal experiments on the control of liver hemorrhage by split-thickness skin grafting. Clinically, they had observed that grafts placed on a raw surface whose granulations had just been surgically débrided would act as a hemostatic agent as well as a skin coverage. This observation suggested that a split-thickness dermal graft might be used in a similar manner to control hemorrhage from the cut liver surface, thus removing some of the previous limitations to liver resection and opening the path for removal of extensive primary and metastatic liver tumors. Traumatic injuries to the liver with hemorrhage could be better handled surgically if bleeding could be controlled by covering the raw liver surface with split-thickness dermal grafts.

Fifteen dogs were operated on, and 2 weeks after the original operation all the wounds were re-examined to determine the fate of the grafts. It was found that the grafts over a resected lobe or within a puncture wound or a liver laceration "took" readily and thus gave a permanent capsulelike covering to the liver. After the graft has taken, this new capsule showed no evidence of replacement by liver tissue. There was no secondary hemorrhage, nor were any biliary fistulae observed. The only abnormality found in the experimental animals after grafting was a small cyst formation in areas where the graft overlapped the parietal or visceral peritoneum.

The advantages of the use of skin as a hemostatic agent in liver surgery are its availability and its ease of application. Grafts may be secured from any adjacent skin area, and if taken prior to resection, the graft is ready for instant use. Since the graft adheres readily to the raw liver surface, simple running sutures between the graft and the liver surface are sufficient, and the time-consuming use of multiple mattress sutures in friable and highly vascular liver parenchyma is avoided. Drainage is unnecessary, and biliary fistulae, extensive adhesions or abscess formation have not occurred.

HYDATID DISEASE OF THE LIVER

RECOGNITION OF HYDATID CYST

One of the recent successful applications of hepatolobectomy is that of removal of hydatid cyst. Previous editions of this book used only 7 lines to describe this disease and said nothing whatever concerning diagnosis or preferred ways of handling it. It is unlikely that medical graduates of the past decade would now be content with such summary dismissal of what has become an important topic in any discussion of hepatic pathology.

Though long endemic in Iceland, Greece, Australia, New Zealand and certain parts of South America, hydatid disease was practically unknown in the United States before the early years of the 20th century. Since then, war on a global scale and vast improvements in international transportation have made us all too familiar with pathologic conditions once regarded as peculiarly "tropical diseases," with proportionate increase in the perplexities of differential diagnosis.

Echinococcus disease (Cysticercus, "hydatid cyst") is caused by a small tapeworm, *Taenia echinococcus,* an intestinal parasite of dogs, but it is readily transferable to cattle and sheep, which are the usual intermediate hosts. It enters the various human organs in the larval stage, giving rise to the so-called hydatid cyst. The liver is the site of predilection, though the lungs are frequently invaded also, and the infestation is not unknown in the kidneys and the bladder.

ERRORS IN DIAGNOSIS

The diagnosis is frequently missed simply because the examining physician does not consider the *possibility* of hydatid cyst. Points helpful in establishing diagnosis are: (1) a history of having originated or resided in a region where echinococcus is prevalent; (2) an urticarial rash giving evidence of hypersensitivity to the hydatid fluid or an anaphylactic shocklike reaction due to the sudden rupture of a hydatid cyst; (3) eosinophilia, together with sepsis and obstructive jaundice; (4) roentgenographic characteristics of the condition are "doming" of the right diaphragm and the shadow of a rounded mass in the parenchyma of the liver.

Clinically, there is usually pain in the right upper abdominal quadrant, elevation of temperature and evidence of sepsis, but only a moderate leukocytosis.

Hepatic hydatid cysts may rupture into the biliary system, the peritoneal cavity, the thorax and—less commonly—into the vascular system, the alimentary canal or the urinary tract. The rupture will be intrabiliary in from 5 to 10 per cent of liver cysts, and in some

30 per cent of these, the intrabiliary rupture will lead to obstruction of the common bile duct. While the majority of writers on this subject consider biliary contamination (bilirrhagia) after marsupialization to be indicative of the existence of a communication between the cyst cavity and the biliary tree, Dagher and Hovnanian[3] of Beirut, Lebanon (where hydatid disease is very common), believe that the presence of daughter cysts or chitinous membranes in the bile ducts is the only positive proof of intrabiliary rupture. In their opinion, the bilious discharge after surgical intervention is probably due to a sudden change in the local hydrodynamics. The constantly elevated pressure of the endocyst exerts a tamponlike action on the actually or potentially eroded bile canaliculi. When the endocyst is removed, releasing the pressure, a free flow of bile takes place into the cyst cavity; this is manifested as bilirrhagia. Thus, the chance of error in diagnosis is emphasized.

Lung Involvement

As soon as there is reasonable certainty of the presence of echinococcus disease in the liver, roentgenograms should be taken of the chest, because daughter cysts frequently invade the lungs and may be detected early enough to safeguard against wholesale involvement of the thoracic cavity.

Cautions to be Observed in Marsupialization of Hydatid Cysts

Before resection of the liver became a feasible operation, marsupialization was the usual method employed in dealing with hydatid cysts. If this technic is to be followed, make the abdominal incision as low down and as far forward as possible and deliver the cyst into the wound *without puncturing it;* pack gauze about it to favor the formation of adhesions. Open the cyst only after adhesions have formed and at no time permit any of the contained fluid to escape into the peritoneal cavity. In cases that are not urgent, the formation of adhesions may be encouraged by painting the serous surfaces with a 5 per cent iodine solution. Suture of the diaphragm to the thoracic parietes may be desirable, but this is difficult to carry out effectively. Owing to the loss of support when the adjacent cyst is

evacuated, the sutures often pull through, producing a "sucking wound" with all its attendant risks.

Protection of the Pleural Cavity

It is all-important to avoid opening the pleural cavity if by any means it can be left intact. The hydatid that communicates with liver and lung transdiaphragmatically may tax the ingenuity of the surgeon and often offers long and difficult operative problems. The pulmonary part can usually be handled without much trouble and hazard, as thoracic surgery has made great strides within the past half century, but the time required to obliterate a large, often multilocular hydatid abscess may extend the procedure beyond the limits of the patient's endurance. At best, prolonged hospital treatment is the only safeguard against remote sequelae.

HEPATOLOBECTOMY FOR MALIGNANT NEOPLASMS

Chief among the uses of hepatic lobectomy is for the removal of neoplasms, both benign and malignant. Because such operations are not performed often, only a small number will be found to have occurred in any particular surgical center or service.

Diagnosis

Though malignant growths are often discovered in the liver, the majority found there are metastatic from a primary focus in some other—often distant—organ or tissue. Consequently, the diagnosis is frequently difficult and often made only at operation or autopsy. Multiple growths and those which are deep-seated or far advanced are inoperable from the outset, but, occasionally, some malignant lesions which are located near the inner edge of the *right lobe* of the liver can be surgically extirpated with a good prognosis.

Safeguards in Removal

It is possible to remove the left lobe almost entirely, if proper precautions are observed. As the left triangular ligament will have to be divided, care must be taken to ligate all large vessels encountered to prevent profuse bleeding. Preliminary hemostasis of the left lobe may be obtained by placing overlapping interrupted mattress sutures. A straight anteropos-

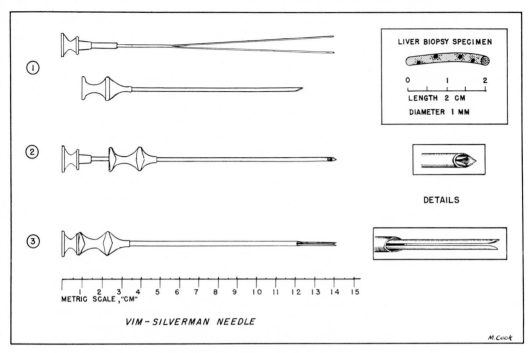

① ② ③

LIVER BIOPSY SPECIMEN

0   1   2

LENGTH 2 CM

DIAMETER 1 MM

DETAILS

METRIC SCALE,"CM"
1 2 3 4 5 6 7 8 9 10 11 12 13 14 15

VIM – SILVERMAN NEEDLE

M. Cook

FIG. 349. Needle-biopsy apparatus.

terior transection is recommended, as this avoids leaving liver tissue from which bile drainage will have been interrupted when the bile ducts which drain it are ligated. A drain should be placed at the site of the liver resection and brought out through the wound to permit escape of any bile which may be excreted from the cut surface; this lessens the danger of *bile peritonitis*. Should there be no bile drainage, the drain can be taken out on the third or fourth day, but in the event of leakage of bile, the drain should be allowed to remain until it ceases. This is an extra safeguard which does not interfere in any way with postoperative healing.

A necessary condition for good results from surgery of a liver growth is *absolute hemostasis*. This can be effected satisfactorily by electrocoagulation. Attempts at tamponade, application of different kinds of hemostatic substances and reduction of the blood flow by constriction, ligation or other means have all proved to be of doubtful value. The indications for operation are the shape, the size and the location of the tumor in relation to the large bile ducts and the blood vessels in the hilus of the liver.

EVALUATION OF NEEDLE BIOPSY OF THE LIVER

The increasing frequency with which needle biopsy is being used in the diagnosis of hepatic diseases makes it of particular interest in connection with any discussion of the errors and the hazards of surgery in this most important organ (Fig. 349). Needle biopsy is now employed to determine both the presence and the character of some pathologic condition of the liver and the existence and the extent of possible injury to the cells of the hepatic tissues. Attempts have been made to correlate the results of liver-function tests with reports of the pathologist on specimens obtained by needle biopsy. However, in my personal experience, the results have not been sufficiently convincing to warrant using the needle method to the exclusion of all other diagnostic procedures. It *supplements* but does not *supersede* those which we are making use of at present. In conjunction with liver-function tests, the needle-biopsy method may provide a more complete picture of the extent and the severity of a disease, as well as its progress (when more than one puncture has been made), and in this way provide a more accurate prognosis. If the hepatic disease is of a diffuse type, it will be possible to secure a fairly accurate histologic picture of the entire gland. On the other hand, if the disease is limited in extent or varies in severity in different sections of the hepatic tissue, biopsy by the needle method will serve no useful purpose.

Negative findings after needle biopsy are most often inconclusive if the condition is not a diffuse one, because the puncture may have been made in an area of tissue which had not been invaded by the pathologic process. On the other hand, a *positive result may be extremely valuable* if the needle has entered the main extent of the growth.

The surgeon should be cautious about accepting the results of diagnostic puncture as a contraindication to exploratory operation. This is particularly true of tumors. Time was when there was no possibility of removing a growth in the liver, so that the patient was regarded as doomed from the outset. This is no longer true, for greater surgical skill and experience have made it possible to resect the liver—especially the left lobe—with relatively good prognostic possibilities. However, the information which needle biopsy puts at the surgeon's disposal may be of the utmost value in the planning and the carrying out of such an operation.

Risks of Needle Biopsy

In May, 1952, Richard Terry of St. Bartholomew's Hospital, London, compiled statistics showing that more than 10,000 liver biopsies had been reported in the literature since 1939.[12] He published a table showing that the *over-all mortality rate* had been 0.12 per cent and the complication rate 0.32 per cent. *The actual number of deaths was 13.* Analyzing these cases, Terry points out the errors which he believes to have been responsible for them. In 11 cases, the direct cause of death was given as *hemorrhage.* In all these patients, a "hopeless" prognosis had already been made. As the case reports on the 2 remaining patients gave no information on this point, we can assume that in more than 10,000 biopsies there were only 2 fatalities in patients whose prognosis was good.

In 5 cases, the error appears to have been

failure to ascertain the prothrombin levels or disregard the fact that they were too low for safety. One patient was "too ill to co-operate," and several more would seem to have been moribund, which most surgeons would regard as a contraindication to biopsy under any circumstances.

Liver biopsy probably should not be undertaken in *undoubted cases of obstructive jaundice* unless secondary deposits are being sought in cancer cases.

Penetration of Abdominal Viscera. This is an error which has not been widely reported, though it probably has happened many times. The discovery of intestinal, pancreatic or renal tissue in the histologic preparation was usually the only evidence of this accident. However, in one case, death followed puncture of the colon.

Biliary Peritonitis. This is an occasional occurrence complicating liver puncture—at least one fatal instance having been reported. It can occur only when biliary obstruction exists, so that the practical safeguard against it is to refrain from employing liver puncture in patients with jaundice unless it has been proved to be nonobstructive.

Safeguards Against Complications After Liver Puncture

The most important precautions against complications are as follows (Terry):

1. Observe Recognized Contraindications. Particularly observe (a) hemorrhagic states failing to respond to treatment, including prothrombin levels below 70 per cent, thrombocytopenia, polycythemia vera and Weil's disease; (b) pyogenic infection in the liver; (c) inability of the patient to co-operate; (d) absence of superficial liver dullness; and (e) moribund, senile or anemic patients.

2. Choice of Operator. Some think that liver biopsy should be performed by a physician rather than a surgeon, while its numerous clinical aspects render it an unsuitable procedure for the pathologist. I cannot concur with this. A surgeon who knows anatomy and pathology well and is properly trained in his specialty is the most suitable person to carry out this procedure.

3. Size of Needle. Do not use too large a needle; one in which the bore is between 1.5 and 1.8 has proved to be safe and satisfactory in most cases. Too large a needle may cause hemorrhage, and one that is too small may fail to obtain a specimen, and even if it does get something, the pathologist may complain that the material is too scanty.

4. Anesthesia. Adequate infiltration of the diaphragm and Glisson's capsule is essential. If the puncture is made without local anesthetization, the "gasp" which the patient will give as the needle passes may cause so sharp a descent of the diaphragm that it might tear the liver capsule. General anesthesia, in order to produce apnea, must be so deep that recovery may be slow and postanesthetic vomiting distressing and capable of hindering hemostasis (if hemorrhage takes place).

5. Duodenal Intubation. If there is any possibility of active cholangitis, particularly if jaundice be present, duodenal intubation should be carried out before doing a puncture. If the specimen obtained by intubation contains pus and micro-organisms, puncture of the liver is contraindicated.

6. Selection of Route. The intercostal route is to be preferred; the subcostal route is applicable only to the cases of gross and undoubted hepatomegaly. But, even under these circumstances, some prefer the intercostal approach, since it permits better perception of the position and the progress of the needle. Unless the physical signs of hepatomegaly are clear-cut, it is wiser to avoid the subcostal route.

7. Depth of Puncture. The deeper the liver is penetrated, the greater the danger of damaging blood vessels of significant size; if a guard is mounted on the needle and adjusted to a distance of 5.5 to 6.5 cm., an adequate specimen will be obtained and penetration of the liver will be limited to about 3.5 cm.

8. Deep Pressure Over the Biopsy Site. Immediately after the biopsy is completed, *firm pressure should be applied to the puncture site* in order to control both bleeding and leakage from the liver wound. It should be maintained for 15 minutes, or, in cases of jaundice or if any cause for concern exists, for one half hour. Terry emphasizes that "this simple and obvious precaution," though barely mentioned in the literature, is of fundamental importance in the prevention of complications, and it should also be used in the treatment of bleeding. The puncture is best done with the patient

in bed; for the 15 to 30 minutes of deep pressure on the biopsy site, he should remain at the edge of the bed, then be lifted gently back into its center. He should remain flat for 6 hours and rest in bed until the following day. Pulse and blood pressure should be recorded frequently. Deep pressure should again be instituted at any evidence of hemorrhage, and blood transfusion should be used if indicated. Compatible blood should be kept immediately available for this purpose. If peritoneal irritation appear, antibiotics should be administered early.

The most recent publication regarding the errors and the safeguards of needle biopsy of the liver which has come to my attention is that of Dennis A. J. Morey and colleagues of the McGuire Veterans' Administration Hospital, Richmond, Va. They made 139 punctures in the livers of 119 patients during an 8-year period. There were 19 failures to establish a correct diagnosis (13.8%). There were 31 cases in which primary or metastatic carcinoma was ultimately demonstrated at autopsy, operation or subsequent needle biopsies, an error of 45.2 per cent.

Hemorrhage. The only severe complication encountered was hemorrhage. One patient died. He suffered from a severe Laennec's cirrhosis, and the biopsy specimen was obtained by the transthoracic route. His prothrombin time had been 33 per cent prior to biopsy, but he died of severe intra-abdominal hemorrhage and irreversible shock. Autopsy showed a well-defined puncture hole in the liver, without evidence of laceration. The patients who survived were given whole blood and vitamin K_1 daily until all evidence of hemorrhage had ceased. In one case, a single transfusion of 500 cc. of fresh, whole blood caused bleeding to cease immediately. Low prothrombin consumption time was implicated in 3 of the 4 cases of hemorrhage; these authors regard its correction before and after biopsy as being very important. It should be determined whenever a blood dyscrasia is suspected. The transthoracic route should not be followed if it can be avoided. Its use appears to be a significant factor in the appearance of complications.

This same advice—to avoid the transthoracic route whenever possible—is also offered by Zamcheck and Klausenstock. They felt

FIG. 350. Diagrammatic drawing illustrating the most frequent locations for subphrenic abscesses, viz., in the right posterior superior and right inferior spaces. Key to figure. (1) Visible abscess areas. (2) Abscesses invading peritoneal cavity. (3) Invisible abscess areas. (a) Right inferior abscess is shown through the liver. Right posterior superior abscess is shown as abscess invading the peritoneal cavity above the liver and behind the right lateral ligament. (b)

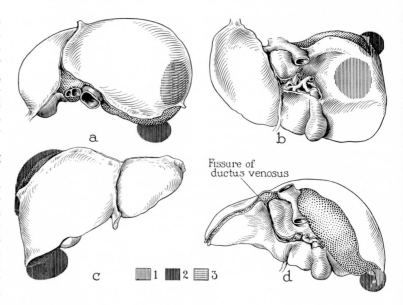

Liver viewed from below, showing right inferior space abscess and abscess from right posterior superior space invading the peritoneal cavity. (c) Liver viewed from in front, showing right inferior space abscess below liver and the right posterior superior abscess above the liver and behind the right lateral ligament. (d) Liver viewed from behind, showing typical location of right posterior superior space with abscess above the liver and behind the right lateral ligament. (Ochsner, A., and Graves, A. M.: Ann. Surg. 98:961)

that giving vitamin K_1 *before* making the puncture, with transient restoration of the prothrombin time to above 60 per cent, created a false sense of security. In patients with low prothrombin time before operation, vitamin K_1 should be continued after the operation or biopsy until all danger of hemorrhage has passed.

This survey indicated that the transthoracic approach was a significant factor in the hemorrhages encountered after needle biopsy of the liver:

This might well be anticipated in view of the proximity of the intercostal vessels and the lung tissues, the dependence upon the patient's ability to control his respiratory movements during the procedure, and the dangers of laceration of diaphragmatic vessels. This approach should be reserved, therefore, for those cases in which the abdominal approach is impossible, and in which the diagnostic worth of the biopsy outweighs the risk. The advantages of this mode of approach over that of exploratory laparotomy should be carefully considered.[13]

SUBPHRENIC ABSCESS

About 75 per cent of subphrenic abscesses occur on the right side and are due, in most cases, to appendicitis, perforated duodenal ulcer or cholecystitis (Fig. 350). The right posterior space is the one most commonly involved. Left-sided abscesses may result from perforation of a high gastric ulcer or from leakage after gastrectomy. A perforation in the wall of the stomach or the duodenum may lead to an abscess in the left postero-inferior space, i.e., in the lesser sac.

An extraperitoneal abscess (in relation to the bare area of the liver) is rare. It may result from lymph-borne infection or from direct spread, as in the case of a retrocecal appendicitis or of suppuration in the region of the right kidney.

DIAGNOSIS

In the main, diagnosis of a subphrenic abscess is difficult. The condition should be suspected whenever pyrexia (especially if septic

FIG. 351. (a) Illustration showing the method of approach to an
abscess in the right posterior superior space. By means of the finger, the peritoneum is peeled from
the undersurface of the diaphragm
until the abscess cavity is reached.
By plunging the finger through the
abscess wall the abscess may be
drained without contaminating the
pleural or peritoneal cavity. Insert
(b) shows location of a right inferior space abscess which may be
drained simultaneously through the
same incision. (Ochsner, A., and
Graves, A. M.: Ann. Surg. 98:
961)

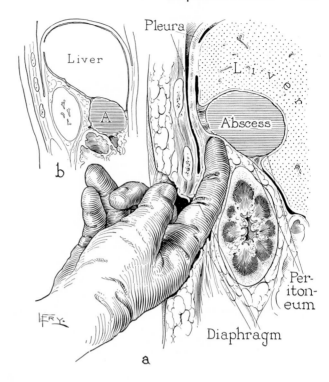

in character) persists after the treatment of
any inflammatory condition within the abdomen. Pain and tenderness over the lower ribs
and roentgenographic evidence of an elevated
fixed diaphragm are *confirmatory signs* but
are by no means consistently present. Often
roentgenographic and laboratory examinations
are of little help. Exploration with an aspirating needle is now generally condemned, since
it entails a very real danger of spreading the
infection to the pleural or the peritoneal cavities. Yet, some surgeons maintain that diagnostic aspiration is permissible provided that
it is carried out on the operating table and
that, if pus is obtained, the surgeon is prepared to proceed immediately to a drainage
operation. The longer the condition remains
undetected, the more likely are chest complications to ensue and to mask the diagnosis.
Therefore, there is a serious risk that, even
after consultation, the pyrexia and the toxemia
which are present may be ascribed to some
pulmonary condition alone and that valuable
time may be lost while treatment is directed
to this end.

TREATMENT

Chemotherapy is often successful in the case
of early subphrenic *infection,* but it should
not be persisted with for more than 4 or 5
days if the infection shows no signs of subsiding. When a *definite abscess* has formed—
as is likely to be the case if the temperature
is high—chemotherapy will be valueless and
indeed may actually be harmful since it masks
the clinical features of the condition.

The treatment of a subphrenic abscess is
essentially operative. The surgeon in charge
must accept full responsibility in making the
diagnosis and should be prepared to carry out
an exploratory operation solely on *suspicion.*
He should not be deterred from operation because lung changes are present, unless he is
convinced that these alone are likely to be
responsible for the patient's condition. There
is no serious reproach if operation fails to disclose a subphrenic abscess. It is a far worse
mistake that the condition should be missed,
for in such cases, a fatal outcome is very likely
to result.

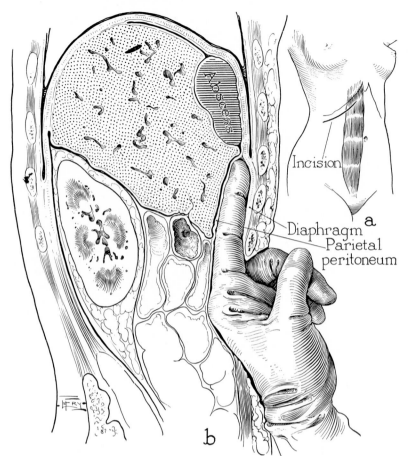

Fig. 352. Illustration showing the method of draining extraperitoneally an abscess in the right anterior superior space. As shown in (a), an incision is made below and paralleling the right costal margin, passing through the flat abdominal muscles and the transversalis fascia. (b) By means of the finger, the parietal peritoneum is peeled from the undersurface of the diaphragm until the abscess cavity is reached. The abscess is then drained extraperitoneally without contaminating either the pleural or the peritoneal cavity. (Ochsner, A., and Graves, A. M.: Ann. Surg. 98:961)

LOCATING THE ABSCESS

In the absence of definite roentgenograhic signs, localization of the abscess is likely to be conjectural. As most such abscesses arise on the *right side,* some guidance as to the space involved may be obtained from the site of maximum tenderness. If this is located over the lower ribs posteriorly, the abscess may be expected to occupy the right posterior space (by far the most common situation). Tenderness under the costal margin *in front* suggests infection of the right anterior space, while tenderness and resistance in the flank may also denote infection of the right anterior space.

If possible, the surgical approach should always be extraperitoneal. In addition, the approach should not be made anywhere which will involve the general pleural cavity because the greatest of all surgical errors is contamination of that area. *The incision must always be made through an area of peritoneum with which the walled-off abscess is in contact. The transpleural approach has now been abandoned.*

DRAINAGE

The safest method of drainage of an abscess on the right side posteriorly (where the great majority arise) is to remove the greater part of the twelfth rib, then to make a transverse incision at the level of the first lumbar spinous process—across the center of the bed of the rib. This incision avoids the pleura and divides the diaphraghmatic fibers arising from the periosteum of the rib (Fig. 351). The surgeon's finger is introduced to explore upward and locate the abscess, which—if and when found—is drained in the usual way. Every precaution should be taken not to injure the duodenum.

Anterior Extraperitoneal Approach. An anterior approach may be considered when the abscess is thought to be situated in front of the liver, or after exploration by the posterior route has been fruitless. An incision is made one half inch below and parallel with the costal margin, and all structures are divided down to, but not through, the peritoneum. The sur-geon's finger is then passed gently upward, separating this from the diaphragm until the abscess is located by touch (Fig. 352). An incision can now be made through the ad-herent peritoneum and the pus evacuated with-out risk of contaminating the general peri-toneal cavity.

Part Two: The Biliary Duct System

CONGENITAL ANOMALIES

ANOMALIES AS A CAUSE OF ERROR

Anomalies in the arteries of the biliary sys-tem may be of great importance to the sur-geon. Therefore, it is desirable that he be well acquainted with the possibility of their ex-istence before undertaking operation. The anomalies having the most surgical significance are those occurring in the terminal branches of the hepatic artery. The relations of these blood vessels to the neighboring bile ducts may follow almost any conceivable pattern (see Figs. 331-345).

The Right Hepatic Artery. This artery may cross anterior to the common hepatic duct—a position in which it is more likely to be injured during a surgical operation than if it followed a normal course. It may also follow along the cystic duct, where it is easily mis-taken for the cystic artery. It may even origi-nate as a separate artery and run along the right side of the common bile duct. Two or even more cystic arteries may take their origin from the right hepatic artery. But the sur-geon should keep in mind that the cystic artery often takes origin from structures other than the right hepatic, e.g., the *left* hepatic artery or the gastroduodenal artery (it takes its course along the common bile duct and the cystic duct to the gallbladder). The right hepatic artery may course along the cystic duct for a considerable distance up the bed of the gallbladder before entering the liver.

The Main Hepatic Artery. This has been found running along the cystic duct. If such an anomalous blood vessel should be ligated, the arterial blood supply to the entire liver would be largely cut off, and death would be likely to follow because of impairment of the hepatic circulation. Normally the hepatic ar-tery lies to the left of the common bile duct, and both structures are anterior to the portal vein.

Anomalous Hepatic Arteries. Should the right hepatic artery or the common hepatic artery be ligated during operation, the result may be fatal. Hemorrhage from an anomalous or accessory vessel which is unexpectedly di-vided may obscure the field, and blind at-tempts to control the bleeding may occasion damage to the bile ducts. Ample and meticu-lous dissection should always precede any operation in this region, so that anatomic variations may be recognized and proper safe-guards established.

SURGICAL TREATMENT OF CONGENITAL ANOMALIES

Torsion of "Floating" Gallbladder. The cystic duct may possess a distinct mesentery, while the gallbladder is free except for a com-plete investment of peritoneum, or the gall-bladder and the cystic duct may both be suspended from the liver by a normal ap-pearing mesentery. Either abnormality gives no evidence of its existence unless it under-goes *torsion*. The symptoms of torsion are a sudden attack of acute pain below the right costal margin, increasing in severity without letup. Rise of temperature, increased pulse rate, vomiting and often complete collapse rapidly ensue. Though the pain is mainly in the right epigastrium, it may be referred to a point below the right shoulder blade. There may also be tenderness and rigidity over the gallbladder.

From these manifestations a diagnosis of acute obstructive cholecystitis is usually made and operation advised and carried out. As the condition is found only in middle-aged or elderly persons, even the most alert surgeon is not likely to think of a *congenital anomaly,* yet prompt operation is the only possible means of relief, so failure to make a correct preoperative diagnosis is of no moment. When surgically exposed, the gallbladder will be found to be greatly edematous, hemorrhagic or even necrotic—depending on how long a time has elapsed since the torsion took place. Twisted pedicle and infarcted gallbladder present so characteristic a picture that even a tyro would recognize it immediately.

Treatment is simple, and the only error likely to impede the surgeon is failure to isolate the cystic duct and artery completely before tying and dividing them. The loose attachment between liver and gallbladder must be clamped and secured for cutting, after which the gallbladder is removed. In some cases, it may be necessary to guard against bile leakage, and the judgment of the surgeon may dictate the type of operation—classic or electrocoagulation (see pp. 487-493, "Electrosurgical Obliteration of the Gallbladder").

Anomalous Right Hepatic Artery. If the right hepatic artery lies parallel with or very close against the cystic duct, it is liable to injury during cholecystectomy. Again, if it forms a loop in front of the common hepatic duct or projects far forward, making a "knuckle" close to the upper margin of the gallbladder neck before its normal backward turn to the portal fissures, it is very vulnerable during removal of the gallbladder. If the right hepatic artery lies across the common hepatic duct, it may also be clamped or divided accidentally during a difficult excision of the gallbladder or in a secondary operation on the bile ducts. If the communication between gallbladder and bile duct is unusually wide and no cystic duct is present, and the right hepatic artery lies—as it frequently does—*behind* the gallbladder, it may be traumatized or even entirely severed when the broad isthmus is clamped or divided.

Anomalous Accessory Cystic Artery. Where an anomalous accessory cystic artery exists, it can always be traced to where it passes in front of the bile ducts. If the surgeon is unaware of the ever-present threat of anomalous cystic arteries, he may be surprised by a severe hemorrhage while doing the preliminary dissection for cholecystectomy or common duct exploration.

Ligation of the Hepatic Artery. This is perhaps the most serious error that the surgeon who undertakes cholecystectomy can commit. Three out of 4 patients will die as a result of such a mistake.

In general, the greatest safeguard against accidents resulting from congenital malformations is a very thorough study of the normal anatomy of the gallbladder, its blood supply and ducts (see Fig. 329) and a working knowledge of the most common congenital anomalies. To this must be added skill in dissection and a cautious approach, taking plenty of time to trace each vessel or duct and to identify it throughout its course.

TREATMENT OF INJURIES TO THE GALLBLADDER AND THE BILE DUCTS

Traumatic Injuries

Modern conditions, especially automobile and industrial accidents, have increased the incidence of traumatic injuries to the gallbladder and the bile ducts as well as to all other parts of the digestive tract. Occasionally, the gallbladder alone will suffer rupture or even complete severance when other abdominal organs have escaped serious injury. More often, the gallbladder damage will be but part of wide abdominal trauma, so that it may be overlooked entirely and put in evidence only by an exsanguinating hemorrhage which rapidly proves to be fatal unless heroic measures are instituted. The clinical picture is the same for all parts of the injured biliary tract: shock, more or less profound; on recovery from shock, constant pain over the right costal margin; evidence of fluid steadily increasing within the abdomen; a jaundiced appearance; rise of temperature and pulse rate; finally, profound toxemia and death. Paracentesis of the abdomen will produce large amounts of bile-stained fluid which will furnish a reliable clue as to what has occurred. Immediate operation offers the only chance for saving the patient's life.

The biliary passages are best approached through a right paramedian or oblique subcostal incision. As soon as the peritoneum is opened, bile will pour out of the wound. A suction tube must be introduced into the abdomen and the bile-stained ascitic fluid drained off. Effusions of bile do not usually cause peritonitis, so it may be possible to clear the field and make a systematic search for the wound. In the common hepatic duct, a tear is most likely to take place high up, close to the junction of the right and the left hepatic ducts. Identification is difficult, and when the wound is finally located, it presents a surgical problem to tax the skill of the most expert. Some surgeons have succeeded in closing such a rent with interrupted sutures placed transversely or a continuous suture of No. 000 medium chromic catgut, thereafter making a small opening in the anterior wall of the common duct through which a T tube is inserted. The upper limb of this tube serves as a splint for the injured duct, while the bile-stained fluid in the peritoneal cavity is being aspirated and the subhepatic region drained with a sheet of soft corrugated rubber. The patient's condition is often too desperate to permit of such manipulations, so nothing more than the insertion of a cigarette drain down to the rent can be done.

However, lacerations in the common bile duct are more easily dealt with than those in the hepatic duct, as most of them occur on the anterior wall of the duct. The duct may be torn in either direction, or it may be completely severed. If only the anterior wall has suffered injury, it is a comparatively easy matter to insert a T tube, as directed above, closing the walls of the ducts around the projecting limb of the tube. In cases of complete severance of the duct, with the patient in fairly good condition, the severed ends should be picked up, freshened and joined by a single row of sutures. The T tube can be inserted *above* or *below* the suture line, but it is a grave error to bring it out *through the line of anastomosis*.

If the lower end of the common duct is badly lacerated or pulpified, or if the surgeon cannot isolate it, it is better to tie and invaginate the proximal end of the duct and to anastomose the gallbladder to the pylorus, to the proximal duodenum or to the proximal jejunum, whichever seems to be easiest and safest under the existing conditions. *Safeguard the anastomosis by being sure beforehand that the cystic duct is patent.*

INJURIES REQUIRING REOPERATION

Aside from traumatic injuries where the gallbladder and the bile ducts are involved in widespread crushing of the abdomen and the pelvis, *benign stricture* of this area is usually due to errors and accidents during cholecystectomy or related operative procedures. Several reports have recently been issued from the St. Lukas Hospital, Copenhagen, Denmark, stressing the increasing frequency of "reoperation" for injuries to the bile ducts incurred in cholecystectomy.[7] Most of these injuries were concentrated in an area about 3 cm. in diameter, at the angle between the cystic duct and the hepatic duct, the very place where aberrant arteries and other anomalies are most likely to be found. The causes of surgical injuries incurred in this particular area may be divided into 4 groups:

1. Profuse and uncontrollable bleeding from the cystic artery or from the right hepatic artery has led to improper and erroneous placing of hemostatic forceps, causing injury to the hepatic duct. As the cystic artery is shorter than the cystic duct, the artery can be torn (sometimes involving the hepatic artery as well) merely by a strong pull on the gallbladder while it is being detached. This error can be guarded against by beginning the operation for cholecystectomy by ligating the artery.

2. Too strong a pull on the cystic duct may draw up the common bile duct into a tip which is ligated, or the common bile duct may become constricted because the cystic duct has been ligated too close to it.

3. If the cystic duct is anomalously absent, the common bile duct may be mistaken for this duct, or if the cystic duct is very short, the same mistake may be made; in either case the common bile duct will be exposed to injury. In addition, a not inconsiderable risk exists if the common bile duct runs parallel with the cystic duct when the latter follows a spiral course, in which case sometimes the two structures are matted together. These sources of technical error can be avoided by a careful exposure by dissection of the bile ducts, so that the surgeon is fully oriented before he ligates the cystic duct. Undoubtedly the risk is greater in those cases where the cystic duct opens into the right hepatic duct or enters the common

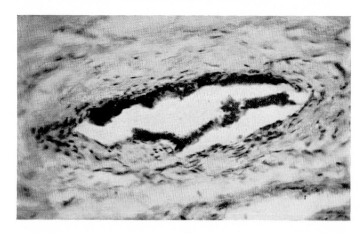

Fig. 353. Shows bile duct in gallbladder bed ($\times$ 90).

bile duct together with both branches of the hepatic duct. In such cases, even with careful dissection of the structures involved, it is easy to mistake the left hepatic branch for the common hepatic duct and to ligate the cystic duct and right hepatic duct together, believing that only the cystic duct is being ligated.

4. Anatomicopathologic changes are a frequent source of error and consequent injury. The migration of gallstones—especially if they are good sized—down into the cystic duct may block it completely, so that a correct survey of the operative field will be very difficult and injury to the underlying bile ducts will be more liable to occur. Inflammatory processes and their sequelae—only too well known to every surgeon who specializes in the biliary system— are a frequent cause of error.

Reports published in this country indicate similar observations. At the Lahey Clinic over a 31-year period, reoperations were performed on 280 patients suffering from stricture or destruction of the bile ducts as a result of operations for gallstones. A very complete study of these cases by Lahey and Pyrtek, published in 1950, points out the errors in various types of gallbladder operations which make such reoperation necessary and also suggests some relatively simple safeguards against injury to the patient's biliary system and to the surgeon's reputation.

Two types of duct injury can occur at the time of a surgical operation on the gallbladder or the bile ducts: (1) crushing of the duct by grasping it with a clamp or (2) the excision of part of the duct—common, common and hepatic, hepatic or sections of anomalous he-patic ducts.

Most of the *crush injuries* to the bile ducts are related to hemorrhage, either from the cystic or the right hepatic artery. These hemorrhages are deep in the wound where it is difficult to keep the blood sponged out, so that the anatomic structures are obscured and attempts to control the bleeding must be made without clear visualization of the field. In several of these cases, the history of the previous operation showed that serious bleeding had been encountered, which was controlled during the operation only by the application of a clamp which had been left in place, to be removed 3 or 4 days later.

When the gallbladder is removed from above downward, and undue traction is exerted on it, such traction will be almost entirely on the cystic artery, and if it is continued, the artery will tear—usually at its point of origin from the right hepatic artery. *Such an emergency can be avoided by careful dissection of the cystic artery before the cystic duct is clamped and cut, and by taking great care not to exert too much traction either on the mobilized gallbladder when it is removed from above downward or on the ampulla of the gallbladder when it is removed from below upward. Never clamp the cystic duct until the artery has been found and divided.*

Treatment of Bile Duct Injury. This should begin with prophylaxis. In performing cholecystectomy, in addition to a sufficiently large incision, adequate anesthesia, excellent illumination and the like, one of the principal points in prophylaxis is to avoid any large hemorrhage. Commence with isolation and ligation of the cystic artery. The cystic duct should never be divided until the surgeon is fully oriented as to all the components of the bile passages in the area (Fig. 353). In cases where there are anatomic variations, it is often better to work from above downward, gradually laying bare the cystic duct as a stem, even though retrograde cystectomy is the method most commonly employed.

If, despite every care and attention to surgical detail, injuries do occur, the next requirement is to discover them and make repairs as soon as possible—*before the operation is concluded*. At no time will conditions for complete and adequate repair be as favorable as at the time the injury takes place. If delayed until fistulae and scar tissue have formed, the difficulties will be greatly increased. It is surprising how few surgical injuries to the bile ducts are recognized during the course of operation, for oozing of bile invariably takes place from the upper lumen of the divided duct. It should be an absolute rule to make a careful inspection of the operative field for oozing of bile at the conclusion of *every* intervention on the biliary system.

As regards the technic to be employed when it is necessary to correct errors made in an earlier cholecystectomy, good results have been obtained by union of the bile passages through an end-to-end suture as well as by anastomosing operation. Choice of method and divergences in technical details are not as important as (1) union of mucosa with mucosa (whether by end-to-end suture or anastomosis) and (2) sure safeguarding against recurrent stenosis by sufficiently protracted use of a suitable tube.

SURGICAL CONSIDERATIONS

Exposure of the Gallbladder

While it is safer to remove the gallbladder from above downward, the operation is bloodier than when working upward. On the other hand, while working from below gives a "dry field," this technic is often beset with many difficulties and dangers. Therefore, the surgeon of limited experience will do better to begin with cholecystectomies from above downward; thus he will be sure to find the cystic artery about the lower third of the gallbladder, at Callot's triangle, where it may be ligated. On the other hand, the more experienced surgeon who prefers to begin dissection in the cholecystoduodenal ligament, there ex-

posing the cystic artery and the cystic duct, may continue in the same direction if the work is progressing satisfactorily. However, if he encounters difficulties, e.g., hemorrhage, adhesions or anomalies, he may abandon operation at that point and proceed with the dissection from above downward.

Incision for exposure of the gallbladder and the biliary passages should always be adequate. Efficient work cannot be done in this area without adequate exposure, good illumination and, above all, meticulous dissection of the structures. Complicated incisions should be avoided.

Closure of the Incision

This is of great importance. I personally prefer catgut for the peritoneum and muscle approximation and some nonabsorbable suture material such as cotton for the fascia. The skin may be closed with the material with which the surgeon has had best results.

Dangers to Avoid

Ligation of the Hepatic Artery. Occasionally the hepatic artery may be mistaken for the cystic artery. In such cases, ligation is likely to prove to be fatal. Therefore, it is essential to dissect meticulously and identify *every* blood vessel before ligating it. The course and the size of the cystic artery are often very confusing. Before ligating, it is best to trace it both upward and downward and to identify its branches on the gallbladder.

Injuries to the Common Duct. There are no "easy" cases in biliary surgery! The experience of the surgeon, his attention to detail and to minutest dissection and identification of structures are of paramount importance. A very short cystic duct may pull up a loop of common duct; if the common duct happens to be small, the surgeon may not recognize it and divide it or inflict some injury on it. He should also always keep in mind the possible anomalies of the duct structure as well as those of the blood vessels. Half a century ago, Austin Flint called this to the attention of the profession. Later observations have proved that the vast majority of cases do not duplicate the textbook picture of what is considered to be "normal" in these structures but, instead, will present variations which the surgeon must be able to recognize and identify properly during operation.

CHOLANGIOGRAPHY. In well-appointed hospitals, equipment is at hand to enable the surgeon to obtain roentgenograms of the biliary duct system during operation. When cholangiography is performed properly, anomalies, stones and obstructions due to pancreatitis or to tumors can be visualized. Thus, if cholangiography is employed routinely, injuries to the common duct can be avoided in many instances.

Sphincterotomy. This operation should be performed only when considered imperative by the diagnosis of a surgeon of mature experience. The procedure is difficult and is accompanied by high morbidity and, on occasion, will be followed by fatal pancreatitis.

It is well to stress here again that those who engage in biliary surgery should have mature experience in dissections and be fully conversant with the complications that may follow operations in this region. Also, if an injury to the common duct is discovered during the operation, it should be repaired there and then. If not, the more time that elapses between injury and repair, the more difficult is the procedure and the less likely are good results to follow.

CHANCES FOR ERROR IN MANAGEMENT OF BILIARY TUMORS

Tumors of any sort are not common in the biliary system. Three types of benign growths have been described: epithelial polyp, adenomyoma and fibroma. *Polyps* of the gallbladder contain gallstones in about 68 per cent of cases. *Adenomyomas* have a tendency toward cyst formation when they occur in the extrabiliary tract, with calculi forming in the cystic spaces, and occasionally intramural abscesses may develop. In the majority of instances, cholecystitis or cholelithiasis will be observed. *Fibromata* are very rare and are seen only in conjunction with chronic cholecystitis. The diagnosis of these benign growths is practically never made before operation. If they cause any symptoms, these will be attributed to the cholecystitis which is regularly present at the same time. A possible exception is, perhaps, the occurrence of pain and colic due to obstruction of the cystic duct by the pedunculated variety of tumor.

Workers at the Mayo Clinic more than 20 years ago claimed that these benign growths could be diagnosed preoperatively by intelli-

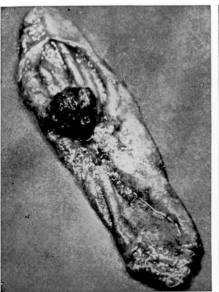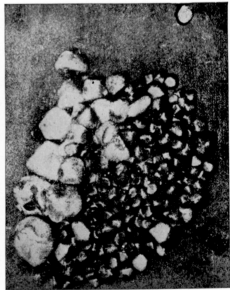

FIG. 354. Gallbladder undergoing malignant degeneration. (*Left*) Carcinoma probably caused by irritation from biliary calculi. (*Right*) Same case; stones removed from gallbladder.

FIG. 355. A question in differential diagnosis; (arrow at 2) is this calcified gallbladder or large gallstone? (Arrow at b, diverticulum of duodenum.)

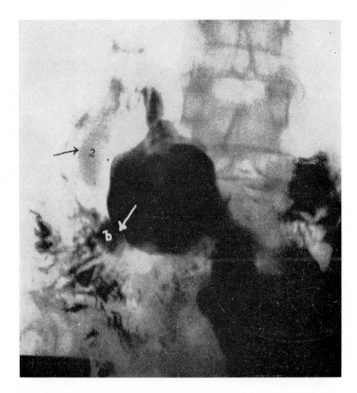

gent use of the cholecystogram. The filling defect caused by a benign tumor maintains the same relative location when the patient's position is shifted, while the shadow cast by a stone is apt to shift as the patient's body is moved. Therefore, *cholecystography* is an aid in avoiding diagnostic mistakes.

Carcinoma of the gallbladder is the neoplasm most often encountered Its incidence in women is almost 4 times as great as in men. Dissemination takes place early, both by metastasis and by direct extension, the liver being the organ most often invaded. Tumor implants at the porta hepatis frequently induce jaundice, and in advanced cases the duodenum may be involved, leading to intestinal obstruction. As gallstones have been found in from 65 to 90 per cent of adenocarcinomas located in the gallbladder, the inference of etiologic relationship is very strong (Fig. 354). It is reasonable to assume that the prompt removal of stones from the gallbladder would do much to lessen the occurrence of cancer of this area. Such surgery is undoubtedly the greatest safeguard at our disposal, and the failure to employ it when the condi-

tions warrant is a grave surgical error. Intravenous cholangiographic studies are useful in establishing early diagnosis, particularly of those growths arising in the bile ducts. Wide resection en bloc is not feasible, owing to the location in the immediate vicinity of such structures as the hepatic artery, the portal vein and the vena cava. Especially in the upper half of the duct system, local resection is the only possible procedure. After resection, continuity is re-established by end-to-end anastomosis (if the gap is not too large) or by joining the duct to the duodenum or the jejunum. Some good results from surgical excision are on record, but, in general, the outlook in any malignancy of the biliary system is poor. If too great a section of the duct wall is removed with a benign lesion, there is real danger of a stricture of the duct. Surgeons should be on their guard against such an error.

GALLSTONES

ROENTGENOGRAPHIC DIAGNOSIS

Though one of the first medical uses of Roentgen's discovery was the detection of stones in the biliary tract, the surgeon of today

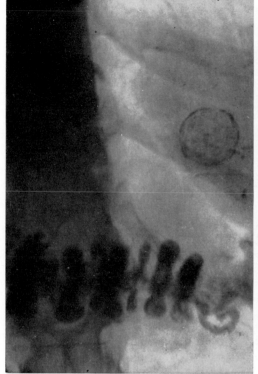

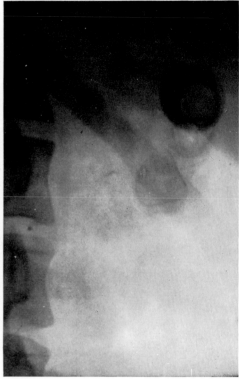

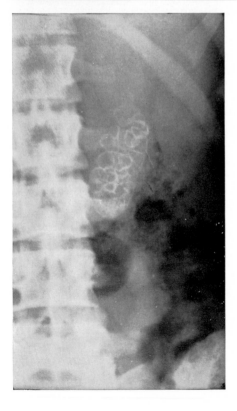

FIG. 356. Examples of opaque gallstones of varying densities easily demonstrable roentgenographically.

knows that too much reliance cannot be placed on the findings of this diagnostic aid. As more and more has been learned about gallbladder disease, the fact that many of the concretions found in the biliary tract are not radiopaque or, at best, are only partially so has shaken the faith of even the most ardent exponents of cholecystography. In some respects, this is unfortunate, but the wisdom of looking out for errors of interpretation (Fig. 355) by both roentgenologists and surgeons is self-evident, and the need for surrounding the establishment of roentgen diagnosis with every possible safeguard may very well be continually emphasized.

The symptoms of chronic cholecystitis are so characteristic and universally recognized that a diagnosis can be established by them alone, without mechanical aids. But differential diagnosis is none the less not always reached without such aids. Chronic peptic ulcer or appen-

FIG. 357. Cholesterin stone made visible roentgenographically by administration of opaque material.

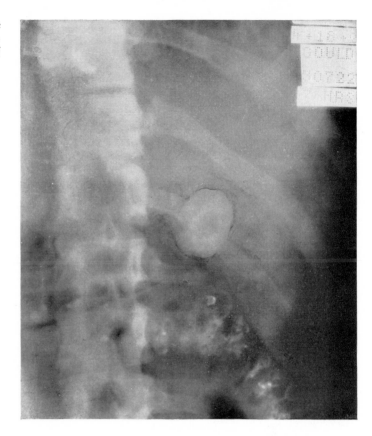

dicitis, chronic relapsing pancreatitis, renal disease and especially carcinoma of the intestines may cause and have caused the most experienced diagnostician to make mistakes, and the man to whom this mishap has once occurred will make full use of all the help roentgenology can offer him.

ROENTGENOGRAPHIC TECHNIC

It is well to begin with plain roentgenograms of the entire gallbladder region (Fig. 356), then follow these by cholecystography. Administer the opaque medium either by mouth or intravenously and use the regular technic for the barium meal with the surgeon's preferred method of administration (Fig. 357). The dye is excreted in the bile and is carried to the gallbladder, where it is concentrated. As the concentrated bile will be radiopaque, the gallbladder will be clearly outlined and the presence or the absence of stones at once indicated. The character, the number and the position of the stones may also be indicated, but with varying degrees of accuracy.

Warning. Do not administer dye to a patient who is jaundiced. If a stone chanced to be impacted in the ampulla of Vater, it might cause a direct communication between the common bile duct and the pancreatic duct, giving the dye opportunity to activate an acute hemorrhage and pancreatitis with rapidly fatal results.

DIFFERENTIAL DIAGNOSIS

Gastric Disturbances. Biliary lithiasis is responsible for a variety of gastric disturbances; these, in turn, may be due to still other causes. Perforation of a gastroduodenal ulcer may be mistaken for gallstone colic because the site and the sudden onset of pain are similar. Also, heart disease and aortic affections, such as angina pectoris, abdominal angina or thrombosis of the coronary arteries, frequently simulate the symptoms of cholecystitis. Biliary

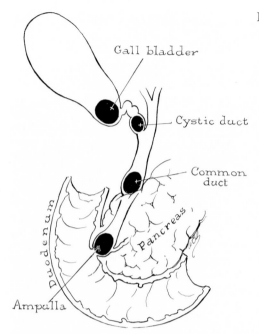

Gall bladder

Cystic duct

Common duct

Duodenum

Pancreas

Ampulla

Fig. 358. Diagram showing common sites for obstructions in biliary system.

characterized by a complete absence of pain. A diagnosis of gastric or duodenal ulcer is often made in such cases. Three factors may be responsible for these errors: (1) embryology (common origin of nerves responsible for reflex gastric reactions usually observed in lithiasis); (2) anatomy (adhesions, periduodenitis); (3) physiology (contraction of the gallbladder, causing pain during the passage of the duodenal contents). Here, roentgenograms, analyses of gastric secretions and duodenal catheterization may be helpful. The results of these must be correlated in order to arrive at a correct diagnosis. Pain may be fleeting and diffuse. Elevation of temperature speaks for the presence of infection. Occult blood suggests ulcer, but its presence does not exclude cholelithiasis.

Obstruction of the Common Bile Duct. It must be determined whether the obstruction is due to a stone or to malignant disease. This is by no means easy and often can be ascertained only through exploratory laparotomy.

At this point, it would be well to recall the

colic is not always due to stones; it occurs in various types of inflammations as well. Gallstone colic may also be simulated by spasm of the ducts stemming from a variety of causes.

Chronic Biliary Lithiasis. This is sometimes

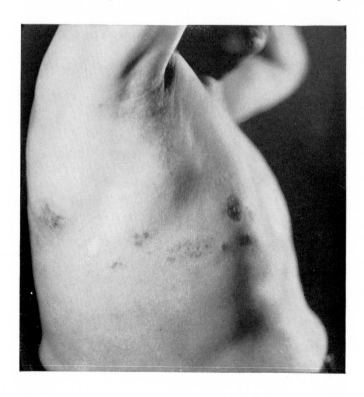

Fig. 359. Truly a case of "mistaken identity"; herpes zoster simulating disease in the right hypochondrium, possibly gallbladder disease.

salient features of biliary obstruction (Fig. 358); many diagnostic and therapeutic errors will be avoided by keeping these facts in mind:

1. LARGE SINGLE STONE OR NUMEROUS FACETED STONES IN THE GALLBLADDER. These will produce no symptoms if there is no active inflammation. When there is inflammation, there will be attacks of biliary colic and symptoms of cholecystitis. There will be no jaundice, and the color of stools will be normal. X-ray examination will indicate the condition; dye will enter the gallbladder.

2. STONE IN CYSTIC DUCT. This is not accompanied by inflammation of the gallbladder. There will be hydrops but no jaundice, and stools will be normal in color. In the presence of inflammation, there will be empyema of the gallbladder. Roentgenograms may be of value in differential diagnosis.

3. STONE IN UPPER PART OF COMMON BILE DUCT. This usually causes colic; with inflammation, symptoms will depend on the degree of obstruction. "Ball-valve" action of the stone may cause the symptoms to alternate. Jaundice, clay-colored stools and a positive van den Bergh test also will depend on the degree of blockage. In these cases the gallbladder is often small. No symptoms of impaired pancreatic function will be present. If not relieved, there are likely to be frequent attacks of pain in the right hypochondrium (Fig. 359), usually accompanied by fever. If the obstruction is due to a tumor, jaundice and clay-colored stools are apt to be constant.

4. STONE IN LOWER PART OF COMMON BILE DUCT. Again, symptoms depend on the extent of blockage and are practically the same as those noted when the stone is in the upper part of the duct. Here, however, pancreatic digestion may occasionally be impaired. If the obstruction is due to tumor or inflammation, symptoms will be more marked and persistent.

In obstruction of the common duct, prompt intervention is indicated. Resort may be had to a prophylactic regimen for a limited time, but the effect of this is never curative. Expectant treatment is permissible for only a short period.

5. STONE IN PANCREATIC DUCT. Symptoms of blockage will depend on the degree of the obstruction, reflected by intensity of pancreatic damage.

Removal of Stone from the Common Bile Duct. When operating for stone in the common bile duct, it is advisable to pass a sound through the lumen, especially the lower segment, to make perfectly sure that no calculi remain. Sometimes, though a probe is passed into the duodenum, it will miss a lurking stone. If the duct is thickened, especially about the head of the pancreas, a calculus should always be suspected. Nodular enlargement of the pancreas at this point usually means a stone. The need for thorough exploration is apparent from experience gained in a very large number of biliary operations done in the Mayo Clinic some years ago, in which postmortem examination revealed that in nearly one third of the deaths following operation for common duct stone, all the stones had not been removed. Hence, all accessible biliary passages should be carefully explored.

After complete removal of the stones from the common bile duct, some resort to primary suture of the incision in the duct, after first verifying the patency of the ampulla of Vater. Cholangiography during operation will also serve to demonstrate the degree of patency of the ampulla. In some cases, delayed passage of the opaque material will be due to stricture of the distal portion of the duct at the level of the pancreas. In these cases, cysticoduodenostomy may be used to complement primary suture, if the caliber and the vascular system of the cystic duct are normal.

The common bile duct has defensive properties which make it more resistant than other structures of the biliary tract. The results of systematic study of the bacterial flora of the biliary tree and of neighboring structures indicate that the bile of the hepatic and common ducts is sterile (in the absence of lithiasis), notwithstanding the proximity of these ducts to structures which may be involved in focal infection. Though primary suture of the common duct has been resorted to without apparent ill effects by some, I do not recommend it. Some form of drainage is good practice.

READING CHOLECYSTOGRAMS

Appearance of the Normal Gallbladder. Following a fat meal, a normal gallbladder will contract satisfactorily and give a good, uniform shadow; it will show definitely that the liver can excrete the dye, that the bile ducts are patent and that the gallbladder walls are intact. *Good outline with negative shadows within it* shows that the dye mixed with bile has entered the gallbladder freely but gives no information as to whether or not the walls are inflamed. Negative shadows *may* or *may not* be due to nonopaque concretions. Again, the gallbladder may have concentrated the dye normally, and the stones will be clearly visible in it (see Fig. 357). In cases of cholesterol stones of small size, the gallbladder may have concentrated the dye normally, but the contrast medium has concealed them. If *there is no shadow*, the gallbladder is so obstructed that the dye cannot pass into it, the lining mucosa may be so diseased that it cannot concentrate the dye, or severe liver disease—toxic or chronic cholangitic hepatitis, for example—has cut off the flow of bile.

Extrinsic Causes for Nonvisualization. It is well to question the patient. It may be that he "forgot" or otherwise failed to swallow the dye capsule; it may have caused him to vomit or may have set up a profuse diarrhea, which prevented proper absorption. Even when these possibilities have been ruled out, the surgeon will have to decide whether failure of visualization is due to disease *within* the gallbladder or to *extrabiliary factors* which acted to prevent dye absorption, such as inflammation of the posterior duodenal wall caused by an ulcer or inflammation of other portions of the intestinal canal immediately adjacent, hitherto unrecognized.

However, in some 96 per cent of patients with a history of previous gallbladder disease, whenever one or more dye tests of the gallbladder failed to visualize, cholelithiasis was found at operation. Even this should not be taken as an unqualified indication for resort to surgery. It requires the best judgment of a thoroughly experienced surgeon who specializes in the biliary system. In more than half the proved cases of cholelithiasis, no shadow was obtained by cholecystography. The combination of "faint shadow" and "poor emptying" in the radiologist's report *does not necessarily* mean an organically diseased gallbladder, though he may be perfectly honest in making a diagnosis of chronic cholecystitis. In the absence of evidence of calculi, such a diagnosis is likely to prove to be in error.

Where the *outline of the gallbladder is irregular,* filling defects may suggest the presence of a neoplasm such as a papilloma. A safeguard in such a case is the taking of a regular barium-meal examination of the stomach and the large bowel in order to exclude duodenal ulcer and chronic appendicitis, as suggested by the Beelers in 1953.

OPERATIONS

The surgeon who undertakes any operation on the gallbladder or the biliary ducts must be thoroughly familiar not only with the normal anatomy of the parts involved but also with the possibilities of anomalous structures which will need to be dealt with should they be uncovered when the surgical field is exposed. Hemorrhage is an ever-present menace. All modern safeguards against this should always be at hand.

CHOLECYSTECTOMY

This operation has been done with steadily increasing frequency during the past half century, so that "operation for gallstones" has become a familiar phrase among lay persons of all social levels. A diagnosis of *cholecystitis* is often made and permission for operation sought and granted, only to have the real condition prove to be *choledocholithiasis* or *neoplasm* of either gallbladder or ducts, requiring operation of a different type and carrying a far graver prognosis. The chances of error are very great and the necessity for erecting safeguards even greater. The surgeon should not allow himself to be "stampeded" into operating. If his incision exposes a malignant growth, the patient's enthusiasm about her "gallstone operation" may undergo a change. The word "cancer" still carries a grim significance to the average layman. Great care in establishing the diagnosis is imperative. Asymptomatic presence of gallstones is not, in itself, a justification for surgical interference.

BILIARY CALCULI FRAGMENTS

In operating for gallbladder calculi, great care should be exercised to make sure that there are no stones or fragments in the common or hepatic ducts that might later work down.

FIG. 360. Contrasts effects of electro-coagulation with those of carbonization. (a) Shows extensive, gradually decreasing area of affected tissue when subjected to bipolar current. (b) Shows charring and generally inefficient results from improper application of current.

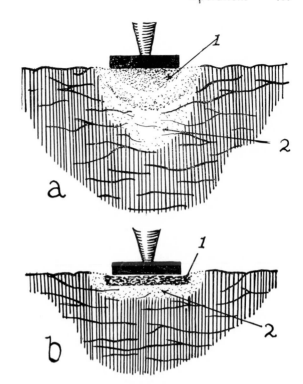

ELECTROSURGICAL OBLITERATION OF THE GALLBLADDER; AUTHOR'S METHOD

In competent hands, removal of the gallbladder by means of the scalpel yields a mortality of about 1 or 2 per cent in uncomplicated cases. Mortality increases with age and is greater in males than in females. It ranges around 10 per cent in unselected cases. Taking into consideration the unreported results of general surgeons, on occasion it may be as high as 20 to 30 per cent or even higher, depending on the incidence of complications.

Analysis of fatalities following classic cholecystectomy affords food for the following reflections:

1. Between 15 and 25 per cent of these patients have enlarged bile capillaries and small bile ducts running in the gallbladder bed, which cause bile leakage when the gallbladder is removed from the bed with a knife (see Fig. 353).

2. When sterile, bile in the peritoneal cavity acts as a chemical poison; when infected, it can cause septic peritonitis.

3. A properly ligated cystic duct does not leak; leakage is usually from the gallbladder bed. Bile has been observed issuing from the wound 230 times in 346 cases of simple cholecystectomy.

4. The gallbladder bed cannot always be obliterated by sutures. Drainage must then be resorted to; this invites leakage. Following the classic procedure, open, unprotected bile and blood channels in the gallbladder bed offer a favorable point of entry for micro-organisms.

5. Drainage can cause trouble in a number of ways, e.g., augmentation of bile seepage, thrombosis and embolism, hemorrhage from eroded vessels, cholemic bleeding, embarrassed cardiac action, particularly in the aged, pneumonia, acute dilatation of the stomach and biliary fistula. To put it differently, many patients die following gallbladder operations not because they were not drained but because of drainage. Nevertheless, though many dangers may be eliminated by omitting drains, drainage following the classic operation may save lives.

Rationale of Author's Method. In seeking to determine how the evils of drainage could be avoided and leakage from divided capillaries and small bile ducts frustrated, I thought that if a dry, nonleaking surface could be substituted for the discharging cavity represented

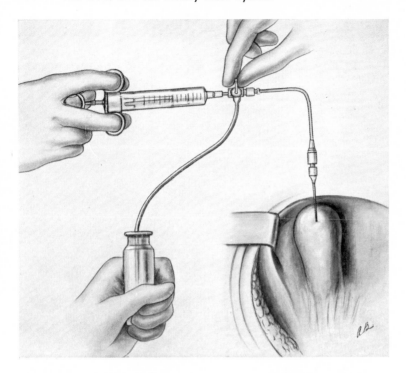

FIG. 361. Author's aspirator evacuates contents of gallbladder, permitting introduction of antiseptic solution, in preparation for removal of gallbladder by author's method.

by the gallbladder bed left by the classic cholecystectomy, it would be an important step in the right direction. Animal experimentation showed that this may be accomplished by proper *electrocoagulation*. When accurately performed, this converts the tissues into a hyalinelike, dry, aseptic, inert tampon. Unfortunately, electrocoagulation is still confused by the uninitiated with *fulguration* and *carbonization,* which actually are entirely different in their actions and effects. *It is important to understand these differences* (Fig. 360).

If a flat electrode of a bipolar current is applied firmly to a tissue surface and a current of proper voltage and sufficient amperage is permitted to pass through it, dehydration and coagulation of the tissue proteins result in a few seconds, and the tissue turns white. This is true electrocoagulation. On the other hand, if this same electrode is not applied firmly or if it is used as a unipolar instrument, a small air space (dielectricum) intervenes between the electrode and the tissue surface, and sparking, fulguration, carbonization and black discoloration of the area results. The carbonized surface stops further penetration of the

current and prevents coagulation. In cauterization, the heat is brought to the tissues from the outside through the heated instrument; in bipolar or short-wave electrocoagulation, the heat is generated within the patient's own tissues, the amount depending on the type of apparatus used.

Definite changes take place when liver tissue is subjected to the electrogoagulating bipolar current. Electrocoagulated surfaces *within the abdomen do not slough,* as do surfaces on the outside or in open cavities (mouth, vagina); in such places, coagulated areas will be eliminated by extrusion. Within the abdomen they become encapsulated and are absorbed. Electrocoagulated surfaces on parenchymatous organs develop an affinity (positive chemotaxis) for serous surfaces, attracting contiguous viscera that are covered with serosa (omentum, stomach, intestines). I have observed such agglutinations only 3 hours after electrocoagulating the surface of the liver. Firm union takes place in a comparatively short time; capillaries and blood vessels of an electrocoagulated area do not thrombose, but a recession of the column of blood is formed within the vessel, above and below the point

FIG. 362. Removal of gallbladder (author's method); inset shows electrocoagulation.

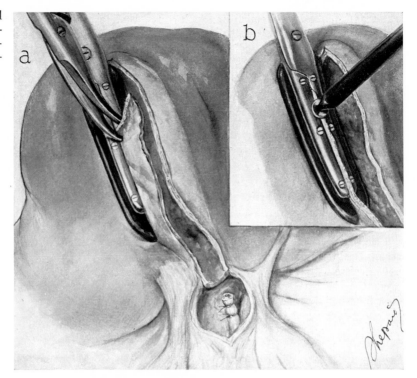

of contact with the electrode; the vessel walls coalesce with the contiguous, homogenous hyaline structures mentioned.

Another important fact to remember is that electrocoagulation of the tissues of the gallbladder frustrates secondary hemorrhage because of the pressure exerted by the sequestered coagulated segment against the contiguous tissues. Thus, electrocoagulation substitutes a secure sterile tampon for an insecure open cavity at the site of the gallbladder bed resulting from the classic cholecystectomy.

I have now been using this method (Figs. 361-364) for many years with entire success, not only in my personal practice, but also on surgical services of friends and colleagues to whom I have recommended it. Nearly 20 years ago, on my recommendation, the eminent British surgeon Hamilton Bailey tried it and has used it consistently in cases suitable for surgery of both gallbladder and biliary tract disease. The technic continues to give Bailey satisfaction and has been used successfully in South America and in many countries of Europe, because the factor of a dry, sterilized operative field, needing no drainage, is everywhere appreciated.

Author's Conclusions. My operation, when carefully followed, may be used in both simple and complicated cases of gallbladder disease without resorting to drainage. It reduces mortality to a minimum and cuts time in the hospital. The much dreaded age factor in these operations loses its terrors. Shock is usually absent.

Failures and fatalities following the classic cholecystectomy are often due to bile leakage as a result of inability to obliterate and cover the gallbladder bed which contains bile capillaries and often larger bile ducts in 15 to 25 per cent of cases. Drains invite bile seepage. My method seals off these openings by electrocoagulation. A sterile, hyaline, dry, protective layer is substituted for a raw, unprotected surface. The falciform ligament or omental graft is superimposed over this area and drainage is omitted entirely.

A prerequisite to achievement of satisfactory results is a patent common duct. An occluded cystic duct from any cause is an indication for this operation.

Experimental studies have shown that any method of carbonization, such as fulguration or electrocauterization, predisposes to hemorrhage, thrombosis and embolism. Such cauterization will not destroy pathogenic microorganisms in the depths of the affected gallbladder wall. Electrocoagulation is free from these drawbacks and effectually destroys the entire thickness of the gallbladder wall and, if desired, the gallbladder bed also. The surgeon has the degree of penetration completely under his control.

The ligamentum falciforme hepatis, or an omental segment, is used as a free graft; its serous structure covers sutured or raw surfaces to advantage, reinforcing and protecting the areas against seepage and safeguarding the processes of repair (Fig. 365).

Electrocoagulated areas of intra-abdominal organs tend to heal by encapsulation. They do not interfere with wound healing; on the contrary, they heal promptly when the wound is closed securely. Therefore, drainage is not only unnecessary, it is distinctly deleterious. As noted earlier, many patients have died as a direct result of drainage. It prolongs the healing process and predisposes to complications. Electrosurgical obliteration of the gallbladder eliminates the necessity for drainage and its unpleasant sequelae.

It should also be pointed out that where choledochostomy or hepaticostomy are indicated, these may be done in conjunction with my procedure. Experimental studies have shown that the implanted falciform ligament or omental graft over the obliterated gallbladder bed forms sufficient protection and does not interfere with a Kehr, Orr or similar drainage tube.

Whereas global mortality for removal of the gallbladder by scalpel methods, in unselected (including complicated) cases, still ranges around 10 per cent or more, the mortality in a series of over 5,000 unselected cases operated on by my method, electrosurgical operation of the gallbladder, was $\frac{1}{3}$ of 1 per cent.

CLASSIC CHOLECYSTECTOMY; DRAINAGE

In the standard procedure, the question of

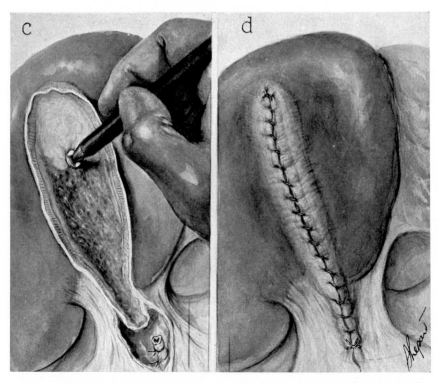

FIG. 363. Removal of gallbladder (author's method) continued. (*Left*) Electrocoagulation of gallbladder bed. (*Right*) Strip of electrocoagulated and crushed tissue united with continuous suture.

whether or not to institute drainage is of the first importance. Experience in the past has appeared to show that wound infection was at least as common with drainage as without. The same was true of hematoma. General results up to about 20 years ago showed a mortality percentage in favor of cholecystectomy with drainage. In scalpel surgery, in spite of the temptation to omit drainage, it seemed wiser to include it.

The type of drain to be used in biliary surgery depends on the nature of the operation being performed. In cholecystectomies, 1 or more cigarette drains may be needed. For dependent drainage, 2 or 3 cigarette drains in Morison's pouch are effective (Fig. 366)

Do not be alarmed if no bile drains from the tube for a few days following cholecystostomy; swelling of the mucous membranes is commonly responsible for this. The flow will soon start if one does not meddle. Should there be excessive flow of bile, this may be due to a stone in the common duct that was overlooked.

Never push a drainage tube too far into the gallbladder. By so doing, the very object for which the tube was introduced may be defeated.

Never try to invaginate an inflamed, thickened gallbladder; it cannot be done. The stitches will simply cut out.

Do not forget to attach a receptacle to the drainage tube and avoid kinking the tube. Drainage tubes introduced into the common bile duct for external drainage are usually sutured in place. Instances have been reported of broken tubes, with a portion left in the duct, necessitating choledochotomy. Carefully avoid

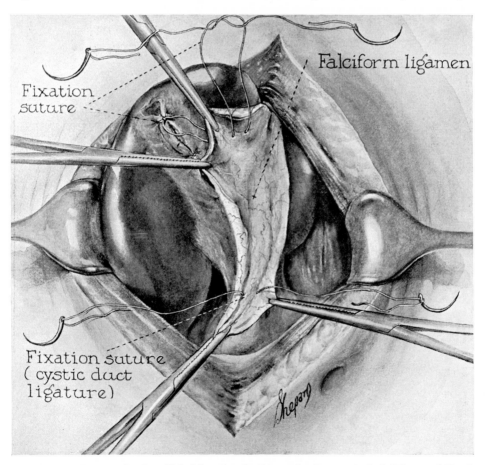

FIG. 364. Removal of gallbladder (author's method) concluded. The mobilized falciform ligament is fixed over the closed, electrocoagulated surface. Note placement of sutures.

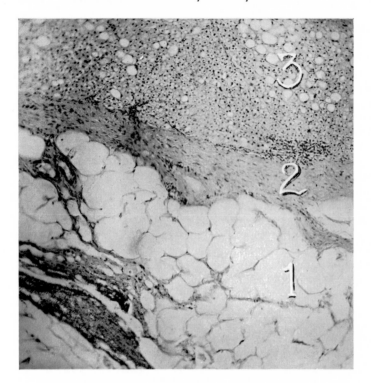

Fig. 365. Histologic study of results after electrosurgical obliteration of gallbladder (author's method), made 10 months after operation. Note excellent preservation of transplanted falciform ligament at 1. Gallbladder bed represented by fibrous band is at 2; normal liver structure at 3.

any pull on a tube from the common bile duct. After cholecystectomy with drainage, a small percentage of patients discharge bile from the wound in spite of the cystic duct having been ligated. This begins at once or a few hours after the operation and is obviously from the raw surface of the gallbladder bed or possibly from an accessory duct. Only rarely

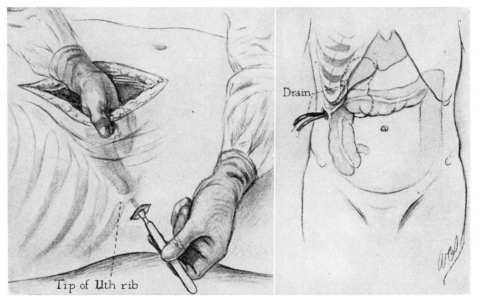

Fig. 366. Drainage through Morison's pouch. (*Left*) Method of incision. (*Right*) Point of emergence for drains.

will a ligature slip off the cystic duct; there is little pressure behind such a ligature to force it off.

Some surgeons may give small thought to the possible presence of accessory ducts—the subject is seldom brought up in this connection—but to close the abdomen with one of these ducts cut and left open may lead to disaster. In all probability, such an accident would be explained as leakage from the cystic duct, the argument being advanced that if it had occurred, bile would flow from the cut end during the operation and that use of a tube would make closure of the abdomen safe. I do not believe that this is necessarily true in view of the aforementioned fact that bile often does not flow at all for many hours after an operation. Though this is not common after cholecystectomy alone, there is no doubt that in cases complicated by severe hepatitis, secretion of bile is temporarily suspended. Moreover, there is no serious objection to leaving a soft rubber drain in place for 2 or 3 days through an incision which displaces the rectus muscle outward; hernia very seldom results, and occasionally a life may be saved.

Quite a large number of injuries to the bile ducts have been reported by various writers; however, these probably represent only a small fraction of the total number of such accidents, for surgeons are understandably sensitive about having committed such errors. As long as surgeons continue to clamp and ligate structures in this region en masse, accidents are bound to occur; they can be avoided only by seeing everything and never forgetting the frequency of abnormalities.

Safeguards. If a patient in whom a cholecystectomy has been performed is the victim of division of an aberrant hepatic duct that has been left unligated, the results may be disastrous. Death in such instances is commonly due to leakage of bile into the general peritoneal cavity, with resulting peritonitis. Expose all ducts and inspect them before cutting and remember that inflammatory changes may so alter their appearance that they may be hard to isolate. Nevertheless, if the possibilities are kept in mind, meticulous dissection will avoid much trouble from this source.

When injury to a duct is discovered during the operation, the manner of repairing it must be considered immediately. End-to-end anastomoses are not likely to be as successful as are junctions of the stump with the duodenum, but if the division is a clean one and other conditions are favorable, end-to-end union may be feasible.

When *postoperative drainage* is used, several points should be kept in mind:

1. Drains should not be removed before the seventh day. If Penrose drains and gauze have both been used, remove the Penrose drains first.

2. If gauze sticks, it should never be twisted or forceably removed because of the danger of hemorrhage.

3. If bleeding into the extrahepatic biliary tract occurs, it may obstruct ducts and T tube. Irrigate the T tube with saline or introduce fluid by the drip method.

4. If drainage appears from the wound, cultures should be made to determine the type of infecting organism and appropriate antibiotics administered.

OPERATIVE PRECAUTIONS AND COMPLICATIONS

To determine the presence of stones in the common bile duct it is of value to withdraw a sample of bile by means of a hypodermic needle. Normally, bile is clear and of a golden yellow color. If, instead, it is black and cloudy, containing flocculi, stones will almost always be found at the lower end of the common bile duct.

IDENTIFICATION OF THE COMMON BILE DUCT

Difficulty in recognizing and locating the common bile duct may arise because, in the presence of old inflammatory conditions, the foramen of Winslow and other landmarks may have been obliterated by adhesions. A structure which may later prove to have been the superior mesenteric artery may be incised in the belief that it is the common bile duct. Avoid this mistake by first aspirating the duct.

EXPLORATION OF THE COMMON BILE DUCT

This operation should *not* be done routinely; opening and exploration should be reserved for those cases where the need for it is clearly indicated. When *palpating the common bile duct,* the surgeon should be careful not to confuse an enlarged lymph node lying next to the duct with a calculus within its lumen; neither should a calcareous plaque on the aorta or the superior mesenteric artery be mistaken for a biliary stone. Such errors could, of course, scarcely occur when the duct is traced between thumb and forefinger.

The common bile duct should be explored at the time of cholecystectomy if the following signs are present: (1) contracted gallbladder; (2) jaundice present during attacks of gallstone colic; (3) stones in the gallbladder; (4) possibility of the presence of a stone when the ducts are palpated. Besides, the ducts should always be explored, even if these indications are lacking, whenever there is marked evidence of long-standing infection, such as thickening or fibrosis, or if the bile is thick, black and tenacious. The mere suspicion of a stone in the common bile duct should be sufficient reason for exploration, a factor in about 50 per cent of all gallstone cases; if such stones are not removed, there are apt to be serious complications.

Injury to the Common Bile Duct

The common bile duct may be injured and the damage discovered during the operation. Repair it promptly under direct vision. Better yet, try to avoid such accidents by avoiding ligation of the cystic duct close to the common bile duct.

Perforation of the Gallbladder

When this occurs, bile tends to collect in the right loin region beneath the kidney pouch (Morison's pouch). A tube introduced here through a stab wound affords satisfactory drainage (see Fig. 366).

Laceration of the Liver

If the liver be lacerated during manipulations of a cholecystectomy or a choledochostomy, bleeding must be carefully arrested before the abdomen is closed. If the laceration is slight, sponge pressure is usually enough; when it is large, interlocking catgut sutures should be employed.

Injury to the Cystic Artery

This may cause severe hemorrhage. This vessel should be looked for, as it is often in an anomalous position and therefore likely to be cut. Also, frequently there will be an accessory cystic duct. Generally speaking, the danger of encountering anomalies of the vascular supply in this region is so great that the surgeon should make every stroke of his knife under direct vision and with utmost care.

Accidental Section of the Cystic Artery. When this occurs, the proximal end may retract into a position where it is nearly impossible to find it again. In attempting to grasp it, the surgeon may include the common or hepatic ducts and injure them also.

Injury to the Hepatic Artery

While rare, injury to the hepatic artery has nevertheless been responsible for some fatalities. The right branch of this artery may be erroneously ligated. The *portal vein* may be injured in some instances owing to its proximity to the common bile duct and also because it may be in an anomalous position. In clamping off the *cystic duct* during a cholecystectomy, any damage to the common or hepatic ducts may result in a biliary fistula or a partial obstruction of the common bile duct from stricture.

Traumatic Injury

Trauma to the bile ducts, either operative or otherwise, will be revealed by the appearance of free bile. The injured spot must be searched for and repaired. Injury to the *pancreatic duct* is not recognized so easily and therefore is likely to pass unobserved. If left untreated, it results in fat necrosis.

Preparation for Closure

In all operations in this area, before closing the abdominal incision, a very careful arrangement of the viscera should be made. The small intestine should not be allowed to come in contact with any infected area, first, because peristalsis might carry the infection throughout the abdomen and, second, if adhesions were to form they would induce ileus. The stomach and the duodenum depend on motility for their functions and must be prevented from coming in contact with denuded areas and forming adhesions. This protection can be furnished by the upper edge of the omentum and the transverse colon. These structures are carried upward and placed between the gallbladder and the ducts and the abdominal cavity; if necessary, they may be held in place by 1 or 2 catgut sutures.

POSTOPERATIVE COMPLICATIONS

If the patient has suffered from biliary colic, he should be kept under direct medical supervision for a considerable period following surgery in order to detect and forestall possible complications. The most common of these are:

1. Persistence or recurrence of symptoms
2. Postoperative adhesions
3. Operative or postoperative hemorrhage
4. Fistula
5. Postoperative peritonitis
6. Postoperative shock
7. Hepatic insufficiency
8. Cardiac affections

These conditions may strike suddenly, even in patients who have received every care. Therefore, constant vigilance is essential.

Postoperative Pain

Attacks of postoperative pain not due to calculi are caused by tearing or kinking of the ducts resulting from adhesions. At present there is no known way of preventing adhesions under these conditions. One of the most important factors in the recurrence of pain following biliary operations seems to be damage to the innervation of the area, especially following removal of the gallbladder (postcholecystectomy syndrome).

Pyloric and Duodenal Adhesions

Postoperative pyloric and duodenal adhesions in the vicinity of either the gallbladder or the extrahepatic biliary passages may produce symptoms. This is more common following operation with drainage. A second operation may be necessary when adhesions become troublesome.

Biliary Fistula

Persistent discharge of bile following gallbladder operations will be due to some condition that prevents healing of the tissues concerned. An overlooked calculus, injury to the common or accessory ducts or some foreign body, e.g., sutures, sponges, drains, may prevent a fistula from closing. Elimination of such an underlying cause will allow closure of the abnormal tract.

Fistula Due to Injury of Common Bile Duct. Fistula may be the first indication of injury to the common bile duct, demonstrated by discharge of bile from the opening left after the drainage tube is removed—a discharge which does not diminish. At first, the surgeon may regard this as being caused by (1) slipping of a ligature from the cystic duct because it was not properly tied; (2) bursting of the cystic duct because of increased pressure in the common bile duct due to an overlooked stone in the ampulla of Vater; or (3) division of an anomalous duct. It will not occur to him that it may be due to an injured common bile duct. Therefore, he waits for the discharge of bile to clear up, thus losing valuable time. *Discharge of bile persisting beyond the eighth or ninth day after a cholecystectomy demands investigation as to whether there has been some injury to the common bile duct.* A ligature does not readily slip off the cystic duct if the common bile duct is patent, because pressure in the biliary system is low. However, if there is obstruction of the common bile duct, causing the pressure to rise, the ligature is very likely to be forced off the cystic duct. *Therefore, persistent discharge of bile usually means an obstruction or an injury to the common bile duct.*

At this stage then, injury must be excluded for the following reasons:

1. If an injury to the common bile duct is allowed to remain for some time, the proximal portion will retract into the portal fissure and become fibrosed and contracted.

2. The liver enlarges as a result of biliary obstruction from the strictured duct.

3. Much fibrosis and firm adhesions to neighboring organs form around the sinus.

All these conditions make operation for repair of the damage extremely difficult and often unsatisfactory. *The whole secret of successful repair of the common bile duct depends on early recognition of the injury, which, in turn, hinges on correct diagnosis of the cause of a persistent discharge of bile after a cholecystectomy.*

Fistula from Overlooked Stone. Not uncommonly a discharging fistula remains after cholecystostomy (carried out perhaps for acute cholecystitis). As a rule, such a fistula will be due to the presence in the cystic duct of a stone which had been overlooked or could not be removed because of an acute fulminating inflammation of the gallbladder. For a time, such a fistula will discharge mucus, then muco-pus and finally pus. In such cases the gall-bladder must be removed.

Postoperative Jaundice

This may appear even after the most careful procedure. It may be due to an overlooked cal-culus or to an injury to the common bile duct. If slight and transitory, it is usually caused by compression by packs or drains or by a mild degree of postoperative pancreatitis or chol-angitis.

Biliary Leakage

Although biliary leakage is common, it is not due, as is often believed, to slipping of a ligature on the cystic duct. More often, bile issues from the gallbladder bed; such discharge is usually transitory, unless due to some of the more serious complications already cited.

Postoperative Biliary Peritonitis

This may be due to the escape of bile into the peritoneal cavity, to soiling of the opera-tive field, to oozing from the bed of the re-moved gallbladder or to improperly repaired or injured ducts. Sometimes the cystic duct is insecurely ligated. Great care must be taken to peritonealize securely all raw bleeding sur-faces and to provide drainage in the presence of any infection.

Hepatic or Renal Insufficiency

Not infrequently we are confronted with patients who, even after the most painstaking intervention on the biliary tract, develop fatal hepatic or renal insufficiency. The conscien-tious surgeons spends many a sleepless night pondering over the reason for such a failure and, all too often, the unavailing effort to save the patient's life. How may we avert such catastrophes? A good laboratory, a reliable corps of assistants and a well-trained sero-chemist are great aids in establishing pre-operatively the status of the patient's blood chemistry, its changes immediately after the operation and the appearance of dangerous manifestations, i.e., changes in the normal con-stituents of the blood plasma. If we can fore-stall or reverse these changes we may be able to tide such a patient over this critical period.

Reflex Postoperative Anuria

So-called reflex postoperative anuria is due to a sudden hepatorenal insufficiency and is occasionally observed in patients with jaundice or infection.

Cholangitis

This is occasionally encountered in the post-operative period. If the infection spreads into the hepatic substance, recovery may be seri-ously retarded. Suitable antibiotics and chemo-therapy should be administered.

Cardiac Insufficiency

This may cause death following operations on the biliary system. Some experts advise digitalis even when the heart appears to be perfectly normal.

Thrombosis of the Portal Vein

This may be mistaken for peritonitis or pancreatitis.

PROGNOSIS

Age

In any operation on the biliary tract, age is an important factor. Generally after the age of 40 there is an upturn in the death rate, as against a practically negligible mortality in younger individuals.

Sex

In the presence of complications, mortality is higher in men than in women. This is due, in part, to the fact that the organs are located deeper in the body in the male (approximately 11 cm. from the anterior abdominal wall in men as compared with 7.5 cm. in women). Also, in males, the liver is situated deeper, the thorax is more rigid, and the spinal column is less flexible, making access to the organs more difficult than in women. Women also have the advantage of higher resistance to hemorrhage and operative shock.

REFERENCES

1. Couinaud, C.: Ou en est la chirurgie hépat-ique?, Rev. prat. **5**:1131, 1955.

2. Crile, G., Jr.: Errors in surgery of the biliary tract, Cleveland Clin. Quart. **21**:90, 1954.

3. Dagher, I. K., and Hovnanian, A. P.: Intrabiliary rupture of hydatid cyst of liver, Ann. Surg. **141**:263, 1955.

4. Healey, J. E., Jr.: Clinical anatomic aspects of radical hepatic surgery, J. Internat. Coll. Surgeons **22**:542, 1954.

5. Honjo, I., and Araki, C.: Total resection of the right lobe of the liver; report of successful case, J. Internat. Coll. Surgeons **23**:23, 1955.

6. Iason, A. H.: Variable patterns in surgical treatment of gallbladder, J. Internat. Coll. Surgeons **24**:233, 1955.

7. Lehmann, K.: Accidental injuries to the deep bile ducts in cholecystectomy (Parts 1-4), Acta chir. scandinav. **105**:195, 1953.

8. Pack, G. T., *et al.*: Total right hepatic lobectomy for cancer of the gallbladder; report of 3 cases, Ann. Surg. **142**:6, 1955.

9. Quattlebaum, J. K.: Massive resection of the liver, Ann. Surg. **137**:787, 1953.

10. Steeper, J. R.: Tumors of the extrahepatic biliary tract, J. Internat. Coll. Surgeons **24**:180, 1955.

11. Stone, P. W., and Saypol, G. M.: Partial hepatectomy, Surg., Gynec. & Obst. **95**:191, 1952.

12. Terry, R.: Risks of needle biopsy of the liver, Brit. M. J. **1**:1102, 1952.

13. Zamcheck, N., and Klausenstock, O.: Liver biopsy; risk of needle biopsy, New England J. Med. **249**:1062, 1953.

19   The Pancreas and the Spleen

PANCREAS

TRAUMA

Acute traumatism to the pancreas may occur as a result of deep lacerating wounds of the upper abdomen, deep penetrating wounds with sharp objects or in the course of bullet wounds. When, for these reasons, laparotomy is performed and the region of the pancreas is explored, the area is carefully inspected and bleeding vessels are secured. Any lacerated or comminuted portion of the pancreas that seems to be partially or completely separated from the main body of this organ is removed. No attempt should be made to suture such fragments into place.

Partial resection of the tail of the pancreas is easily performed after mass ligation of the gland proximal to the injured portion. Care must be exercised to avoid injury to the splenic artery and vein which lie posterior and above the gland. In emergency, ligation of these vessels need not be followed by splenectomy unless otherwise indicated. Silk sutures and ligatures are always employed on or about the pancreas. Penrose drains are always placed in the area.

Lacerated or comminuted wounds to the head of the pancreas are best treated conservatively at first. When hemorrhage is arrested, careful inspection is made to discover perforations in the stomach or the bowel. These are closed. If possible, choledochostomy is performed. No further operative interference is indicated; the region is widely drained (Penrose drains), with closure of the abdominal wound.

Pancreatic fistulas of traumatic origin are always treated conservatively at first. Most of them will close spontaneously. If there is copious discharge, continuous suction drainage is instituted. Attention is paid to possible electrolyte disturbances incidental to such fluid losses. Appropriate care of the adjacent skin surfaces is necessary to avoid digestive action on the part of the pancreatic enzymes in the juice. Application of tincture of benzoin to the surface, and over this a liberal use of aluminum dusting powder, is an effective treatment.

Persistent pancreatic fistulas necessitate excision down to and including that portion of the pancreas from which they arise.

ACUTE HEMORRHAGIC PANCREATITIS

The diagnosis of acute hemorrhagic pancreatitis is based on the clinical history and findings, but as the situation develops, differentiation from other conditions is necessary, because in these other conditions immediate operation is indicated, whereas in acute pancreatitis, the modern treatment is nonsurgical, at least at the outset. This condition is always serious and the mortality is high, but experience in recent years clearly indicates a lower mortality by conservative management than by early operative interference.

For the differentiation of acute hemorrhagic pancreatitis from other acute upper abdominal accidents, the possibility of acute perforation of peptic ulcer is the first consideration. In the latter event, air under the diaphragm will be indicated by appropriate roentgenograms and, of course, if present, indicates perforation. An important sign strongly suggesting pancreatitis is to have the patient lie flat on his back and the examiner place the fingers of each hand against the costovertebral angles and exert sudden upward pressure. If this elicits a sudden sharp increase in pain, the diagnosis of acute pancreatitis is strongly suggested.

Another feature of the diagnosis of acute pancreatitis is the history of rather sudden explosive onset of symptoms, with rapid appearance of shock (rapid thready pulse, marked weakness, cold clammy perspiration and fall in blood pressure). Two laboratory findings are helpful in the diagnosis: rapid elevation of the leukocyte count to 25,000 or 30,000 per cu. mm. and high titer of blood amylase (Samogy units). High blood amylase levels are not always present in acute hemorrhagic pancreatitis and may be missed if the determinations are made early in the attack, or if there is transitory occlusion of pancreatic secretion due to the passage of common duct calculi.

Recent studies in various centers do not confirm the earlier reliance on elevated blood amylase findings as being strong evidence of acute pancreatitis, for it is becoming more clearly realized that this condition may be present *without* elevated blood amylase. Thus, more importance must be attached to the history and the physical findings in these patients.

The treatment of acute hemorrhagic pan-

creatitis, as stated above, is now conservative. Measures are instituted to combat shock, e.g., blood transfusions, appropriate parenteral fluids, continuous gastric aspiration and sedation. The use of antibiotics has been debated, inasmuch as the importance of infection as a prime etiologic factor is questioned. However, it would seem that such therapy can do no harm, and, in some quarters, chlortetracycline has been regarded as being specifically beneficial in this condition.

If the surgeon is not fully convinced that acute pancreatitis is the correct diagnosis and performs laparotomy because of fear that some other condition is present, and finally does find acute pancreatitis, i.e., edematous, enlarged pancreas with petechiae, bloody exudate in the upper abdomen and in the lesser

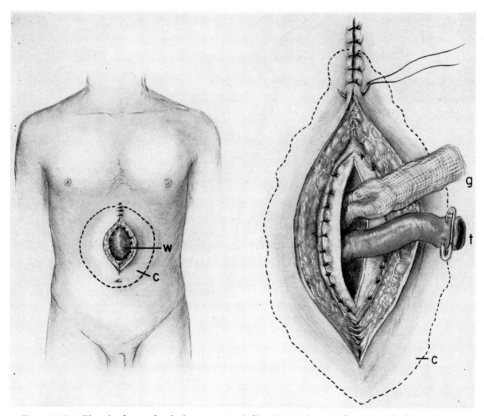

FIG. 367. Classical method for marsupialization of pseudocyst of the pancreas. (C) Cyst wall. (W) Partially closed laparotomy wound with pseudocyst wall sutured to it. (G) Gauze pack that fills collapsed cyst. (T) Soft rubber drain. The whole procedure may be carried out in one operation, but 48 to 72 hours may be permitted to elapse between stage 1, at the left, and stage 2, at the right. (Breitner: Chirurgische Operationslehre, Vienna, Urban)

peritoneal cavity and typical "white spots" on the visceral and parietal peritoneal surfaces of the upper abdomen, certain procedures would seem to be indicated:

1. Aspiration of the exudate

2. Careful inspection of the extrahepatic biliary tract and search for concretions, especially an impacted one in the ampulla. If this is present, an attempt should be made to dislodge it, first, by choledochotomy, with passage of sounds into the duodenum, and, if this fails, by duodenostomy and direct incision into the papilla of Vater. If calculi are *not* found, cholecystostomy is performed.

3. Two or 3 soft rubber drains are placed in the pancreas, but multiple incisions into the latter are not done, as was the custom years ago.

Sequelae. In acute hemorrhagic pancreatitis sequelae include abscess formation and pseudocysts. In patients recovering from acute hemorrhagic pancreatitis the surgeon must be aware that abscess formation may sometimes occur. Such abscesses develop in the lesser peritoneal sac or under the left diaphragm. Once the diagnosis is established, drainage is instituted. This is carried out with minimal disturbance of viscera during exposure of the site to be drained. Pseudocysts may occur not only after acute hemorrhagic pancreatitis but also as a result of injury to the pancreas incident to a dull blow in the upper abdomen or as a result of a crushing injury, such as the passage of a vehicle wheel over the body.

The classic mode of treatment is drainage, with or without marsupialization (Fig. 367). In recent years there have been a number of published reports of successful drainage of these cysts and their anastomosis with either the stomach or a segment of upper jejunum for internal drainage. Such internal drainage may prove to be satisfactory, but, prior to its execution, the surgeon must ascertain that the pseudocyst is truly unilocular. If multilocular, the individual loculated cysts should be broken down. The writer has had occasion to reoperate on patients with multilocular cysts, only one large loculus of which was anastomosed to the bowel, leaving the other separate loculi intact to continue to increase in size. In the case of true cysts (blastomas), their excision should be envisaged rather than drainage by one method or another. If this is not possible, they

are marsupialized and the lining destroyed by cauterization, if possible, with phenol or the actual cautery.

CHRONIC RELAPSING PANCREATITIS

Often this condition is accompanied by calcification of varying degrees. In the past these calculi were often regarded as being in the ducts, so surgical removal was envisaged under certain circumstances. At present, it is realized that the calcification is essentially intraparenchymal, and pancreatic duct lithotomy is no longer carried out.

Conservative management for the pancreas itself and the elimination of disease of the external biliary passages—including the gallbladder—are the modern approaches to the problem.

Aggravation of symptoms and repetition of acute exacerbations are treated in several ways: division of the sphincter of Oddi (in some instances); appropriate sympathetic neurectomies; dietary supervision; and absolute prohibition of alcohol. It must be admitted that no one form of treatment is entirely satisfactory, and in the extreme form, total pancreatectomy, with its accompanying hazards and disadvantages, must be carried out as a method of desperation. Good results have been achieved by the latter.

CARCINOMA

Cancer of the head of the pancreas should be excised by pancreatoduodenectomy. The question arises as to how to be sure that the lesion in the head of the pancreas *is* cancer and not chronic interstitial pancreatitis. The writer is of the opinion that, where such a question arises, one can never be absolutely sure, so the surgeon must rely entirely on his own judgment. The harder the lesion, the more likely that it is cancer.

Incision into the head of the pancreas in order to secure tissue for frozen section does not constitute good judgment because (1) there is danger of hemorrhage—the extent of which may become a major problem; (2) tissue which may appear to be cancerous macroscopically, may, in frozen section, prove to be only chronic inflammation; (3) a zone of pancreatitis may surround a carcinoma, and incision into this zone may mislead the surgeon.

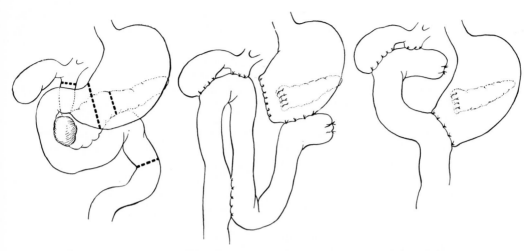

Fig. 368. (*Left*) Incisions for pancreatoduodenectomy. (*Center and right*) Two current methods for reconstituting the alimentary canal. The author ligates the pancreatic stump. Some surgeons reimplant the stump into the jejunum in an endeavor to return pancreatic secretion. This implantation may be carried out at any point of convenience, usually between the choledocho-enterostomy and the gastroenterostomy. (Breitner: Chirurgische Operationslehre, Vienna, Urban)

In view of the purported poor results from pancreatoduodenectomy for cancer of the head of the pancreas, there has been some discussion as to its justification. With the passage of time, however, increasing numbers of 5-year survivors from this procedure for cancer of the pancreas are being recorded. In this writer's personal series there are 4 "over-5-year" survivors, in 2 of whom there are regional lymph node metastases.

In the aged or the poor-risk patient, cholecystogastrostomy or enterostomy or a choledocho-enterostomy may be performed for palliation. Survival for many months, with relief from jaundice, may be secured for such patients. On the other hand, in poor-risk or deeply jaundiced patients, such short-circuiting procedures may be a preliminary step to final excisional surgery 3 or 4 weeks later.

With increasing experience, several types of reconstitution of the alimentary tract have been described following excision of the head of the pancreas and the duodenum (Fig. 368). One popular method is to bring up the first loop of jejunum, anastomose it to the common duct end-to-end and then anastomose the transected end of the stomach into the side of this loop. At a point lower in the loop, the transected end of the pancreatic stump is implanted

into the bowel. Another method described is to implant "tamponlike" the transected stump of the pancreas into the upper (open) end of the jejunum, at a lower point implant the common duct and at a still lower site anastomose the transected end of the stomach. In these situations, it is anticipated that pancreatic secretions will be returned to the bowel. In most instances, however, it would appear that eventually cicatrization will occur at the pancreatic stump with occlusion of secretions.

The writer continues to pursue the principles of his originally described technic, i.e., Billroth II gastroenterostomy and implantation of the common bile duct into the jejunum, distal to gastrojejunostomy. If the cystic duct and the gallbladder are preserved, the fundus of the gallbladder is also anastomosed to the jejunum, thus affording two routes for biliary enteric drainage. The pancreatic stump is ligated by a mass ligation and also by a row of interlocking interrupted mattress sutures. In all ligatures and sutures about the pancreas, silk is employed. In this manner the pancreatic secretions are occluded because the pancreatic stump is not implanted into the bowel. Penrose drains are placed to the site of pancreatic stump ligation and remain for a week. In some instances, no pancreatic fistula results, though in most instances such fistulas develop. They must be expected and accepted. They do not prolonged hospitalization, and the patient must be taught to change dressings as needed. In the course of a few weeks or months they close spontaneously. Their presence does not constitute a basis for limitation of general normal activity.

Exclusion of pancreatic secretion from the alimentary canal is well tolerated in most patients. The stools are usually bulkier than normal, tend to be "fatty" and may be slightly more numerous. Experience has shown that essentially normal nutritional status may be maintained indefinitely under these conditions. However, if "steatorrhea" does occur, powdered pancreatin is given, to be ingested with each meal, i.e., 3 or 4 heaping teaspoonfuls suspended in a glass of milk or water. After a period, this may be discontinued, to be resumed if and when necessary.

There is also the question of total duodeno-pancreatectomy for carcinoma of the head as well as the body of the pancreas. This is a formidable operation with considerable risks. The reason for advocating this operation is that cancer arising anywhere in the organ is more radically removed than would be the case if only portions of the gland were excised. The diabetes resulting from total pancreatectomy is not severe; usually it is controlled with 15 to 30 units of insulin a day. Even if the patient is already diabetic, the operation will not result in much—if any—aggravation of the diabetes.

Following total pancreatectomy, control of the diabetes is the responsibility of the collaborating internist. However, the surgeon must be cognizant of certain principles in this problem. High blood-glucose levels must be expected and accepted for the first 24 to 48 hours. During this period the patient may exhibit insulin hypersensitivity. Urinalysis will show "4-plus" sugar, but this in itself is not important at the moment. The presence of diacetic acid at *any* time *is* important and is indication for proper insulin therapy forthwith.

SPLEEN

TRAUMA

Excision of the traumatized spleen is usually an emergency operation for the arrest of hemorrhage. Excision is envisaged rather than suture repair of the lacerated or comminuted organ because the latter is often not feasible. Rapid mobilization of the spleen is carried out by inserting the right hand over the diaphragmatic curved surface, grasping the organ and elevating it outward and to the left with rotation, so as to bring the posterior aspect of the hilum into view. This maneuver exposes the splenic artery and vein with their branches. Hemostats are applied rapidly and these vessels are transected. With further exposure of the organ, the gastrosplenic vessels are exposed and similarly clamped, divided and ligated. The ligamentous attachments to diaphragm, splenic flexure of colon and other peritoneal reflections are severed, and the organ is removed, either in toto or in fragments, as the case may be. Injury to the tip of the tail of the pancreas in the hilum is to be avoided, but often the hemostats are applied so rapidly that the tip is included by them. In itself, this is not important. The tip of the pancreatic tail is included in the mass ligature of the splenic vessels. The stumps of the ligated splenic vein and artery are carefully inspected to ascertain whether or not they may be retracted; they are not completely secured. A good precaution is to ligate these vessels a second time when the spleen has been excised and all obvious bleeding arrested.

ENLARGED SPLEEN

In recent years, the indications for the excision of the enlarged spleen have changed quite a bit, and are now usually posed by the collaborating internist. In splenocytic hemolytic jaundice and in thrombocytopenic purpura, splenectomy may yield spectacular results. The operation in these patients is not carried out in the presence of shock and hemorrhage; thus the procedure may be more deliberate than when the spleen is ruptured. The hilum may be exposed by the anterior approach, first securing and dividing the gastrosplenic vessels and finally the larger splenic vessels in the hilum. Of special interest and importance is a careful inspection of the whole region, especially the hilar region, to ascertain whether or not small spherical or oval accessory spleens are present, all of which must also be excised lest the desired effects of splenectomy in thrombocytopenic purpura and congenital hemolytic jaundice fail to be secured after "splenectomy."

In excision of large spleens for one reason or another, the organ may be found to be very fragile and easily ruptured. Gentle handling is of the utmost importance, and where accidental rupture or laceration is feared, the direct anterior approach to the hilum is especially indicated in order first to occlude the blood supply to the organ.

Division of the splenic artery before the splenic vein may result in some reduction in the size of the organ when and if this may be especially desirable.

20 Hernia

Operations for hernia are generally regarded —by patients as well as physicians—as being relatively unimportant. It is true that when carried out with skill and under proper surgical safeguards they are less dangerous than many other major procedures. Nonetheless, they are by no means entirely free from risk, for there are certain circumstances attended by special dangers against which the surgeon should always be on his guard.

DIAGNOSIS

Errors in the diagnosis of hernia are easily made, thus it is essential that the surgeon be certain of his diagnosis before selecting the method of treatment. A mass in the scrotal sac, in the inguinal or the femoral region is not necessarily a hernia (Fig. 369). A fat-covered femoral hernia may not be palpable, so, if one is suspected, the more common types of hernia must first be excluded. When uncertainty still remains, all available diagnostic methods should be employed before undertaking operation for some other suspected abdominal condition. Do not forget, however, that it is often impossible to recognize a hernia without first opening the abdomen.

According to Hamilton Bailey,[1] *Malgaigne's bulgings* (Fig. 370) are more than suggestive of weak abdominal musculature which predisposes to hernia, particularly *direct inguinal hernia*. The following is his procedure: Ask the patient to cough (while he is standing erect with his abdomen and inguinal region bared) and closely observe the external abdominal ring, noting whether there is an impulse. Ask the patient to cough again and thereafter compare the ring of the opposite side.

When neither a swelling nor an impulse can be seen, ask the patient to point to the

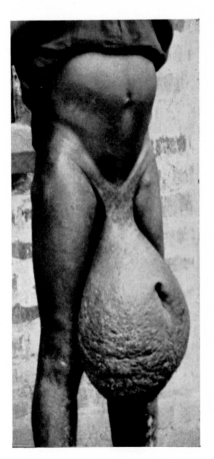

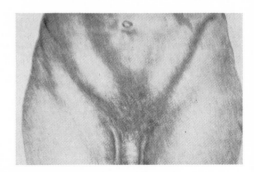

Fig. 369. (*Left*) Elephantiasis of scrotum.

Fig. 370. (*Above*) Malgaigne's bulgings. (Bailey, Hamilton: Demonstrations of Physical Signs in Clinical Surgery, ed. 12, Baltimore, Williams and Wilkins)

place where he experienced pain or noticed a swelling.

If there is no obvious lump, invaginate the scrotum upon the little finger, then rotate the finger so that the nail lies against the cord and follow the cord upward. This will lead the pulp of the finger, with its tactile sensibility, to the external abdominal ring. If the finger is not introduced in this way, it is more than likely that the nail will abut against the ring, and the point of the examination will be missed. *A normal ring feels like a triangular slit; it barely admits the tip of the little finger.*

If more than this is possible, it is not normal. Have the patient cough again and note if there is a *palpable* impulse.

In the female, when there is no obvious lump, the surgeon should lay 2 fingers over, immediately below and to the inner side of the external abdominal ring and test for an impulse when the patient coughs. As it is impossible to explore the ring in a female patient by invaginating the skin (as in the male), this is a very valuable diagnostic test.

If there is an obvious lump (in either sex), and if the surgeon can "get above the lump,"

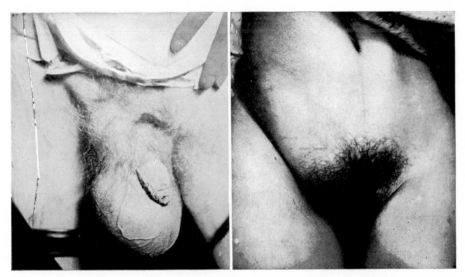

FIG. 371. Neither of these was hernia. (*Left*) Tuberculosis of testis (tuberculous epididymitis; lymphadenitis; hydrocele). (*Right*) Lipoma. (See Fig. 372.)

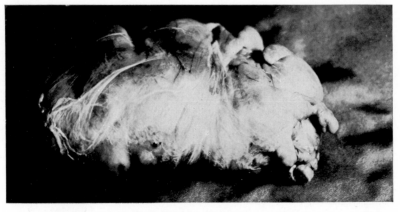

FIG. 372. Same patient as in Figure 371. At operation the true condition turned out to be lipoma.

it is manifestly *not* issuing from the inguinal canal and therefore cannot be a hernia (Figs. 371 and 372). If he cannot get above the lump, he should ascertain the relationship of the neck of the sac and its continuity with the inguinal canal. Grasping the neck of the sac between his thumb and finger, he again asks the patient to cough and notes whether or not there is an impulse. If no impulse is visible, the hernia is probably irreducible, so the surgeon must now decide (on data other than purely local) whether or not the protrusion is strangulated.

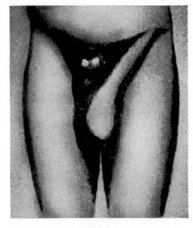

FIG. 373. Infantile type of hydrocele. (After Bazy)

CLINICAL PICTURE

In its *very earliest stage,* when the hernia begins to force its way through the internal inguinal ring, there will be no obvious swelling, even though there may be considerable pain over the ring. The pain will be increased during exercise but will be relieved by rest. There may also be pain in the epigastrium, or referred to the back or, again, indefinitely all over the abdomen.

In the *second stage,* vague pains in the groin may attract the patient's attention to this area, and there a swelling will be found. As swelling and pain are relieved on lying down, if a physician is consulted at this stage, *he may make an erroneous diagnosis or none at all*—which in itself is a serious error. So long as an inguinal hernia remains reducible and uncomplicated, any external swelling will be soft and easily compressible, but if the examiner's finger invaginates the scrotum when the patient coughs, the finger tip will receive an expanding impulse and the hernia can be detected as a *bulge.*

Examination must always be done in both upright and prone positions. *Many errors have resulted from failure to observe this rule.*

If the hernia is *inside* the scrotum, the inguinal canal will give a sensation of "fullness" to the palpating finger, and with the patient in the erect position, the intrascrotal mass will be larger, often lying above and in front of the testicle, with the elements of the

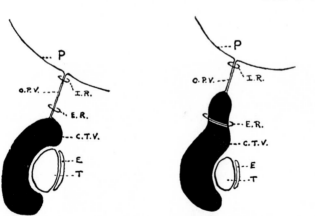

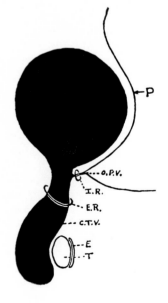

FIG. 374. Forms of hydrocele. (*Left*) Simple or vaginal. (*Center*) Infantile. (*Right*) Abdominoscrotal. (Key: P, peritoneum; E, epididymis; T, testis; IR, internal inguinal ring; ER, external inguinal ring; OPV, obliterated processus vaginalis; CTV, cavity of tunica vaginalis.)

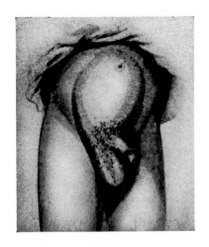

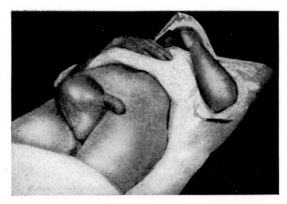

FIG. 375. Two views of patient with abdominoscrotal hydrocele.

FIG. 376. Showing layers of abdominal wall and peritoneum in relation to abdominal hydrocele. (Key: PA, abdominal wall; PPA, peritoneum covering abdominal wall; PI, peritoneum covering iliac fossa, compressed by tumor; PaH, wall of hydrocele; AF, femoral arch; CSP, peritoneal cul-de-sac; SH, scrotal portion of hydrocele; T, testis; AH, abdominal portion of hydrocele; PeH, pelvic portion of hydrocele.) (After Bazy)

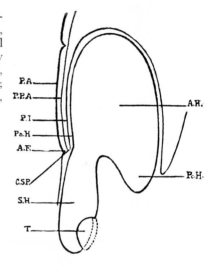

cord in the rear. If this mass is reduced, the abdominal rings, as well as the canal itself, will be found to be dilated, while the cord beyond the external ring where the sac is located will feel abnormally thick. Let me repeat Bailey's dictum: *The swelling is not a hernia if thumb and finger can be brought together with only cord and external skin intervening.*

Hydrocele. In infancy and early childhood, a hernia is so frequently associated with a hydrocele that it is never safe to operate on a child for either condition unless a *positive* differential diagnosis has been made. Most hernias in children reduce themselves when the child reclines, but hydroceles (Fig. 373) never do, except on the rarest occasions when a pinpoint opening exists between the hydrocele and the accompanying hernial sac, as this allows the fluid to empty slowly into the abdominal cavity (Fig. 374).

Once herniation has taken place, the size of the hernia tends to increase steadily unless active measures are applied to halt its progress. Often the patient will "push it back" himself and fail to consult a physician until *incarceration* or *strangulation* compel him to do so. Even then, diagnosis may be difficult.

When the surgeon has excluded hydrocele of the cord, a possible inguinal adenitis or funiculitis, *abdominoscrotal hydrocele* must still be kept in mind, though it is decidedly rare (Fig. 375). In this type of hydrocele, fluid accumulates in the cavity of the tunica vaginalis, causing scrotal enlargement and extending through the region of the inguinal canal into the abdomen or the iliac fossa (Figs. 376-378). A full description of hydrocele is given in Chapter 21, page 550. As a hydrocele has frequently been mistaken for a hernia, or vice versa, the danger which accompanies this error is that a trocar may be plunged into the hernial mass (bowel), giving rise to peritonitis.

Case Report. A young man brought to the hospital with a fulminating peritonitis gave a his-

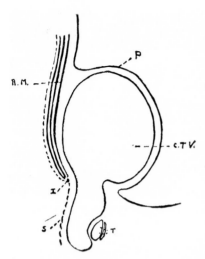

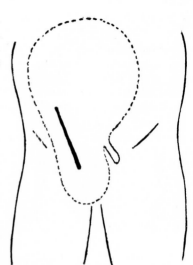

Fig. 377. (*Left*) Diagram showing relation of peritoneum and abdominal musculature to abdominoscrotal hydrocele. (Key: AM, abdominal muscles; P, peritoneum; CTV, cavity of tunica vaginalis; T, testis and epididymis; S, scrotal wall; I, level of inguinal ligament.) (*Right*) Diagram of incision used for correction of abdominoscrotal hydrocele. (After Prather)

tory to the effect that the surgeon who had treated him made a diagnosis of hydrocele and had attempted to evacuate it by forcing a trocar into the supposed accumulation of fluid in the scrotum. The patient died, and necropsy revealed a punctured bowel, with resulting peritoneal infection.

Psoas Abscess. On one occasion I saw a patient operated on for a supposed inguinal hernia, when, on incision, a psoas abscess was found. Such a diagnostic error in the practice of an experienced surgeon should not have

occurred. The surgeon must be able to distinguish inguinal hernia, bilocular or communicating hydrocele and a burrowing abscess. If intestine is present in the mass (as evidenced by tympany) or if the omentum is palpable, the diagnosis of hernia is evident and will be positive if the mass is reducible.

Strangulated Hernia. In order to avoid error and guard against therapeutic neglect, the surgeon should always keep in mind the possible locations of strangulated internal hernia, which are:

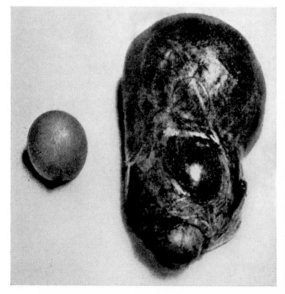

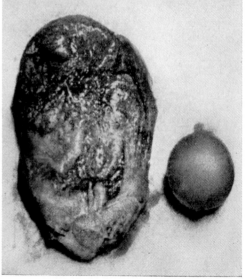

Fig. 378. (*Left*) Excised hydrocele mass (note large lemon shown for comparison of size). (*Right*) Sac after being opened and emptied, with small testis at lower end. (After Prather)

1. Retroperitoneal:

   A. In the neighborhood of the duodeno-jejunal flexure

   B. In the neighborhood of the cecum

   C. In the mesentery of the pelvic colon

2. Hernia of the foramen of Winslow

3. Through the transverse mesocolon after a posterior gastrojejunostomy

4. In gastroenterostomy Roux-en-Y

5. Obturator hernia

One should never wait for the cardinal symptoms and the signs of intestinal occlusion (complete obstipation, vomiting) which usually appear in strangulated hernia. Herniotomy should always be performed under direct vision during all stages of the intervention. Incisions should be large and reach beyond the upper pole of the hernia in order to see the anatomic conditions present; avoid injury to important structures such as blood vessels and nerves.

Hernia Laparotomy. This is indicated in cases of voluminous inguinal hernias with adhesions or femoral hernia embedded in fat tissues. In large umbilical hernias of adults, particularly in fat women, the omentum should be resected. Mayo's oval incision permits the surgeon to withdraw from the abdominal cavity the hernial sac and its contents en bloc. The affected loops of bowel should be carefully scrutinized both above and below the hernial sac and gently manipulated, particularly in patients over 50 years of age. Bear in mind the possibility of *retrograde strangulation.* Avoid displacing the sac and its contents into the subperitoneal tissues. This is a rare error, but it does happen occasionally.

Secondary Necrosis in Gangrene of the Bowel. This is particularly serious. Affections of the circulation (stasis, infarcts) are more dangerous than the evident symptoms of mechanical strangulation (Fig. 379). Such vascular lesions involving structures beyond the

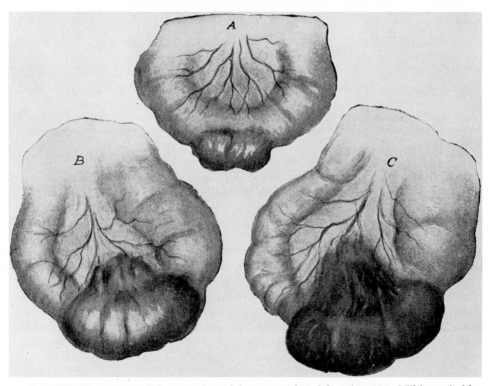

FIG. 379. Degrees of injury to bowel in strangulated hernia. (A) Mild, probably reversible injury. Bowel may be reposited safely. (B) Marked circulatory changes without irreversible damage. Use of hot packs *before reposition* should restore circulation. (C) Irreversible gangrenous changes; resection must be done.

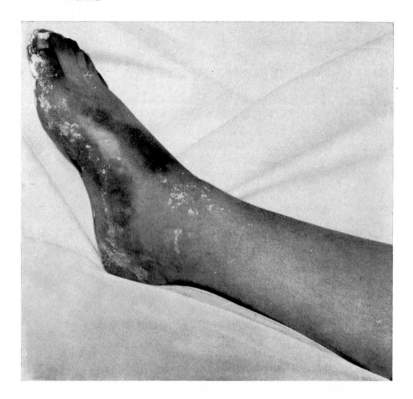

FIG. 380. Gangrene following injury to femoral artery during hernia operation.

apparently necrotic portions of the bowel have an importance which all too often goes unrecognized.

Direct Observation of the Bowel Condition. To allow such direct observation, some surgeons resort to partial operations such as lateral suture, exteriorization of the affected loop of bowel or keeping it in place under warm compresses. In doubtful cases, however, many prefer to do an enterectomy in addition to the herniorrhaphy. If this plan is followed, safeguards against any possible peritoneal infection must be rigidly maintained. Various complications are likely to be followed by fistulization and the formation of adhesions.

Incarceration Without Obstruction. This is often associated with minimal systemic disturbance, but operation should be advised and carried out because of the risk of later strangulation. If the patient's general systemic condition is good (no evidence of gangrene or peritonitis), treat as for uncomplicated inguinal hernia. In freeing the adhesions which have caused the incarceration, *safeguard the herniated viscera, making sure to return them intact and untraumatized to the abdominal cavity.* Leave any adherent peritoneum which

is attached to the bowel as a margin or "cuff" after cutting away the redundant section. This part of the operation may be safeguarded by leaving a "fringe" of peritoneum to cover any traumatized or irritated places on the wall of the intestine. This prevents the formation of fresh adhesions when the loops of bowel are replaced in the abdomen; it also reduces the possibility of perforation.

Obstruction Without Strangulation. Obstruction may exist before strangulation takes place. Surgical intervention is none the less imperative. The constricting mechanism must be freed so that the obstruction will be reduced, making possible the return of the herniated viscera to their normal place. In inguinal hernia, the constriction may be at the pillars of the external ring, or a band of thickened peritoneum may be compressing the neck of the sac. In other varieties of hernia, ligaments or fascial structures in the area may be responsible for the constriction.

The errors most likely here are failing to keep the anatomy of the parts in mind—perhaps forgetting the presence of important great vessels. Avoid opening the bowel which may be within the sac or cutting a vessel in the mesentery. If the constriction is due to thickening of the peritoneum at the neck of the sac, there is especial danger of damaging vessels or bowel wall. If part of the contents is omentum, it will usually be found to be fibrosed and should be cut away with the sac. Dissect away each adhesion, severing it between clips and ligating with care. Transfix the omentum with each ligature to prevent slipping. It is an easy matter to damage the vas in the inguinal canal during such dissection and, in dealing with a *femoral hernia,* beware of injuring the femoral or saphenous veins at this point in the procedure (Fig. 380).

Diagnosis of Strangulated Hernia

Strangulation is more frequent in femoral and umbilical hernia because of the unyielding nature of the femoral canal and the fibrous ring of the umbilical defect. The small intestine is more likely to be the structure herniated when strangulation has occurred, so the symptoms will differ somewhat from those of lower bowel obstruction. Upper abdominal distention and subsequent vomiting begin earlier. This means that toxemia develops rapidly, and imbalance of electrolytes and fluid takes place suddenly. If the condition has advanced to the stage of gangrene, fever and leukocytosis are more prominent features than when the large bowel is the part involved. With strangulated hernia, too, severe pain and local tenderness are more prominent manifestations; rebound tenderness and rigidity are more marked, and the position of the sac opening can usually be palpated as a tender mass. Once the diagnosis is established, if there is distention and there has been any vomiting, it is extremely important to "decompress" the intestine as rapidly as possible. Insertion of the Miller-Abbott tube is useful here. Fluid and electrolyte status should be investigated if there is time, but, under emergency conditions, it is usually possible to dispense with elaborate tests and within a few hours give sufficient fluids and electrolytes (and moderate degree of digitalization if the heart condition demands it) to permit successful repair of a strangulating obstruction. *Waiting for "decompression" may turn out to be a serious error.*

In both direct and indirect inguinal hernias, it should be a matter of routine to open the peritoneum at the internal ring. *Failure to do this is one of the commonest errors in the treatment of direct hernia.* Through this error the hernial sac may not be completely eliminated, so the additional presence of an *indirect* or femoral hernia might not be detected. *Opening the peritoneum at the internal ring is the best safeguard against injury to the bladder, as well as making certain that any indirect hernia (if it exists) will be exposed.*

In direct hernias the transversalis fascia often will be found to be thinned out and redundant. In carrying out the Bassini procedure (or one of its modifications), the conjoined tendon and the internal edge of Poupart's ligament can sometimes be approximated only by exerting extreme tension, which may cause the ligament to give way. To prevent this accident, methods have been devised to include Cooper's ligament in the suture or to carry the suture through the pectineus fascia in order to lessen the strain on Poupart's ligament. *However, none of these procedures takes the place of proper utilization of the transversalis fascia, if this structure is well preserved.*

INJECTION TREATMENT OF HERNIA

The treatment of hernia by sclerosing injections was introduced in 1835 by the French surgeon, Velpeau. About a year later the method was employed by the American surgeon, Pancoast, who was apparently unaware of what had already been done in France.

As no satisfactory operative procedure for the cure of hernia had been devised up to that time, it is not surprising that the idea received quite wide acceptance during the 1840's. The popularity of the injection method continued during the second half of the 19th century, but as it was taken up by unlicensed practitioners and widely advertised in the lay press, reputable physicians abandoned it as "quackery" without giving its real merit in selected cases any just consideration. When Bassini and, a little later, Halstead published their procedures for the repair of hernia, operative treatment of this lesion became possible in many cases where it previously had been out of the question, and even the suggestion of injection treatment was regarded as "unethical,"

Yet, a case for the use of sclerosing injections in certain instances of inguinal hernia may still be made out. About the year 1930, a number of surgeons of unquestioned standing and ability undertook to revive the procedure, and their results were sufficiently favorable to entitle injection to consideration as an *alternative* to operation in situations where the classic procedures are inadvisable or out of the question. At present, however, interest seems again to have waned. No authoritative publication concerning the injection treatment of hernia has appeared in medical literature for at least 3 years.

During the height of the popularity of the injection method, it was claimed that any reducible hernia could and *should* be treated by it, except for these contraindications: (1) incarceration or strangulation; (2) active venereal disease; (3) diabetes mellitus; or (4) active or quiescent tuberculosis. The patient should be safeguarded by most careful preinjection treatment, beginning with a complete physical examination to rule out the above-named contraindications and any other physical defects not connected with the hernia. When the solution to be used has been selected, the patient must be tested to see if there is any allergic reaction. *Never overlook this—to omit this test is a very serious error.*

INDICATIONS FOR INJECTION TREATMENT

No one except a thoroughly competent surgeon should ever attempt to inject a hernia of any type. He must be familiar with the anatomy of the parts involved and have practiced the operation many times. It is no work for tyros. *The most common error in using the method is failure to make absolutely certain that reduction is possible.* No hernia should be injected unless it can be kept constantly in reduction by the use of a properly fitted truss. The patient lies prone while the injection is being made; the truss must be removed during the actual injection but put on again before he arises. The truss must be worn night and day for at least 2 months after the last injection. If all goes well, thereafter it may be removed at night and then gradually discarded altogether.

The injection treatment has many times proved to be a means of cure after operation has repeatedly failed. Nevertheless, the decision to make use of it should be reached only after most careful consideration. There is no form of treatment of hernia where errors in judgment are so likely to be made and none which must be more carefully safeguarded every step of the way. The worst error of all is to look upon injection as a "quick and easy" form of treatment.

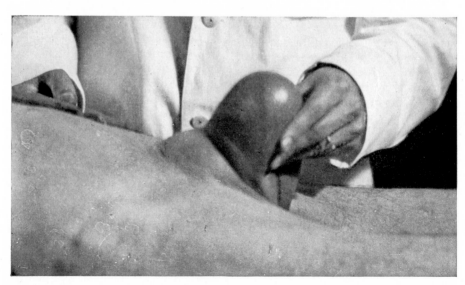

FIG. 381. Large strangulated hernia. Resistance is encountered when strangulated mass is pressed against external inguinal ring. (See Fig. 382.)

COMPLICATIONS

Complications of the injection technic would seem to be rare. Many of those reported might have been avoided by careful co-operation of the patient and good judgment on the part of the physician. In a few cases there has been swelling of the spermatic cord and the scrotum, but, as a rule, this has cleared up with the application of an icebag, elevation of the scrotum and loosening of the truss while the patient is in bed for 48 hours. Treatment is delayed for a week and then resumed in the usual manner.

Atrophy of the Testicle. Though rare, occasionally atrophy of the testicle has been found in patients who had worn an improperly fitted truss *prior to treatment*. It is probably a pressure atrophy. Skin infection may occur because of chafing by the truss and improper hygienic care by the patient.

Other possible complications of the injection method are accidental bowel perforation by the needle, intestinal obstruction due to adhesions from inadvertent intraperitoneal injection or strangulation from failure to maintain reduction, perirectal abscess, fecal fistula and thrombosis of deep epigastric, iliac or femoral vessels.

In general, injection treatment should be employed only by the specialist. It involves less danger than surgery only in selected cases of small, reducible, indirect, inguinal hernias and when given by those skilled in the injection of suitable standardized solutions which are nonirritating. I had to perform orchidectomy because of gangrene of the testicle following injection by a "hernia specialist." Adequate truss support for a sufficient length of time is essential.

GENERAL OPERATIVE CONSIDERATIONS

TAXIS

In every case of simple hernia, taxis should be tried, but *it must be done gently* (Figs. 381 and 382).

Case Report. A patient with a diagnosis of strangulated hernia was brought to me by a physician who, in his zeal to reduce it, had tried taxis rather vigorously. The man was in poor condition because of shock, but, under local anesthesia, the tissues were liberated and the intestine was found to be ruptured. Intestinal repair was carried out and drainage instituted, with no attempt to repair the hernia. The condition of the patient was precarious; I had to resort to rapid, incomplete clo-

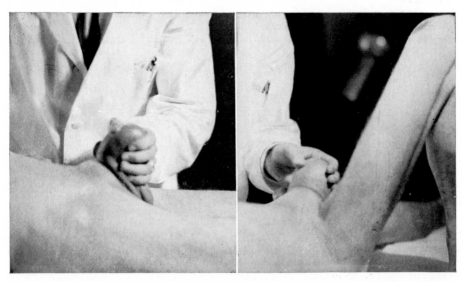

FIG. 382. Right and wrong methods of applying taxis to strangulated hernia. (*Left*) With legs flat, patient's abdominal muscles are not relaxed. Pressure is being applied against resistance of inguinal ring. *This is a dangerous procedure.* (*Right*) With legs drawn up, abdominal muscles are relaxed, and gentle manipulations are being used to coax the hernial contents past the inguinal ring.

sure. Hypodermoclysis and stimulating measures failed to restore him, and death occurred 14 hours later. The forcible taxis undoubtedly was responsible for the loss of his life.

Again, beware of forcible taxis! If everything goes smoothly and well, gently continue such efforts. If not, desist without hesitation. Transport the patient to a well-equipped hospial and operate immediately.

Remember that *gangrene of the bowel* may occur at any time after 6 hours subsequent to the beginning of strangulation, for the application of force is especially dangerous when there is a possibility of beginning gangrene of the intestine. This is particularly true of *obturator hernia.* Gangrene of the incarcerated intestine begins early; therefore, errors in diagnosis—especially those which hinder prompt resort to surgery—are very prone to prove fatal. In the abdominal operation, when the loops of intestine relating to the neck of the sac have been clearly identified, *gentle traction* may be made upon them, but *no vigorous traction* should be exerted for fear of damaging the intestinal wall. If at first reduction fails, gently dilate the restricting ring with the finger, or use a grooved director, along which hemostatic forceps may be passed and the ring stretched by opening the blades. In dealing with this type of hernia, the relation of the vessels to the neck of the sac must be kept in mind, and, if possible, the obturator artery should be identified by palpation or even dissection. Following this, traction upon the strangulated loops may be repeated, and if it still proves to be obstinate, an assistant may exert outside pressure over Scarpa's triangle, while from within the ab-

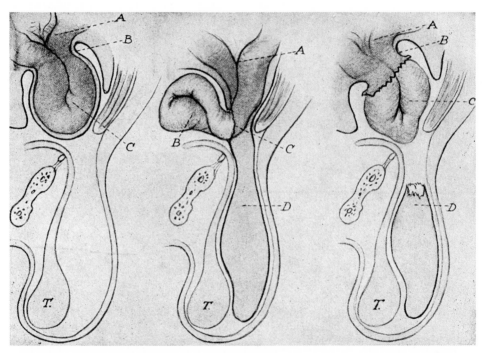

Fig. 383. Reduction en masse. (*Left*) The whole mass may be reduced, carrying the constricting ring with it (B). A sense of false security that satisfactory reduction has been accomplished will result. Guard against it. (C) Shows both the strangulated mass and the sac pushed above the internal ring. (*Center*) During the reduction the sac may be ruptured and its contents (intestine, omentum, etc.) pushed into the extraperitoneal cellular tissue. The strangulated loop is displaced at (B) through the tear in the sac (C) into the extraperitoneal cellular tissue. The empty sac is shown in (D). (*Right*) Through a circular rupture of the sac below the neck a false reduction may ensue. Note the neck reduced with the strangulated loop and strangulation persists. (B) Neck. (C) Strangulated loop. (D) Empty sac. (After Lejars)

domen the surgeon exercises traction upon the hernia itself. At best, however, taxis is a blind procedure which may result in irreparable injury to the strangulated, distended loops of intestine; if reduction is effected, it may be *reduction en bloc* with vascular injury or it may be a "false" reduction (Figs. 383 and 384). In fully half the cases where previous strong taxis has been exerted, intestinal hemorrhage has occurred.

Never attempt to replace the bulk of the hernial protrusion all at once when applying taxis. Exert continuous *gentle* pressure, allowing the bowel to slip back slowly and reach the abdominal cavity uninjured. A patient who for years has been doing his own "replacing" will be able to co-operate by suggesting how and in which position he can be relieved most quickly and easily.

INJURY TO THE SPERMATIC CORD AND THE TESTICLE

In children especially, the spermatic cord may be injured when isolating the hernial sac, which usually lies anteriorly and on the inner side of the cord. Indirect inguinal hernia in children and infants is not due to muscular weakness—as is usually the case with an adult patient—but rather to the failure of the *processus vaginalis* to atrophy following normal descent of the testicles into the scrotum during the final weeks of intra-uterine life. The testicle and the cord are enfolded after entering the scrotum by the processus vaginalis, but it never completely covers them. As fetal development continues, the processus is pinched off, thus forming the ensheathing *tunica vaginalis*, while the upper part normally atrophies. Should it fail to atrophy, however, it remains as a preformed hernial sac which at birth will be manifest as a recurrent reducible mass in the inguinal area. The protrusion may not be evident until the child is several months old and then will be in evidence only when he screams or strains. Incarceration occurs most commonly during the

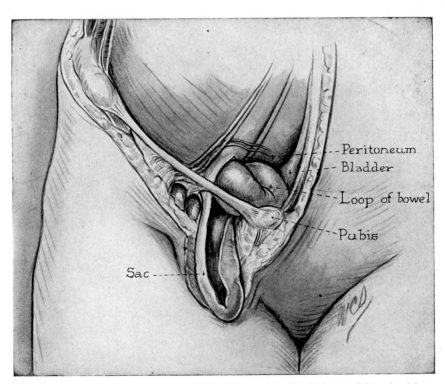

FIG. 384. "False reduction" after incision of neck of femoral hernia. Note intestine lodged between pubes and peritoneum, and empty hernial sac. Unless hernial contents are definitely reposited into abdominal cavity, there can be no assurance of successful reduction. (After Farabeuf)

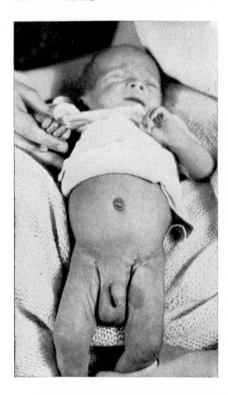

FIG. 385. Infant aged 6 weeks, shown at time of discharge from hospital following operation for strangulated hernia. Never assume that a condition is *not* hernia simply because the patient is very young!

first 6 months, the symptoms being swelling, which persists in the inguinal region, vomiting and abdominal cramps.

The surgeon should attempt to reduce an incarcerated hernia in an infant because of the associated tissue edema and the friability of the sac. A suitable narcotic should be given, the foot of the crib elevated and an icepack applied to the swollen groin. If the incarceration can be reduced by these measures, surgery may be postponed for 2 or 3 days. *Otherwise, immediate surgery is the only safe course.* In children, do not employ a technic which involves transplantation of the cord. For the very young it is not necessary and only makes the operation longer and more difficult. *Hematoma* and *atrophy of the testicle* are more likely to follow.

No matter what technic is employed in operating for inguinal hernia on an infant (Fig. 385) or young child, only a very small incision will be necessary. The chief risk is trauma to the vas deferens, which at this age is a very delicate structure and easily torn. In older patients, keep in mind the possibility of injury to the plexus paminiformis and to the spermatic artery, which might bring about necrosis of the testicle. The vas is more likely to be injured than are other structures, but the cord may be completely severed, producing internal hemorrhage and resulting in destruction of the testicle of that side.

In operating for hernia be sure that, after repairing the inguinal canal, no undue pressure has been exerted on the cord. Before closing the skin, the surgeon should introduce the tip of his little finger into the inguinal canal and make sure that there is no interference with the circulation as the result of excessive pressure on the spermatic cord by the tightly superimposed structures.

Avoid strangulation of tissues by too tight ligatures. *Approximation is what is wanted, not strangulation.*

Never ligate omentum near the bowel. A piece of intestine may be inadvertently included. *Hematoma of the scrotum* is a not unusual complication following hernia operations. This is due to injury of the vessels of the spermatic cord and also to failure to ligate vessels in the adjoining tissues. A hydrocele may result from injury to the spermatic veins and lymphatics.

BLADDER INJURY

Take care not to injure the bladder; it may not be recognized when the hernial sac is freed, or it may present itself as a cystocele or as a diverticulum. Though urine may flow from such bladder injury, it will often be unnoticed. Even if such an injury is very slight, it may be sufficient to induce uremic shock, and leaking urine may be responsible for acute peritonitis. Many cases are on record where a portion of the bladder was included in ligating a hernial sac, and doubtless a great many more have never gotten into print.

Identification of Bladder. A strange-looking mass may be discovered at the inner side of the hernial ring, and the cautious surgeon will bear in mind the possibility of its turning out to be the bladder. He should not incise it or start to dissect it until he is positive it is *not* the bladder. The ureter of that side may not be readily recognizable and may suffer injury in both inguinal and femoral hernia operations. This accident happens more often on the right side than on the left.

THE SAC

Always remove the sac, however small it may be. Remove a small sac and close the transversalis fascia in exactly the same way as you would a large gaping sac, for a small sac often tends to enlarge, separating even a well-performed muscular reconstruction. *Every sac must be completely removed to ensure against recurrence of the hernia.* Whenever possible, cut the sac flush with the peritoneal surface, obliterating it entirely. *Open the sac with the greatest caution,* especially if the contents are bound together by adhesions. As the contents usually consist of intestinal loops and omentum, if they are held together by adhesions which cannot be readily severed and there is no gangrene of the bowel, it is often best to return the mass en bloc into the abdominal cavity. However, it must be remembered that if adherent loops of bowel in a hernial sac are inverted into the abdomen, *they may remain kinked,* causing possible obstruction of the bowel. For the same reason, the loops of bowel still in the abdomen, but in the immediate vicinity of those herniated, should be examined with care, as they are sometimes thickened and their lumina diminished, so that they have become a potential source of stricture.

Suturing. When suturing the orifice of a hernial sac, be sure that a loop of intestine has not been included in the suture. It is not good surgery merely to reduce the contents of the sac and suture the orifice. Before final closure, consider all the possibilities which might arise from the condition. If a loop of intestine is accidentally included in the suture, it may cause a local or even a general peritonitis or set up some form of intestinal obstruction. The following case is an example from my personal experience.

Case Report. Some years ago I was doing a herniorrhaphy, and, when at the point of bringing the respective structures to Poupart's ligament, I acceded to the request of an assistant that he be permitted to conclude the operation. The following day I was called out of the city. On my return, 3 days later, I found the patient in the throes of intestinal obstruction and advancing peritonitis. He died that night, and necropsy revealed that the assistant had picked up a portion of the bowel, which resulted in intestinal occlusion, peritonitis and death.

Every surgeon should be impressed with the necessity for the closest possible scrutiny in the placing of sutures and the care with which the needle should be guided while working in close proximity to important structures. The suturing of the hernial orifice should always be carried out under full vision. *When a large indirect sac must be dealt with,* close the sac high and use a purse-string suture of quilting cotton, or the surgeon's preferred suture material; then permit it to retract beneath the internal oblique muscle, *but do not transfix it.* After the neck of the sac has retracted, a defect in the transversalis fascia will become apparent at the internal ring. This should be closed tightly around the cord structures, using interrupted quilting sutures and carefully inverting the preperitoneal fat.

This closure of the transversalis fascia at the internal ring is extremely important, as failure to effect it completely is a frequent cause of recurrence in indirect hernia, quite as much as failure to remove the entire sac is in other types of hernia.

High Amputation of Sac; Obliquity of Canal. *Two underlying factors in hernia operations must always be kept in the surgeon's mind:* high amputation of the hernial sac, with reconstruction of the transversalis fascia, and restoration of the obliquity of the inguinal canal. In some cases of inguinal hernia the obliquity of the canal cannot be restored, owing perhaps to pronounced weakness of the abdominal wall with general abdominal ptosis, or the structures forming the hernial boundaries have become stretched and thinned through failure to seek treatment promptly, so that the canal has been destroyed to such an extent that it is impossible to restore its obliquity. In the management of such a situation, the inguinal canal must be so dealt with that there is little opportunity for the hernia to recur, while, at the same time, the closure must not be so tight as to strangulate the cord and its vessels.

Vascular and Neural Complications. *Avoid*

compression of the venous plexus and subsequent venous stasis. Thrombosis of the plexus pampiniformis is manifested by a painful swelling of the testicle, which may not appear until weeks or months after the herniorrhaphy. Severe vascular stenosis is likely to bring about "neuralgic" pains in the region of the vas deferens which will demand relief. Inclusion of nerves in sutures or ligatures will have similar results. There is also the possibility of *injuring the ilio-inguinal nerve* which traverses the fibers of the internal oblique and the region of the external ring. The course of this nerve is such that it may be sectioned or easily included in the suture. The *iliohypogastric and the genitocrural nerves* may also be injured. Such nerve damage is illustrated by the following case.

Case Report. A man was operated on by a very capable surgeon for a right inguinal hernia. After the operation the patient suffered from neuralgic pains which prevented him from attending to his business and brought on a severe postoperative neurosis. All known methods of treatment failed to restore him to health, so, as a last resort, a second herniorrhaphy was performed. The ilioinguinal nerve was located, but it was embedded so strongly in adhesions that it was deemed impossible to liberate it. I severed the nerve, after which prompt recovery followed.

Gangrene of Strangulated Intestine. After freeing strangulated intestine, each loop must be examined individually and minutely for signs of impending gangrene. The vitality of every part of the intestine involved in a hernia must be fully proved before its return to the abdominal cavity. The examination should include the portion of the intestine immediately outside the sac and that still in the abdomen. Contractility of the intestinal wall, its response to pinching, is a positive sign of viability. Other signs are bleeding, a shiny appearance, elasticity and absence of apparent gangrenous patches. One will sometimes be surprised to find a gangrenous patch or a minute perforation where one least suspects it. This is particularly true of the area which was constricted at the neck of the hernia.

Caution Before Resecting Intestinal Loops. The surgeon should not be too hasty in resecting loops of intestine which *appear* to be devitalized. Frequently such loops become viable after persistent treatment with hot saline solution. Nevertheless, it must be remembered that perforation is a possibility up to the seventh or eighth day after strangulation. In addition, the reduced loops may be so thickened and their lumina so diminished that stricture results.

When there is no doubt as to gangrene, resection becomes inevitable and should extend well into unchanged tissue. *Resect only in perfectly sound tissue.* Occasionally, because of the danger of hemorrhage, it may be wiser not to remove a richly vascular sac, but to close it with sutures and leave it in place. *Never resect the intestine at the hernial opening!* Put a laparotomy sponge into the wound; cover with sterile towels; open the abdomen from above (as in any other celiotomy); deliver the bowel through the laparotomy wound; resect. Close the inguinal region, or the femoral, as the case may be. Provide drainage in cases that have been much handled or when one is not absolutely certain of asepsis.

Case Report. I vividly recall the tragic death of a patient on whom I operated many years ago for a voluminous, direct inguinal hernia. Nothing unusual was found at operation. The procedure was comparatively simple, and everything went well until the third postoperative day, when the patient experienced a sharp chill, followed by a rapid rise in temperature and pulse rate. Septic manifestations ensued in quick succession, and, despite desperate efforts to save him, the patient succumbed.

A thorough investigation into the cause of this tragedy revealed that our assistant had been in contact with septic material on the previous day.

The surgeon should be sure of himself, of his assistants and of his operating room personnel.

Another—only slightly less serious—error which may arise because of imperfect coordination between the surgeon and his assisting staff is operating on the wrong side! In a busy surgeon's life, this may happen if he entrusts the history taking to careless assistants and interns. In order to avoid such mistakes, it is a wise precaution to instruct the person who takes the history and makes the preliminary examination to leave a spot of silver nitrate or mercurochrome on the affected side, in addition, of course, to noting carefully on the history sheet the side on which the hernia exists. Also, the surgical

TABLE 3. RESULTS FROM DIFFERENT TYPES OF OPERATIONS IN 978 TRACED CASES

TYPE OF OPERATION	OBLIQUE HERNIA		DIRECT HERNIA	
	OPERATIONS	RECURRENCES	OPERATIONS	RECURRENCES
Bassini	532	17— 3.2 %	185	29—15.67%
Bassini with rectus	13	0	35	4—11.4%
Cord not transplanted	112	3— 2.67%	25	7—28%
Extra-aponeurotic transplant of cord	8	1—12.5%	64	10—15.62%
Atypical repair	0	0	4	2—50%
Total	665	21— 3.0%	313	52—16.61%

supervisor should be notified as to where the hernia is located, in this way securing a double check.

RECURRENCES

In simple oblique inguinal hernia, recurrence is estimated at about 3 per cent. In direct hernia, the percentage is about 16 per cent, which may be greatly increased in the aged (Table 3). Permitting a patient to return to full activity after a hernia operation is a common reason for recurrence. "When can I get back to work, Doctor?" is demanded by the vast majority of those who have undergone herniorrhaphy. I endeavor to keep my patients at comparative rest for about 3 weeks. If the patient's vocation demands much exertion, he should not resume it within 3 weeks to 2 months. However, if he is a person of leisure or if his occupation is not physically arduous, an earlier resumption of regular duties may be permitted.

The causes of recurrence of inguinal hernia after operation have been listed as follows:

1. Patient unsuitable for operation in the first place because of the type of hernia and the poor condition of the parts which had to be utilized

2. Unwise selection of original operative procedure which failed to meet the indications of the particular case

3. Sac was not removed or not ligated high enough; or a *double sac* was not recognized nor removed

4. The inguinal canal was under tension during the repair

5. The nerve supply of the inguinal region was injured during the original operation

6. Postoperative infection

7. Repaired structures separated postoperatively—either because the sutures failed to hold or the strain of postoperative vomiting was too great

8. Rent in transversalis fascia was not repaired

SUBSTANCES USED IN REPAIR OF HERNIAS

As far back as the beginning of World War II, surgeons seeking means for repairing large defects of the abdominal wall with loss of substance were turning to metallic implants for solution of the problem. *Tantalum mesh* and *Vitallium plate* have been most commonly employed, either alone or in combination with dermal grafts. Fascial transplants, pedicled muscle or fascial flaps used alone have all had their advocates recently, but, though exact figures are not available, recurrence after the use of such material is not entirely eliminated.

Dermal Grafts. Errors which have contributed to the failure of dermal grafts are insufficient advanced planning and lack of care in sterilizing the skin used, so that infection rendered the attempt useless and—in some instances—set up septic conditions at the remote site whence the grafts were removed. Lack of surgical cleanliness is, of course, inexcusable under any circumstances, save accidental emergencies, but repair of hernia where there is extensive loss of substance offers especial chance for bacterial invasion. Technical errors appear to have been the chief cause of failure in the employment of dermal grafts. When wound infection had been warded off, the grafts appear to have "taken" well, and recurrence of the hernias was rare. Only a well-trained surgeon should attempt this type of hernial repair. Dermis has been found to be better than fascia as a material for grafts because it is exceedingly strong in all directions of pull, in contrast with fascia wherein most of its strength is in the longitudinal direction of its fibers. Moreover, skin grafts are readily available in different parts of the body in almost any quantity, size or shape, whereas the sources of fascia are limited. Dermis is more readily replaced by live connective tissue with blood and nerve supply to form an integral living part of the abdominal wall.

Tantalum Mesh. Even more than dermis, tantalum mesh is always at hand for use in any hernia when, in the course of an operation for repair of hernia, it develops that additional substance is needed to complete closure of the abdominal wall. The mesh is supplied in sheets from which pieces of any shape or size can be cut with scissors; its flexibility permits it to be readily approximated to any surface, and it can be autoclaved repeatedly without affecting its consistency.

As a safeguard against recurrence of a large defect, a layer of tantalum gauze has proved to be satisfactory in many reported cases. Usually another layer of peritoneum can be interposed between the abdominal viscera and the metal implant. Sometimes, however, the bowel may be accidentally opened during the attempt to close the abdominal wall, hazarding delayed healing or even peritonitis. If the skin overlying such a large defect is not opened at all, but tantalum mesh applied directly over it, the bowel would be safeguarded and an additional layer of tissue would be available to strengthen the wall further. Moreover, the mesh induces a fibroblastic response which will fill it up by the end of 3 weeks, as has been shown by animal experiment as well as clinical observation in reoperated cases. The graft strengthened by the mesh becomes homogeneously fused by fibrosis to the surrounding tissues.[4]

Dangers of Using Metal Implants. This subject has not been dwelt upon by those recently reporting in the literature. Enthusiasts are likely not to expatiate on their failures. I have seen one report of a case where continuous drainage from a wound infection made it necessary to remove the mesh. Several

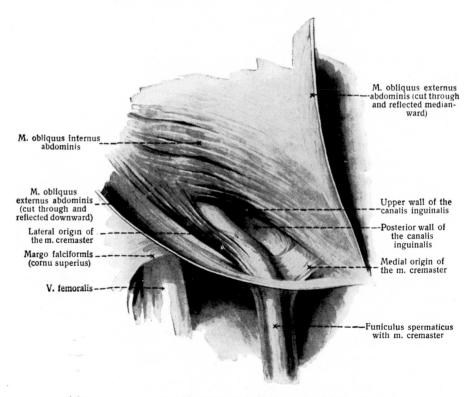

M. obliquus externus abdominis (cut through and reflected medianward)

M. obliquus internus abdominis

M. obliquus externus abdominis (cut through and reflected downward)

Lateral origin of the m. cremaster

Margo falciformis (cornu superius)

V. femoralis

Upper wall of the canalis inguinalis

Posterior wall of the canalis inguinalis

Medial origin of the m. cremaster

Funiculus spermaticus with m. cremaster

FIG. 386. Anatomy of right inguinal canal in male. (After Spalteholz)

authors have told of wound infections and purulent postoperative drainage, though the end-results were satisfactory. In a large series of experiments on dogs, from which segments of the abdominal wall—rectus abdominis, internal and external oblique muscles down to the peritoneum—had been removed and metal implants used for repair, fragmentation of the implant was observed in every animal after the lapse of 6 months or longer.

In the clinical cases of these experimenters, fragmentation occurred once with tantalum and once with stainless steel. When stainless steel was used, recurrence was attributed to fragmentation, as it took place in the central portion of the mesh. Four other recurrences were attributed to errors in technic. In 3 cases the sheets of mesh used were too small to cover the defects adequately; in another, 2 sheets of mesh were overlapped, causing necrosis and sinus formation.

As the use of metal implants in the repair of large hernias becomes more general, such technical errors should be eliminated.[8]

INGUINAL HERNIA

As inguinal hernia is a relatively common condition, every practicing physician should have a thorough knowledge of the normal inguinal canal and be familiar with its abnormal anatomy and the variations in hernial types that he is likely to encounter. A study of the accompanying illustrations (Figs. 386 and 387) will be of assistance. The methods of diagnosis described on pages 504-507 usually suffice to detect incipient inguinal hernia, but complicated cases demand special investigation. Differentiation between *direct, indirect* and *femoral hernia* can usually be established when the patient is in the upright position with the inguinal region bared. The surgeon uses his right hand for a right inguinal hernia and his left for a left-sided hernia (Fig. 388), placing his first, second and third fingers over the inguinal region with the index finger on the "weak spot," the middle finger extending along the inguinal canal, with the tip at the external inguinal ring, while the third finger controls the femoral canal and fossa ovalis (Fig. 389). Coughing or straining will make possible the perception of a peculiar sliding movement of a viscus under the fingers, *permitting determination of the type of hernia present.*

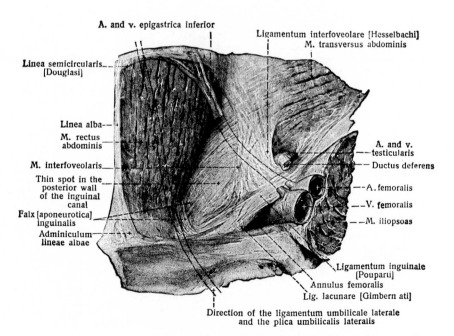

FIG. 387. Anatomy of posterior wall of right inguinal canal in male, rear view.
(After Spalteholz)

Direct vs. Indirect Hernia

Origin. Indirect inguinal hernia is of *embryologic origin*. Direct inguinal hernia is *acquired* (Fig. 390). By "embryologic" we mean that a previous embryologic path has been reopened; when we speak of inguinal hernia, we mean the path taken during the descent of the testicle. Two layers of peritoneum which should have fused during descent of the testicle did so only very loosely and

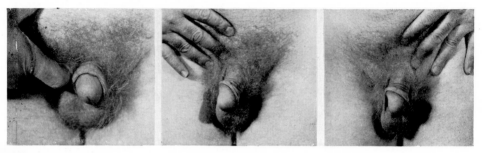

Fig. 388. Methods of examining for hernia. (*Left*) Conventional method. (*Center and right*) Zieman's method, using right hand for right side, left for left.

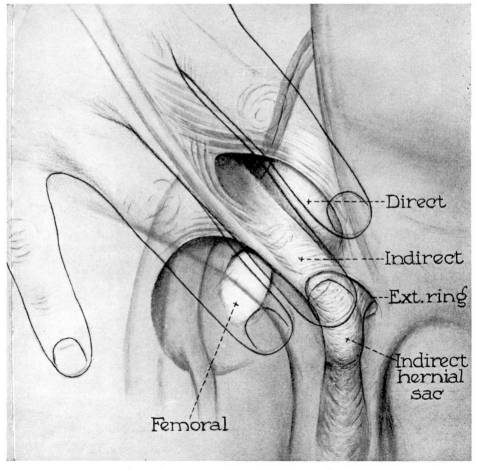

Fig. 389. Schematic drawing showing relations of various types of hernia to examining fingers. (After Zieman)

were reopened during stress and strain. There-fore, every congenital inguinal hernia is embryologic, but every embryologic inguinal hernia is *not* congenital.

A *direct hernia* has nothing to do with embryologic paths or congenital defects. It is "acquired" because of a weakening in the transversalis fascia. The differentiation is important in view of treatment, for there is no form of management which can be carried out routinely for all types of hernia.[5]

Important Differential Points. These are as follows:

1. Age of onset: indirect hernia is usually seen in those under the age of 40; direct hernias in those over 40.

2. Appearance on standing: an indirect hernia does not appear immediately when the patient is upright; the direct hernial bulge appears at once when the patient stands.

3. Reduction: an indirect hernia must usually be pushed back by the patient or else reduces itself slowly; a direct hernia disappears as soon as the patient lies down.

4. Scrotal: An indirect hernia may become scrotal, but I have never seen a *direct* scrotal hernia.

5. Strangulation: indirect hernias may strangulate, but I have never seen a strangulated direct hernia. One must differentiate between *incarceration* and *strangulation*.

Treatment of Indirect and Direct Inguinal Hernia. Radical operation only is indicated for the treatment of inguinal hernia because of the lasting results and comparative safety. But, before undertaking any operative procedure, it is most important that the surgeon understand the internal oblique muscle and its "shutterlike" action. By contracting, the internal oblique approximates itself to Pou-

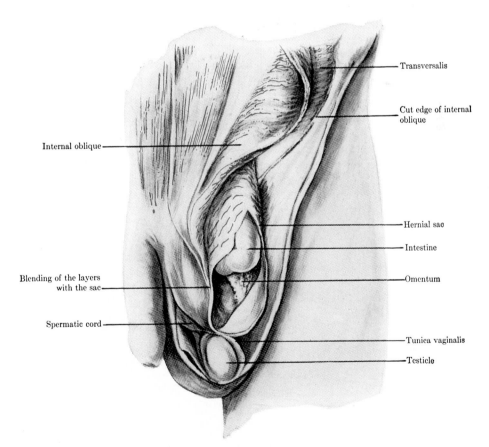

Fig. 390. Drawing from actual dissection of acquired oblique inguinal hernia.
(Davis: Applied Anatomy, Philadelphia, Lippincott)

part's ligament, thus fortifying Hesselbach's triangle. Therefore, it stands to reason that this muscle should not be sutured, but rather left alone to carry on its own function. Comprehension of this fact probably accounts for the lessened popularity of the Bassini operation.

ANESTHESIA. Improvements in methods and materials have made the use of spinal and regional anesthesia almost universal in hernia operations. Even in the aged, if the relatively few contraindications (see pp. 33, 35, 43 and 334) are carefully observed, results will be satisfactory. The oldest patient on whom I have operated was 90 years of age—the father of a physician. The condition was urgent; a large loop of bowel was strangulated. Resection was carried out under procaine anesthesia (which I was using regularly at that time), and the outcome was completely successful.

FEMORAL HERNIA

The anatomic structures concerned in fem-oral hernia are well shown in Figures 391 and 392. The surgeon should refresh his memory now and then, unless he is very frequently called on to diagnose femoral hernia. The femoral ring is a rigid or semirigid opening bounded in front by Poupart's ligament, behind by the iliopectineal line of the os pubis, the pubic portion of the fascia lata and Cooper's ligament, laterally by the femoral vein and medially by Gimbernat's ligament, from which it extends downward to the upper part of the saphenous opening.

The *saphenous opening* or *fossa ovalis* is a deficiency in the fascia lata where the saphenous vein passes through it, at the upper medial part of the thigh, just below the medial end of Poupart's ligament. The *saphenous vein* runs superficial to the deep fascia of the leg up to the last and shortest division of its course. It is the longest vein in the body. About an inch from its junction with the femoral vein, the saphenous penetrates the deep fascia at the fossa ovalis, its passage

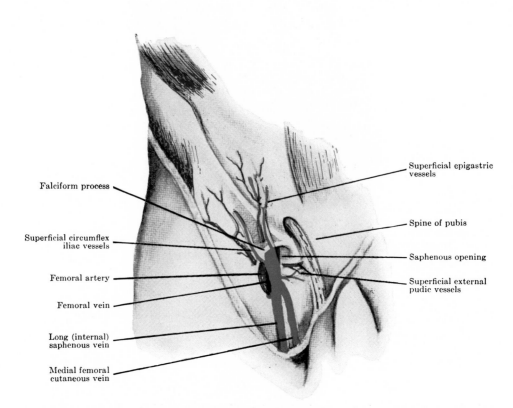

Falciform process

Superficial circumflex iliac vessels

Femoral artery

Femoral vein

Long (internal) saphenous vein

Medial femoral cutaneous vein

Superficial epigastric vessels

Spine of pubis

Saphenous opening

Superficial external pudic vessels

FIG. 391. Anatomy of saphenous opening (fossa ovalis). (Davis: Applied Anatomy, Philadelphia, Lippincott)

making a comparatively weak area in the deep fascia close to the femoral canal, thus presenting a line of least resistance to any hernia which might penetrate the canal and—increasing in size—exert pressure for expansion.

If a portion of peritoneum protrudes through the femoral ring, it will soon provide itself with an investment from the extraperitoneal fascia and fat and at the fundus will be overlaid by the femoral septum. Thus equipped, it will descend through the femoral canal as far as the fossa ovalis, where it will be deflected in a superficial direction by the attachments to the margins of the fossa, eventually emerging superficial to the fascia lata of the thigh. Here it would again change its direction so as to pass upward over the inguinal ligament and the aponeurosis of the external oblique, to be overlaid by superficial fascia and skin.[7]

DIFFERENTIAL DIAGNOSIS

Femoral hernia must be differentiated from other types of hernia, from varix of the saphenous vein and, occasionally, from cold abscess. Such abscesses, though rare in this location, occasionally cause great confusion. Careful examination of the spine should be made, even though cold abscesses often arise when there is no obvious spinal disease. The swelling caused by an abscess gives no impulse on coughing and is more prominent when the patient stands upright.

Saphenous Varix. This disappears when the patient lies down; when he arises, its return may be prevented by applying pressure over the femoral vein. If a swelling due to varix of the saphenous vein is palpated when the patient is coughing, the "thrill" characteristic of a varix will be felt, in contrast with the "impulse" of a hernia.

Inguinal Hernia. The chief differentiation is, of course, that between *inguinal* and *femoral hernia* (see Fig. 392). To tell them apart, it is important to locate the pubic tubercle. In femoral hernia, the swelling is medial to this bony protuberance. Inguinal hernia may also be somewhat lateral to the pubic tubercle, but the femoral is much further toward the side. If the condition is reducible, there is less chance of confusion; none the less, irre-

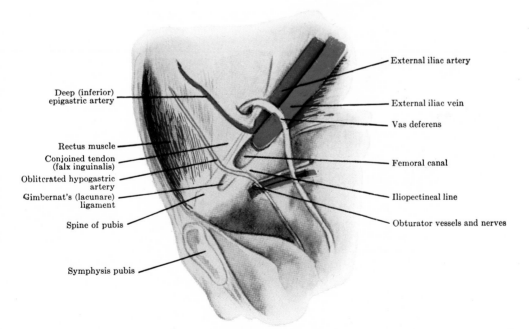

FIG. 392. Anatomy of inguinal and femoral regions viewed from within (peritoneum removed). (Davis: Applied Anatomy, Philadelphia, Lippincott)

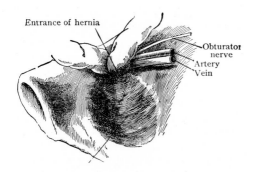

Fig. 393. Right obturator hernia as seen from within through obturator membrane. (After Piersol)

ducible inguinal hernia may be difficult to differentiate from femoral hernia, especially in the female.

In femoral hernia the usual signs and symptoms of intestinal obstruction develop slowly in approximately a third of the cases. This is because the ilium or the colon is involved low down or only a section of the bowel's circumference has been caught. So much emphasis is now being laid on *cancer* that the vague intestinal upsets due to hernial obstruction are often regarded as being indications of intestinal malignancy. *Complicated femoral hernia should be suspected in any patient with vague and undiagnosed gastro-intestinal complaints.* Pain and vomiting are the most common symptoms associated with strangulation.

OPERATIVE SAFEGUARDS

Remember that in a femoral hernia, strangulation is not commonly due to Gimbernat's ligament, as is generally believed, but to a relatively thickened and rigid band of tissue at the neck of the sac. This should be divided quite independently of Gimbernat's ligament. Indeed, both Gimbernat's and Poupart's ligaments should always be respected if possible because they are supporting structures of great importance, and if they are sectioned, there will be a predisposition to recurrence of the hernia.

There are two ways of treating the femoral sac: (1) cut away its terminal portion and stitch up the remainder; (2) free the sac and some of its parietal peritoneum and convert it into an intra-abdominal pad.

Danger to Contents of Sac in Strangulation.

In an incarcerated femoral hernia there is the same danger to the contents of the sac when opening it as has already been mentioned for inguinal hernia. *Always do this under full vision and verify the precise nature of the sac contents.* There may be a secondary incarceration of part of the contents within the original hernial sac, and, when opening the outer sac, this possibility should be kept in mind. One portion of the intestinal contents may form a typically crural incarceration. and another portion may be strangulated in a properitoneal hernial sac.

If, when operating on a femoral hernia, resection of a part of the intestine becomes necessary, *a median or a paramedian laparotomy is a prerequisite,* as it may be extremely difficult to replace the anastomosed intestine through the hernial incision. If a large segment of bowel has to be resected, the whole procedure is perhaps best performed through the laparotomy wound.

In order to obtain success in femoral herniorrhaphies, the sac must be entirely obliterated. Many methods of closure have been advised, but the simplest is the best. Avoid complicated procedures. Remember that in a thin patient, while operating on a femoral hernia, the surgeon must guide his scalpel with great care lest he open the bowel as well as the hernial sac because of the thinness of the superimposed skin. If the patient is fat, the panniculus adiposus may cause great difficulty. A small strangulated hernia, even though it contains gangrenous bowel, may, under such conditions, be difficult of access, and, through careless dissecting, one may enter the bowel, with subsequent peritonitis and death.

Always safeguard the femoral vein! It is an easy matter to injure it while closing the hernial opening. Both femoral and saphenous veins can be easily traumatized at this step in the operative procedure.

OBTURATOR HERNIA

Obturator hernia is relatively rare, about 500 cases having been reported in the literature. It is seen most often in women 60 years of age or over, no more than 20 per cent of the patients being males. The herniation takes place in the obturator foramen and canal in the innominate bone on the anterolateral surface of either side of the pelvis (Fig. 393). The structures which surround the *internal* obturator opening are very dense and unyielding, while *externally* the canal opening is beneath the pectineus, the adductor longus and the obturator externus muscles. This strong, dense muscular encasement offers maximum protection to the obturator canal, probably accounting for the rarity of obturator hernia. On the other hand, if herniation does take place, there is greater likelihood of *strangulation*—an important point in both diagnosis and treatment.

Symptoms and Diagnosis

The symptoms are those of acute intestinal obstruction. *Pain along the course of the obturator nerve* is the important symptom suggesting obturator hernia. Pressure of the hernial sac and its contents on the obturator nerve is the probable cause of this lancinating pain, which is known as the *Romberg-Howship sign.* Actually, no more than half the cases present this sign, but frequently the patient may complain that extension of the thigh or any motion of the hip is very distressing, and he will keep the leg flexed so as to relieve the pull on the nerves. The presence of a detectable bulge over the upper medial part of the thigh, in the external obturator region —especially if it is associated with tenderness—will provide a valuable diagnostic clue. Vaginal or rectal examination may reveal a tender mass on the anterolateral surface of the pelvis at the location of the internal obturator foramen. An erroneous diagnosis of acute appendicitis is frequently made when obturator hernia occurs on the right side, especially if the patient is seen early before signs of intestinal obstruction become apparent.

Confusion between strangulated femoral hernia and obturator hernia is a serious error, because the only satisfactory approach to obturator hernia is through the abdomen, whereas there are 3 or possibly 4 routes which have been used satisfactorily in order to reach the femoral variety. The abdominal approach gives a better view of the operative field, which facilitates reduction of the hernia, while if any intestinal resection or other extensive procedure is later found to be necessary, it can be performed more readily.

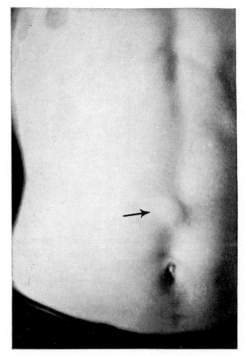

Fig. 394. Hernia in linea alba.

Because most of the victims of obturator hernia are elderly and often in a much debilitated condition, special safeguards must be provided before, during and after operation. The anesthetic must be selected with particular view to safety and *should always be administered by a skilled and experienced anesthetist* who is fully aware of any cardiac or vascular deficiencies that the patient may have. Unfortunately, this is not always possible, because the patient may not reach the hospital until he is in extremis, his condition so desperate as to make preliminary examination hasty and superficial. The mortality is high and will probably remain so. Nonetheless, every effort should be exerted to lower it.

OTHER HERNIAS

Diagnoses of gastric disturbance or disease of the biliary passages are often made and patients treated for long periods without benefit, when the repair of a small, but unnoticed, epigastric protrusion would have cured them speedily.

Case Report. A man of affairs, aged 57, was sent to me by his physician, with a diagnosis of

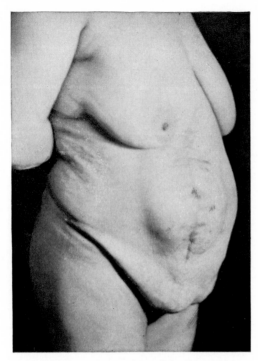

FIG. 395. Incisional hernia.

ulcer of the stomach and a request that I operate on him. The diagnosis was said to have been definitely made by roentgenography and other clinical methods. Thorough examination of the patient revealed an *epigastric protrusion,* the size of the end of the little finger, which was tender to pressure. An exploratory operation showed nothing abnormal in the stomach. The hernial sac was in the linea alba and adherent to its surroundings. A herniorrhaphy brought about disappearance of all symptoms.

Epigastric Hernia. When other causes for *tenderness in the linea alba region* have been excluded, one should think of an *epigastric hernia.* Hernia of the linea albo is not at all infrequent (Fig. 394). In young children the condition may disappear with age, but older patients should always be subjected to operation.

Hernia in Operation Scars. Hernias often occur in operation scars (Fig. 395). If the surgeon has difficulty in repairing a hernia of this type, he should try making a *transverse incision* and, in closing, *unite the tissues transversely.*

Hernia Through Petit's Triangle. This may be the cause of an otherwise inexplicable backache.

Sciatic Hernia. This may also give rise to confusion (Figs. 396 and 397).

Sliding Hernia. These hernias offer particular problems. A thorough knowledge of anatomy is of the utmost importance. They offer operative difficulties and, on occasion, tax the ingenuity of the surgeon.[6]

Hernia in Poor-Risk Patient. The aged, the debilitated and those suffering from metabolic diseases, cardiovascular abnormalities or other devastating conditions require special preoperative care, meticulous operative procedures and watchful postoperative nursing.[10]

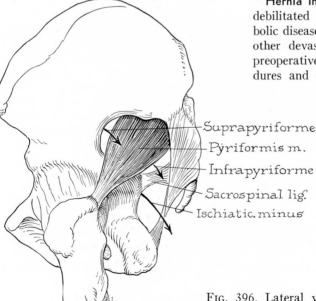

Suprapyriforme
Pyriformis m.
Infrapyriforme
Sacrospinal lig.
Ischiatic. minus

FIG. 396. Lateral view of pelvis, showing openings through which sciatic hernia may occur.

UMBILICAL CORD HERNIA

A word of warning to those who practice obstetrics! Be on the lookout for hernia into the umbilical cord while delivering the child. Look carefully before cutting the cord. I know of two cases in which the peritoneal cavity had been opened and a loop of intestine incised in the act of cutting the cord when such hernia existed. Umbilical cord hernia has a double danger in the newborn: (1) gangrene of the intestine and (2) infection.

In dealing with an umbilical cord hernia, there is likely to be added danger from *adhesions* which have formed between the intestine or other abdominal organ and the outer abdominal wall. The liver, as well as the intestine, may be in the hernial sac and will complicate resection of the bowel if, because of difficulty in restoring it to its proper position, bowel resection becomes necessary. It must be remembered that in the hernial sac of an umbilical cord hernia there is no separate peritoneal sac, and during the incision the bowel can be injured very easily. There is a tendency for the original pouch to divide into a number of sacs communicating with one another, though they may have separate septa and diverticula, and there may be distinct peritoneal openings into the different sacs. The most unusual combinations may be encountered, such as prolapsed omentum asso-

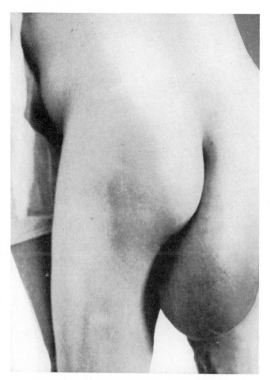

Fig. 397. Sciatic hernia (Surgical Service, Cook County Hosp.).

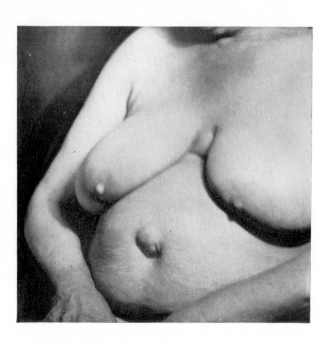

Fig. 398. Small strangulated umbilical hernia in female. Subjective symptoms were mild. At operation, a piece of strangulated bowel was found.

ciated with chronic peritonitis in the hernial sac, preperitoneal fat, etc.

Under these difficult conditions, the surgeon should open the abdominal cavity just above the protruding mass and work downward from this starting point. *Never incise directly over the hernial mass.* A transverse incision is better than a longitudinal one because most of the fibers of the abdominal aponeurosis run transversely, and the hernia is the result of the thinning and weakening of these fibers (Fig. 398).

Because the contents of the hernial sac of an umbilical cord hernia are often so voluminous (Fig. 399), it may be very difficult to replace the herniated organs in the abdomen, and they are likely to be injured during manipulation. In addition, the resultant great compression and tension lead to excitation of the vagus, with functional disturbance of the organs and the blood vessels which it innervates. In patients already subject to cardiac disturbance, the heart action may be weakened.

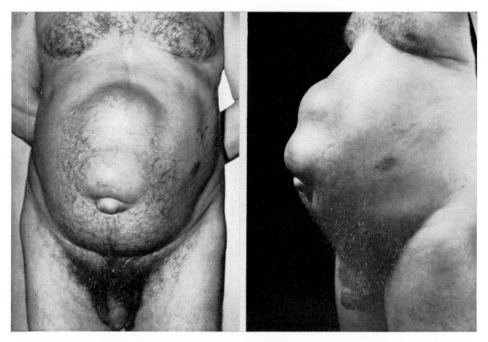

Fig. 399. Two views of patient with ventral hernia. Pain was diagnosed as incipient bowel obstruction, but proved to be due to herpes zoster.

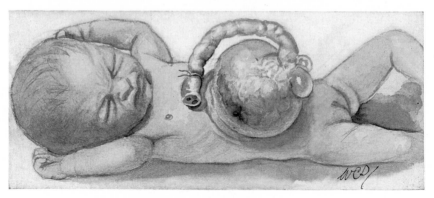

Fig. 400. Amniotic hernia.

SYMPTOMS

The symptoms of a strangulated umbilical cord hernia are often only an exaggeration of those of long-standing, uncomplicated hernia. Delay in operation accounts for the high percentage of unfavorable results after surgery finally has been resorted to. The danger of herniorrhaphy is far less than that of postponing this procedure. Though sometimes, when exposed by incision, the loops of intestine in the principal sac of an umbilical cord hernia may be unchanged in appearance, there are more likely to be all the changes due to incarceration of one of the subsidiary sacs, or a strangulated loop may be in a deep-lying diverticulum, or a protrusion of the chief sac. Torsion of a loop or loops may be found in or between sacs.

RECURRENCE

Umbilical cord hernias are more likely to recur after surgical repair than are either the inguinal or femoral types. This is because permanent changes have taken place in the constituents of the abdominal wall so that it is no longer able to withstand pressure. This is especially true in elderly fat women, in whom this type of hernia is most frequently observed.

AMNIOTIC HERNIA

This has been defined as a primary amniotic hernia of the linea alba with secondary actual herniation. It is also known as *congenital umbilical hernia, omphalocele congenitalis,* *ectopia viscerum* and *hernia funiculus umbilicalis* (Fig. 400). There are two varieties of amniotic hernia, the *embryonic* and the *fetal,* the fetal being usually the smaller. Usually giving no symptoms, the child at times will give evidence of transitory umbilical pain. Small hernias of this variety usually disappear before the age of 3 years, spontaneously or aided by abdominal strapping. An amniotic hernia may vary in size from a slight protrusion as small as the finger tip to one as large as a fetal head.

DIAGNOSIS

Amniotic hernia is readily recognized, though it may be confused with hydrocele of the umbilical cord. In hydrocele, however, bladder symptoms are absent, and needle aspiration will demonstrate that the contained fluid is *not* urine. It differs from *postnatal hernia* in that the postnatal variety has a location excentric from the cord. Amniotic hernia has a ring situated at the center of the umbilicus. It is covered by amnion and a thin layer of peritoneum, with a thin layer of Wharton's jelly in between. There may be no defined ring. In one reported case, the amnion was fused with the peritoneum and formed the covering of the hernial sac.

TREATMENT

Surgery is the only sure means of preventing peritonitis or paralytic ileus. The approach may be either intraperitoneal or extraperitoneal. The intraperitoneal approach is used

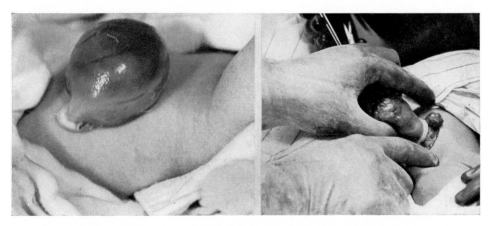

Fig. 401. (*Left*) Amniotic hernia in infant 10 days old. (*Right*) Same patient— exposure of sac.

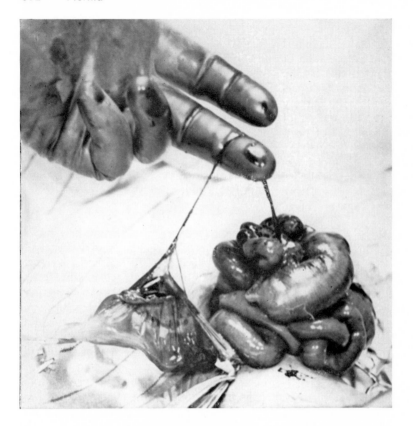

Fig. 402. Amniotic hernia; dissection of sac and exposure of hernial contents.

when it is necessary to open the abdomen to examine the viscera or deal with peritonitis. The dangers of this type of surgery have been greatly reduced by the introduction in recent years of chemotherapy and antibiotics. The earlier the operation, the better are the infant's chances of recovery. Operation has been performed successfully a half hour after de-

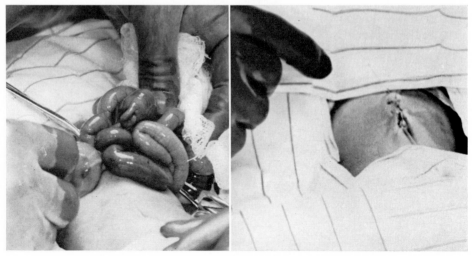

Fig. 403. Amniotic hernia. (*Left*) Contents separated from sac. (*Right*) Abdomen closed.

Fig. 404. Enormous ventral hernia.

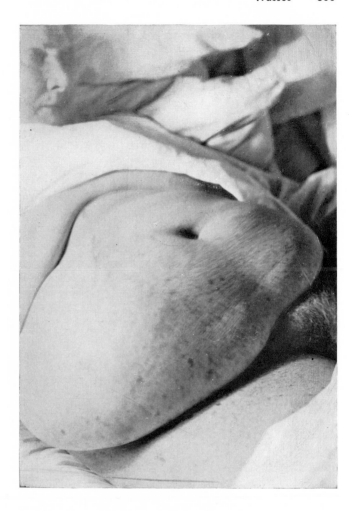

livery and satisfactory recovery reported for a number of operations within 2 to 12 hours after birth (Figs. 401-403). With the extraperitoneal approach there is less danger of shock, and the mortality rate is lower.

SAFEGUARDS IN TECHNIC

After opening the sac and examining its contents, *do not attempt to reduce the hernia into the cord*. Liberate all adhesions and ligate the umbilical vessels in the falciform ligament; ligate the urachus. If possible, dissect out the layers of the abdominal wall and suture each separately.

TRUSSES

Trusses after herniorrhaphies are abominations. They weaken instead of strengthen the structures. However, in the infantile type of umbilical hernia, cure from treatment by a truss may commonly be expected. It is wrong to subject these children to operative treatment before attempting cure by means of a truss. After 4 years of age, however, such treatment is only palliative.

CRITERIA OF A PROPER TRUSS

A truss should not cause pain when worn and should be so constructed as to prevent compression of the spermatic cord or important vascular structures. *An ill-fitting truss is worse than none*. The infant must wear it day and night, and it should not be removed, even when he is being bathed. The truss must exert precisely the proper degree of pressure and must fit exactly. The surgeon must understand what is needed and supervise the work of the truss maker, making sure that he is

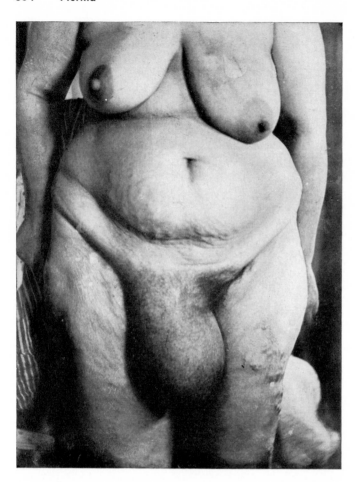

FIG. 405. Enormous inguinal hernia complicating pregnancy.

competent and capable of supplying the patient's needs. All attempts to improve a hernia by mechanical measures will be frustrated if the herniated organs are constantly permitted to slip out of the abdomen and enter the sac.

Contraindications to the use of trusses are irreducible hernia, inflamed hernia, hydrocele, cryptorchidism and interstitial hernia.

VOLUMINOUS HERNIAS

With increasing public health education and the establishment of well-equipped medical centers in most of the centers of population, the voluminous hernias (Fig. 404) which used to be brought to the surgeon quite regularly are not often seen. But, when they do come, they demand the highest skill and best surgical judgment for their management, posing a problem that is often difficult or even impossible of solution. Often they are complicated by an associated pregnancy, so it would be folly to advise operation in such cases before labor has been terminated.

Case Report. A woman carrying an enormous hernia (Fig. 405) came to me 40 years ago, well advanced in pregnancy. It would have been most ill-advised to attempt operation before she gave birth to her child, so she was carried through to full-term delivery and informed that she would be operated on when she had recovered sufficiently to withstand such a procedure. About a year after her delivery I operated on her, and a large amount of abdominal contents was found in the hernial sac. The usual reposition of the hernial contents into the abdomen, the resection of the hernial sac and repair of the inguinal canal led to complete recovery. Fortunately, I did not have to resect the intestine, but the intense distress suffered by this patient would have warranted it had it been otherwise impossible to return it to the abdomen.

Case Report. A man, about 45 years old, came to me for operation after carrying a hernia (Fig. 406) for more than 15 years. Other surgeons previously consulted had refused to operate for fear that there might be too much eventration and that thinning of the abdominal wall, coupled with the long duration of the hernia, might preclude the possibility of successful reposition. Though this argument was well founded, a beginning ulceration of the skin had now made it impossible for him to pursue his occupation as a billposter and rendered him bedridden much of the time, so that operation became imperative.

When the abdomen was opened it was found that small and large bowel, as well as a great portion of the omentum, formed the hernial contents. I was very fortunate in being able to reposit them without much difficulty and to close the inguinal canal with a modified Bassini procedure. The patient left the hospital in excellent condition, the wound having healed by primary intention. He returned to his work after thorough cicatrization of the tissues.

Individualization of Operative Technic

In operating on a large hernia we must not be enslaved by any one particular technic. The surgeon doing this type of work must be versatile; he must be thoroughly familiar with the Bassini procedure and its modifications, the Andrews' operation and perhaps Ferguson's method so as to command a number of operative procedures that will be suitable for the respective cases. Do not be in haste to resect the bowel. No matter how skillful the surgeon, haste increases the mortality total. Resect only those portions of the bowel that are hopelessly diseased, or when forced to eliminate a mass which cannot be reposited successfully in the abdomen.

Full-thickness skin grafts and whaleskin grafts may be used in certain cases, particularly when the surgeon is thoroughly conversant with the technic and the use of the grafts.[3, 8]

Preoperative Management

If the hernia is a large one, prepare the patient thoroughly before operating (except in cases of extreme urgency). During such period of preparation, urge the patient to remain in bed much of the time. Reduce the hernia frequently and thus endeavor gradually to accommodate the abdomen to its additional contents after reduction.

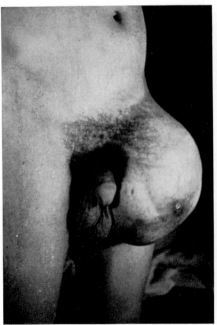 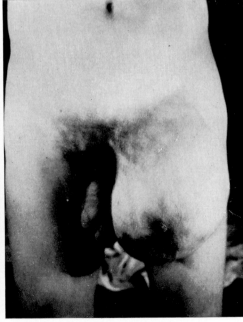

Fig. 406. Two views of patient with direct inguinal hernia of enormous size.

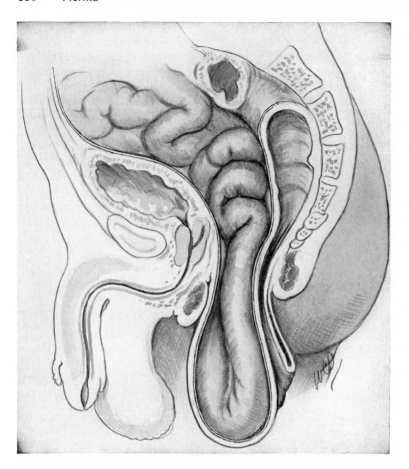

FIG. 407. Perineal hernia with prolapse of rectum; sagittal section. (After Sultan)

The fact that surgical intervention is dangerous in such cases, and the further fact that hernias are likely to occur following the defective closure of any abdominal surgical wound, means that one should pay particular attention to measures for their prevention by assuring, so far as possible, good consolidation of the abdominal wall. Proper primary closure is the principal preventive measure. It is not in postoperative hernias alone that difficulties arise when the hernia is unusually large. Inguinal and femoral as well as other voluminous hernias (Fig. 407) are occasionally seen, the treatment of which is a source of perplexity to the surgeon. Radical surgery offers a serious problem not alone on the grounds of surgical technic but also from the viewpoint of the patient's safety. Such are those cases in which a large part of the intestine—if not all—or of the stomach, the uterus or some other organ has descended into the inguinal hernial sac. This renders the hernia partly or wholly irreducible because of the seeming inability of the abdomen to accommodate the herniated organs.

In such voluminous hernias, we find them either wholly irreducible or reducible to only a very limited degree. The carriers of such sizable sacs have often had them for so long a time that they are taken for granted, and there is no great tendency toward strangulation or other cause of acute symptoms. In a very fat woman a voluminous hernia may be unnoticed because it is hidden in a mass of fatty tissue, but eventually, reflex phenomena—nausea, vomiting, etc.—may cause great and continued distress, for which the patient will seek surgical relief.

Careful examination of such a hernia will reveal anatomic changes that suggest the utter impossibility of returning the hernial contents to the abdomen without using extreme force and thus causing great damage to the intestines and other viscera. There may be such a

Fig. 408. Recurrent inguinal hernia in female. This patient had been operated upon *7 times* for this condition. The author believes insufficient rest following operation, to allow for thorough cicatrization, was the cause for recurrence.

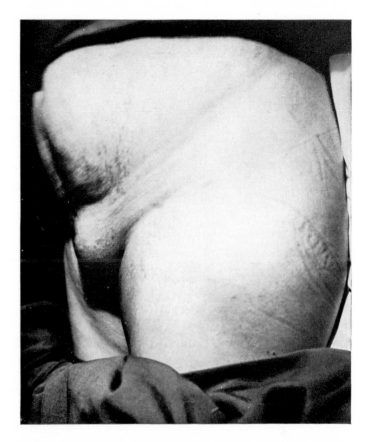

pronounced retraction of the diaphragm, when the displaced organs are forced back, that the functions of lungs and heart may be impeded, killing the patient by asphyxia. However, it has been shown in the two personal cases related above that the well-trained and careful surgeon can meet and overcome all these difficulties by individualizing the plan of treatment for each patient.

POSTOPERATIVE REST

As a final word of caution, let me emphasize once more the necessity of the patient remaining at rest for a sufficient time following any hernia operation. A woman came to us who had been operated on 7 times for inguinal hernia, recurrence having followed each attempt to cure the condition (Fig. 408). Close questioning disclosed that she had never remained at rest for a sufficient time following the operations. While the technic was undoubtedly sound in most of the operations she had undergone, I was of the opinion that she had not given her tissues the necessary

rest for regeneration. We operated on her under spinal-block anesthesia and found the structures very much thinned. The patient was instructed to rest for at least 2 months. I believe that it was because of this longer period of rest that our operation proved to be successful, for after the lapse of 2 years there has been no recurrence.

REFERENCES

1. Bailey, H.: Demonstrations of Physical Signs in Clinical Surgery, ed. 12, pp. 194-205, Baltimore, Williams & Wilkins, 1954.
2. Bradford, B., Jr., and Jarrett, J. T.: Inguinal hernia in infancy and early childhood, Am. Surgeon **18**:1023, 1952.
3. Behrend, M., and Behrend, R.: Full thickness skin grafts in the repair of voluminous hernias, J. Internat. Coll. Surgeons **13**:41, 1950.
4. Guy, C. C., and Werelius, C. Y.: Use of tantalum mesh in hernia repair, A. M. A. Arch. Surg. **62**:867, 1951.
5. Hashimoto, E. I., and Clark, J. H.: Utilization of the aponeurosis transversus ab-

dominis, Cooper's ligament and the iliopubic tract in the repair of inguinal and femoral hernias, Am. Surgeon 18:690, 1952.

6. Koontz, A. R.: The operation for difficult sliding hernia of the large bowel, Am. Surgeon 18:78, 1952.

7. Mikkelsen, W. P., and Berne, C. J.: Femoral hernioplasty, Surgery 35:743, 1954.

8. Preston, D. J.: Repair of abdominal hernia with steel cloth implant, J. Internat. Coll. Surgeons 18:513, 1952.

9. Strahan, A. W. B.: Hernia repair by whole skin graft, Brit. J. Surg. 38:276, 1951.

10. Warren, K. W.: Hernias in the poor risk patient; their surgical treatment, S. Clin. North America 34:761, 1954.

21 Genito-urinary Surgery

PENIS AND URETHRA

The skin of the penis is loosely attached and freely movable. It contains no subcutaneous fat, and the prepuce has no hair follicles. Because of the absence of hair, the prepuce may be used to advantage in reconstruction procedures of the urethra, chiefly in the repair of hypospadias (Fig. 409). Because the prepuce can be so employed, a child with this condition should not be circumcised, since only a dorsal flap of tissue will be present, which should be preserved for possible later use in repair of the deformity. In avulsion of the skin of the penis, a new covering can be easily obtained by burying the exposed area of the penis under the skin of the scrotum, so that a complete graft with an intact blood supply may be made available. In gangrene of the penile skin or in burns of the penis, *skin grafting* may be necessary.

INJURIES OF THE PENIS

Except for war injuries, trauma to the penis is an infrequent occurrence. The penis may be wounded by the insane as a form of self-mutilation, or such trauma may be inflicted by another individual. Belfield has mentioned a case in which the penis had been completely divided by a knife, only the urethra remaining intact. Considerable bleeding ensued, and the patient was almost exsanguinated within a short time. The cut edges of the corpora cavernosa were reunited, and the wound healed by first intention. However, this proved to be disastrous to the patient, since the scar at the point where the penis had been cut and later sutured prevented erection beyond this point (about the middle of the shaft). The continuity of the circulation in the corpora cavernosa was blocked, and the terminal half of the penis always remained flaccid. The victim's assailant had accomplished his purpose.

The present author observed a complete avulsion of the glans penis as the result of suction from a vacuum cleaner. Bleeding was profuse, but, after the glans had been removed, a functioning organ still remained with the corpora cavernosa intact. The urethral meatus was at the fossa navicularis, and as an end-result the penis was shortened.

Although penile injuries heal very rapidly if they are superficial, deep wounds of the corpora cavernosa result in scar formation; this leads to partial or complete impotence because the scar prevents filling of the venous sinuses of the corpora cavernosa, thus interfering with erection, and causing incurvation.

We have often seen end-results of circumcision in which the operater, apparently unskilled, removed a small portion of the glans penis also. In one case the entire glans had

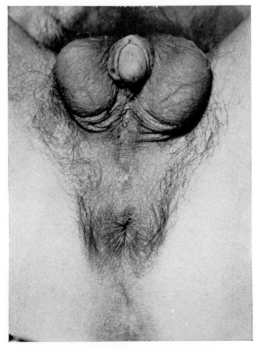

FIG. 409. Scrotal hypospadias. (Rolnick, H. C.: The Practice of Urology, vol. 1, p. 179, Philadelphia, Lippincott)

been cut away. The loss, in this individual, produced psychological disturbances—because of the shortening of the phallus—when he reached sexual maturity.

When giving local anesthesia for circumcision, it is a mistake to inject the corpora cavernosa deep under Buck's fascia. Considerable hemorrhage may follow in this highly vascular structure, with possible secondary infection.

The so-called castration injury from land mines in the recent war occasionally produced disastrous results due to damage or complete destruction of the testicles and the penis. The lesions are rare in civilian practice. It is indeed surprising that the external genitalia, which are exposed and therefore apparently easily subject to trauma, are so seldom injured in falls, contusions, lacerations to the perineum or when the pelvis is fractured.

INJURIES TO THE URETHRA

Open Injuries. These are penetrating wounds most frequently resulting from injuries to the perineum, particularly those due to high explosives. They may be extensive, requiring considerable effort to effect repair. Preliminary diversion of the urine by cystotomy is usually necessary. If possible, the urethra should be splinted over a retention catheter inserted retrograde through the cystotomy. This can be done if the defect in the urethra is not large. The urethra will readily regenerate over the splinting catheter if its ends can be brought close together. However, if the injury is extensive, *débridement* and excision of tissue may be necessary, followed by reunion over the splinting catheter. This may be difficult,

because in some cases there is a large defect which does not bridge itself over very readily, and the ends of the torn urethra cannot be brought together.

Closed Injuries. These are the most common. If not severe, and if the tear of the urethra is incomplete, a retention catheter may be all that is needed for control of bleeding and rapid healing. These closed lesions are usually a result of falling astride some hard object, or of a blow against the perineum, producing the tear in the perineal urethra. Rupture of the urethra is frequently associated with fracture of the pelvis and is not uncommon in traffic and industrial accidents (Fig. 410). In these cases, repair must be done by open operation. When the tear is not too extensive, this is best accomplished by means of a cystotomy followed by retrograde insertion of a urethral catheter as a splint. When there is marked extravasation of blood and urine, perineal drainage must also be instituted. The perineum should be incised to promote drainage and to help locate the distal urethra in order to pass the catheter. More extensive incisions will result in considerable scarring and later will interfere with potency, due to injury to the perineal muscles.

INCURVATION OF THE PENIS

This condition usually accompanies hypospadias and must be corrected before any attempt is made to repair the defect in the urethra. Repair of this incurvation, which is congenital, is not always simple, for unless a deep cut is made on the ventral surface of the penis just below the corona to relieve the adhesions, the incurvation will not be corrected.

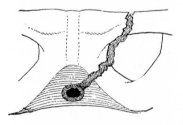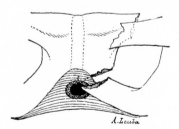

FIG. 410. Diagrams to show (*left*) how the urethra can be torn in fracture of the pelvis by extension of laceration of tissues alone. (*Right*) How a fragment of bone can tear the urethra. (Papin) (Rolnick, H. C.: The Practice of Urology, vol. 1, p. 188, Philadelphia, Lippincott)

Considerable bleeding may occur during this procedure because the vascular bodies of the corpora cavernosa may be incised as a result of deep dissection beyond the fascial bands, and much time and effort must be consumed for hemostasis. When the operation is completed, the penis should be kept under tension by means of a suture attached to the skin of the abdomen so that it remains straight.

HYPOSPADIAS

Minor degrees of hypospadias do not require operation. Extreme degrees of this condition at the perineoscrotal junction are occasionally associated with pseudohermaphroditism. Hypospadias of the midportion of the urethra and farther down do require repair.

Many procedures have been recommended, which is an indication that the problem is difficult and that none of them has proved to be entirely satisfactory. In some clinics this operation is done by the plastic surgeon, for it requires painstaking care and adherence to the general principles of plastic repair throughout the body. Unless meticulous precautions are taken in doing this operation, the results will be unsatisfactory. At present, the most useful procedure for developing a new urethra with a minimum of tension on the tissues is the Dennis-Brown operation, which makes use of the prepuce brought down at the time of repair of the incurvation. It is an error not to correct the incurvation of the penis as a preliminary procedure. It is also necessary to divert the urine with a urethrotomy or a cystotomy previous to any attempt at repair. Some patients have been subjected to repeated operations before a successful result could be obtained.

DORSAL SLIT

A dorsal slit is occasionally necessary for acquired inflammatory phimosis or paraphimosis (Fig. 411). In most cases the swelling can be reduced by hot applications, irrigations and antibiotics. In paraphimosis, the injection of hyaluronidase may bring about rapid subsidence of the swelling, permitting the prepuce to be brought back to normal. However, when the inflammation does not subside, a dorsal slit should be made. In doing this it is a necessary safeguard to cut not only the area of the phimotic prepuce but also the band of tissue at the coronal junction. This is particularly necessary in order to relieve the constriction

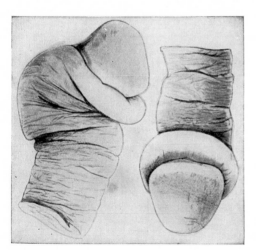
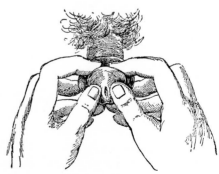

FIG. 411. (*Left*) Lateral and dorsal views of a paraphimosis. (Kaufmann) (*Right*) How to reduce a paraphimosis. The glans is grasped on each side by the thumbs and index fingers. Pressure is steadily made by the thumbs in a backward direction so as to reduce the edema of the glans until it slips into the edematous prepuce, which is gradually pulled over the glans. If unsuccessful after repeated efforts, a dorsal slit must be done immediately. (White and Martin) (Rolnick, H. C.: The Practice of Urology, vol. 1, p. 198, Philadelphia, Lippincott)

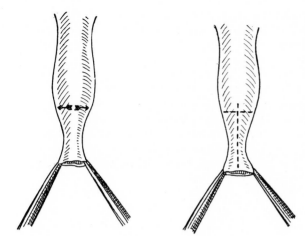

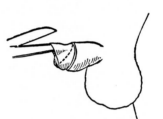

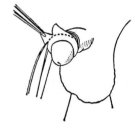

FIG. 412. Step 1 of circumcision by the dorsal slit method. The edges of the prepuce are grasped by forceps at the mucocutaneous junction. The vertical dotted line indicates the dorsal slit, and the transverse double arrow or dotted line indicates where prepuce should be divided at level of base of glans penis. (Rolnick, H. C.: The Practice of Urology, vol. 2, chap. 48, Philadelphia, Lippincott)

FIG. 413. (*Right*) Step 2 of circumcision by the dorsal slit method. Trimming edges of prepuce so that the skin flap is divided at a higher level than is that of the mucosa, so that latter will be everted when healing occurs. (Rolnick, H. C.: The Practice of Urology, vol. 2, chap. 48, Philadelphia, Lippincott)

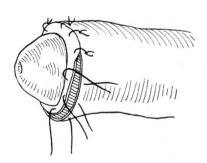

FIG. 414. Step 3 of circumcision by the dorsal slit method (see Figs. 412 and 413). Note how mucosa is everted because level of division of the skin is higher than is that of the inner layer of the prepuce. (Rolnick, H. C.: The Practice of Urology, vol. 2, chap. 48, Philadelphia, Lippincott)

of the paraphimosis. Some bleeding may ensue. If bleeding is active, the mucosa and the skin may be sutured, otherwise bandaging of the incision is sufficient for control.

CIRCUMCISION

Although circumcision (Figs. 412-414) has been practiced for thousands of years, and is considered by some to be a simple operation, errors are likely, and certain safeguards are necessary. If too much mucosa and skin are removed it may be difficult to unite them, and a constricting fibrous ring may develop around the glans penis upon healing. One must be careful to obtain complete hemostasis,

particularly at the frenulum, for the frenular artery is often cut during the procedure.

When hemostasis is not complete, considerable bleeding may follow, and it may be necessary even to return the patient to the operating room. If bleeding has not been well controlled, the penis and the scrotum may become edematous and disclored as a result of extravasation of blood, with possible later secondary infection. Priapism, which often occurs early after circumcision, particularly in the adult, should be controlled by the administration of estrogenic hormone for the first few days. If this is not done, a subcutaneous hematoma may follow and separation of the wound take place. The patient may develop an incurvation of the penis after circumcision if too much skin has been removed. In doing a circumcision, it is well to remember that preputeal adhesions to the glans and the corona are common and may prevent retraction of the prepuce. These adhesions must be broken up or severed in order to obtain a successful result. If this is not done, aside from an unsuccessful result, the glans may be cut accidentally, because of poor exposure, with considerable resultant bleeding.

PAPILLOMATA OF THE PENIS
("VENEREAL WARTS")

These usually occur on the glans about the corona, probably due to irritation from the secretions of the prepuce. They can be cauterized, but the patient should also be circumcised to guard against recurrence. Balanoposthitis, inflammation of the mucosa of glans and prepuce, is also a result of irritation; circumcision is indicated for the cure of this condition.

IMPOTENCE

As previously stated, surgical or traumatic injuries to the penis will result in scar formation that may interfere with the blood supply and result in either partial or complete impotence.

In injuries to the urethra, where rupture has caused extravasation of blood and urine into the perineum, evacuation and drainage must be done perineally. However, it is unwise to do extensive dissection unless absolutely necessary for repair of the urethra. Considerable scar formation will frequently follow and interfere with erection later. The muscles of the perineum are important in maintaining erection, and also the highly vascular bulbous urethra itself; therefore, these fibers should be traumatized as little as possible.

CARCINOMA OF THE PENIS

This is a rare condition occurring only in individuals who have not been circumcised. When the condition is diagnosed early, it will respond to local irradiation or partial amputation. When it is advanced, total removal of

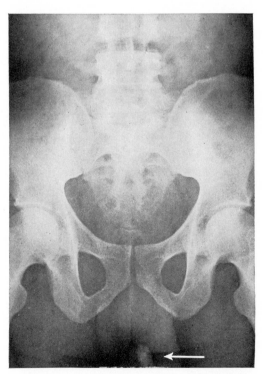 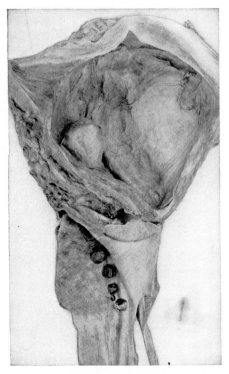

FIG. 415. (*Left*) Calculus in the penile urethra. (*Right*) A necropsy specimen showing a number of calculi in the posterior urethra. (Rolnick, H. C.: The Practice of Urology, vol. 1, p. 195, Philadelphia, Lippincott)

the penis and the inguinal glands is necessary, but it is then usually too late for complete eradication and cure.

Urethral Calculi

These are practically always secondary. Most commonly, calculi (Fig. 415) found in the urethra are renal calculi which have passed down along the entire urinary tract and finally reached the urethral orifice but, proving too large to pass the narrow meatus, are detained at that point. Thus, one finds that occasionally a urethral calculus must be extracted from this opening. Prostatic calculi and prostatic or bladder incrustations may block the urethra on their way out, anywhere along the course of the urethra, causing considerable difficulty in the attempt at their removal. If the stone or incrustation is deep in the posterior prostatic urethra, it is best to push it back into the bladder with a sound and then evacuate it through a large cystoscope or urethroscope sheath. If it is still too large, it should be crushed within the bladder.

Most urethral calculi may be removed by nonsurgical methods. However, if they are too large to pass the meatus, or too firmly impacted to be dislodged transurethrally, surgery must be undertaken.

Internal Urethrotomy

Internal urethrotomy belongs to the historic past; it is rarely indicated today. Once it was done for strictures of the anterior urethra. The stricture is incised with the urethrotome in the urethra or with a knife inserted deep through the urethral meatus. Ventral incisions cut the unsupported urethra, and a fistula which can be permanent may result. In internal urethrotomy the incisions are made on the dorsal surface, and when too deep they extend into the corpora cavernosa. Incurvation of the penis is frequently a sequel and may persist for a long time. Urethrotomy, whether external or internal, does no more than permit for the later dilatation of the stricture with sounds.

External Urethrotomy

External urethrotomy, although occasionally necessary, is a relatively rare operation at present. Cutting of a stricture merely permits one to dilate the so-called impassable stricture. Dilatation is necessary as a follow-up procedure within a few days after the urethrotomy is done. If dilatation is not done shortly after the urethrotomy, the patient is much worse off than before because of the additional scar tissue which the operation has produced. When dense strictures are present, the occasional operation of urethrectomy, with end-to-end anastomosis of the urethra, should be done if not too great a portion of the urethra has been cut away. *Never do an external urethrotomy on the anterior urethra and never do an internal urethrotomy on the posterior urethra.* If an external urethrotomy is done on the anterior urethra, a permanent urethral fistula may result.

Perforating, penetrating or instrumental injuries to the anterior urethra often result in permanent urethral fistula. When an internal urethrotomy is performed for stricture of the posterior urethra, urinary extravasation may follow, for this portion of the urethra is thin and is not protected by any other structures.

Urethral Fistula

When a small urethral fistula is still present following an apparently successful repair of hypospadias or as a result of a periurethral abscess, the fistulous tract can be repaired by dissecting it carefully down to the urethra and tying and inverting its base as a safeguard against recurrence.

External Urethrotomy for Temporary Diversion of Urine ("Boutonnière")

External urethrotomy of the perineal urethra is frequently done in order to divert the urine before repairing a hypospadias. It is occasionally done in transurethral prostatic resection when the phallic urethra is too narrow to permit passing a resectoscope. This is not a difficult procedure, but certain precautions are necessary. The patient should be in the lithotomy position. Considerable bleeding may follow if the incision is too close to the scrotoperineal juncture, for the bulb of the urethra, which is highly vascular, may be incised by mistake. After the urethra has been located and incised over a metal guide, it is very important to place guy sutures on each side of the opening, so that one may direct a catheter into the bladder (Fig. 416). If this precaution is not taken, and the urethra is

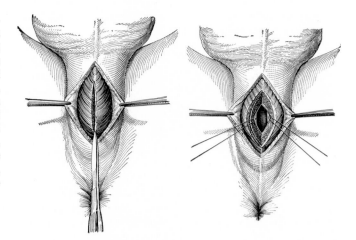

FIG. 416. External urethrotomy. (*Left*) Shows how urethra is divided in midline while a grooved sound or filiform in the lumen of the urethra is held firmly against the perineum. (*Right*) Note how the urethra has been divided over guide and edges of urethral mucosa held apart by traction sutures. (Duval) (Rolnick, H. C.: The Practice of Urology, vol. 2, p. 1002, Philadelphia, Lippincott)

allowed to retract, the operator can become almost completely "lost" in the perineum and encounter considerable difficulty in finding the prostatic urethra, even after the urethrotomy has been completed.

After the catheter has been inserted, it should be well tested in order to make certain that it is in proper position and draining well. It should then be sutured to the external skin in order to keep it in place for a number of days. A Foley catheter may also be used. When there is no further need for bladder drainage, the catheter may be removed, permitting the incision in the urethra to heal and close spontaneously.

THE SCROTUM AND ITS CONTENTS

EDEMA

Chronic, "brawny" edema of the scrotum is usually the end-result of urinary extravasation with multiple abscesses and fistulae in the perineum, characterized as "sprinkling pot" perineum (Fig. 417). It is necessary to differentiate between edema of the scrotum and urinary extravasation. Superficial urinary extravasation is the result of rupture of the urethra or of erosion in "periurethral phlegmon," and its spread is limited to Colles' fascia. Periurethral phlegmon is rarely seen in private practice. It is even infrequent in general hospitals, for it is almost always due to long-neglected, impermeable urethral stricture with erosion and fistulae.

The surgical treatment of acute urinary extravasation should consist either of cystot-omy or external urethrotomy for diversion of the urine, with multiple free incisions of the infected edematous areas and through-and-through drainage. Chemotherapy and antibiotics will control infection. Mortality in these patients is still quite high, if operation has been delayed.

TRAUMATIC INJURIES

Lacerations and extensive injuries to the scrotum by land mines in time of war—the so-called castration injuries—may produce considerable damage to the scrotal tissues. Transplantation of skin may be necessary for

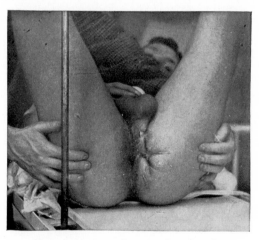

FIG. 417. A perineum that has been operated upon for fistula several times and one opening that still exists. (Guiteras: Urology, New York, Appleton) (Rolnick, H. C.: The Practice of Urology, vol. 1, p. 256, Philadelphia, Lippincott)

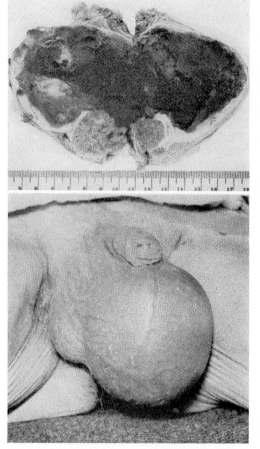

Fig. 418. (*Top*) Old hydrocele with a recent hematoma. (*Bottom*) A large, infected hydrocele, with marked redness of the scrotum. (Rolnick, H. C.: The Practice of Urology, vol. 1, chap. 20, Philadelphia, Lippincott)

repair. When damage is not so extensive, regeneration will be spontaneous, since the regenerative capacity of the scrotum is rather remarkable.

HEMATOMA

This is usually the result of a penetrating injury to the scrotum. The hematoma may attain rather extensive proportions, with marked discoloration. Treatment is surgical, consisting of careful evacuation of clots and control of all bleeding points, with drainage of the wound to control infection. It is interesting to note that, even when a hematoma is quite large, the testes are usually not in-

volved. It is important to differentiate between hematoma of the scrotum and hematocele (Fig. 418), an accumulation of blood within the tunica vaginalis testis; the latter is usually a result of hemorrhage within an old hydrocele sac.

Complete hemostasis is of great importance in all operations on the scrotum and its contents, for the loose cellular tissue of the cord, the tunica and the scrotum has no inherent capacity for hemostasis. Therefore, painstaking care is necessary to control bleeding. All bleeding areas should be clamped and ligated, and much time may have to be consumed, in scrotal operations, for this purpose. If bleeding is allowed to continue, a hematoma may form, with later development of secondary infection and a prolonged convalescence. In many instances it is a wise safeguard to drain the scrotum for 1 or 2 days after a scrotal operation.

SCROTAL ABSCESS

This is most frequently secondary to an abscess of the epididymis. In the aged it is not uncommon for a severe, acute epididymitis to break down and form an abscess, followed by the formation of a suppurating scrotal fistula. In younger men scrotal abscess following epididymitis is usually indicative of tuberculosis of the epididymis.

In tuberculous epididymitis the involved scrotal area with its fistulous tract should be well resected and the epididymis removed. It may also be necessary to remove the testis since it also is frequently involved. In non tuberculous epididymitis with abscess the area should be drained. The abscess will then heal, and the epididymitis will usually gradually resolve. In the aged patient a suppurative epididymitis is best treated by complete orchidectomy.

INGUINAL ADENOPATHY

Except in cases of carcinoma of the penis. it is rarely necessary to remove the inguinal glands. However, it is sometimes necessary to excise a small portion of an inguinal node for diagnostic purposes. Any procedure for removal of inguinal glands must be done carefully, for they are located around the saphenous vein. Injuries to the saphenous vein, or even to the femoral veins, during such operations have occurred and may require ligating of these vessels, with possible interference with the blood supply to the leg.

UNDESCENDED TESTICLE

Cases of arrested or aberrant descent of one testis require operation in order to bring the gland to its normal position in the scrotum. Moore demonstrated, some years ago, that spermatogenesis will occur only when the testis is in its normal location because it requires a lower temperature than that to which it is subjected when in the inguinal region or the abdomen.

Opinion varies considerably as to when the operation of orchiopexy should be done. Some recommend that the testis be brought down at the age of 4 or 5 years; others, including the author, think it wise to wait until the boy is 8 or 9. A course of injections of anterior pituitary hormone may be given before operation, as these may cause the testis to pass a little farther downward, thus making the ultimate procedure less difficult. The testis may also pass all the way down spontaneously; however, this occurs infrequently when the condition is unilateral. When one testis is in the scrotum and the other undescended, the cause of the anomaly is either a mechanical obstruction or aberrant descent; therefore, surgical relief is usually necessary.

Operation. The operative incision is the same as that used for inguinal hernia. Thorough hemostasis is necessary. Practically all of these young patients have an associated congenital hernia. This must be located and the sac separated carefully from the cord, particular care being taken of the vessels of the cord to which it is adherent. This is often a tedious procedure but must be done conscientiously. It is necessary to make a simple hernial sac of the congenital hernia by dividing it, thus separating it completely from its continuation as the tunica vaginalis of the testis. Separate the sac carefully from the adherent vessels and then free it upward to the inguinal ring. This sac is very thin and tears easily, yet it must be accurately ligated.

Following this, extreme care must be taken to lengthen the cord. The vas is an elastic structure and rarely gives any trouble; the chief difficulty is likely to be with the blood supply for the testis. This part of the procedure requires every safeguard when removing tissue about these structures to obtain added length. The thin bands of tissue about the vessels of the cord must be removed, particularly at the internal inguinal ring. They must also be freed along their entire length, particularly at their insertion into the testis. Thus, the two points where length may be obtained are near the abdominal ring and at the testis. The vessels should not be cut or injured in the attempt to bring the testis down. If the vessels were to be cut, sufficient length could readily be had, but the purpose of the operation would be defeated, for the testis would atrophy. The meager blood supply accompanying the vas deferens is insufficient for the testis. Care must also be taken not to cut or injure the vas, for again the purpose of the operation would be defeated, as the testis would then have no outlet for its sperm.

If the testis is under tension after it has been brought down, it may retract upward again into the inguinal canal during the process of fibrosis and healing. This will be unsatisfactory in the end, for, when the testis is retracted upward tightly against the inguinal ring, atrophy may follow.

In order to avoid such later tension and retraction, a 2-stage (Torek) operation will give the best results in most cases (Figs. 419-421). In this procedure, after sufficient length has been obtained—or as much length as is possible at that time—the testis is sutured to the fascia of the thigh through a small incision on the inside of the thigh at the level of the scrotum. The testis is then covered by suturing the scrotum to the incision. The patient is sent home after a week or 10 days with the testis in this position and is able to be up and about normally. After a period of about 6 weeks, the testis is separated from the fascia of the thigh, when it will be found that the vessels have lengthened permanently. The incisions in scrotum and thigh may then be closed.

This operation is satisfactory for the immediate purpose of bringing the testis down. However, tension on the blood vessels supplying the testis, or on the gland itself, during the period when it is attached to the thigh may interfere with its proper functioning later on. Many urologists question whether the undescended testis which has been thus brought

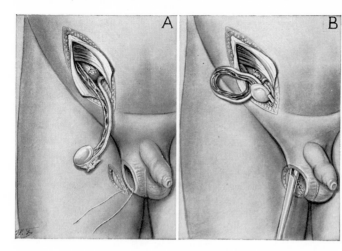

Fig. 419. Technic of Torek operation for undescended testis (see Figs. 420 and 421). (A) Placing of testis on thigh to prove sufficient length of vessel. Mode of suturing posterior lip of thigh and scrotal incision is shown. (B) It is completed. In this drawing, the testis is being pulled down through the scrotal incision before being placed in its new bed on the fascia lata of the thigh. (Rolnick, H. C.: The Practice of Urology, vol. 2, p. 1099, Philadelphia, Lippincott)

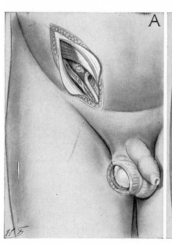
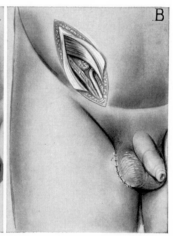

Fig. 420. Technic of Torek operation for undescended testis (see Figs. 419 and 421). (A) The testis is anchored to the fascia lata by several sutures. (B) Closure of the anterior lips of the scrotal and thigh incisions. (Rolnick, H. C.: The Practice of Urology, vol. 2, p. 1099, Philadelphia, Lippincott)

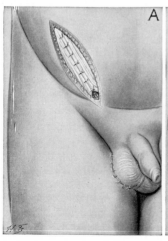
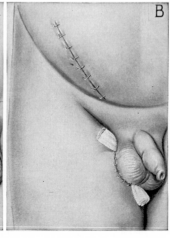

Fig. 421. Technic of Torek operation for undescended testis (see Figs. 419 and 420). (A) Closure of inguinal canal with or without transplantation of the spermatic cord. (B) A rubber dam or gauze drain is shown introduced through both extremities of the scrotal-thigh incisions which have been sutured. No attempt should be made to replace the testis in the scrotum until 2 months after the primary operation. (Rolnick, H. C.: The Practice of Urology, vol. 2, p. 1100, Philadelphia, Lippincott)

down surgically, with or without tension, will function properly later on in any event.

Acute Orchitis

This condition may occur in conjunction with mumps and, occasionally, in older patients with severe suppurative epididymitis. Mumps orchitis should be treated by aspiration of the associated hydrocele and puncture of the tunica to help reduce the swelling. Small incisions for the purpose of releasing the fluid within the tunica vaginalis, which will be under extreme tension, together with administration of pooled plasma and estrogenic hormones, constitute another form of treatment which is advised by some.

Biopsy of the Testis (Charney)

This is a simple procedure which can be done under local anesthesia and is of considerable value in determining fertility. The technic may be found described in any standard text. It is necessary only to point out here that difficulties may arise unless care is taken to suture the tunica vaginalis propria after the excision of a small amount of the testicular tissue. Unless this safeguard is taken, the parenchyma of the testis, which is usually under some tension, may protrude. Healing would then be delayed, and secondary infection might occur.

Subcapsular Orchidectomy

Although many urologists advise total orchidectomy in the treatment of carcinoma of the prostate, a subcapsular orchidectomy is all that is actually necessary to remove practically all of the gonadal tissue. Removal of the parenchyma of the testis can readily be accomplished in this manner through a simple incision in the median raphe and secures the purpose of the operation, viz., control of the prostatic carcinoma by removal of androgenic tissue.

The choice of this operation over complete removal is very important psychologically, for, when it is finished, the patient usually does not realize that his gonads have been removed; the tunica of the testis and the epididymis with the spermatic cord are still left in the scrotum, and he is aware only that a mass of more or less normal size is still present in the scrotal sac.

Tumor of the Testis

For clinical purposes, tumors of the testis should be divided into two classifications: (1) the relatively benign seminomas and teratomas, and (2) the highly malignant teratocarcinomas, embryonal carcinomas and chorioepitheliomas. Fortunately, most of these tumors prove to be seminomas or dysgerminomas, for the prognosis is good in the great majority of these cases. For the malignant forms, the prognosis is poor indeed.

Diagnosis. This may be difficult. Tumors of the testis are usually seen in those from 18 to 30 years of age, and they must be differentiated from epididymitis and periorchitis. In early cases the Aschheim-Zondek test is of value, but only when the result is *positive*. It is not reliable in most cases of seminoma, for it will usually be negative even in the presence of a tumor. An associated hydrocele often adds to the confusion. However, with experience, one comes to recognize a suspicious nodule or hardness in the testis. Even if there is no more than serious doubt, operation is indicated.

Operation. A simple orchiectomy with high ligation of the cord is usually all that is necessary. This is the procedure of choice and should be followed later by extensive irradiation, both local and general. It is important to avoid operative or preoperative manipulation of the tumor in order to avoid spreading the tumor cells. The tumor should be removed through a high inguinal or a scrotal incision. The cord should be approached directly, clamped, cut and ligated before the testis is brought out. Secure ligation of the highly vascular cord is important. The vas may be separated from the cord and ligated individually, but this is not necessary. It is a wise precaution to drain the scrotum for a few days postoperatively.

As previously stated, simple orchiectomy is usually all that is necessary for relatively benign growths. Although it is important to follow up with irradiation, it is questionable if this improves the prognosis. In over 80 per cent of cases, the patient remains well; if no metastases have occurred within 2 or 3 years after an orchiectomy for tumor, it is extremely unlikely that such will appear later.

During postoperative irradiation, the remaining testis must be carefully protected, for these patients can later beget normal children.

The highly malignant teratocarcinoma, embryonal carcinoma or chorio-epithelioma metastasize early into the retroperitoneal space. The radical operation has been recommended for these growths, with extensive dissection of the lymph nodes high up into the region of the kidney and followed later by very extensive deep irradiation. Lloyd Lewis and others with broad experience report better results in cases of highly malignant tumor from the radical operation followed by later extensive irradiation. In most instances, however, the writer questions whether anything more than simple orchiectomy should be done, for, even with a radical operation, some of the metastatic nodes are likely to be missed or simply cannot be removed. This makes it evident that the *type* of tumor is of the greatest importance in prognosis.

Hydrocele

Congenital hydrocele usually clears up spontaneously within a few months after birth, but when it persists, there is usually an associated hernia, in which case operation will be required for relief. However, a hydrocele may persist for many years without causing discomfort or requiring attention. When and if it finally does, it may be aspirated as often as is needed—which may be no more than 2 or 3 times a year. Injection with a sclerosing solution (still recommended by some) may cause severe reactions and result in later atrophy of the testis; therefore, it should definitely be avoided. If the hydrocele is to be eradicated, the best procedure is the "bottle" operation. Or, if the hydrocele is not too large, its edges may merely be sutured and everted.

An old man with a large, chronic hydrocele usually has a large, redundant spermatic cord with a poor blood supply to a nonfunctioning testis. In these patients, rather than a hydrocelectomy, it is often better to do an orchiectomy, for the devitalized tissues of the testis frequently undergo some degree of necrosis, with subsequent infection and a long postoperative convalescence. Also, it is often wisest to do an orchiectomy when operating on an older man for an inguinal hernia because a much better result can be had when there is no need to transplant the cord.

Caution. In operations for repair of inguinal hernia, it is necessary that the inguinal canal be not too tightly closed about the cord, for interference with the blood supply of the testis may result. Failure to observe this safeguard is one reason why it is not uncommon for hydrocele or atrophy of the testis to follow operative repair of an inguinal hernia.

Spermatocele

These cysts of variable size are frequently found in the adult. Usually they are of no significance; occasionally they are large enough to be mistaken for a supernumerary testis. They are practically always located above the testis and transilluminate the same as a hydrocele.

For purposes of differential diagnosis, it should be noted that the fluid from a spermatocele cyst is either pale gray or soapy in appearance, and contains spermatozoa, whereas that from the hydrocele is yellow. A spermatocele cyst must be excised; it cannot be everted, as in the "bottle" operation for hydrocele, for it will then recur. In the process of such excision, care must be taken not to injure the blood supply to the testis, for the spermatocele is usually close to the spermatic vessels at the head of the epididymis.

Epididymitis

In nearly all cases, treatment of epididymitis is nonsurgical, but, when complicated, may require surgery. It is often a complication or a sequel of prostatic affections. It also often follows urethral instrumentation. Complications, other than scrotal abscess, may be an abscess of the testis itself, or the so-called chocolate cyst of the testis, which requires treatment by orchiectomy. When hardness and induration persist or the epididymitis itself does not subside, orchiectomy is also indicated in aged patients.

Epididymectomy

Due to the greatly decreased incidence of tuberculous epididymitis for which epididymectomy was chiefly indicated, this operation is now done infrequently. Care is required in this procedure since the spermatic vessels may easily be cut, making orchiectomy necessary.

The vessels of the spermatic cord enter the testis somewhat posterior and lateral to the head of the epididymis. Therefore, the head of the epididymis must be dissected off with extreme caution and the vessels kept under constant observation. The tail of the epididymis peels very readily off the tunica vaginalis. The operation may be started either at the scrotal vas or at the head of the epididymis.

Vasectomy in Prostatectomy

This operation should be routine for patients undergoing prostatic surgery, provided that they have reached an age (e.g., 60 years) when there is reduced sexual life. Bilateral vasectomy, done at the same time as prostatectomy, will prevent epididymitis in the vast majority of cases; otherwise, an incidence of epididymitis as high as 20 or 25 per cent may be expected. In the aged epididymitis can cause considerable morbidity or, at the least, a delay in convalescence.

Reunion of the Vas Deferens

When a patient has been sterilized by vasectomy, continuity may *sometimes* be restored at a later date by reuniting the two cut ends. However, this is not a simple procedure, for the 2 ends may be widely separated, and success is always doubtful.

SPERMATIC CORD, VAS DEFERENS AND SEMINAL VESICLES

Varicocele

This is such a common condition that it might be said that *most* men have it in some degree. It is nearly always found on the left side, because the left testis is lower than the right, and the left spermatic vein inserts into the renal vein rather than directly into the vena cava. Thus, the blood supply reaches the vena cava only indirectly, in contrast with that of the right side where the connection is direct.

Most patients, even with a large varicocele, are not aware that anything is amiss; when symptoms of heaviness and discomfort arise, these are usually relieved by the use of a scrotal support. Operation is rarely indicated and should be done only when the varicocele

is very marked or is causing considerable distress or persistent pain.

In spite of the fact that a high incision in the inguinal region will permit direct access to the spermatic vein, it is questionable whether this approach is satisfactory, since cutting and ligating the spermatic vein cuts off the chief return blood supply to the testis, and leaves only the vessel accompanying the vas, which is usually insufficient. Atrophy of the testis and hydrocele are not uncommon sequelae of this type of varicocelectomy. A better approach is to make an incision high in the scrotum just below the inguinal ring. It is neither necessary nor desirable to ligate all the vessels of the pampiniform plexus because of the danger of atrophy of the testis. One portion of the plexus may be separated, ligated and cut, leaving the remaining veins intact. The severed ends of the vessels should then be tied together in order to help lift and support the testis. With only some of the vessels resected, a considerable blood supply is

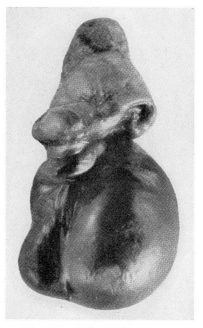

Fig. 422. Photograph showing gangrene of the testis owing to acute torsion of the spermatic cord. (Rolnick, H. C.: The Practice of Urology, vol. 1, chap. 19, Philadelphia, Lippincott)

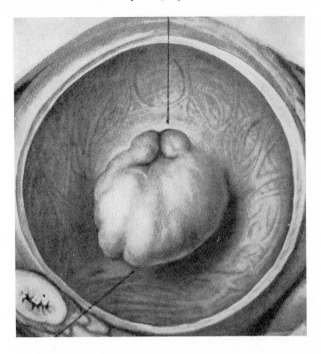

Fig. 423. Vesical aspect of a prostatic hypertrophy illustrating the intravesical type of enlargement. Note the large middle lobe and the two hyperplastic nodules on either side of the ventral (anterior) edge of internal orifice. (Tandler and Zuckerkandl) (Rolnick, H. C.: The Practice of Urology, vol. 2, Philadelphia, Lippincott)

left for the testis, and a good end-result is assured.

Injuries of the Spermatic Cord

These injuries are rare except in connection with surgery. In operating for varicocele, care must be taken to ligate thoroughly. If this is not done, severe bleeding may ensue and a large hematoma develop. In hernia operations, bleeding from the cord may follow incautious manipulation and dissection. Unless hemostasis is complete, hematoma may follow, with discoloration of the entire inguinal region, followed later by secondary infection. In herniotomy, also, a tight inguinal ring at the close of the operation, particularly if the cord has been transplanted, can later cause compression of the cord and atrophy of the testis, as well as development of hydrocele.

Torsion of the Spermatic Cord

This condition is relatively rare and has received much more attention in the literature than it deserves (Fig. 422). It is difficult to diagnose and may be mistaken for acute epididymitis, strangulated hernia or even injury to the testis and cord. It usually occurs early in life and, when first brought to the physician's or surgeon's attention, has almost always been present for some time, so that irre-

versible damage has already been done to the testis; and orchidectomy, with rare exceptions, is necessary. In those few cases where the condition is seen within the first 2-3 hours and diagnosed accurately, the cord may be unwound and the testis will then return to normal.

It has been assumed that torsion is the result of a loose gubernaculum. Therefore, in order to prevent torsion on the opposite side, the lower pole of that side should be sewed down firmly to the scrotum.

Infections of the Spermatic Cord

These may arise in cases of severe epididymitis and cause more pain and discomfort than the primary condition, but they usually subside at the same time. It should be noted that tuberculosis of the epididymis involves the vas deferens. Therefore, when an epididymectomy is done for the tuberculosis, the vas should also be removed as high up as possible.

THE PROSTATE GLAND

The surgical importance of the prostate lies in its anatomic position astride the neck of the bladder and in the fact that the changes which it undergoes during a man's lifetime can produce a variety of untoward symptoms. As a man grows older, even though his health be excellent otherwise, he is likely to have at least some difficulty due to interference with urination as a result of enlargement of his prostate.

PROSTATIC CALCULI

These are of extremely frequent occurrence, especially in men over the age of 40. They rarely require operative intervention for they usually produce no symptoms. When prostatectomy is otherwise indicated, any prostatic calculi should also be removed.

"Dumbbell" Prostatic Calculus. Fortunately, this condition has grown increasingly rare of late years since we have learned better how to control infection in the prostatic bed after suprapubic prostatectomy. It can occur if we fail to relieve the obstruction at the bladder neck, thus leaving almost an hourglass bladder in which infected urine collects in the prostatic bed, with development of incrustation and formation of the stone.

HYPERTROPHY OF THE PROSTATE

Much of the treatment of the enlarged prostate, as it occurs in the middle-aged or elderly patient, revolves around medical management. Often this is all that is required over long periods of years. However, the possibility of a need for surgical intervention must be kept in mind, especially with reference to the poor surgical risk. Mere *enlargement* of the gland is not by any means always an indication for surgery, as such enlargement may be almost entirely in the intravesical lateral lobes (Fig. 423) and produce no significant degree of obstruction with few subjective symptoms. The patient who complains of frequency, urgency and difficulty on urination, with residual urine, is most likely to be a candidate for surgery, in direct contrast with the patient with a relatively asymptomatic though often markedly enlarged prostate. The latter may be worse off following operation, and particularly transurethral resection, unless practically complete removal is accomplished.

An episode of acute urinary retention is not necessarily an indication for surgery. The aged patient, confined to bed following surgery somewhere in the lower abdomen, frequently develops this complication. Intermittent catheterization, or a few days with a retention catheter, will often return such a patient to normal. Prostatectomy should be considered only if one or more of the following criteria are met.

1. Acute Urinary Retention. As stated previously, this condition is an indication for surgery *only* when it does not yield promptly to the catheter. Repeated episodes of urinary retention or increasing urinary difficulty make prostatectomy imperative.

2. Chronic Urinary Retention. The amount of residual urine is the guiding factor here, but the actual amount must be considered in the light of the age and the general condition of the patient. A quantity which may be an indication for surgery in an otherwise normal man of 60 would be of little significance in a somewhat debilitated man of 80.

3. Other Urinary Symptoms. The presence or absence of residual urine alone is not a definite indication for surgery unless the amount is large. Other factors to be considered are the presence of anatomic enlargement of the prostate—as determined by rectal examination and cystoscopy—together with marked subjective symptoms. Prostatic obstruction with subjective symptoms is a definite indication for surgery, even though there be no significant amount of residual urine.

4. Hematuria. Occasional, mild initial or terminal hematuria (usually due to benign prostatic hypertrophy) is of no great importance, but the more severe forms, requiring an indwelling catheter for control, may require early cystotomy and prostatectomy.

5. Associated Conditions. The presence of bladder calculi or diverticulae with chronic infection indicates a significant degree of obstruction at the bladder neck and should be corrected at the time of operation.

Preoperative Preparation

Preoperative studies and preparation of the patient for prostatectomy routinely should include the following.

1. Flat X-ray Plates of Kidneys, Ureters and Bladder—also of the Chest. These will indicate the presence of bladder calculi and give evidence of possible bony metastases from carcinoma in the prostate, also the general condition of the lungs.

2. Intravenous Pyelogram. This frequently corroborates other evidence of disturbances of

kidney function, being sometimes even more specific than nitrogen metabolism studies. Chronic urinary retention with back pressure produces dilatation of the ureters and pyelonephritis. "Fish-hooking" of the ureters where they enter the bladder is extremely significant. The pyelogram also shows the outline of the bladder, indicating the size of the prostate. *Retrograde pyelogram* is rarely necessary and, in fact, is usually contraindicated because of the rather formidable difficulties that may be encountered; cystotomy is often simpler and safer than insertion of the rigid cystoscope.

3. Air Cystogram. This is done in some clinics to eliminate the need for cystoscopy.

4. Other Tests. These should include electrocardiograms and determinations of blood nitrogen metabolism and blood sugar.

5. Catheterization. When there is a history of chronic urinary retention, and partial or complete retention is currently present, together with a disturbance of the nitrogen metabolism, a catheter should be inserted and left in place until the patient's nitrogen metabolism has returned to normal. In acute retention the catheter should be left in place for several days, until the acute symptoms have subsided, before operation is undertaken. However, if the patient does not tolerate the catheter, or there is undue difficulty in passing it, then a preliminary cystotomy should be done. If the patient does tolerate instrumentation and the prostate is not too large, cystoscopy can be done before operation and will yield considerable information. An indwelling catheter causes no loss of time in preoperative preparation, and it has long been recognized that a smoother and shorter convalescence follows. It is also of great value in resolving the associated prostatitis and fever.

Operative Procedures

Of the various open operations for the relief of prostatic obstruction, suprapubic prostatectomy is the most common (Fig. 424). Since this is done through an open bladder, it is actually a transvesical procedure; therefore, it is necessary first to consider the suprapubic opening or cystotomy.

Cystotomy. In performing a cystotomy, it may on occasion be necessary to place the patient in the Trendelenburg position, but this should be avoided if possible since, in an

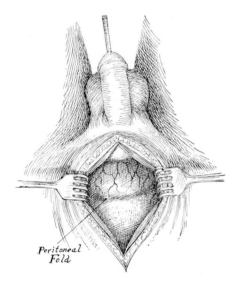

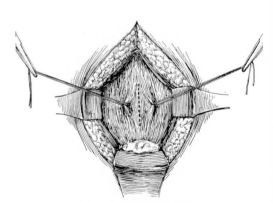

Peritoneal Fold

Fig. 424. (*Left*) Operative field in suprapubic cystotomy. The bladder has been distended with fluid so that the venous plexus on its vertex and anterior wall help to identify the structure as the bladder. The peritoneal fold is shown passing transversely across bladder. It must be pushed toward umbilicus (with gauze) before opening bladder (*right*). (*Right*) Second step of suprapubic cystotomy. The peritoneal fold (*left*) has been well retracted, and two traction sutures have been inserted through wall of bladder before incising latter along dotted line as close as possible to upper end of bladder. Instead of traction sutures, some prefer to use Allis forceps. (Rolnick, H. C.: The Practice of Urology, vol. 2, p. 1108, Philadelphia, Lippincott)

elderly patient, with the head down, the heart and the respiratory action may be embarrassed to a point that could spell the difference between a successful and a fatal outcome. *Never forget that the margin of safety for the old man is always small.*

In preparation for this operation, the bladder should be distended with fluid so that it may be approached and opened without entering the peritoneum. A midline incision is then made, beginning at the symphysis pubis and extending upward about 10 cm. The perivesical fat and fascia are separated away from the bladder and the peritoneum peeled off and separated upward until the bladder is exposed. Thus one may readily avoid the peritoneum. Next, the bladder is grasped with 2 Allis forceps, one on each side, and opened in the midline between them, after which the incision is extended upward as high as possible.

In our experience, the Allis forceps has proved to be the most important single instrument in urologic surgery. Tissues can be exposed and secured readily with this instrument. Trauma is minimal. Needless to say, they are much too useful to be employed as towel clips!

When a cystotomy is done for drainage, i.e., as the first stage of a 2-stage prostatectomy, a mushroom (Pezzer) catheter is inserted and should emerge at the *upper* end of the incision when the bladder is closed. This is necessary in order to prevent the catheter from resting against the symphysis and lying on the prostate and the bladder neck. If this simple safeguard is not observed, much trouble may arise later.

With the exception of transperitoneal nephrectomy and transplantation of the ureter into the bowel, all operations on the urinary tract can and should be done extraperitoneally. While it is true that there is less danger today of infection with a transperitoneal approach, it is still possible for a severe or fulminating peritonitis to develop following spillage of infected urine. If the peritoneum should be opened accidentally, it must be closed with extreme care before the completion of the operation in order to avoid this danger.

Secondary cystotomy, when it becomes necessary, is often difficult and requires painstaking care because of the scarring and the distortion of the suprapubic space and the perivesical tissues. The peritoneum frequently is adherent to the scarred areas over the symphysis, making it difficult even to locate the bladder. When the wall of the bladder is thickened and hypertrophied as the result of long-standing prostatic obstruction, cystotomy, which is usually a simple procedure, may occasionally be extremely difficult. One may cut tangentially into this thickened bladder wall and miss the bladder cavity entirely. When this or similar problems arise, distending the bladder with additional fluid may help.

After the cystotomy has been done, the bladder, when empty and collapsed, may obscure the area of the opening and much difficulty may ensue. Careful use of the Allis instruments can avoid this. If the bladder cannot be refilled, a sound inserted through the urethra may help in relocating the cystotomy opening.

It should also be pointed out that the valid surgical principle of *good exposure* is as useful here as elsewhere. Nothing is to be gained by a "buttonhole" incision, since an adequately large opening heals as fast as a little one.

Trocar Puncture of the Bladder. This should be done only in an emergency. It is indicated for the patient who is extremely ill or in shock with overdistention, where a catheter cannot be passed and where a cystotomy would be too great a risk. A trocar inserted into the bladder above the pubis allows for the insertion of a small Foley catheter through its lumen; the trocar is then removed. However, trocar puncture is apt to be unsafe because of the danger of entering the peritoneum, which can extend lower than expected. It is also possible to puncture the bowel.

If the patient be irrational, he may get out of bed and pull the catheter out. If this should occur during the first or second postoperative day following cystotomy or trocar puncture, it is usually impossible to replace it and all the previous efforts will have gone for naught.

Two-stage Prostatectomy. PRELIMINARY CYSTOTOMY. When prostatectomy is required for a patient who is a poor risk, it is well to divide the procedure into two stages. It may be very tempting, once the bladder is open, to go ahead and complete the whole operation at once, but in these questionable situations, it is much wiser to postpone the actual removal of the prostate till a later time when the cystot-

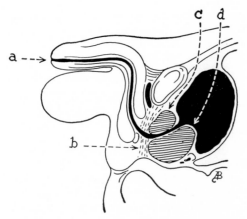

FIG. 425. Diagrammatic representation of the various routes of attack on the enlarged prostate. (a) Transurethral approach; (b) perineal approach; (c) retropubic extravesical approach; (d) suprapubic transvesical approach. (Rolnick, H. C.: The Practice of Urology, vol. 2, chap. 50, Philadelphia, Lippincott)

omy has had a chance to serve its purpose as a sort of "safety valve." Continuous urinary drainage through a cystotomy puts the bladder completely at rest ("splinting the bladder"). The prostatic urethra—the most absorptive portion of the urinary tract—is also thus allowed to rest. The kidneys become decompressed. The blood pressure stabilizes, and edema and infection in the prostate subside; sometimes the prostate will be found to have shrunk by half, when the second stage is done 1 to 2 weeks later.

Permanent Cystotomy. This may occasionally become necessary in a patient with a "neurogenic bladder," who has been suffering from chronic retention and cannot tolerate a retention catheter. In the past, permanent cystotomy was done to relieve chronic retention due to carcinoma of the prostate, but relief of obstruction in these patients is now accomplished by transurethral resection.

Suprapubic Prostatectomy. Many variations of this operation have been recommended, some of which are valuable (Fig. 425). The actual technic of this and other procedures to be mentioned later are to be found in any standard text; here it is necessary only to point out certain precautions.

Gentleness should be one's rule here as elsewhere. "You don't tear out a prostate; you enucleate it." If some force is required, a finger in the rectum will often aid in enucleation. Again, let me stress the importance of adequate exposure. It is true that some parts of this operation must be done "blind," but good visualization should be had as far as is practical. Also, bear in mind that, though a cystoscopy may have been done just prior to the operation, it is still quite possible to miss a tumor or a diverticulum in the bladder unless the entire bladder is carefully inspected.

CONTROL OF HEMORRHAGE. This still remains the most important problem during and after any type of prostatic surgery. With good exposure, arterial bleeding at the bladder neck may be visualized and the vessels transfixed and sutured. Venous bleeding and bleeding from the sinuses in the capsule cause blood to well up from the prostatic bed during and immediately following the enucleation. Unless this is controlled as soon as possible, much blood may be lost. A large sponge may be inserted into the "bed" to act as a tamponade for temporary control. A bag catheter is then passed through the urethra into the bladder and the sponge removed. A large bag with a capacity up to 100 cc. should be used. Some urologists employ traction on the catheter as a further help in control of bleeding, but we believe that this involves danger of some degree of later incontinence because of traction on the external sphincter. It is occasionally best to fill the bag of the catheter while it is still deep in the bladder and then bring it down against the bladder neck. This may accomplish hemostasis, since most of the active bleeding is likely to occur at this point.

PACKING THE CAVITY. This was done routinely in the past, but, today, with the use of larger sizes of bag catheters, it is rarely necessary. However, there are times when even one of these larger catheters will not control hemorrhage, particularly when the cavity is unusually large. Therefore, it is well to remember that, when all other methods fail, a large gauze pack will usually accomplish the desired purpose. Absorbable thrombin is of doubtful value and, since it is not always absorbable, can cause complications by acting as a foreign body. Some patients develop severe bladder spasm from gauze packing, especially if it has been put in too firmly; later removal may be a major undertaking in some instances. The best practice is to leave such packing in place for 2 to 3 days, then to remove it in stages over a similar period. Even so, bleeding may recur with the removal of the pack.

It might be well to point out that in almost any urologic surgery gauze packing can often be a "lifesaver" for the control of bleeding. One or more 5-yard rolls of gauze inserted quickly and firmly, upward, inward and forward into the renal bed will compress a "lost" renal pedicle after nephrectomy and completely control bleeding. Similarly, a torn internal iliac vein which can be neither ligated nor sutured, or the vena cava in a like condition, may be packed. Whenever we have a difficult nephrectomy, we like to have several such rolls of packing at hand.

RECURRENT BLEEDING. The recurrence of bleeding after prostatectomy may be controlled by the urethral catheter and frequent irrigation of the bladder to remove clots. The retention catheter must be watched and irrigated frequently until bleeding subsides; however, if it cannot be controlled in this manner, the patient should be returned to surgery and the bleeding points fulgurated through a resectoscope in the urethra.

SHOCK. If the bladder becomes filled with clots, shock may follow, not only because of the loss of blood and the extreme pain and discomfort from distention, but also because of a reaction, not too well understood, of the bladder itself to the presence of the clots. Apparently, they also act as a foreign body. When these clots have been evacuated (using either the Ellik evacuator or the Toomey syringe), inspection of the bladder will usually reveal no further evidence of bleeding from the prostatic bed. It seems possible that, with the relief of distention, the tissues return to a normal state of contraction and the vessels are closed off.

Bleeding may occur as late as 2 or 3 weeks after the operation. A patient sent home a bit too early may have to return to the hospital if bleeding is severe. However, urine which is only blood-tinged (initial or terminal) is of little significance and is relatively normal when it continues for several days or even weeks following prostatectomy. The patient should be limited as to activities after return home for 2 or 3 weeks. Following suprapubic prostatectomy, a large mushroom catheter is inserted into the bladder for drainage. Nothing is gained by primary closure of the bladder without this drainage, since this means depending solely on a urethral catheter for both drainage and hemostasis. As previously indicated, the suprapubic catheter is a "safety valve," especially during the first few days following operation. The following seems to us to be a satisfactory routine, though considerable variation is possible.

For the first few hours after the operation, the urethral bag catheter may be kept under slight tension. Next day, the Foley bag should be emptied, and, if there is no bleeding, the catheter is removed the following day, giving the urethra a chance to heal. At the end of 5 to 7 days, the suprapubic catheter is removed, after which the urethral catheter may be reinserted to expedite closure of the cystotomy wound.

If the cystotomy fails to close within a reasonable length of time, and a persistent urinary fistula develops, this is usually an indication that obstruction at the bladder neck is still present. In these cases a resectoscope may be inserted, the contracted bladder neck resected and any tags removed.

In doing a planned 2-stage prostatectomy, some surgeons make a practice of suturing the bladder to the rectus fascia in the first stage in order to bring the prostate closer to the surface to facilitate enucleation during the second stage. However, it has been our observation that this "hooking up" of the bladder close to the surface tends to produce a permanent urinary fistula, necessitating, in some cases, a later, secondary closure of the bladder. When such secondary closure is necessary, a careful dissection of the fistulous tract is done, the bladder freed from the fascia, followed by complete closure of the bladder wall. A urethral catheter should be inserted for drainage.

ADMINISTRATION OF BLOOD AND FLUIDS. This is probably the single factor that has done most to lower the mortality and the morbidity from prostatectomy in recent years. Since blood loss is the greatest individual

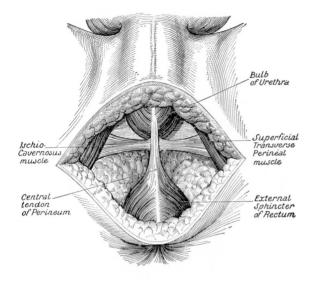

Bulb
of Urethra

Ischio-
Cavernosus
muscle

Superficial
Transverse
Perineal
muscle

Central
tendon
of Perineum

External
Sphincter
of Rectum

Fig. 426. Perineal prostatectomy. Dissection to show position of transversus perinei muscles and of bulbous portion of the urethra. (Rolnick, H. C.: The Practice of Urology, vol. 2, p. 1056, Philadelphia, Lippincott)

problem in all these operations, regardless of procedure, administration of blood at the beginning of the operation should be practically routine. If blood is replaced as rapidly as it is lost, the patient's condition will remain satisfactory. It is not wise to wait until he is nearly exsanguinated before beginning transfusion, for he may go into shock. The possibility of late-appearing hemolytic jaundice with hepatitis should not be minimized—we have seen several instances of this sequel and some deaths have been reported—but there is no question that in the past many deaths following prostatectomy resulted from the fact that blood was neither readily available nor freely given.

Five hundred cc. of blood is usually sufficient in these cases. If the patient has any cardiac limitations, it should be given more slowly than normal. In situations where bleeding is persistent and not readily controlled, additional amounts of blood may be needed.

Perineal Prostatectomy. Although this is a direct anatomic approach, it has a number of serious drawbacks and is done relatively infrequently at present (Fig. 426). There may be injury to the rectum during this operation. The ischial tuberosities limit exposure, and in some individuals working space is restricted and the entire operation must be done practically "blind." It is difficult to visualize the bladder neck; also, bleeding vessels may slip out of sight because of the upward retraction of the bladder neck. Injury to the nerves and the

muscles of the perineum almost always produces incontinence, at least temporarily, and since permanent impotence also usually follows, this procedure should be ruled out for any man under 60, or even the man beyond this age who is still sexually active.

In doing this operation, if it is preferred over those now more commonly used, extreme care must be exercised to avoid injury to the rectum. If it should be injured at the beginning, before the prostatic capsule has been opened, the operation should be stopped and the damage repaired, with a suprapubic prostatectomy or transurethral resection undertaken at a later time. If the opening in the rectum is discovered only at the end of the operation, the result can be disastrous, for recto-urethral or rectovesical fistula may develop, requiring later plastic repair of both rectum and urethra.

Several safeguards may help the surgeon toward success with this approach. Careful separation of the central tendon and of the muscles aids visualization. Be sure that the rectum is fully exposed to view and adequately protected throughout the operation. Bleeding is controlled with a bag catheter, but it may also be necessary to maintain tension on it for some hours if hemorrhage persists. Compression on the perineum may also help to control bleeding.

Retropubic Prostatectomy. This is also a direct or anatomic approach to the prostate and is now a standard procedure. The prostate is best visualized by this procedure, and bleeding is least difficult to control, though here, as in all other operations on this organ, hemorrhage may be a serious problem. One late complication that has been reported is osteitis pubis, though it is not peculiar to this method and may occur even after simple cystotomy. Danger of infection of the suprapubic space is now minimized by chemotherapy and antibiotics.

In this operation the prostate is approached directly as it lies distal to the bladder neck. The bladder is first emptied, then retracted downward and forward. Occasionally the Trendelenburg position is employed, but it is usually better simply to elevate the pelvis on the back rest.

Considerable bleeding may develop at the beginning from vessels on the surface of the capsule. The plexus of Santorini, the vessels supplying the prostate, is located on the anterior surface. The vessels in the midline must be ligated before incising the capsule. The lateral superficial vessels may also bleed considerably when manipulated; these may be packed off temporarily.

When enucleating through a transverse incision in the capsule, care must be taken not to tear it farther, as such large tears can be very troublesome. In contrast with transvesical prostatectomy, enucleation is carried from the apex upward toward the bladder neck. Arteries and large veins, bleeding in the capsule, should be clamped with Allis forceps, then sutured or ligated. All tags should be removed and a wedge resected from the bladder neck. A similar wedge must also occasionally be taken from this interureteric ridge in order to eliminate any possibility of later obstruction.

The bladder itself is not opened in this method, unless some pathologic condition is evident, but it may be inspected through a retractor placed in the bladder neck. The capsule is then closed carefully over a large urethral catheter (preferably a No. 24 Tieman coude). Here, as elsewhere, a careful watch must be kept for bleeding, and the catheter should be irrigated, or changed, as often as necessary. Bleeding occurs from the venous sinuses and can be severe. Here, as in the transvesical method, the patient occasionally may have to be returned to surgery and clots evacuated from the bladder.

Vasectomy in association with prostatectomy is advisable in patients who are no longer sexually active, since it will reduce the possibility of the epididymitis which follows removal of the prostate in some 25 per cent of all patients. In younger men, the risk of epididymitis is more than overbalanced by the mental and physical hazards from ligation of the vas.

Transurethral Resection. The details of this technic are fully covered in monographs on this subject by Nesbit and Barnes, as well as in standard surgical texts, and will not be discussed here.

Complications

1. Results of Incomplete Removal. It is important not only to enucleate the prostate but also to cut the bladder neck rather widely. In suprapubic prostatectomy, the contracted bladder neck is sometimes overlooked. The prostate must be completely removed, regardless of the type of operation performed. Partial enucleation, as done in the early days of open prostatic surgery, has proved to be unsatisfactory; and the same is true in transurethral resection when only a channel is cut. Merely "cutting a groove" in transurethral resection may even aggravate existing conditions since the supports of the gland are disturbed. *When the floor is removed, the walls cave in; if the walls are removed, the roof caves in.* In transurethral resection, if residual tissue remains it often has a poor blood supply, resulting in slough, secondary infection and recurrent bleeding. The presence of such devitalized tissues may cause symptoms which persist over a long period of time. In many instances a second operation to remove such tissues may become necessary.

2. Hemorrhage. Since the advent of the sulfonamides and antibiotics, *urinary-tract infection*—once paired with hemorrhage as main hazards in prostatic surgery—can be fairly well controlled and today is rarely a problem. Therefore, hemorrhage remains as the single most cogent hazard, regardless of the type of procedure chosen. Any improvements in operative technic should be aimed at improving hemostasis. One advantage of the *retropubic approach* is that the improved exposure of the prostatic bed which it provides enables the surgeon to see any bleeding vessels and suture them. Blood loss, during these operations, can be very severe if not properly controlled. At best, there will be a loss of from 300 to 500 cc. of blood during and immediately following the operation. For this reason, we feel that, as previously indicated, administration of at least 500 cc. of whole blood is mandatory.

3. Intravascular Hemolysis in Transurethral Resection. Much has been written on this complication which occurs when the venous sinuses in the prostatic capsule have been opened during the operation, thus permitting the water medium to enter the general circulation and cause hemolysis. If, instead, an isotonic solution, such as glycine, is used, this will not happen. Intravascular hemolysis, of itself, even when marked, does not cause renal damage; it is only when the factor of *shock* is added that lower nephron nephrosis may result. Lower nephron nephrosis or the "kidney of shock" may result from marked blood loss, prolonged operation time, severe or too deep anesthesia and particularly from the surgical accident of perforation with extravasation.

4. Perforation of the Bladder and Prostatic Capsule. This may occur in either the fundus or the neck of the bladder during transurethral resection and also in the prostatic capsule. Perforation of the bladder is usually retroperitoneal, rarely intraperitoneal. The first indication will be slowly rising blood pressure, usually accompanied by substernal and shoulder pain, with considerable suprapubic pain and rigidity. In doing a transurethral resection, there is an advantage to the use of *spinal anesthesia* here for many reasons and also in that the patient who is awake will complain immediately if this complication materializes. A slight perforation may be controlled by an indwelling urethral catheter, but, in most instances, immediate cystotomy and the institution of suprapubic and perivesical space drainage are required to avoid spread of infection along the fascial planes which may extend upward into the perirenal space.

5. Impotence. Decrease or loss of sexual vigor may follow any type of prostatectomy. However, since impotence practically always follows use of the perineal approach, it is obvious that it should not be used on patients who are still potent. Also, following any of these operations, though potency may be normal, there may be no ejaculation. This can be due to any of several factors: (a) the ejaculatory ducts may have been torn and thus have become occluded later by scar, or (b) ejaculation may be retrograde into the bladder, due to nonfunctioning of the bladder neck or the internal sphincter. (The bladder neck actually serves as an accessory sexual organ, in that, at the height of orgasm, it contracts so that the ejaculate may be expelled only in a forward direction.)

6. Incontinence. This may follow any type of prostatic surgery if the external urethral sphincter has been damaged. It may follow a *rough* enucleation, whether performed suprapubically or retropubically. Actual section of the sphincter has occurred in transurethral resection, particularly in the past. The surgeon, at all times, must be keenly aware of his anatomic landmarks, especially of the relation between the verumontanum and the external sphincter, when doing transurethral resection. In the perineal approach, another factor which may induce incontinence is also present, even though careful and proper enucleation has been done. This is the fact that the perineal muscles and nerves play an important part in urinary control, and these are unavoidably disturbed to a varying degree. While the incidence of incontinence following perineal prostatectomy is low in experienced hands, it is still likely to be higher than when some other approach is used. *Radical* prostatectomy, whether performed perineally or retropubically, tends to have a higher incidence of incontinence because of the extensive nature of the surgery, in which the external sphincter may be injured.

CARCINOMA OF THE PROSTATE

Diagnosis and Incidence. In its early stages, carcinoma of the prostate is best detected by the index finger in the rectum; however, a statement made many years ago still holds true: "By the time carcinoma of the prostate may be diagnosed by the rectal finger, it is already too late to operate!" Not more than 2 to 3 per cent of those patients in whom a diagnosis is made are discovered early enough before extension to be suitable for radical

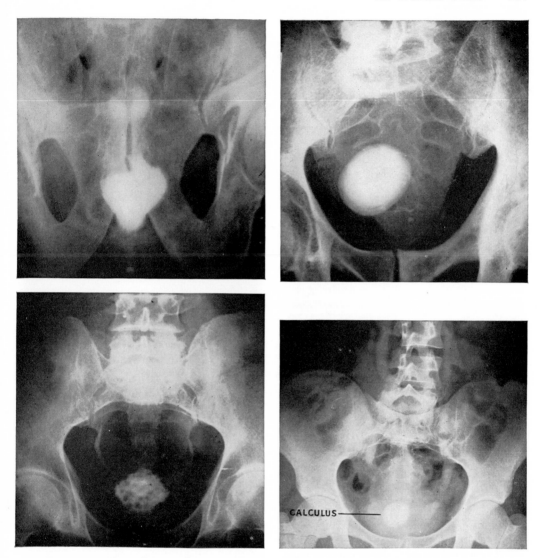

FIG. 427. (*Top, left*) Large dumbbell calculus—prostatic bed (postprostatectomy) showing the stone which occupies the entire prostatic bed, filling the bladder neck and extending partly into bladder. (*Top, right*) Large laminated bladder calculus. (*Bottom, left*) Multiple small bladder calculi, originally prostatic calculi, which present a negative shadow on the cystogram following intravenous pyelogram. (*Bottom, right*) Bladder calculus with bladder neck obstruction producing bilateral hydronephrosis. (Rolnick, H. C.: The Practice of Urology, vol. 1, facing p. 504, Philadelphia, Lippincott)

prostatectomy. A prostate which, when enucleated, appears to be grossly benign may show a small carcinomatous area, yet this will prove to be all the carcinoma the patient has, and he may remain well thereafter.

Statistics on the incidence of carcinoma of the prostate vary considerably. It is seen more frequently in general hospitals than in private practice, possibly because of the higher average age of general-hospital patients. Some statistics appear to indicate an incidence as high as 20 per cent, others no higher than 5 to 10 per cent. It is probable that approximately 1 out of 10 who come to

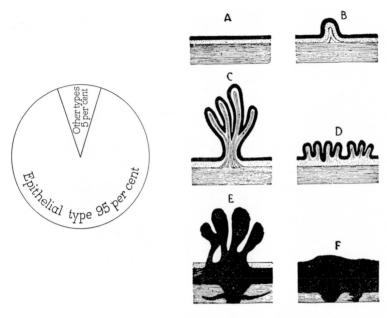

FIG. 428. (*Left*) Diagram to illustrate the relative frequency of the various types of tumors of the bladder. Note predominance (95%) of those of the epithelial type. (*Right*) Diagrammatic representation of mode of origin of various types of bladder cancer. (A) Normal bladder wall. Epithelial layer shown as solid black line. (B) Elevation of epithelial layer (mucosa) with its underlying submucous layer and blood vessel. (C) How a simple (benign) papilloma with long narrow pedicle evolves from B. (D) Multiple sessile (benign) papillomata arising in similar manner. (E) A pedunculated or sessile benign papilloma has undergone malignant changes and invaded pedicle as well as submucous and muscular coats of bladder wall. (F) How an infiltrating (nonpapillomatous) cancer invades all of the coats with but little protrusion of tumor into the bladder lumen. (Rolnick, H. C.: The Practice of Urology, vol. 1, p. 511, Philadelphia, Lippincott)

operation have carcinoma. Figures based on necropsy findings are not satisfactory, since anatomic evidence of carcinoma may be present in the very aged subject, when there was no evidence or symptoms during life and the growth was biologically inactive.

Radical Perineal Prostatectomy for Carcinoma. This approach seems preferable to radical retropubic prostatectomy, for the prostatic and membranous urethra are better exposed and more adequate removal of tissue is possible.

THE BLADDER

BLADDER CALCULI

Diagnosis. Diagnosis of bladder stones is made, in most cases, by x-ray examination (Fig. 427). However, a small percentage, including some stones of large size, will yield no x-ray shadow and must be identified by cystoscopy. Even positive x-ray findings should be confirmed by cystoscopy, which will also help to determine the type of operation needed for removal.

In the female, bladder stones are uncommon, since they occur chiefly in conjunction with bladder-neck obstruction, a condition relatively rare in women.

If stones are small, they may be evacuated through the sheath of the cystoscope or resectoscope, unless there are indications that they may pass of themselves. Another method is to use a cystoscopic forceps through the resectoscope sheath.

Some bladder calculi are large, soft, white or grayish stones which can occasionally be broken up for removal merely by the resectoscope loop. Small, round or cuboidal stones, yellowish or dark brown in color, often seen in the bladder, are actually prostatic calculi which have passed into the bladder. These often evacuate spontaneously. However, if stones of either type are too large to pass or too hard, they must be removed either by crushing and evacuation or by cystotomy.

Litholapaxy. This procedure may be done either by means of the cystoscopic lithotrite or the "blind" lithotrite. We prefer the blind lithotrite, as it seems to be somewhat the less dangerous instrument.

Cystotomy. When a large stone is associated with obstructive prostatic hypertrophy, when there is an associated bladder diverticulum, when much inflammation or infection is present, or when the bladder wall is thin and the stone adherent to it, cystotomy must be done for removal of the stone. When a single, large, fixed stone is removed, what promised to be a relatively simple procedure is sometimes followed by a stormy postoperative course, because the eroded bladder surface allows for rapid systemic absorption. However, this is less likely today than formerly, before the introduction of the sulfonamides.

Bladder Tumors

In the main, these may be classified as (1) papilloma or noninfiltrating, which are relatively benign, and (2) infiltrating or malignant (Fig. 428). Microscopically, the papilloma, in most cases, shows some evidence of low-grade, transitional cell carcinoma, though clinically it is benign. However, some of these clinically benign growths may "bridge over" to become infiltrating and malignant. Therefore, they should be removed as soon as possible.

For clinical purposes, the distinction between the benign and the malignant type of tumor is quite evident. In most instances it can readily be determined by cystoscopy. The papilloma usually has a soft, noninfiltrating base or may be attached to the bladder wall by a fibrous stalk or pedicle. These growths may be solitary or multiple and when removed have a tendency to recur; therefore, a patient who has once had a papilloma removed should be frequently re-examined by cystoscopy over a 3- to 4-year period in case of such recurrence.

Diagnosis. Except for the large papillomata, cystoscopy is the only means of diagnosis. Large benign papilloma will produce a filling defect on the cystogram. Infiltrating tumors also are diagnosed in this manner.

Removal of Papillomata. Except when very numerous, removal can be effected by fulguration by means of a cystoscopic electrode. In some cases this is simple enough to be done as an office procedure on the ambulatory patient and can be repeated as necessary. Often it is not even necessary to use an anesthetic, unless the growth is located near the bladder neck. The fundus of the bladder is so poorly supplied with sensory nerves that simple fulguration of a few small areas in this region is relatively painless.

Infiltrating Bladder Tumors. These present a serious problem, for they indicate the presence of carcinoma with some degree of extension. Although they may be controlled, complete eradication usually is not possible.

EXAMINATION. This is done on the anesthetized patient. With a finger in the rectum and the opposite hand on the suprapubic region, evidence of the presence and the degree of infiltration may be elicited (Jewett). Also, in many cases the extent of infiltration may be determined at the time of transurethral resection for removal of the growth. It is then possible to see if the infiltration extends deep into the muscle tissue or beyond.

TREATMENT. In infiltrating bladder tumors treatment varies. Some urologists recommend cystotomy and deep surgical diathermy; others, cystotomy with implantation of radium. Surgical resection or segmental resection of both the tumor itself and a large portion of the bladder may be done if the tumor appears to be limited to the dome of the bladder. In these relatively favorable situations—they are few in number—a subtotal cystectomy may be done; even here, however, infiltration may already have gone far beyond what is indicated by the *gross appearance* of the tissues.

Cystectomy

This is a major procedure with a relatively high percentage of mortality. The problems that it raises are, for all practical purposes, almost as serious as those that it solves. It is necessary to transplant the ureters into the bowel or skin, neither of which is satisfactory. Within the past few years, transplantation into an isolated ileal loop has given better results, for the problem of hyperchloremic acidosis is practically eliminated through this ileal conduit. Man cannot retrogress a hundred million years to his reptilian forebears in having a cloaca without paying a tragically high price in the form of disturbed body chemistry and progressive or recurrent infec-

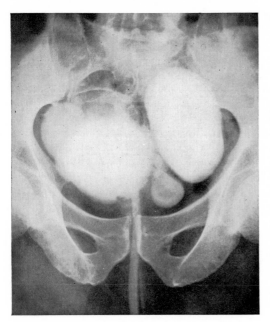

Fig. 429. Multiple bladder diverticula, with the diverticulum as large as the bladder itself. The sac of the diverticulum shows a smooth outline, whereas the bladder itself shows irregularities indicating chronic severe infections. (Rolnick, H. C.: The Practice of Urology, vol. 1, p. 482, Philadelphia, Lippincott)

tion. Obstruction to the ureter, due to scarring, with all its attendant sequelae, is not an infrequent complication. For these reasons, the operation of cystectomy with ureteral transplantation into the sigmoid has undergone a rather thorough evaluation and has been discarded by most urologists. The ileal conduit has also proved to be unsatisfactory. It is our impression, therefore, that these infiltrating bladder tumors are better treated by cystotomy with either deep diathermy or radium implantation, or by transurethral resection.

TRANSURETHRAL RESECTION

This type of operation, performed on the closed bladder, has proved to be satisfactory in our hands not only in prolonging the lives of these patients but also in making them more comfortable. Many of them are even able to resume fairly active lives. This pro-

cedure may also be repeated at intervals, as needed, unless and until the condition develops to a point where this treatment is no longer beneficial. It seems to us that transurethral resection has an even more important place in the treatment of bladder tumors than it has in treating prostatic or bladder-neck obstructions.

DIVERTICULUM

With respect to this type of abnormality, two points require special notice. The first is the necessity for differentiating between *cellules*—the result of muscular hypertrophy which follows long-standing bladder-neck obstruction and the development of trabeculation—and *true diverticula* (Fig. 429). Cellules are of no importance and require no treatment. A diverticulum may or may not require surgical intervention, depending on its size, shape and location.

Diagnosis of the specific type of sac encountered is governed by many factors, such as the age and the sex of the patient (they are extremely rare in females and somewhat unusual in males under 40), the presence or absence of bladder neck or prostatic obstruction and whether or not the sac is, of itself, causing urinary retention.

The second point, associated with the matter of the size and the location of the sac, is the fact that when it is large and extends downward, laterally and inferiorly, it is most apt to be deeply adherent, frequently to the bowel behind and, in some cases, even to the iliac vessels. This is especially likely following long-standing infections.

A markedly trabeculated bladder looks like the thickened cordae tendinae of the compensated heart. These conditions may be found in patients who have had a long-standing obstruction at the bladder neck to which the bladder has compensated itself by hypertrophy and thickening of its musculature. The shallow spaces between the hypertrophied layers of muscle are the cellulae referred to previously.

Diverticula usually occur near the ureteral orifice on either or both sides. These areas are, embryologically, the weakest points in the bladder wall. They occur most frequently in men over 50 and are practically always

FIG. 430. Exstrophy of the bladder associated with complete epispadias and bilateral nondescent of the testes. (Rolnick, H. C.: The Practice of Urology, vol. 1, facing p. 436, Philadelphia, Lippincott)

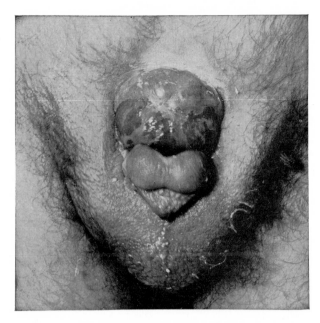

associated with bladder-neck obstruction, usually bladder-neck contracture; also, although less frequently, with simple hypertrophy of the prostate. They are sometimes found in younger men affected with *congenital* bladder-neck obstruction. They may be demonstrated on the cystogram and seen with the cystoscope.

If the neck of the diverticulum is wide, so that the floor may be readily seen, and when the cystogram indicates little or no urinary retention, it does not require operation. When the opposite conditions obtain, it can in many cases be successfully operated on by transurethral resection of the neck of the diverticulum, thus making it a nonretaining sac.

A large retention diverticulum, which shows failure to empty on the cystogram, requires open operation for its removal. This is the type of sac which usually shows some degree of chronic infection and is frequently adherent to adjacent structures. When this situation is found, the sac must first be separated from the bladder and then removed. In some cases it may be satisfactory merely to remove the endothelium of the cavity, and to deal appropriately with the opening in the bladder wall, where the neck of the sac has been resected. Since the continuity of the sac with the bladder has been severed, there should be no recurrence.

The orifice or neck of a diverticulum is frequently very close to the ureteral orifice, and in some cases the ureteral orifice is actually inside this opening.

Removal of diverticula is done by a cystotomy with extension of the incision laterally to the neck of the sac. The orifice is then completely circumcised and the sac separated from the bladder, the opening in the bladder wall being closed later. An attempt is now made to remove as much of the sac itself as possible. It is not necessary, as indicated previously, to remove the entire sac, particularly if it is very adherent posteriorly.

For this operation, good exposure may be had through a low midline incision, which may be extended upward as far as needed. The suprapubic space is opened, the same as for a retropubic prostatectomy, thus giving a direct approach. The vesical arteries, being relatively large, may be cut and hemorrhage must be carefully controlled. Drainage must be instituted in both the suprapubic space and the lateral cavity.

TRAUMA

Rupture of the bladder (Fig. 430) may be subcutaneous or nonpenetrating, or penetrating. Spontaneous rupture, which falls into the first category, is extremely rare, and it results from fatty degeneration of the bladder muscle. The bladder will withstand enormous distention without rupture. Traumatic, subcutaneous rupture, occurring with a distended bladder, may result when the victim falls against some blunt object, as during a drunken stupor, or in a traffic or industrial accident. Penetrating wounds resulting in rupture are most frequent in connection with battle injuries. Even these types of damage are much less likely to produce rupture if the bladder is empty when the blow is struck.

These patients are often in shock when first seen. Attempts to urinate produce only a few drops of blood. Attempts to pass a catheter often fail since the urethra may also be torn; this is most frequent when there has been a severe or crushing fracture of the pelvic bones. So much surface discoloration may have occurred that it is often difficult to estimate the extent of the internal damage.

When the patient is not in shock, an intravenous pyelogram may be enlightening. If a catheter can be inserted, indicating that the urethra is not involved, yet little or no urine and some blood is obtained, this also suggests rupture. Most ruptures will be found to be extraperitoneal.

When in doubt, or when there is direct evidence of a torn urethra, a cystotomy should be done—provided, of course, that the extent of the injuries to adjacent structures permits. Through the cystotomy opening the ruptured bladder wall may be repaired. A cystotomy tube should be left in place for drainage.

In penetrating wounds, such as war injuries, the damage may include tearing of the rectum and the sigmoid as well. In such cases extensive repair is required, and a colostomy must be established, together with prolonged suprapubic and perineal drainage. In such instances repair of the urethra may have to wait until later.

In cases of intraperitoneal rupture, it is surprising to note how well the peritoneum will tolerate the contact with sterile urine; large quantities can sometimes accumulate with little reaction, either local or systemic. This has been observed in cases of both subcutaneous bladder rupture and accidental cutting of a ureter (during hysterectomy). On the other hand, peritoneal shock will occasionally follow operative injuries to the bladder which have been overlooked, in which

situation the patient may die within 24 to 48 hours.

INJURIES IN CONNECTION WITH ABDOMINOPERINEAL RESECTION

Occasionally the prostatic urethra may be cut or, still more rarely, the bladder itself injured during extensive surgery on the large bowel, with a resulting perineal fistula. Following abdominoperineal resection for carcinoma, especially in the male, urinary retention is a not uncommon complication. This is especially likely in those who have some degree of prostatic hypertrophy prior to the resection. Urinary retention results here from disturbance of the sympathetic nerves—also to the fact that a large cavity has been produced, into which the bladder, deprived of part of its natural support, falls (as in cystocele in the female). Most of these patients recover from the retention within a few weeks, with the aid of drainage by catheter; for those who do not, prostatic surgery may be required.

Transurethral resection is the operation of choice here since the recent abdominal wound often is markedly inflamed, and the presence of adhesions will not permit a suprapubic or a retropubic approach. However, in doing a transurethral resection on a patient whose rectum has been closed, extra care is needed as to the extent and the depth of the resection since no finger in the rectum may be used as a guide. When the prostate is large, the otherwise less desirable perineal approach may be the safer choice.

INJURIES IN CONNECTION WITH PELVIC AND GYNECOLOGIC OPERATIONS

Two situations in particular may lead to injuries in this category. The first is in operations on large scrotal hernias. Occasionally a portion of the bladder will be incorporated into the hernial sac and may be opened accidentally. If in doubt as to the identity of a structure encountered under such conditions, a catheter should be inserted. If the bladder has already been penetrated before one's suspicions are aroused, insertion of a finger will reveal the bladder neck, in which case the opening must be sutured and the bladder drained with a urethral retention catheter.

The most common situation in which the

bladder may suffer is during hysterectomy, either abdominal or vaginal; injury may occur when attempting to find a line of cleavage in the presence of large fibroids, or where there is marked inflammation with scarring and distortion of the bladder; this is especially likely when the operation is a secondary one. In vaginal hysterectomy the bladder may be difficult to separate and may be perforated during the operation—or considerable denudation of the bladder wall may reduce the blood supply, with resultant slough and some degree of later necrosis. When injuries are discovered during the course of the operation, the bladder wall should be sutured and a retention catheter inserted, in which case there usually will be no further trouble. However, if the injury is not discovered, the patient may begin to pass urine through the vagina, indicating the development of a vesicovaginal fistula, a somewhat difficult condition to correct. Such a fistula may also develop some 5 or 6 days after operation, if the bladder wall has been inadvertently incorporated in some of the suture lines, due to sloughing.

Vesicovaginal Fistula

Much has been written about this condition, both as to its causes and the methods for its cure. The principle involved in its repair is complete mobilization of the bladder with respect to its attachment to the vagina. If this is achieved and the openings in the two structures are closed separately, they should heal and remain closed; but to accomplish this is not simple. There are many cases on record where several or even a large number of operations have been required before success was attained. The most important single safeguard is to wait until all the tissues involved have completely healed from the original operation before repair is attempted. This may take several months. The same is true if, as happens occasionally, the rectum is also involved and must likewise be repaired.

To avoid this type of injury in the first place, all patients being prepared for pelvic surgery should be catheterized routinely to obtain the empty bladder which is so much less subject to any sort of damage. If this is not done, and in cases where the bladder is

atonic, it is possible to err by diagnosing as a fibroid what is really only a distended bladder.

Bladder Symptoms after Hysterectomy

In the presence of fibroids, some gynecologists recommend removal of an asymptomatic uterus as a means of relieving patients with some urinary discomfort. However, it has been our observation that the opposite result is more likely to follow. In fact, some patients who have not had such difficulties before develop urgency and frequency following hysterectomy, possibly due to loss of some of the supporting structures of the bladder after this operation.

THE URETERS

Diagnosis

Pathologic disturbances which demand surgical intervention for their correction usually

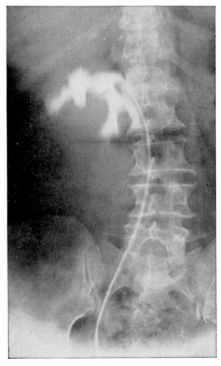

Fig. 431. Marked displacement of ureter mesially with resultant urographic deformity in a case of retroperitoneal sarcoma in an adult. (Rolnick, H. C.: The Practice of Urology, vol. 2, p. 868, Philadelphia, Lippincott)

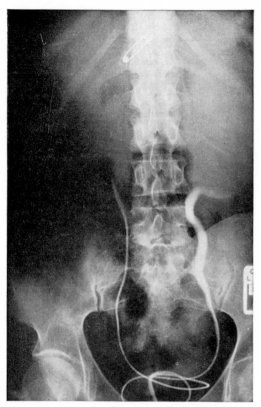

FIG. 432. Large hydronephrotic sac due to congenital obstruction at the ureteropelvic juncture by bands and aberrant vessels. There was a large mass in the abdomen, and the contrast medium could not be injected into the renal pelvis. Nephrectomy was done with considerable difficulty. (Rolnick, H. C.: The Practice of Urology, vol. 2, p. 697, Philadelphia, Lippincott)

are diagnosed only roentgenographically. The functioning ureter undergoes peristalsis; therefore, it may vary somewhat in its position and diameter due to the contraction and the dilatation along its course. However, the circular and the longitudinal muscles of the ureter may become permanently lengthened as a result of obstruction or atony. The ureter then will become dilated and elongated and vary somewhat in position; it may also become kinked, though this, of itself, is of no diagnostic importance.

Sharp *angulation* of the ureter at the ureteropelvic junction may occur with a "dropped" kidney, but, unless there is definite evidence of hydronephrosis on that side, this sign also is of no clinical importance. With a movable kidney, a sharp kink may also appear but, alone, is not an indication for nephropexy. In some individuals a ureter may be redundant; in the presence of ectopic kidney, it will be quite short. Thus the length of the ureter may be a diagnostic criterion between a congenitally ectopic and a "dropped" kidney.

Deviation of the ureter from what may be considered to be its normal course is most likely to be caused by a retroperitoneal tumor or other retroperitoneal masses (Fig. 431). Intraperitoneal masses, unless extremely large or infiltrating into the posterior peritoneum (e.g., carcinoma of the cecum), usually do not cause deviation of the ureter. Occasionally a large fibroid may cause a spreading of the ureter at its vesical end; also, an enlarged spleen with perisplenitis can sometimes obscure the outline of the kidney and also produce a deviation in the ureter.

One anomaly which is observed occasionally is the retrocaval ureter. This is limited to the right side and is a situation in which the ureter passes under the vena cava and winds around it.

All such findings of deviation, based on roentgenograms, must be carefully interpreted to determine whether the observed condition is pathologic or merely a variation within normal limits.

URETERAL STRICTURE

As a clinical entity this condition is rare, although it has been stated by some authorities to be relatively common, particularly in the female. Many patients have been subjected to periodic dilations for the relief of a myriad of symptoms supposedly arising from the presence of this condition, but we believe, with Schreiber, that the only type of stricture which actually occurs is due either to (1) a long-standing stone with ureteritis and periureteritis, or (2) injury, usually surgical. We do not do dilation for so-called "ureteral stricture," for, as stated above, this condition does not exist.

CONGENITAL OBSTRUCTION AT THE URETEROPELVIC JUNCTURE

These patients gradually develop a hydronephrosis which becomes more marked as they approach maturity; when not relieved, in an appreciable proportion of cases, complete hydronephrotic atrophy of the kidney follows. These congenital obstructions result from (1) ureteral stricture at the ureteropelvic juncture, (2) aberrant vessels, or (3) congenital bands. The intravenous pyelogram is diagnostically valuable here; the renal pelvis will fill out, but there will be no visualization of the ureter, or it will be visible for only a few centimeters downward.

Congenital stricture at the ureteropelvic juncture (Fig. 432) is the most usual cause of this condition, with aberrant vessels next in order. When the hydronephrosis is not marked, and there is still sufficient renal parenchyma present, a plastic operation may be done with satisfactory results. Minor degrees of congenital ureteropelvic obstructions, usually bilateral, require no treatment. Among the various procedures that have been devised, the best appears to be the Foley-Y plastic operation, in which the strictured ureter is incised lengthwise and a wedge-shaped portion of the pelvis is brought down and united to the ureter over the incision. In many cases, merely cutting the stricture lengthwise in a manner akin to the Ramstedt operation (for congenital pyloric stenosis) is enough. In thus cutting the stricture, only a small band of tissue may be left posteriorly to maintain continuity, for the ureter will bridge over the defect in front, restoring complete continuity. In our experience, it has been necessary to leave a ureteral catheter in place for 4 or 5 days only, as a splint; after that time, it may simply become a foreign body which interferes with healing.

When the obstruction is due to an aberrant vessel at the lower pole, a more complicated problem exists, regardless of whether the vessel is the sole cause or if it is associated with the congenital stricture already described. The vessels supplying the kidney are end-arteries having no collateral circulation; if any one of them is severed, that portion of the kidney supplied by it will undergo atrophy and fibrosis. It is essential to determine the amount of kidney parenchyma which the aberrant vessel supplies. This may be done by temporarily occluding the vessel with a rubberized clamp; the portion deprived of its blood supply will blanch, giving an index

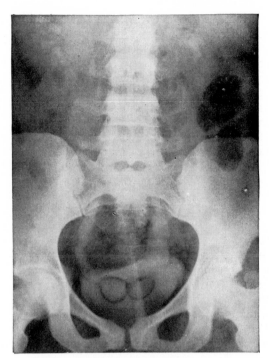

Fig. 433. Bilateral ureterocele. Intravenous pyelogram showing typical outline of the ureteroceles which appear like the thickened end of a baseball bat. (Rolnick, H. C.: The Practice of Urology, vol. 1, p. 567, Philadelphia, Lippincott)

to the amount of renal damage which will result from cutting the vessel to relieve the obstruction. A small vessel may be cut with a reasonable degree of safety, but severing a large one may compromise too much of the parenchyma; the vessel must be preserved in the majority of cases.

If the size of the aberrant vessel is such that it cannot be spared, it is perfectly practical, in most cases, to cut and reunite the ureter. Many urologists recommend resecting the strictured portion of the ureter and reuniting it in all cases rather than the other plastic operations. No hydronephrosis nor hydro-ureter will develop above the point where this was done. To demonstrate, we have inadvertently separated a ureter from the renal pelvis while operating for stones, and reunited it, obtaining normal pyelographic findings later. Therefore, we believe that if the plastic operation referred to cannot circumvent the aberrant vessel, the ureter should be divided and reunited.

Following operation—either pyelostomy or nephrostomy—the renal pelvis or the kidney should be drained for a few days. End-results of plastic operations on the renal pelvis are often unsatisfactory because, in most cases, there has already been marked progression of the hydronephrosis. In other cases, infection persists, or the operation itself may have been improperly done. Such patients may later require nephrectomy.

URETEROCELE

This consists of a dilatation of the intramural vesical ureter; it is congenital in the vast majority of cases; occasionally acquired in the adult, it may vary considerably in size (Fig. 433). This terminal portion of the ureter dilates to become a sac which fills with urine and does not completely empty, *the result of a congenitally narrow ureteral meatus.* The wall of the ureter becomes thin

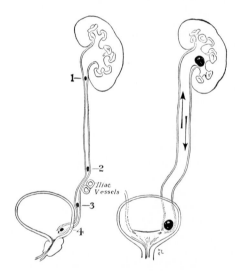

FIG. 434. (*Left*) Diagrammatic representation of most common levels at which ureteral calculi are impacted. (1) Just below ureteropelvic junction. (2) In iliac ureter. (3) In juxtavesical portion of ureter. (4) Just proximal to vesical orifice. (*Right*) Diagram to show how a calculus can migrate from the renal pelvis to the lowermost portion of the ureter and vice versa, if the ureter is dilated. (Rolnick, H. C.: The Practice of Urology, vol. 1, p. 590, Philadelphia, Lippincott)

and balloonlike. The sac is frequently infected and stones are common findings.

Some urologists also give the name of ureterocele to a small, nipplelike elevation of the meatus, but, in reality, this represents little more than a variation from the normal that is of little clinical significance.

Any one of several methods of treatment may be employed, depending somewhat on the size and the condition of the sac. Formerly, they were often treated by cystoscopic cutting and insertion of a fulgurating electrode into the ureteral meatus, followed by enlargement of the orifice and cutting of the sac. This procedure has now been almost wholly replaced by one making use of the resectoscope loop to remove the thin sac on the "roof" of the ureter to establish a wide ureteral orifice. When stones are present, they may be removed with the loop after the mucosa of the sac has been cut away. Occasionally a large stone may fall into the bladder and have to be crushed before it can be removed.

If the ureterocele is very large, especially in a child, it is best to do a *suprapubic cystotomy* and remove the sac by cutting with scissors. In *transurethral resection,* it is unwise to fulgurate, except at points of bleeding, since a stricture of the ureter may develop, with the possibility of ascending infection and hydronephrosis; if this occurs, nephrectomy may later become necessary. Except for the unusually large ureterocele, "de-roofing" with the resectoscope loop is the treatment of choice.

URETERAL CALCULUS

It is well to bear in mind that ureteral stones far more often than not will be passed spontaneously. Even if the stone, in the course of its travels, blocks the ureter completely for a time, with complete anuria of that side, the patient may suffer no permanent ill effects since the kidney has remarkable powers of taking care of itself during such temporary blockage. If there are no marked symptoms, in the known presence of a stone in the ureter with complete block, we can afford to wait for several days or even a week or more, in the hope that it will become dislodged and renal function return. If this does not happen, or if the patient has repeated colic or develops fever, operation is indicated for its removal.

There are two places in the course of the ureter which will most frequently obstruct the passage of calculi (Fig. 434). One is at the *ureteropelvic juncture,* or a few centimeters below it; the other is at the *uretero-vesical juncture* where the ureter naturally narrows. *High ureterotomy* is done for stone in the upper third of the ureter, at about the level of the third, fourth or fifth lumbar vertebra; *low ureterotomy* is employed for stone in the lower ureter. A so-called mid-ureterotomy, actually an extension of one of the other two technics, may occasionally be necessary.

High Ureterotomy. The patient is placed in the lumbar position, on his side, as for nephrectomy. An incision is made below the twelfth rib, below the region of the kidney. This should be extended downward and forward, rather than posteriorly, and should be adequate but need not be large. The peritoneum is retracted forward from the psoas muscle until the ureter is exposed. The portion of the ureter which harbors the stone should now be located so that it may be felt and removed through a small lengthwise incision.

In doing a ureterotomy, it is an error to strip the ureter from its sheath for any distance since the ureteral sheath contains most of the blood and lymph supply to the ureter; if the ureter is drawn far out, some of its blood supply may be cut off and slough may occur later.

When a marked periureteritis is found to be present, it is best to make the incision immediately above or below the inflamed area, after which the stone is gently coaxed down or up to the incision. Cutting directly into a severely or chronically inflamed ureter may result in some degree of later sloughing, with possible stricture. A necessary safeguard is to have a routine flat x-ray plate made immediately before the operation, for the stone may have moved during the interval since the previous roentgenogram, even if that were made no longer ago than the previous evening. The stone may also move *during* the operation itself, particularly if spinal anesthesia, with its marked relaxation of tissues, is being used. This is more likely to occur in the female ureter since it is usually of greater caliber than that of the male.

Whenever possible it is best not to place the patient in the Trendelenburg position at the beginning of this operation, particularly for the low approach. Rather, wait until after the ureter has been exposed.

For all ureteral operations we prefer to use the Allis forceps. One is placed on the ureter above the stone, the other below, after exposure has been made for the very important purpose of preventing the stone from moving up or down the ureter and out of the operative field. Also, to prevent the stone from moving out of the field before it is located, during the operation, one Allis forceps may be placed *below* the stone in high ureterotomy or *above* it in the low procedure.

When the stone is located close to the renal pelvis, some urologists prefer to push it up into the pelvis and remove it through a pyelotomy. If the incision is not large, the ureter need not be sutured. Instead, a Penrose drain is inserted and left in place for 6 or 7 days to permit urinary drainage. If removed sooner, urine draining from the incision in the ureter may extravasate into the retroperitoneal space.

The incision in the ureter will heal spontaneously. In rare instances, where there is marked periureteritis, it may be of assistance to insert a ureteral catheter as a splint. This will guard against later stricture formation. Even here, however, if there is adequate drainage to the outside, inflammatory processes will usually subside more readily when there is no interference from a foreign body in the lumen of the ureter. When the incision in the ureter has been large, 1 or 2 fine intestinal gut sutures may be placed, through the serosa only, on each side, and tied lightly to assure coaption of the cut edges. Deep sutures in the ureteral wall may cause obstruction and slough, with later formation of a stricture.

All incisions in the ureter for the purpose of removing stones should be made parallel with its long axis, not transverse.

Low Ureterotomy. This is a far more difficult procedure than high ureterotomy. A number of different types of incisions have been recommended as an avenue of approach to the lower ureter for removal of a stone; we have even seen the old Kraske approach employed for the purpose. In our own experience, the median suprapubic, the midrectus and the pararectus incisions have all proved to be good in some instances, while occasionally they have been extremely difficult. It seems to us that the best approach is the so-called Gibson-Pfannenstiel incision, exposing the iliac vessels, which then serve as landmarks for locating the ureter. (The greatest difficulty is usually this very problem of locating the ureter.) When the external iliac vessels have been exposed, the peritoneum is gradually retracted forward, whereupon the ureter should be found closely attached to it and crossing the iliac vessels at their bifurcation. Although the ureter, as located by this method, is almost at the junction of its lower with its middle third, and therefore well above the diagnosed position of the stone, much time may be saved through finding it quickly. From this point, very little more time is needed to follow it downward to where the stone is located. Actually, much time may be consumed with any of the recommended approaches, but the Gibson incision seems to be the fastest.

CAUTION. One frequent source of error in this operation is to mistake the obliterated hypogastric or other vessels or the vas for the ureter, since they may look and feel much the same.

In low ureterotomy, the approach is downward along the ureter, where it becomes deeply seated posterior to the bladder and close to the bowel. This area is so bounded by bony structures that there is very little room for adequate exposure, making errors frequent. Exposure may be improved somewhat by cutting the rectus muscle at its tendinous portion. In seeking the stone, it should be remembered that it is usually located lower than it appeared on the x-ray plate; it will usually be found about 3 or 4 cm. above the ureteral meatus.

When using retractors in order to improve exposure, the best type to use are Deaver retractors. These should be placed above, below and in front but *not* behind, since a posteriorly placed retractor might compress or injure the iliac vessels. The iliac artery is thick and stout, but the iliac vein is thin. Altogether, although adequate exposure can be had, it is difficult, for retractors may not be used precisely where they would be the most help.

When making the low approach, the deep epigastric vessels will be encountered, but they may usually be retracted out of the field. Only occasionally is it necessary to cut them. The same is true of the spermatic cord or round ligament; these may be retracted upward. As mentioned previously, the ureter should not be pulled out of its sheath because this may cause it to become devitalized.

In the female, the uterine artery crosses the ureter low down; in most cases, when it is necessary to approach the subvesical ureter, this must be clamped, ligated and cut. Because of the large size of this vessel, severe bleeding may follow if this is not done well. *In the male,* the artery supplying the seminal vesicle also crosses low, near the ureter, and, though not so large as the uterine artery, must be similarly handled and with the same degree of care.

Where the ureter passes under the bladder, it must be separated from the vesical fascia in order to expose it in that area. In attempting to locate and remove the stone, the portion of the ureter where it lies must be kept in view, and the stone should be felt before incising the ureter. During all this time, regardless of the patient's position on the table, an Allis forceps should be in place above the area where the stone has been located to assure that it will not slip upward again and out of the field of operation.

It is an error to cut into the ureter *above* the area where the stone is located and then to probe for it. The stone may be broken up and the fragments distributed, some getting pushed on into the bladder, others becoming imbedded in the wall of the ureter to cause continuing obstruction. A large stone may be plainly palpable before the ureter is well exposed, and it may be possible to cut down on it right then, but there is danger in this, since, working almost blindly, the surgeon may cut the ureter transversely with the chance of later development of an obstinate urinary fistula. Another method that is sometimes used but is condemned is to cut into the ureter higher up and then insert a small scoop or forceps and try to bring the stone up and out; this is most unsatisfactory and may cause severe damage.

All incisions in the ureter for whatever purpose should be longitudinal and as short as is practical. The length of an incision may be accurately regulated by placing an Allis forceps close to either side of the stone before starting to cut. No stricture will follow such an incision, no splinting catheter nor any sutures will be required, and healing will be prompt in the vast majority of cases.

In rare instances, however, and in spite of all precautions, late bleeding and some slough of the ureter may occur; this complication is self-limiting and should clear up without further sequelae. As a precaution, drains should be left in place for about a week and then removed. If the ureter has not closed by that time, the patient will continue to get wet for a few days more through the tract established for the drainage.

Tumor of the Ureter

This is an interesting subject and can merely be mentioned here. It is a well-recognized fact that papillary tumors of the renal pelvis will metastasize down the ureter and into the bladder on the affected side. Nephrectomy is practically always necessary in operating for ureteral tumors. Papillary tumors of the ureter are the most common and squamous cell tumors are the most highly malignant. It is essential to do a complete ureterectomy as well as a partial cystectomy at the same time.

Ureterectomy

When nephrectomy is being done, as mentioned in the preceding section, the kidney incision is first directed downward so as to expose as much of the ureter as may be freed from above. The kidney is removed and a suture placed in the upper end of the ureter for later identification purposes. The ureter is then separated downward as far as it can be reached. Care must be used in doing this because of its proximity to the ovarian or the spermatic vessels and to the occasionally found accessory vena cava. Injury to any of these vessels can cause severe hemorrhage.

Next, the patient is turned onto his back and a separate incision made. Two separate incisions are necessary, because further extension of the kidney incision would cut all the muscles of the abdominal wall and result in permanent weakening of that wall. Through this second incision, the ureter is approached

from below and removed in one piece, together with a portion of the trigone.

Occasionally ureterectomy is necessary for tuberculosis of the kidney, as well as for marked chronic hydronephrosis. If the large hydro-ureter which is frequently associated with hydronephrosis is not removed, it becomes a cesspool for stagnant urine, with frequent urinary reflux and pyo-ureter.

In those cases where a solitary papilloma is found in the ureter, it has been recommended that the affected portion of the ureter be excised and the ureter then reunited. However, with very few exceptions, this is unwise because these growths are seldom solitary; therefore, when they appear, ureteronephrectomy is nearly always indicated.

Injuries to the Ureter

Penetrating ureteral injuries are very rare and only a few were reported in war casualties. More common is damage resulting from surgical interventions upon neighboring structures, the uterus and ovaries, during gynecologic operations.

This usually happens at a point where the broad ligament and the uterine vessels lie close to the ureter. The ureter may be accidentally cut during difficult or complicated operations, especially if it is already markedly distorted; in which connection it should be pointed out that preliminary insertion of a ureteral catheter will not necessarily prevent accidents, even though some gynecologists recommend preliminary ureteral catheterization before all pelvic operations, particularly hysterectomy for fibroids. During simple hysterectomy, the ureter may be readily visualized, and care and experience should prevent injuries in the majority of cases.

However, accidents *do* happen occasionally, even in experienced hands, and it behooves every surgeon to know how to deal with them. If the ureter has been inadvertently ligated, and this is discovered before the completion of the procedure, the suture may be removed, usually with no resulting damage. Even if it has been cut, it can usually be reunited, unless a considerable portion of it has actual'y been removed. If there is not enough length remaining to allow reunion of the cut ends, it will be necessary either to reimplant in another portion of the bladder wall or, in extreme cases,

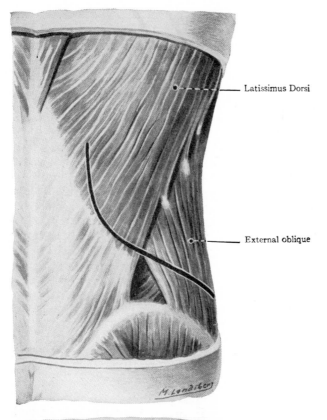

Latissimus Dorsi

External oblique

FIG. 435. First layer of muscles to be divided in lumbar approach to kidney. The incision begins at the angle between the last rib and the erector spinae muscles, passing at first vertically downward and then curving forward, dividing the latissimus dorsi and external oblique muscles almost at right angles to their fibers. (Rolnick, H. C.: The Practice of Urology, vol. 2, chap. 53, Philadelphia, Lippincott)

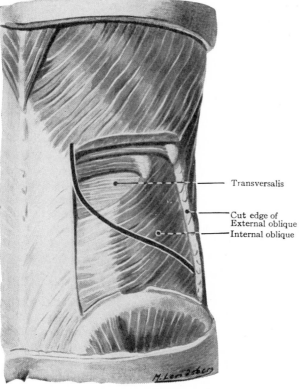

Transversalis

Cut edge of
External oblique
Internal oblique

FIG. 436. Second layer, showing relation of incision in lumbar approach to kidney and to division of internal oblique muscle. (Rolnick, H. C.: The Practice of Urology, vol. 2, chap. 53, Philadelphia, Lippincott)

to do a ureteroneocystostomy by extending a flap from the bladder wall to meet the shortened ureter.

If the accident is not discovered at the time of operation but is suspected immediately or shortly afterward because of anuria, the problem becomes one of judgment as well as action. It is wise to wait from 12 to 18 hours before becoming convinced that a mechanical stoppage exists, since *temporary* anuria may occur immediately following such operations from a variety of causes. If, however, within the first 24 hours following operation, the surgeon does become convinced that some accident has occurred, the wound should be reopened if the patient's condition permits. The urologist should insert a ureteral catheter, upward into the ureter to ascertain the point at which the injury has occurred, thus making repair possible.

If over 48 hours have already elapsed, and the anuria persists, with the cystoscope showing evidence of blockage of both ureters, bilateral nephrostomy will be the lifesaving measure. If there is evidence of urinary extravasation in the abdominal cavity, but the indications point to injury on one side only, then it is wise to do a nephrostomy on that side alone, with the attempt at repair of the ureter delayed until a later time.

In cases where the ureter has been accidentally cut, or clamped and ligated, it is sometimes recommended, because of the difficulty in some instances of repairing and restoring continuity. to tie off the ureter and do nothing further. The kidney will then cease to function, and autonephrectomy will follow. However, although this may seem to be satisfactory, sepsis, with chills and fever, often occurs, and nephrectomy then becomes necessary.

The remarkable powers of regeneration of the ureter have already been indicated. Even if it has been cut or torn nearly through, for example, at the ureteropelvic juncture, it will regenerate with little more aid than an indwelling catheter as a splint. In cases of surgical accident, a T tube may also be used with good results and need be left in place for only a week or 10 days.

URETEROVAGINAL FISTULA

This is usually the result of operative injury, as previously indicated. The patient may or may not have chills and fever, even though constantly retaining a pool of urine in the vagina.

The regenerative capacity of the ureter can come into play here also, permitting spontaneous closure of such fistulae with no aid beyond frequent cystoscopic ureteral manipulations. The catheter should be passed up the ureter to the point of obstruction and an attempt made to bypass it. It is not necessary that the catheter actually bypass the obstruction, for the manipulation will help to soften the occluding scar and permit the ureter to regenerate. However, if the fistula persists after several months of such treatment, a plastic operation should be done to reinsert the ureter into the bladder. If this too should fail, then a nephrectomy may become necessary.

THE KIDNEY AND THE ADRENAL GLAND

It is extremely important that the surgeon who undertakes to operate on the kidney and the adrenals be fully familiar with their anatomy and the peculiarities of their location. Any good standard anatomy text goes into these details far more fully than would be practical or appropriate here; to such the reader is earnestly referred.

SURGICAL APPROACH TO THE KIDNEY

The most used surgical approach to the kidney is the *lumbar incision* (Figs. 435, 436, 437), though occasionally the transperitoneal exposure is employed. As the kidney lies behind and outside the peritoneum, with the patient properly placed in lumbar position, the lumbar incision affords the best exposure for kidney surgery. The boundaries for this approach are a rhomboid defined above by the ribs, behind by the erector spinae muscle, below by the crest of the ilium and in front by the rectus muscle.

Placing the patient properly on the table is important in order to obtain as much room as possible, for this rhomboid is, at best, a limited space which must be enlarged as much as possible before starting the operation. *This point cannot be overemphasized!* If exposure is insufficient, it will be necessary to work blindly when mobilizing the kidney. This is hazardous, for an aberrant vessel may be torn in attempting to free the upper pole. If the

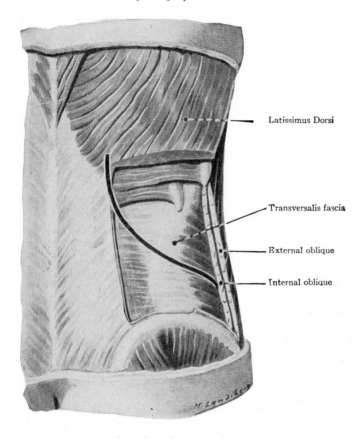

Latissimus Dorsi

Transversalis fascia

External oblique

Internal oblique

FIG. 437. Third layer, showing relation of incision for lumbar approach to kidney and to the transversalis fascia and muscle. (Rolnick, H. C.: The Practice of Urology, vol. 2, chap. 53, Philadelphia, Lippincott)

incision is too low or not wide enough, the renal pedicle is often placed under extreme tension in order to deliver the organ. However, if care is used, the ileoinguinal and ileohypogastric nerves can be safeguarded, for these nerves are usually visible when adequate exposure has been obtained and can be retracted out of the field. If these nerves are preserved and the incision is not extended too far toward the front, postoperative weakness of the abdominal wall can be avoided. Also, if the incision is high enough behind, and the kidney has been well exposed, there will be direct access to the vessels of the renal pedicle. Then, if difficulties arise and excessive bleeding occurs, these vessels are easily accessible.

At best, the area (rhomboid) gives but limited space in which to work. Turn the patient on his side, at the edge of the table, with his lumbar region over the back rest. Elevate the rest as high as possible and "break" the table. Place sandbags in front and supports under the hips, the shoulders and the head. The legs should be bent at the knee, the upper leg being kept in line with the body, and a pillow placed between them. The patient may then be maintained in this difficult position by means of a wide strip of adhesive, long enough to extend over the hips and be firmly attached around the table.

ENDOTRACHEAL ANESTHESIA

Inhalation anesthesia is the best for kidney surgery; and the patient should always be intubated, i.e., it should be administered by the endotracheal route. The endotracheal catheter is the greatest safety device that the anesthetist possesses today.

In placing the patient in the difficult lumbar position, the side on which he is lying is often markedly compressed; only when he has been intubated can the lung thus crowded be well aerated and expanded and the possibility of contralateral pulmonary atelectasis be avoided. Intubation is a most important safeguard in this respect.

CHANGES IN BLOOD PRESSURE

When the back rest is elevated, the patient's blood pressure will change, sometimes dropping considerably. An error frequently made is to elevate the rest too rapidly, which affects the blood pressure unfavorably. Proceed slowly and carefully, raising the rest gradually. This will usually permit the blood pressure to be controlled and stabilized. It is so essential that the patient be in proper position, *elevated high on the back rest*, that even if the blood pressure cannot be stabilized, we should not compromise. Only in this position will the lumbar space be large enough to give the surgeon room to work. It is the job of the anesthetist, to stabilize the pressure with the patient in this extreme lumbar position.

INCISION

The Lumbar Incision. This incision should be as high as possible while still remaining extrapleural and subdiaphragmatic, close to the twelfth rib (or above it), as far back and high up as it can be without entering the pleura. The twelfth rib is frequently resected in order to obtain more exposure. This is a free rib (i.e., not part of the chest cage), thus is readily resected or retracted downward.

The Israel-Mayo Incision. This is a muscle-cutting incision which gives more room than the older muscle-splitting Czerny or Simon incisions which gave inadequate exposure. It is transverse and curving, extending downward and forward, beginning at the costovertebral angle, at the junction of the twelfth rib with the erector spinae muscle, and extending forward to the iliac crest.

The Presman Interspace Incision. We have recently adopted an eleventh interspace incision for surgical approach to the kidney, *retracting the twelfth rib downward* instead of resecting it. When the rib is resected in order to obtain exposure, the sharp stump which remains may be in the way during the operative procedure. Postoperatively, the stump may be painful for a long time. If the rib is permitted to remain, the supports of the chest cage are much firmer and the incision can be closed more accurately. There is also very little weakness of the abdominal wall after this incision.

The Negamatsu Incision. Removing a flap of ribs, known as the "Negamatsu incision," is another device to afford more exposure of the operative field.

The chances for error in selecting the exact spot for any lumbar incision are numerous. Small incisions are inadequate and dangerous. Yet, on the other hand, it is an error to make a very large incision which almost "quarters" the patient. If it is too far forward, very little added exposure is obtained, and the patient is usually left with a weakened abdominal wall because the muscles have been cut too extensively and the nerves have usually been severed. Although adequate exposure is necessary, an inch more room high up in the back, at the costovertebral angle, is worth more than 4 inches in front. With the incisions now employed, there is more chance that the pleura occasionally may be opened, but the peritoneum is invaded far less frequently than in the past. Operation on the patient in the lumbar position can nearly always be carried out without opening the peritoneum. But, with any incision close to or about the twelfth rib, or where ribs have been removed, it is essential to safeguard the pleura. The hissing sound of air entering the pleural cavity gives warning when this accident has occurred; the breach should be closed at once. The anesthetist who has intubated the patient is of great help here, for, if necessary, he can distend the lung on the affected side, exposing the pleura so that it can be readily seen and sutured. Furthermore, with the patient intubated when the pleura is opened accidentally, collapse of the lung can be prevented.

DELIVERY OF THE KIDNEY

It is almost always necessary to mobilize the kidney and deliver it from its bed in order to do whatever may be necessary. If there is a large stone in the renal pelvis, occasionally it is possible to remove it by freeing the lower pole only, but in the majority of cases, the organ should be mobilized and delivered, for, unless this be done, there is danger of injury to the renal vessels and no control of bleeding should this occur. It is most important to *free the upper pole first* (Fig. 438). The liver or the spleen (depending on which side is being operated) is gently retracted when necessary. Avoid the error of mistaking the spleen for the kidney; this may happen if exposure

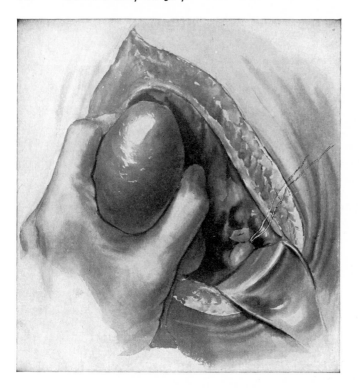

FIG. 438. Search for upper polar vessels before complete mobilization of kidney is attempted. The lower polar vessels are first sought for and then the upper pole is retracted, as shown here, while one palpates for polar vessels. (Rolnick, H. C.: The Practice of Urology, vol. 2, p. 1158, Philadelphia, Lippincott)

is a little far forward on the left side and the peritoneum has been entered.

In order to expose the kidney, the peritoneum is retracted forward and the perirenal fat exposed and entered. A line of cleavage is then readily obtained within the fatty capsule and the upper pole of the kidney freed with an upward sweep of the finger. Begin on the posterior surface of the kidney and work upward toward the upper pole, thus avoiding the vessels, as these are nearly always on the anterior surface. Even if the upper pole is deep and high up, it can be freed under vision if the incision has been adequate and with good retraction.

When the upper pole has been freed, the hand should sweep around and downward posteriorly, freeing the lower pole. If the fascia of the upper and lower poles is firm, scissors may be used. After the lower pole has been exposed, the ureter can readily be found with a little farther downward posterior exposure. When the ureter has been located, it is separated from the fascia and fat and grasped with an Allis forceps, then freed upward to the renal pelvis. With both upper and lower poles free, the hand can sweep around forward and release the kidney from bowel and peritoneum.

Finally, the renal vessels are approached and all loose fat and fascia freed. The kidney is now movable and may be freely delivered into the wound. "Gentleness in the handling of tissues with dispatch is the mark of the surgeon."

The right kidney has a slightly shorter vascular pedicle than the left, but, for practical purposes, this is not important if exposure has been adequate. The kidney should not be under tension when it has been delivered. It is not necessary to work against time; if delivery is managed properly, whatever is necessary may be done with "dispatch." With experience and the necessary "sense of feel," the difference between adhesions and vessels can practically always be recognized. Scissors may be used for cutting dense adhesions, but vessels must be safeguarded. Aberrant vessels are usually found at the upper pole and are often hard to see. Here, as elsewhere throughout surgery, the surgeon "who has a sense of feel of live tissue" usually has little difficulty. Generally speaking, this "sense of feel" makes for a surgeon; skill in cutting, clamping and ligating is secondary.

During exposure of the upper pole of the kidney, the adrenal is usually separated from it without difficulty. However, occasionally all or a portion of the adrenal may be removed accidentally when doing a nephrectomy. This may happen when there is marked perinephritis, or when a large tumor is being removed together with its perirenal fat. No untoward reaction occurs with either partial or total adrenalectomy under these conditions, and no adrenal shock will follow. Under normal conditions, the remaining adrenal will supply all physiologic needs.

ADRENAL SHOCK

Adrenal shock may occur when adrenalectomy is done for *Cushing's syndrome* or for removal of a pheochromocytoma. It is necessary that these patients be adequately prepared before surgery and that supportive measures be carried out during and immediately after the operation. In cases of Cushing's syndrome, cortisone and ACTH will tide the patient over; in those with pheochromocytoma, benzodioxane, Dibenamine and Regitine may be employed. When there is disturbance of adrenal function with pathologic hypersecretion of one adrenal, as it occurs in these conditions, the remaining adrenal ceases to function. If adrenalectomy is performed for relief, and no supportive measures are instituted, the patient will go into shock because of marked hypotension. The remaining gland, which has been dormant, will resume physiologic activity, but this usually does not occur until a period of 24 to 48 hours has elapsed after the operation, during which time the patient must have supportive treatment.

DANGER OF BOWEL DAMAGE

When the pleura has been opened, this must be recognized and closed immediately; but if it is the peritoneum that is invaded, this *can wait* until after the nephrectomy has been completed. There is special danger of injury to the bowel in secondary operations and where marked perinephritis is present. In doing a nephrectomy, there is possibility of damage when the peritoneum and the bowel have not been well freed anteriorly and retracted out of the field before placing clamps on the renal pedicle. Therefore, the clamps must be placed on the pedicle under vision and with their ends free. If the ascending or the descending colon has been injured by the clamp, a fecal fistula may develop later, but this will usually close spontaneously within

a relatively short period of time. Injury can occur to the duodenum, which, on the right side, is very close to the kidney. This is a serious complication, because a duodenal fistula often causes fatal tissue necrosis.

NEPHRECTOMY

When the kidney has been delivered, the ureter is freed downward as far as possible, then clamped, cut and ligated. The portion of the ureter remaining is transfixed, and the upper part, where it is attached to the pelvis, is ligated; the ureter and the pelvis are held upward out of the way so that clamps may be placed on the renal vessels only. The spermatic or ovarian vessels accompany the ureter or lie very close to it. When separating the ureter downward, these vessels may be torn, with resultant severe bleeding.

The safest means of controlling vessels when doing a nephrectomy is the two-clamp method (Figs. 439 and 440). The $7\frac{1}{4}$-inch, slightly curved Carmalt clamps are the most satisfactory, for they will not slip. The lower clamp is applied first, as far down as possible without clamping the vena cava; the upper clamp is applied almost directly above it. It is best to place the clamps on the renal vessels from the upper posterior angle of the wound with points extending anterior beyond the vessels. In order to do this, the upper angle of the skin-and-muscle incision behind should be high enough to give room to apply the clamps at this point. The fat and fascia surrounding the vessels should be freed as much as possible so that the renal pedicle contains only the vessels. This is not always possible but is the ideal to be sought. With good anterior retraction, the points of both clamps can be well exposed; the kidney is then removed with a sharp knife, leaving about $\frac{1}{4}$ inch of the pedicle above the upper clamp. If a tumor or a marked infection is involved—as in tuberculosis—a third clamp may be placed above the second (upper) so that when the kidney is cut off, there will then be no "spill" back into the wound. Under other conditions, the extra clamp may simply be in the way. In any case, the clamps should be held firmly by an assistant, but with no tension on the pedicle.

A doubled No. 2 chromic catgut ligature full length is then placed below the lowest clamp and tied firmly, but without "sawing" against the clamp (which might weaken the

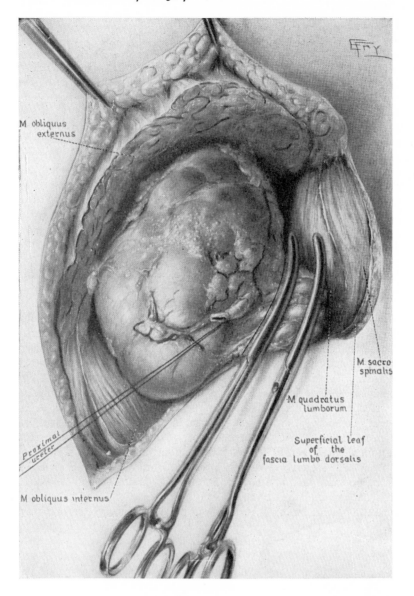

M obliquus
externus

M sacro
spinalis

M quadratus
lumborum

Proximal
ureter

Superficial leaf
of the
fascia lumbo dorsalis

M obliquus internus

Fig. 439. The W. J. Mayo two-clamp method of nephrectomy. See Figure 440 for details of application. (Rolnick, H. C.: The Practice of Urology, vol. 2, chap. 53, Philadelphia, Lippincott)

gut). When the ligature has been firmly applied, the lower clamp is first gently loosened, then gradually removed. The opening and removal of the clamp by the assistant should be done with one hand only. Following this, a similar No. 2 chromic catgut is used as a transfixion suture immediately below the upper clamp and ligature. This clamp is then also slowly loosened and removed. In this manner, proper hemostasis will be obtained.

If aberrant vessels are present, they should be separately clamped, severed and ligated before clamps are applied to the main vessels.

Occasionally, when there is marked peripyelitis and induration of the pedicle, massive clamping of the ureter and the vessels will be needed. It is rarely necessary to use the very large curved, semilunar kidney-pedicle clamp (9¼-inch Herrick clamp), for this is much too long and cumbersome. It is often difficult to apply and must be used blindly; the control that it gives may not be adequate. Sometimes the clamps may be applied, beginning at the lower anterior angle of the wound and extending upward and backward, but it is preferable to place them from the posterior angle, for it is much easier to ligate the pedicle with the points of the clamps free and visible. It is not good to cross the clamps in the two-clamp method by placing one from the upper angle behind and the other from the anterior angle, for then it is difficult to ligate the pedicle securely.

Some surgeons like to use a "safety" ligature before placing a clamp on the pedicle. However, what appears to be a safety device is often actually an added encumbrance, for the clamps frequently cover this ligature and loosen it. Therefore, it is in the way and, when further ligation is done, all the ligatures may slip and the pedicle may be "lost," with marked resultant bleeding.

Injury to the Renal Pedicle

Injury to the renal vessels may occur when doing simple pyelotomy. This is an unfortunate mishap, for nephrectomy may then be necessary. Injury to the vessels may occur when the pelvis is anterior and the vessels posterior. Occasionally the vessels cover the pelvis, and it is then difficult to do a pyelotomy at all. When a nephrectomy is not planned, and a large aberrant vessel has been torn at either upper or lower pole in attempting to deliver the kidney, the vessel should be clamped and ligated immediately. If considerable kidney tissue is compromised by this loss of blood supply, nephrectomy may then become necessary.

When doing a nephrectomy, the main vessels may be torn if they have been placed under too much tension or if clamps have been applied roughly and blindly. Not all of the pedicle may be incorporated in the clamp if it is applied blindly. When this occurs, the kidney will usually become blue, hard and tense, for the artery is frequently what is missed. No harm will result if the surgeon reapplies the clamp incorporating the whole pedicle. When vessels are injured or not ligated properly, this may be a major surgical mishap, for massive bleeding may immediately ensue, requiring prompt, often heroic, action. This is a situation where the surgeon must remain cool, for the patient can *bleed to death very rapidly*.

With proper exposure, the pedicle is always within reach and bleeding may be controlled. A sponge or a finger should be applied immediately with some pressure over the bleeding points. The vessels can then usually be seen and a clamp applied. *Never clamp blindly*, for the bowel or the vena cava can thus be injured. If some exposure can be had after the pedicle has been "lost," clamps can usually be reapplied and the vessels then carefully and securely ligated. Occasionally, after having apparently tied the pedicle securely, one vessel may slip away from the suture and bleeding may appear, but the source of it can usually be located, the clamp (or clamps) reapplied and the vessel ligated.

In doing a nephrectomy, particularly for calculus pyonephrosis, where adhesions are

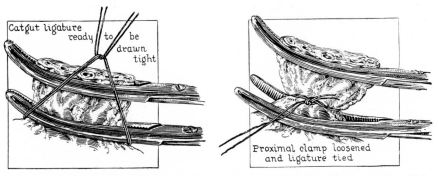

Fig. 440. Two-clamp method of W. J. Mayo for ligation of the renal pedicle. (*Left*) An en-masse ligature is applied between the proximal clamp and the large abdominal vessels. (*Right*) The proximal clamp is being loosened and withdrawn while the first ligature is tightened. Another ligature is next applied en masse before the second clamp is removed. (Rolnick, H. C.: The Practice of Urology, vol. 2, chap. 53, Philadelphia, Lippincott)

marked and where there is considerable indurated peripelvic fat, it may be difficult to apply the clamp securely to the renal pedicle. It is then necessary to incorporate a considerable amount of tissue to permit firm application of the clamp. A transfixion suture below the upper clamp is particularly important for proper hemostasis. Occasionally it may be necessary to place a transfixion suture under the lower clamp, but *this is somewhat dangerous, for bleeding may follow transfixion of large vessels.*

Occasionally it may be necessary to do a subcapsular nephrectomy in calculus pyonephrosis, when the fatty capsule and the peripelvic fat are thick and where it is difficult to mobilize the kidney without leaving some of the pelvis behind.

In advanced cases, where the patient has had perinephritic abscess or fistula, it may be necessary to do a *morcellement,* removing piecemeal as much of the renal tissue as possible, then ligating the pedicle. It is fortunate that in these cases the vessels are usually markedly sclerosed and occasionally already thrombosed. In long-standing calculus pyonephrosis with fistula, we have removed necrotic kidney tissue without even applying a ligature.

Sometimes the pedicle may be very short, and a portion of the vena cava may be incorporated in the clamp. It may not be possible to apply a ligature because it will usually slip off the torn vena cava. When the pedicle has been "lost" and clamps reapplied and bleeding controlled, it still may not be possible to ligate the pedicle because the ends of the clamps may be buried so that they cannot be visualized. If it is not possible to apply a ligature, the clamps must be left in place for a period of 3 to 4 days. This results in a very trying situation for both patient and surgeon; the patient must lie constantly on one side in a very difficult position and with very little movement. The clamps must be supported and tied together on the outside and gauze packing placed in the wound. There is always the danger that if the clamps are disturbed the vessels may be torn or eroded.

When the patient is brought back to the operating room, the clamps are first opened and left in situ for a period of 4 to 6 hours, with no attempt to withdraw them. This is in order to permit the clamped vessels to retract from the teeth of the clamp.

Clamps should never be left longer than 4 days, for secondary bleeding, due to erosion of the vessels, may occur. Fortunately, it is rarely necessary to leave clamps in place after this type of operation.

If the pedicle is "lost" and severe bleeding follows, and it is not found possible to expose and locate the bleeding vessels in order to apply clamps, then recourse should be had to *packing.* Two or 3 large 4-inch 5-yard gauze packs are applied rapidly, by inserting the packs upward, backward, then somewhat forward against the pedicle. This will control bleeding in practically all cases when serious difficulties of this kind have arisen. We have had experience on a few occasions with a "lost" renal pedicle but have always been able to control bleeding with packing. It is well to remember that when serious bleeding occurs in urologic surgery, whether this be from the renal pedicle, the iliac vein or even, as may sometimes happen, the vena cava (also, otherwise uncontrollable bleeding from the *prostatic bed*), packing can be resorted to successfully. It is always well to have a 5-yard roll of gauze open on the table and ready for use should trouble be encountered during any nephrectomy, for there is always the possibility of such severe bleeding.

A gauze pack, when used in this way, should be left in place for a week to 10 days. It may be loosened gradually but should not be removed entirely until at least 8 days have elapsed. Final removal should be done in the operating room, for bleeding may recur if the clot in the vessel is dislodged; this is more likely to happen if the packing is removed too early.

CLOSURE OF THE LUMBAR INCISION

The lumbar incision should be carefully closed in layers. Closure of all three layers of muscle at one time, in a massive ligature with interrupted sutures, is *not recommended.* Too much tissue is thus incorporated into the ligatures and they may not hold; the result is wound separation and hernia. Therefore, it is necessary to close the muscles in layers. The kidney bed is drained with Penrose drains, which should be left in place at the upper angle of the wound for a period of 5 to 7 days.

TRANSPERITONEAL NEPHRECTOMY

This approach is being used more frequently now that danger from infection has been so much reduced. Also, the urologist is now better trained in general surgery and does not hesitate to work in the peritoneal cavity. Ureteral transplantation is done transperitoneally. An ectopic kidney is usually best approached by this route; a low-lying ectopic kidney should always be approached through the abdomen. Thus, when a patient has both biliary and renal calculi on the right side, the gallstones may be removed first, then the posterior peritoneum opened and the kidney stones taken out through the same incision.

In operating on the adrenals, when exploration of the abdomen must be done, the transperitoneal approach may be necessary in order to examine the ovaries and search for aberrant renal structures. Some surgeons routinely perform a transperitoneal adrenalectomy, although the adrenals are located high up and are difficult to reach through the abdomen. However, the value of transperitoneal exposure is that both the adrenals and the abdomen may be explored through the one incision. Also, when doing *nephrectomy for tumor*, direct access may be had to the renal vessels. However, the vessels are usually high and posterior, and it is frequently difficult to approach them immediately. Ligation of the renal vessels before delivering the kidney is the ideal procedure when operating for tumor. In most cases, however, the lower pole must be delivered first, then the ureter found, cut and ligated and the vessels approached from below upward as well as from above. When a nephrectomy has been completed, the posterior peritoneum should be closed, if possible, and the renal bed drained through a stab wound in the flank. The parietal peritoneum and the abdominal wall are closed without drainage.

The *chief benefit to the patient* in the abdominal approach to the kidney is that he lies flat on the table, thus greatly reducing the chance of shock. The difficult position needed for the lumbar approach can thus be avoided; some patients, particularly the aged, have a "fixed spine," so that it may be difficult to bend ("break") them into the lumbar position.

The short, muscular or overweight individual presents many obstacles to kidney surgery. A large abdomen interferes with the transperitoneal approach. When such a patient is placed on his side to be "broken" for the lumbar approach, the space between the ribs and the iliac crest is so small that it is hard to obtain proper exposure. Also, he frequently slides off the back rest. For the obese individual who is not muscular and not too short, the lumbar approach is preferable, since, when placed on his side, the loose, fatty, protuberant abdomen falls downward and forward, so that the lumbar space is actually considerably enlarged and more exposed.

Therefore, to sum up, although transperitoneal nephrectomy is done more frequently today than in the past, and is the routine approach for kidney tumors in the young, this operation should be only an occasional procedure in other situations. Lumbar nephrectomy or the lumbar approach to the kidney is better in the majority of cases.

The abdominal incision for transperitoneal nephrectomy should be either pararectus or midrectus, extending from the ribs downward to below the level of the umbilicus. Usually only a longitudinal incision is necessary; added transverse T or L incisions rarely help. After the peritoneum has been entered, the mesocolon is located and the large bowel is retracted anteriorly and mesially. The posterior peritoneum is then entered and the kidney exposed and mobilized.

TRANSTHORACIC NEPHRECTOMY

The thoraco-abdominal approach to the upper portion of the abdomen and the kidney was first done during World War II (Harper) for extensive injuries to the chest and the abdomen. Many of the surgeons who had had experience near the front lines often operated through the chest and diaphragm in approaching the abdominal organs. The kidney and the spleen can be readily removed in this manner. However, as a *planned approach* for the removal of even large kidney tumors (Chute) it is rarely indicated (Robinson). We have never done a nephrectomy through the chest but in the past have had the experience, when doing an adrenalectomy, of accidentally open-

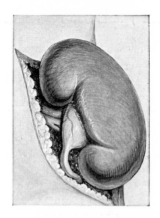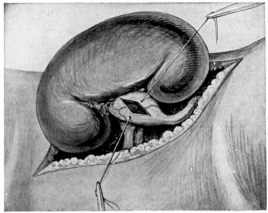

FIG. 441. (*Left*) First step of technic of ordinary posterior pyelotomy. The kidney has been drawn into abdominal incision, laid on its ventral surface and posterior aspect of the renal pelvis exposed. Note avascularity of this surface. (*Right*) Second step of the technic of ordinary posterior pyelotomy. The two traction sutures of fine catgut have been inserted, and the edges of the pyelotomy incision are retracted. (Rolnick, H. C.: The Practice of Urology, vol. 2, p. 1159, Philadelphia, Lippincott)

ing the pleura. The transthoracic operation still presents some hazards. Pneumonitis and collapse of the lung are frequent aftermaths of exposure of the pleura and cutting into the diaphragm.

It is recommended that the transthoracic approach to the kidney be done in cases of marked kyphosis, scoliosis or other severe deformities of the spine and the chest in which the lumbar space appears to be completely covered by ribs. The author can recall three instances of markedly deformed individuals in whom extrapleural resection of the twelfth rib, or the eleventh and twelfth ribs, made it possible to do a nephrectomy without difficulty through the simple lumbar subdiaphragmatic extrapleural and extraperitoneal approach.

PYELOTOMY

This is probably the most difficult of renal operations because the kidney often cannot be delivered well enough to expose its pelvis (Fig. 441). Pyelotomy should never be done blindly, for the vessels are readily injured, so that an operation intended only for the removal of a stone may develop into a hazardous emergency procedure including removal of the kidney. Pyelotomy (cutting in the renal pelvis) is usually done for removal of stones from the pelvis or the calyces.

If the pelvis is large and the renal pedicle long, pyelotomy does not present much difficulty, since the kidney can easily be delivered and the structures readily be identified. However, if the pelvis is small and the renal pedicle short, particularly if there be also an aberrant vessel to the upper or lower pole, exposure of the pelvis may present problems. When these conditions are found, i.e., when the little finger cannot be inserted into the renal pelvis, it is wiser not to persist in attempting to remove the stone by pyelotomy. Furthermore, in endeavoring to enlarge the pelvis, where it is practically entirely intrarenal, the ureter and the pelvis may be considerably torn. In the majority of cases, however, the renal pelvis is of moderate size and only partially intrarenal. When the pelvis is small and somewhat intrarenal, it may be exposed by dissecting upward into the hilus. A small blunt hilus retractor is of assistance here in exposing the pelvis, even when it is largely intrarenal.

The pelvis must be well exposed and under vision at all times. It is frequently supplied with an abundant covering of fat, and in the presence of a stone, there is often marked peripyelitis with induration of this perirenal fat, which must be dissected off. The pelvis is supplied with one or two small peripelvic vessels which, though usually of no importance, occasionally bleed considerably, requiring ligation.

The renal vessels enter the kidney on its anterior aspect and lie rather high up, approaching it from above. The pelvis is usually posterior and inferior to the renal vessels and extends downward to become the ureter. Therefore, in most cases, the renal pelvis can be approached safely from the posterior surface of the kidney. Occasionally the vessels cover either the lower or the upper border of the pelvis and therefore must be carefully safeguarded. Sometimes the vessels may cross over the pelvis; approach is then difficult, for they must be retracted before the pelvis can be opened.

Posterior Pyelotomy

The pelvis usually must be approached from the posterior surface, but sometimes it lies toward the front with its vessels behind it. In this situation, the pelvis must be approached from the anterior surface of the kidney. Variations constantly occur in regard to the insertion of the vessels.

When doing pyelotomy the kidney may be lifted out of its bed and brought up, but frequently it is difficult to approach the pelvis unless the kidney is rotated somewhat, with the lower pole brought upward and outward, higher than the upper pole. Occasionally, after the kidney has been delivered, the upper pole can be pushed downward, deep into the wound, with only the lower pole high up and rotated, in order to expose the pelvis. If it is not possible thus to rotate the kidney posteriorly, the pelvis may be approached from its inferior angle.

In the majority of cases it is best to locate the upper ureter and follow it gradually upward, freeing the pelvis up to its hilus. This is the safest and best way of exposing it. Even though the kidney is rotated and its lower pole finally lifted upward in order to expose the pelvis, the kidney should always be completely mobilized, for then and then only can one have complete control of both the kidney and its pedicle.

The incision in the pelvis may be extended upward to the hilus. It is an error to extend it far downward, for that gives but little room, and unnecessary cutting and tearing of the ureter may ensue. The little finger is inserted in the renal pelvis in search of the stone if it cannot be immediately located. It may be hard to enter the calyces of the kidney because the infundibula are always very narrow. Explore carefully and do not give up too readily when there is trouble in locating the stone.

A stone or stones which have been in the renal pelvis may fall out into the wound with the first gush of escaping urine; watch for this and do not make the error of continuing to explore the renal pelvis when the stone has already come out. Sometimes the stone may actually be on a sponge that has been discarded. In palpating for a stone, the thickened endothelium of the irregular calyces and infundibula will feel hard and may be mistaken for a stone by the inexperienced. Various types of stone forceps are recommended for removing stones through a pyelotomy. These curved instruments are of help but must necessarily be inserted blindly. When the stone has been loosened, an Allis forceps or even a small curved forceps is just as useful. With the finger in place, if the stone is wedged tightly in one of the calyces, it is much better to do a combined pyelotomy and nephrotomy directly over the stone. This does less damage than attempting to extract a fixed stone through the pyelotomy incision.

When the stone in the renal pelvis is large, the incision may be lengthened upward toward the hilus and into the renal parenchyma. Relatively large stones can be removed in this manner through an enlarged pyelotomy or pyelonephrotomy, for serious tears of the renal parenchyma, as well as injury to the vessels, may follow forceful attempts at extraction of a large stone unless this precaution is observed.

Nephrotomy

When a renal calculus is embedded in the calyx or is so situated that it cannot be approached through the renal pelvis, either because the pelvis is intrarenal or because the stone is too large, it should then be removed through a nephrotomy incision. The usual incision in nephrotomy is on the convexity of the kidney (the so-called avascular area). However, if the stone can be felt and has been well localized by roentgenography, a small incision should be made directly over it, a forceps inserted and the stone removed.

When the incision in the kidney is not large, bleeding can be controlled by manual compression. However, if the stone is large, a wide nephrotomy is necessary, and it is best to place a rubberized intestinal clamp on the renal pedicle to control the bleeding. This then becomes a bloodless procedure, and, if done with dispatch, little damage to the kidney results from the temporary stoppage of its blood supply; the total time should not exceed 15 or 20 minutes. During this period the clamp may be loosened at intervals to maintain some degree of circulation.

The procedure known as "needling the kidney" to locate a securely hidden stone, we have found of small value. A clear x-ray plate in full view during the operation is much to be preferred. This is still true, even if additional plates have to be made while surgery is in progress. However, it must be remembered that some 10 or 15 per cent of renal calculi are radiolucent, in which case, if all else fails, it may be necessary to enlarge the incision to a complete nephrotomy. With the pedicle clamped, careful search will then nearly always reveal the stone.

If stones are soft and break up during removal, it is wise to irrigate the kidney with the nephrotomy wound still wide open, for if stones or pieces of any appreciable size are left behind, symptoms may be markedly aggravated, with secondary infection and bleeding, making nephrectomy necessary later. However, if there is one large stone and other very small ones, and if the large one can be removed without difficulty but the very small ones are hard to locate, it is sometimes best not to search for the little ones at all, especially if they appear to be located in the tips of the calyces. With the large stone out of the way and the obstruction removed, the chances are that in time the small stones will pass of themselves.

Roentgenograms as Safeguards. When doing renal surgery, roentgenograms should always be in the room, in the shadow box and visible at all times. It is necessary to check on the organs themselves, the records and the roentgenograms to be sure that the operation *is being done on the diseased kidney*. It is not superfluous to mention that it is essential to make certain that the patient *has another normally functioning kidney*; this fatal omission *has* occurred.

Occasionally it is necessary to make important decisions at the operating table. The patient may have stones on both sides, one side giving more trouble than the other. Considerable infection may also be present. If the renal parenchyma is thin and functions poorly, nephrectomy should be done on the "poor" side, even though the patient is known to be a "stone former." However, if there is considerable sound parenchyma still present, it is best to do only a nephrotomy to remove the stones. Nephrostomy drainage and antibiotics should control the infection.

In this connection we might mention a case of our own in which nephrectomy was done for tumor, where the "good" kidney was functioning fairly well but was small and somewhat hypoplastic. This patient recovered in a sense but was never really well afterward, for, although it is true that not more than one fourth of the kidney substance is needed to sustain life, it is skirting an extremely narrow margin of safety to depend on a single kidney if it is abnormally small.

NEPHROSTOMY

This operation consists of incision and drainage of the kidney. When nephrotomy has been done for removal of stone, the incision is usually closed unless marked infection is present. In order to obtain drainage, it is best to incise the renal pelvis to permit escape of blood from within the kidney. The amount of bleeding may be enough to form a clot, blocking the ureter unless this is done after nephrotomy. A small Mallecot or Pezzer catheter is the best type for nephrostomy. When the wound is closed, the nephrostomy tube should make its exit at the lower anterior angle of the wound in order to permit the patient to lie flat and also to keep the tube from kinking.

Bilateral emergency nephrostomy can be done under local infiltration anesthesia through a muscle-splitting incision. Kidneys whose ureters have been ligated are under marked tension. The lower pole can be readily exposed and incised and the catheter inserted into the renal pelvis. In most cases, however, when doing nephrostomy, it is best to deliver the kidney if the patient is not too ill. The renal pelvis should be opened, a forceps inserted into the renal parenchyma and a mushroom catheter brought into the incision through the renal parenchyma and drawn into the renal pelvis. This is necessary if the pelvis and calyces are irregular, in which case it is often difficult to find the pelvis through a simple nephrotomy incision. In plastic operations at the ureteropelvic juncture, nephrostomy or pyelostomy is needed for drainage.

Patients with advanced carcinoma of the uterus or the prostate who have developed hydronephrosis due to ureteral obstruction may be kept alive a little longer by bilateral nephrostomy. However, incrustations may form within the nephrostomy tube which, therefore, should be changed as often as necessary.

Occasionally permanent bilateral nephrostomy is necessary in order to sustain life, particularly in children who have suffered considerable damage from congenital obstruction at the bladder neck. We have had a few patients who have carried on for a long time with a permanent nephrostomy on a solitary kidney. One patient who had bilateral hydronephrosis due to congenital ureteropelvic obstruction required nephrectomy and permanent nephrostomy on the other side. After this nephrostomy had been in place for a year, the patient insisted on having the tube out because she wanted to be able to urinate normally. Unfortunately, the bladder had become markedly contracted from disuse and could no longer function as a reservoir.

Heminephrectomy

This is a difficult procedure, as the blood supply of the kidney normally varies considerably from one individual to another. In attempting to do a partial nephrectomy at one or the other pole of the kidney, the blood supply of the entire organ may be compromised. A so-called heminephrectomy is done in most cases on patients with double kidneys in which only the upper calyx is involved. In doing heminephrectomy, a wedge-shaped area is cut out from either pole of the kidney, the remaining portion being later carefully secured with reinforced mattress sutures covered with fat or muscle to control bleeding.

Resection of a Solitary Cyst of the Kidney

This should be a simple procedure. When a solitary cyst is found at operation, the thin cyst wall is incised and the fluid aspirated.

Only the portion of the wall which protrudes outward from the kidney should be excised; nothing further need be done, and no bleeding will be encountered. However, if the incision is carried close to the renal parenchyma, bleeding may result and require suture. It is not necessary to peel off the portion of the cyst wall which is attached to the kidney, for when this is done considerable bleeding may follow. Neither is it necessary to cauterize or carbolize the floor of the cyst. It should not recur if the roof has been removed.

Kidney Biopsy

When the kidney has been exposed during operation, cutting out a small portion of the parenchyma with scissors or knife for biopsy is a minor procedure and requires only the precaution of suturing the cut area. Such samples may be of some value.

When biopsy is done alone as a diagnostic procedure, the sample is obtained through the skin with a needle. This method has comparatively little real value; since it may be dangerous, it should be avoided.

Adrenalectomy

Operations on the adrenals are best done via the lumbar approach. The incision is made a little higher than that for the kidney. Occasionally the eleventh rib must be resected in order to obtain adequate exposure. The right side is more difficult to get at than the left because of its intimate relationship to the vena cava. Bilateral simultaneous approach to the adrenals can be had with the patient flat on his abdomen and the table "broken." This is the operation recommended by Young; but, in our experience, it is not as satisfactory as the lumbar approach. If both sides require operation, the patient may be turned to the opposite lumbar position quite readily.

Surgical Aspects of Renal Anomalies

Anomalies of the kidneys, per se, do not require surgery. It is only when they become infected, or otherwise fail to function properly, that they require surgical intervention, and then the only additional problems are those which may be directly due to their unusual character or position and, quite often, to attendant oddities in blood supply or appendages. If they lie unusually low, they may

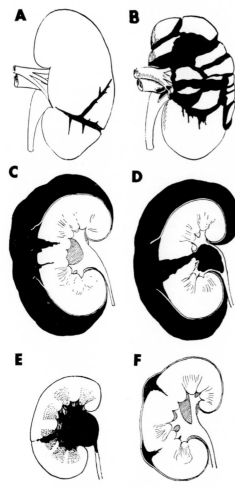

FIG. 442. Diagrammatic representation of the various degrees of injury of kidney. (Papin.) (A) Fissured rupture involving only lower pole. (B) Almost complete destruction of kidney, involving large vessels at pedicle. (C) Small laceration of cortex but large perinephritic hematoma. (D) Same as C, but extending into renal pelvis. (E) Marked accumulation of blood in pelvis from relatively slight injury of parenchyma. (F) Subcapsular tears with localized hematoma. (Rolnick, H. C.: The Practice of Urology, vol. 2, chap. 32, Philadelphia, Lippincott)

sometimes be approached more easily by the transperitoneal route.

INJURIES TO THE KIDNEY

Pyelographic Injuries. In retrograde pyelography, the catheter which is inserted into the renal pelvis may penetrate the parenchyma. This occurs much more often than is generally realized. When too much of the pyelographic medium is injected, it may produce a tear into the renal parenchyma and result in extravasation of the medium. So-called pyelovenous backflow will also occur. These patients may have considerable pain and show bloody urine, together with fever, lasting several days. Usually nothing further happens and the kidney recovers.

Penetrating Injuries. These include stab and bullet wounds which perforate the kidney, and extensive war wounds. When the kidney has been severely damaged, it must be removed, even if the status of the uninjured side cannot be ascertained. Experience during World War II by surgeons at the front, where severe injuries of various organs occurred, showed that the spleen as well as the kidney could be removed through a chest incision. Stab wounds of the kidney, if they are not extensive, like surgical wounds, will heal practically spontaneously.

Subparietal or Nonpenetrating Renal Injuries. These result from falls or blows to the kidney region without open injury to the skin. The mechanism of these injuries is similar to the *contra coupe* in the skull (i.e., an indirect blow to a viscus). The injury may be either of a mild degree, consisting of subcapsular contusions of the parenchyma or superficial tears, or transcapular injury with severe "fracture" of the kidney (see Fig. 442). Aside from the immediate shock resulting from the injury, the one definite finding is that of *hematuria*.

If the injury does not appear to be severe and no hematoma develops in the flank (the patient being kept at complete bed rest), the hematuria will cease in a few days and there will be complete recovery. The majority of such injuries can be treated conservatively and without surgery.

Intravenous pyelography is of assistance in establishing early diagnosis, for function of the kidney is markedly interfered with during the first 24 to 48 hours. Either no secretion is seen, or a "spill" from extravasation due to the injury will be noted. We do not advise retrograde pyelography, for it may promote bleeding and infection and is not helpful in making a diagnosis.

If bleeding persists, and a hematoma develops in the flank, open operation should be resorted to, for in most instances injury will turn out to have been severe and nephrectomy will be necessary.

Tumors of the Kidney

Nephrectomy is indicated in practically all cases of neoplasm of the kidney. If the involvement is not marked and the kidney is movable, removal should not present any special problems. However, if the growth is large, greatly distended veins are usually found on its surface, and much bleeding may follow attempts at mobilization and delivery of the kidney. Incisions should be wide and adequate, and the kidney, together with its fatty capsule, should be removed completely. These operations can be very bloody; therefore, they should be carried out as speedily as possible.

When the growth is in the upper pole and is somewhat adherent, it is often difficult to separate the kidney from the diaphragm. The transperitoneal approach is often valuable in this situation, as it helps eliminate spreading of the tumor cells. Transthoracic and other types of enlarged incisions are also sometimes recommended for removal of *large* kidney tumors.

In Wilms's tumor and other growths in the kidneys of young children, nephrectomy should be done as soon as they are diagnosed, even though it might appear that the operation could be done more easily after preliminary irradiation had somewhat reduced their size. While it is true that they do shrink rapidly under irradiation, it is an error to delay because of the likelihood that some of the tumor cells may be "squeezed" into the circulation.

The transperitoneal approach is preferred. Wherever possible the vessels should be approached from immediately above before attempting to mobilize and remove the kidney. This again is to prevent scattering of the tumor cells. Manipulation should be avoided as far as possible for the same reasons.

Large series of cases indicate that these young patients tolerate these operations well, and, where excision is followed by extensive x-ray therapy, an encouraging proportion recover fully and show no recurrence, *provided* that there have been early diagnosis and prompt intervention.

Papillary Tumors of the Renal Pelvis. Since these are apt to be of small size, they are often difficult to diagnose. When of appreciable size, they show a filling defect in the renal pelvis, or they may produce a negative shadow which could be mistaken for a radiolucent stone. As this type of tumor metastasizes along the course of the ureter and into the bladder, it is necessary to do a complete nephro-ureterectomy and even to remove a portion of the trigone. This entire procedure should be done at one time through two incisions, rather than to delay the ureterectomy until a later time.

Squamous Cell Carcinoma of the Renal Pelvis. This type of neoplasm is *highly malignant*. Diagnostically, the kidney will feel hard; at the time of operation, the pedicle will be found to be infiltrated, though the kidney itself will not be much enlarged as a rule. Prognosis is poor.

Occasionally this type of carcinoma will develop in the patient who has had a longstanding "silent" coral calculus of the kidney.

Nephro-ureterectomy

This procedure has been mentioned earlier; here we only wish to add that when a ureteral tumor is suspected, the ureter *must always be approached first* to determine whether or not such a tumor is actually present. Naturally, if it is not, the nephro-ureterectomy would be entirely unnecessary. In many such cases the "tumor" turns out to be a granuloma or a radiolucent stone. If an infiltrating tumor really is present, then the kidney can be removed secondarily. Or, as indicated above, if a papillary tumor of the renal pelvis is found, then the ureter should be removed for its entire length to prevent later metastasis.

22 Gynecologic Surgery

Failures in gynecologic surgery result from ignorance of the general principles of surgical procedure as well as from lack of knowledge of the physiology and the anatomy of the female pelvis. A surgeon who specializes in gynecology should be prepared to handle intestinal surgery as well, for he frequently meets with problems involving the intestinal tract.

GENERAL CONSIDERATIONS

Knowledge of the anatomy of the pelvis is the *sine qua non* of the qualified surgeon (Figs. 443 and 444). This knowledge may be acquired in an incomplete fashion by the actual doing of operations, but nothing can take the place of formal, didactic instruction combined with operating frequently under

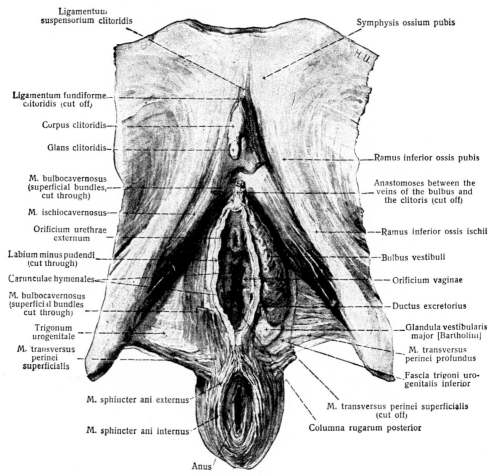

FIG. 443. Bulbus vestibuli and trigonum urogenitale. (Spalteholz: Hand-Atlas of Human Anatomy, Philadelphia, Lippincott)

skilled supervision. A "resident" should not be permitted to undertake surgery in any haphazard fashion but, instead, should receive the benefit of observing well-established technics. Only in this way can the incidence of operative failures be reduced to a minimum.

VARICOSITIES

Varicosities in the legs frequently coexist with and indicate the presence of similar conditions in the pelvis. If possible, varicosities in the extremities should be treated by a specialist in surgery of the peripheral vascular system, whose objective is their obliteration. When such surgery is undertaken, several prophylactic measures against thromboembolic phenomena may serve as safeguards.

Elastic stockings or bandages should be worn prior to the operation, and ambulation should be started as soon after surgery as possible. Anticoagulants are rarely in order. In my own practice, no special measures for the management of varicosities have been employed, and I have had no difficulties.

INCISION

The type of incision to be used for pelvic celiotomy is rarely debatable. When cosmetic considerations are urgent, as in "show people," the Pfannenstiel incision should be employed. In all other patients, an ample midline or para-midline incision should be used for maximum exposure. A precaution which should always be included whenever feasible is palpa-

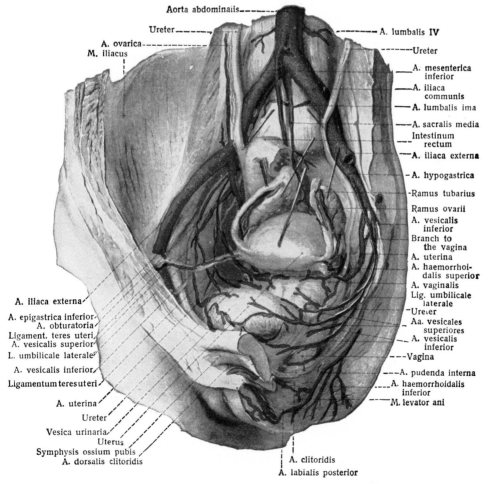

FIG. 444. Arteries of the female pelvis. (Spalteholz: Hand-Atlas of Human Anatomy, Philadelphia, Lippincott)

tion of all adjacent viscera, i.e., gallbladder, liver, stomach, spleen and kidneys. This should be done before the pelvic operation is begun.

PELVIC INFECTION

Whether acute or subacute, this is generally a contraindication to surgery, which should be delayed until the temperature is normal. Then a vaginal examination should be performed. If there is no recrudescence of fever and the blood count remains normal, then it is safe to operate. The surgeon who waits for infection to subside is rewarded by a less vascular operative field, clear planes of cleavage and the prospect of an uneventful convalescence.

OPERATIVE AND POSTOPERATIVE CONSIDERATIONS

PROTECTION OF PERONEAL NERVES

Bear in mind that, during gynecologic operations, flexion and fixation of the legs in the Trendelenburg position may cause injury to the peroneal nerves by compression, with resulting postoperative muscular paralysis. Also, compression of the brachial plexus may produce an Erb's palsy. Severe postoperative backache may plague the patient who has been in the lithotomy position when the legs are markedly abducted. Be sure that the patient's legs are well protected with soft padding at any point where they come in contact with metal parts of the standards.

ELDERLY PATIENTS

The aged woman is frequently enfeebled and deserves extra consideration, both preoperatively and postoperatively. Early ambulation will help prevent hypostatic pneumonia. Generous use of vitamins and fluids should be made.

Gentle handling of tissues is important for any patient; this is especially true of the aged. However, age per se should not rule out surgery; with proper preparation, the elderly patient withstands surgery as well as the youthful one.

INTERNAL HEMORRHAGE

Severe internal bleeding may result from the slipping of a ligature that has been placed upon the uterine or the ovarian artery or other blood vessels. If necessary, use double ligatures. Always be sure that all active bleeding has been stopped before the abdomen is closed.

POSTOPERATIVE ACTIVITY

Today, "early ambulation" is the rule, but this should be applied only to the patient who is physically able to undertake it. Otherwise, changing position in bed, doing mild leg exercises and dangling the legs over the side of the bed will help to prevent phlebitis. Early use of a back rest is also valuable.

LOCAL ANESTHESIA

This has only a limited field of usefulness in gynecologic surgery. In spite of the slight added risk in spinal or general anesthesia, these are usually preferable because they permit smooth and rapid operation.

Local infiltration anesthesia is frequently employed in the senile patient; even vaginal hysterectomy may be performed with surprising ease with only mild preoperative medication. Minor vaginal operations on old women are often done under local anesthesia only.

An exsanguinated patient (as from a ruptured tubal pregnancy) can be rapidly celiotomized under local anesthesia, even while the transfusion is being given. As soon as the bleeding has been controlled by clamps, the patient may be "put to sleep" by inhalation anesthesia. This method keeps operative trauma to a minimum.

REDUCTION OF MORBIDITY AND MORTALITY

For purposes of clarity, it should be stated that the term "morbidity" is used here in reference to *febrile morbidity* (i.e., fever of 100.4° F. or over on any 2 postoperative days, not counting the first). The validity of such a criterion is questionable, but there seems to be none better.

"Mortality" implies death during or after an operation. The time of death after operation cannot be stated arbitrarily; however, to apply, it must be shown that the life of the patient was materially shortened by the operation.

Gynecologic "operations" should be distinguished from *diagnostic procedures*. There is often considerable overlapping. For example, a cervical biopsy or a posterior colpotomy is a gynecologic operation performed for diagnostic purposes. Conversely, diagnostic procedures, such as dilatation and curettage, or tubal insufflation, may also be therapeutic.

Strictly diagnostic procedures, such as culdoscopy, pneumoperitoneoscopy or salpingography, are rarely accompanied by morbidity or mortality.

INDICATIONS FOR OPERATION

The *safety* of a given operative procedure should not be the chief reason for selecting it in preference to some other. Certain difficult operations with a high statistical primary mortality may be "indicated" in certain circumstances; paradoxically, elimination of needless surgery may result in a rise in the morbidity and mortality percentages. Even the pathologic condition of the patient's tissues does not always supply an answer.

SKILL OF THE SURGEON

This encompasses more than mere technical skill. If the patient is considered as a whole, the following should be included under this heading:

1. Preoperative Examination and Preparation:

A. Putting the patient into a proper frame of mind for operation is an obvious necessity. Experience is the best teacher in this respect.

B. A complete physical examination to rule out serious abnormalities is essential. Complete urinalysis and blood count should be done. In older patients, blood chemistry should be determined routinely. Abnormal findings require medical consultation and a re-evaluation of the patient's status, with a view to possible postponement of surgery.

2. Infection:

A. Focal infections, oral sepsis or cystitis should be cleared up as much as possible prior to surgery. Antibiotics should be given prophylactically before any operative procedure, and also during convalescence, to those patients who may be harboring pathogenic organisms, as well as when the surgery may be accompanied by intestinal involvement.

B. Postoperative febrile reactions which appear to be infectious should be treated promptly with appropriate antibiotics. Often

treatment must be empiric until an exact diagnosis can be made. How high the temperature should be allowed to go and how long it should be allowed to persist before giving antibiotics are arbitrary criteria which vary from one gynecologist to another.

3. Obesity or Malnutrition:

A. The obese patient requires special consideration. If possible, elective surgery should be postponed until some weight reduction has been accomplished. Closure of the abdominal wall in these overweight subjects may take extra time, but it must be done with every safeguard. Hemostasis and fascial closing must be as perfect as possible.

B. Malnutrition accompanied by marked underweight should likewise be treated before surgery since healing is often impeded by malnutrition. A high-protein, high-vitamin diet is indicated.

4. Psychic Management:

This has already been briefly stated as "putting the patient in a proper frame of mind." A good *rapport* with the patient is essential. Avoid frightening her with a "bombshell" diagnosis; also, do not be stampeded by any feeling she may have of impending doom. If you honestly believe that one particular operation or a certain special anesthetic is indicated, "stick to your guns." The administration of Nembutal or Seconal the evening before surgery will help to allay nervousness.

5. Anesthesia:

Consult with the anesthetist as to the best method for each individual patient. Most gynecologists prefer spinal anesthesia. Familiarity with the anesthetist's methods is valuable. Especially avoid telling him that you are "almost through," for he may then begin lightening the anesthesia too soon, if you have misjudged your timing.

6. Preparation of the Operative Field:

A. Abdominal procedures require a sterile skin field. A close shave, followed by several soap-and-water washings, should suffice. In the operating room the routine antiseptic preparation must be carried out.

B. For vaginal surgery, a warm tap-water douche is given following the usual shave on the preceding evening. An antibiotic vaginal suppository is then inserted deep into the posterior vaginal fornix. Bacitracin and Terramycin are equally effective in reducing the potential morbidity in vaginal surgery.

7. Transfusion:

A. Marked anemia is a contraindication to surgery, an exception being ruptured ectopic pregnancy. In this condition, transfusion should be started before or at the beginning of surgery.

B. A patient should not be scheduled for surgery with less than 3,000,000 RBC or with an Hb. of less than 11 Gm. However, if surgery must be done, no less than 1,000 cc. of blood (2 units) should be available in the operating room, to be given during the operation and in the recovery ward; the replacement of only 500 cc. (as is sometimes recommended) following surgery seems inconsistent, in view of our knowledge that a normal person can easily withstand a loss of like amount, assuming that he starts with 11 to 12 Gm. of Hb. An anemic patient demands more than 500 cc. of blood, though 500 is better than no blood at all. In radical pelvic surgery, the amount of matched blood to be held available should be no less than 4 units.

8. Fluid Balance:

Usually the patient should receive nothing by mouth for 8 to 12 hours prior to surgery. During the operation, 1,000 cc. of 5 per cent glucose in normal saline should be given intravenously by slow drip. This may be repeated during the day with little fear of overloading the circulation, even if the patient can tolerate fluids by mouth. This method assures a well-hydrated patient.

9. Early Ambulation:

Today, the benefits of early ambulation have been demonstrated beyond doubt. Even the patient with a Foley catheter is gotten out of bed as soon as possible.

10. Specific Surgical Factors:

A. Delicate handling of tissues results in a smoother postoperative course. Also, the anesthesia will not be disturbed if we avoid rough handling of the bowel and the omentum.

B. Accurate hemostasis is the *sine qua non* of all surgical procedures. Pelvic operations are often characterized by considerable oozing from raw surfaces. Hot laparotomy pads will usually stop this oozing if no large bleeding points are visible. Never attempt to make the same suture serve as a ligature and for approximation.

C. The intestines should be gently but positively walled off and kept out of the operative field. If postoperative distention is anticipated, Wangensteen suction should be started the evening before the operation. A patient who has had previous surgery and is anxious and swallowing air will invariably develop more or less tympanites.

D. Appendectomy in conjunction with other procedures is indicated:

1. if the patient is young, or

2. at any age, if the appendix contains fecoliths or show evidence of chronic infection.

E. Appendectomy is contraindicated:

1. in ruptured tubal pregnancy, or

2. if, for any other reason, it is important to conclude the operation as speedily as possible.

F. Drainage of pelvic abscess should always be done through the vagina. The occurrence of this type of complication is infrequent today; insertion of abdominal drains after pelvic surgery is very rarely necessary.

G. Because of the need for frequent catheterization and also the use of the indwelling catheter, urinary tract infections are rather common. Therefore, the prophylactic and therapeutic use of the sulfa drugs and antibiotics is indicated whenever pelvic surgery appears likely to result in disturbance of urinary tract drainage.

CHOICE OF SURGICAL APPROACH

The question frequently arises as to whether a hysterectomy should be done via the abdominal or the vaginal approach. This decision depends on quite a number of factors, the most important being the skill of the surgeon. Other determining factors include the size of the uterus and whether there are associated pathologic conditions in the ovaries and the tubes. The question of the need for exploration in the upper abdominal cavity may also determine the route to be taken. When a plastic procedure on the anterior or posterior wall of the vagina is necessary, and there is no contraindication to vaginal hysterectomy, much time will be saved if the entire operation can be done by the vaginal route. However, if the surgeon's experience with the vaginal route is limited, he would better serve the patient's needs by doing the plastic work from below and the hysterectomy from above.

The advantages of the vaginal approach include:

1. Less shock (making this excellent for the geriatric patient)
2. Less loss of blood
3. Smoother convalescence
4. More rapid convalescence
5. Shortened operating time
6. Fewer circulatory complications
7. Very low mortality
8. Fewer general complications
9. Invariable removal of the cervix

On the other hand, it should be borne in mind that no hysterectomy is complete without an inspection of the ovaries, the tubes and the rectosigmoid. The upper abdominal contents cannot be inspected via the vagina, and if there is reason to believe that pathologic conditions exist there (i.e., they cannot be ruled out by the history and other means of diagnosis, such as roentgenography), it is far better to do an anterior celiotomy and explore the abdomen thoroughly. All pelvic disorders cannot be removed by the vaginal route, and there are some definite contraindications; even so, the greater the surgeon's experience, the more he would use this approach. Such contraindications include:

1. A uterus larger than a normal 3½-month pregnancy
2. History of previous pelvic surgery, particularly if the tissues are fixed
3. The presence of pelvic endometriosis, with fixation
4. The presence of subacute or chronic pelvic inflammation
5. Tuberculosis of the uterus and adnexa
6. Fixation of cervix and parametrium, making it impossible to pull the cervix down to the introitus
7. Lack of familiarity by the surgeon with the anatomy and the required technics.

PITFALLS IN DIAGNOSIS

ERRORS FROM HASTY OPERATION

Errors in gynecologic procedure can and should be minimized. Hunner's admonitions in this respect are worth emphasizing. He regretted, justly, that there are so many unnecessary and ill-advised operations and named some of the factors leading to these errors. Not infrequently, the surgeon is influenced to perform an operation before he has had time to investigate the case thoroughly. Many surgeons undertake procedures for which they have not been trained. Many useless operations are performed for insufficient reasons. Errors in diagnosis may be traced directly to haste, whereas careful preoperative study would have ensured an accurate evaluation and safety for the patients. Patients should always be clearly informed of the character of the treatment necessary to relieve their symptoms. Hunner adds that, in gynecology, the pitfalls in diagnosis may be avoided by keeping in mind the many gastro-intestinal, orthopedic, neurogenic and urologic conditions, the symptoms of which so often are misinterpreted as being of gynecologic origin. Every gynecologist should have thorough urologic training, or at least be in close touch with a urologist.

UROLOGIC CONDITIONS

Urinary tract symptoms often simulate those due to pressure of tumors, to malposition of pelvic organs or to inflammatory conditions in the pelvis. Severe cases of dysmenorrhea may have their origin in the ureteral, rather than in the genital tract. Tender ureters may be responsible for dyspareunia rather than disease in the internal genitalia. Ovarian pain may be diagnosed as ureteritis, leading, in many instances, to unnecessary sacrifice of the ovaries. Symptoms produced by "falling of the womb" may be simulated by jarring and tugging on diseased ureters at the point where they pass through the broad ligament. In cases of menorrhagia, the patients often will be found to have a definite severe dyscrasia, due to their mode of living or to marked constitutional or local disease.

Ureteral Stricture. Because of interference with renal function by obstruction, with resultant toxemia affecting the nervous, mental, gastro-intestinal and other functions, ureteral stricture is a common cause of a dyscrasia. Such conditions may often respond to adequate renal drainage. In young women, persistent menorrhagia may be due to a focus of infection in the tonsils or elsewhere. Uterine or ovarian tumors, accompanied by high lumbar pain in the region of the broad ligament, particularly when accompanied by bladder symptoms, call for a careful survey of the entire urinary tract to determine the possible presence of serious renal stasis. In cases of incontinence, repair of the urethral sphincter often fails because the symptoms are due to impulses from diseased ureters rather than to failure of urethral function. Naturally, gynecologic operations rarely relieve such symptoms; therefore, careful investigation should always be made *before* the patient is promised relief from any gynecologic procedure.

Also, many errors are due to ignorance concerning the comparative frequency of *elusive ulcer of the bladder* and the difficulty in locating this small lesion on otherwise normal-appearing bladder mucosa. The same applies to ignorance concerning the great frequency of ureteral stricture.

The urinary tract may harbor serious lesions, while the urinalyses remain completely negative. With an elusive ulcer, the urine may look clear to the naked eye and show only an occasional leukocyte or erythrocyte microscopically. Again, in ureteral stricture, the urine may be completely negative or show only a few erythrocytes, leukocytes, casts, a varying amount of albumin—or a combination of these. The foreign elements are often reported by the laboratory as "normal" or "so slightly altered as to be insignificant." A secondary pyelitis is found in some cases. With ureteral stricture, one or both kidneys may be hydronephrotic, yet secrete relatively normal urine. The kidney pelvis may be smaller than normal, with chronic interstitial nephritis, yet show negative urine. Even a competent urologist may overlook an elusive ulcer or a stricture of the ureter. *A ureteral catheter without a bulb will pass two thirds of all strictures without noticeable obstruction*; in such cases, a flat roentgenogram commonly reveals nothing of diagnostic value.

Incontinence. One of the reasons for failure in operations for the correction of "stress incontinence" is inaccurate diagnosis of its cause. Many surgeons have tried to correct the incontinence by tightening the urethra and the urethrovesical fascias *before* submitting the patient to varied diagnostic procedures. *Incontinence* may be due to disease of the spinal cord, such as *spina bifida occulta*, pernicious anemia, tabes or multiple sclerosis. The incontinence occurring with these conditions is really a paradoxical one in which the loss of urine is due to overflow. Among other causes, also not due to abnormal muscular conditions, are stricture or diverticulum of the urethra, urethrocele (either congenital or acquired), polyps of the urethrovesical junction and chronic cystitis. Before attempting surgical correction, an endoscopic examination of the urethra, together with cystoscopic examination of the bladder, should be done, since the causes of the incontinence may be either urethral or vesical.

In the aged, a not uncommon cause of stress incontinence is atrophy of the anterior vaginal wall. In many cases this may be relieved by estrogenic therapy.

Passage of *ureteral stones* or "gravel" is often mistaken for pelvic disease, especially if the pain is left-sided. *Twisted ovarian cyst, ectopic pregnancy* and *salpingitis* have all been diagnosed incorrectly. A study of the urine, a good pyelogram and a history carefully taken and as carefully interpreted will lead to a proper diagnosis and avoid unnecessary pelvic surgery.

GASTRO-INTESTINAL SYMPTOMS

These may simulate pelvic disease. Diseases of the intestinal tract which are sometimes diagnosed erroneously in this way are appendicitis, regional ileitis, diverticulitis, spastic colon and carcinoma of the rectosigmoid.

Appendicitis. The appendix, situated close to the right side of the pelvic area and occasionally actually in the pelvis, when diseased, is frequently the culprit when the ovaries or the tubes are being blamed. Similarly, pelvic disturbances may be diagnosed as acute appendicitis. The acute abdominal conditions which occasionally follow rupture of the Graafian follicle, with the spilling of blood into the abdomen, are often diagnosed as appendicitis. Therefore, in taking a patient's history, care should be taken to inquire about the time relationship between the onset of pain and the menstrual cycle; if it were midway between "periods," follicle rupture may be suspected. The differential white count and the sedimentation rate are very helpful here in making a correct diagnosis. However, if it proves to be impossible to distinguish between an acutely inflamed appendix and a ruptured Graafian follicle, then surgery is indicated.

Regional Ileitis. With its tendency to the

formation of abscesses, regional ileitis may very easily be mistaken for pelvic disease. This is especially true when there are masses which lie in the pelvis. Sometimes these masses are bilateral, simulating tubo-ovarian disease. Here, a history of cryptogenic fever, together with the characteristic x-ray findings in the small bowel, will aid in the diagnosis.

Diverticulitis of the Large Bowel. In women over the age of 40, this must be strongly suspected when there is a mass on the left side. The most common diagnosis is pyosalpinx. However, since purulent inflammatory disease is usually bilateral, roentgenograms of the lower bowel should be used to rule out diverticulosis. As the latter is best treated with antibiotics and chemotherapy rather than by surgery, the differential diagnosis is most important.

Spastic Colitis. This may be accompanied by distress in the lower abdomen and is especially likely to be mistaken for pelvic disease, particularly when the pain is observed to be aggravated during menstruation. A very thorough pelvic examination usually will reveal the absence of pelvic involvement. As this is not an emergency, the patient may be treated by the use of a proper diet and the administration of antispasmodics, and she will usually show improvement. Failure to diagnose this condition correctly has been the cause of many unnecessary celiotomies.

ORTHOPEDIC CONDITIONS

Many women are afflicted with *backache*. Most of the time this is not of pelvic origin, even though there be a retroverted or a retrocedent uterus. Before attempting to shorten the round ligament, a therapeutic test should be made. The uterus must be replaced manually and a pessary inserted and worn for several months. If this relieves the pain, but with its removal the uterus again retroverts with a return of the symptoms, then and only then is surgery indicated. In a nullipara, it is very rare for a retroverted uterus to require shortening of the round ligament.

One of the most common causes of true gynecologic backache is *endocervicitis with parametrial infiltration*. This type of pain will disappear on proper medication. If, at the same time, the patient is found to have a posterior malposition of the uterus, it is all too common for her to be subjected to useless surgery. The origin of gynecogenic backache is low, just above or even below the sacral area. If no pelvic findings other than malposition are to be found, the patient should be examined by an orthopedist. Also, such other conditions as presacral lipoma, intervertebral disk rupture, hypertrophic changes in the spine, sacro-iliac disease, sacralization of the fifth lumbar vertebra, myositis, spondylolisthesis and coccygodynia should not be overlooked.

NEUROLOGIC CONDITIONS

These should be constantly borne in mind. They include the "girdle of pain" seen in lues, myeloma and malignant metastasis of the spine.

ENDOMETRIOSIS

This is the growth of endometrial tissue in locations other than the uterine cavity. There are many theories to account for this phenomenon, no one of which can fully explain all these lesions. However, Sampson's transplant or implantation theory and peritoneal metaplasia will explain most of them.

The condition appears in several variants; those described as *internal endometriosis* include the subbasal or intramural (adenomyosis), while the *external* variety covers those lesions found on the serous surface of the uterus or external to it. The external type may also be situated in the tubes, the ovaries, the appendix, the intestines, the vagina, the navel, the abdominal wall, the sacro-uterine ligaments or the rectovaginal septum.

Although endometriosis is not considered to be a neoplasm, it has invasive properties, even to the extent of causing obstruction by obliterating the lumen of the bowel. Because of these tendencies, it is necessary to try to remove all traces of the lesion either by surgery or by cauterization. It goes without saying that in young women management should be conservative; as little ovarian tissue should be removed as is consistent with obliteration of the entire lesion. In nullipara a thorough dilation of the cervix should be done before celiotomy in order to allow freer flow of the menstrual discharge. When the rectosigmoid is involved and has become adherent to the posterior surface of the uterus, the adhesions must be separated carefully and all surface growth cauterized with a nasal-tip cautery. In order to prevent recurrent adhesions, the round ligament must be shortened to keep the raw surfaces apart.

In women beyond the childbearing age, more radical surgery may be indicated. Either the pelvic organs should be removed en masse or the ovaries destroyed by irradiation.

Diagnosis of Endometriosis. This is frequently missed. Unless there are definite symptoms, a diagnosis of some inflammatory condition is usually made. This condition should be kept constantly in mind if this error is to be avoided. Also, remember that the extent of the disease in no way corresponds to the amount of pain that it may produce. The patient with a small lesion in the sacrouterine ligament or the rectovaginal septum may suffer intolerable pain, while one with very extensive bilateral lesions may have no pain at all. In fact, it is quite common for endometriosis to be discovered by chance, while an operation is being done for some entirely different pathologic entity.

When pain is present, it is usually worse during the menstrual period. When a unilateral or bilateral chocolate cyst is present (Sampson's tumor), there may be characteristic pain beginning several days before menstruation and lasting throughout the period and even several days beyond it.

DYSPAREUNIA. This condition is aggravated close to the "period" and is seen when the lesion is located in the rectovaginal septum or the sacro-uterine ligament. The *menstrual cycle may be disturbed,* and the incidence of *infertility* is quite high.

Safeguards Against Endometriosis. Test of tubal patency should not be done close to the time of the menstrual period. Since patients already afflicted with this condition are frequently irregular, it is best to wait to do the test for 4 days after all menstrual flow has ceased.

When doing a cesarean section, care must be taken not to implant endometrial tissue into the abdomen or the abdominal wall. Gauze packs should be so placed as to catch any drippings from the uterine cavity. Although material from a chocolate cyst rarely propagates when implanted, such a cyst should be care-

fully walled off to prevent spillage and avoid chemical irritation.

Some 20 per cent of the young women who have had conservative operations may need additional surgery later. In the meantime, they are able to bear children, which should compensate them for this need of subsequent surgical treatment.

CONGENITAL MALFORMATIONS

These result from errors in development. They frequently go undiscovered. The more common forms are imperforate hymen, septate vagina, absence of vagina, atresia of vagina, uterus didelphys (double uterus, septate vagina), uterus duplex or bicornis with vagina simplex and uterus bicornis unicollis with vagina simplex.

IMPERFORATE HYMEN

It is surprising how often a young girl with an imperforate hymen will be given hormonal and other treatment to bring on menstruation. This may be continued even for years, with all sorts of untoward results, until pain and continuing discomfort drive her to seek advice elsewhere. A simple crucial incision will release the inspissated blood; no matter how distorted the affected organs may have become, they will usually return to normal and menstruation will be established. The only needed safeguard is to avoid introducing infection following the incising of the hymen.

SEPTATE VAGINA AND ATRESIA OF THE VAGINA

These may usually be corrected quite simply, with no more than ordinary care beyond recalling the proximity of the bladder and the rectum.

ABSENCE OF A VAGINA
(With or Without a Uterus)

If the patient is contemplating marriage, it is desirable to develop some sort of vagina (Fig. 445). Many operations have been devised for this purpose, some of which carry a great deal of risk (i.e., constructing a vagina from the bowel). Others make use of an elongated labia minora or of skin from the inner part of the thigh to build a vaginal tube. What seems to me to be a simpler method—

one which I introduced in 1935 and have used a number of times with good results—involves channeling a space between the bladder and the rectum, followed by the use of a prosthesis made of glass or plastic to keep the raw surfaces separated until a new surface membrane has developed. As long as the neovagina is used, or the prosthesis worn, it will remain patent and serviceable.

DUPLICATION OF UTERUS AND VAGINA

This malformation often leads to diagnostic and therapeutic errors (Figs. 446 and 447). Because of the poor development of both uteri, spontaneous abortion is very likely. Occasionally the uteri are unequal in size; when pregnancy takes place on one side, the underdeveloped side may prevent normal expulsion of the fetus at term. Again, both uteri may become pregnant and each prevent the emptying of the other. Fortunately, it is sometimes possible to operate on such a condition when the patient is not pregnant and make a single organ

from the two. I have done this successfully a few times; one of these patients has had 3 pregnancies. All of these patients required cesarean section.

PSEUDOHERMAPHRODITISM

So much has been said and written on the physical aspects of this unfortunate situation that here it remains only to say that, to do his full duty, the surgeon who is called on to try to render the patient definitely of one sex or the other should consider the subject's ultimate happiness *first* and the mechanical features only secondarily. This, of course, applies to reasoning adults; when the paradox is discovered in infancy, the situation is somewhat different, though, again, the psychological aspects should come first in making any ultimate decision. The teen-ager who has been raised, let us say, as a boy may be driven even to suicide if suddenly confronted with the legal fact of being a girl. Similarly, a man who has proudly proclaimed that he has a son is

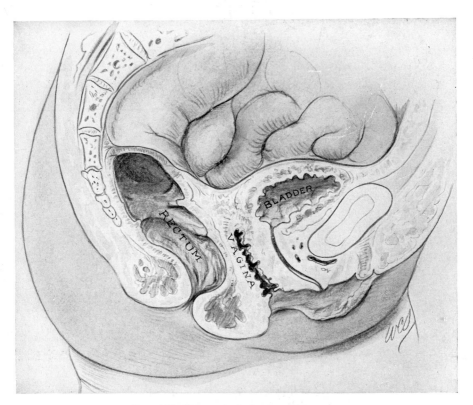

FIG. 445. Congenital absence of uterus.

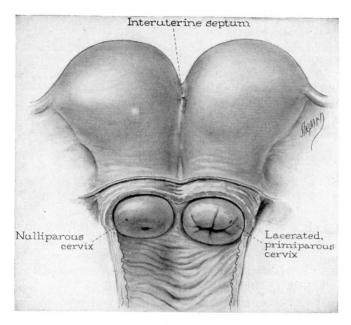

FIG. 446. Double uterus with single vagina.

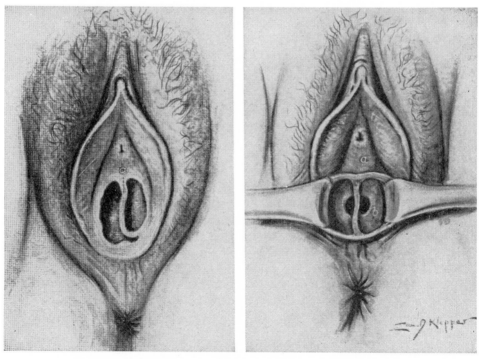

FIG. 447. (*Left*) Double uterus with double vagina. (a) Septum. (*Right*) Double uterus with double vagina. (a) Septum. (b) Uterus bilateralis.

not readily going to admit that the new arrival is really a girl, especially if "he" has several older sisters!

OTHER AFFECTIONS

Bartholin's Gland

An acutely suppurating Bartholin gland should be drained *but not removed.* A pack should be placed in the cavity and allowed to remain for 72 hours to keep the incision open. Later, if a Bartholin cyst should form, causing distortion of the labium so that sexual contact is prevented, the cyst should be completely removed.

Hymen

Occasionally, tags of the hymen (carunculae myrtiformes) will be long enough to induce dyspareunia. These should be removed, care being taken to observe strict asepsis.

Vulva

It is extremely important to do a biopsy on *every lesion* found on the vulva, particularly in older women. The decision as to whether or not the lesion is malignant depends on the findings of such an examination. *Benign lesions* may be removed locally or by simple vulvectomy. *Malignant lesions* must be treated by *radical vulvectomy,* with removal of all the superficial and deep lymph nodes in both groins, as well as those under and above Poupart's ligament.

In *leukoplakic vulvitis* and *kraurosis vulvae,* all that is indicated is a simple vulvectomy. If this were carried out routinely in such conditions, the incidence of malignant lesions of the vulva would be markedly reduced. The only real caution here is care in the differential diagnosis; leukoplakic vulvitis may be confused with a monilial infection or vitiligo.

OPERATIVE PROCEDURES

Operations on the Vulva and the Vagina

Perineal Repairs. If the extent of the lesion is determined before operating, perineal repairs will not fail. The rectum should be freed from the posterior surface of the vaginal mucous membrane so that the levator muscles and the fascia may be interposed between the two. The rectum must not be included in the sutures, as this error might lead to infection of the whole field of operation.

Rectocele. Again, failure to determine in advance the extent of the lesion is a likely source of error in posterior colporrhaphy. For example, it is of little benefit to attempt to treat a high rectocele and an enterocele by a procedure adapted only for the low rectocele. Dissection of the vaginal mucous membrane must be as high as the point where the levator muscles separate, even if the dissection must extend up to the vault of the vagina. If an enterocele is also present, the sacro-uterine ligaments must be brought together in the midline, and the depth of the posterior cul-de-sac must also be shortened. The entrance to the vagina should admit at least the width of the surgeon's 2 fingers.

Pelvic Abscess. This is a localized collection of pus in the posterior cul-de-sac, which causes bulging of the posterior fornix and encroaches upon the floor of the vagina. If there is any question of the existence of an abscess, a posterior colpocentesis should be done. If pus is obtained, a colpotomy should be performed to drain it. Not only must drainage be carried out, but the opening into the cul-de-sac must also be retained to allow it to be complete. In carrying out these procedures the rectum must be carefully safeguarded. An excellent "rule of thumb" is to use the same care in entering the pelvic cavity *through the vagina as through a laparotomy.*

It is dangerous to drain an abscess from above because of the chance of permitting upward spread of the infection, although occasionally it may be necessary. Wherever possible, drain the abscess through the vagina; chemotherapy should also be prescribed.

Verruca Acuminata. If small, verruca acuminata may be removed by applications of podophyllin; but if there is a very large pedunculated mass, it should be removed either by excision or by the use of the heavy-bladed cautery. As these lesions are *always infected,* do not expect primary union following excision or simple vulvectomy. Biopsy is mandatory because of the chance of carcinoma.

Urethral Caruncle. This resembles carcinoma of the urethra with prolapse, ulceration and bleeding. Biopsy should precede any treatment. Caruncles may be treated with podophyllin or may be removed with the nasal-tip cautery under local anesthesia.

OPERATIONS ON THE CERVIX

Microscopic studies should precede cauterization or any other procedure on the cervix. These may take the form of Papanicolaou smears or of biopsies of one or more cervical areas. Gross appearance will not indicate whether any lesion is benign or malignant. Even a small lesion, if it is malignant, should not be treated by simple cauterization or an amputation of the cervix; but if it is diagnosed as benign, then whatever procedure will best serve the patient's interests may be carried out.

Dilatation of the Cervix. Certain types of dilators may very easily cause lacerations. This may be avoided by using a graduated set of dilators and by working slowly. When this procedure is done for dysmenorrhea or sterility, a glass Baldwin pessary should be sewed into the cervix and allowed to remain until just before the next menstrual period. This has the effect of keeping the canal dilated far beyond its normal physiologic limits and prevents it from returning to its prior status.

Amputation of the Cervix. This should include removal of *all* diseased tissue, not merely *part* of it. This may necessitate reflecting the bladder flap upward. Be sure to see that there is no atresia of the cervical canal, with its attendant accumulation of menstrual blood in the body of the uterus, as this will cause severe dysmenorrhea; it may be avoided by leaving a Baldwin pessary in the repaired cervix for a week to 10 days. Postoperative hemorrhage may be avoided by being certain to tie the descending rami of the uterine vessel *above* the point of amputation. Also, it is good practice to pass sounds into the uterus when the patient returns for a check-up.

Fibroids and Cervical Polyps. Whether they have their origin in the body of the uterus or in the cervical canal, fibroids and cervical

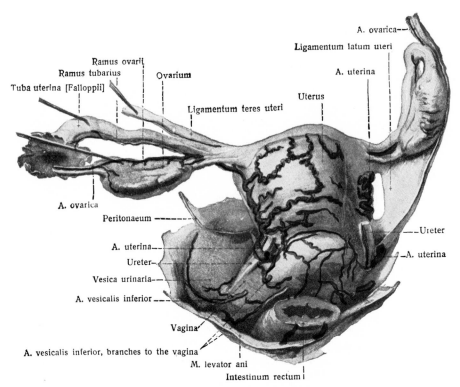

FIG. 448. Arteries of the uterus and the surrounding structures. (Spalteholz: Hand-Atlas of Human Anatomy, Philadelphia, Lippincott)

polyps should, on removal, be subjected to microscopic study. Polyps are rarely malignant, but even these should be subjected to such examination.

OPERATIONS ON THE UTERUS
(Fig. 448)

Suspension and Fixation Operations. The old Kelly suspension of the uterus to the abdominal wall has no place in modern surgery; it does nothing to correct the basic weakness always present in acquired *prolapsus*. Shortening of the round ligament should not be done unless it is definitely indicated, and should always be accompanied by shortening of the sacro-uterine ligament as well, to assure increase in flexion of the uterus. Either the abdominal or the vaginal approach may be used. There are many good technics, but keep in mind that the shortening must be accomplished under direct vision. The Baldy-Webster procedure is ideal since it provides support for both uterus and ovaries in one operation.

There are very few real indications for shortening of the round ligament. These are:

1. In a multipara, a retroversion producing backache, leukorrhea and menorrhagia, when these symptoms are relieved by placing the uterus manually in its proper position, followed by insertion of a Smith-Hodge pessary. If, after wearing the pessary for several months, the uterus falls back when the pessary is removed and there is a return of the former symptoms.

2. When, in operating for endometriosis, there are lesions on the posterior surface of the uterus which may adhere, or have already adhered and been separated, shortening of the round ligament will lift the uterus away from the sigmoid.

3. In a young nullipara with retroversion with prolapse, shortening of both round and uterosacral ligaments may be combined with repair of cystocele and rectocele in order to preserve menstrual physiology and ability to bear children.

4. In doing celiotomy for pelvic disease and where the uterus is in extreme retroversion, provided that further surgery is not contraindicated

5. In some unusual cases of repeated spontaneous abortion which have occurred in spite

of raising the uterus and the wearing of a pessary

6. Where a retroverted uterus is bound down by adhesions following inflammatory disease or endometriosis, in conjunction with celiotomy. The vaginal round ligament shortening should be done only when sterilization may be done at the same time.

By no means can *uterine prolapse* always be corrected by the same type of operation. A procidentia, or third-degree prolapse, requires different treatment than a first- or a second-degree prolapse. Insistence on treating them all alike will lead only to many failures. The choice of procedure must be guided by such considerations as the *age* of the patient, the *degree* of the prolapse, the amount of *surgical risk* and the amount and kind of *associated pathologic conditions*. A diseased uterus may have to be sacrificed. It should also be borne in mind that prolapse is usually associated with other conditions resulting from weaknesses of the pelvic floor, such as cystocele, rectocele, enterocele and inversion of the vagina.

Types of Operation

Celiotomy and Vaginal Repair. This is best adapted to young women in whom normal reproductive ability must be conserved.

Interposition. This is seldom done today because of the bladder disturbances produced. It was originally devised as a cure for a large cystocele. The patient should be sterilized, as it leaves the uterus in a bad position for normal pregnancy.

Vaginal Hysterectomy and Plastic Repair. These are indicated only when the uterus must be sacrificed because of disease or when the patient is beyond childbearing age. There are many good technics; among the best is the Heaney clamp procedure.

Manchester Type of Operation. This is an anterior and posterior vaginal plastic repair, with amputation of the cervix, using the cardinal ligaments to hold the stump of the uterus high in the vault of the vagina. This procedure is applicable only to first- and second-degree prolapse and shows a *high rate of recurrence*.

Le Fort-Neugebauer Operation. This should be reserved for women who are *very poor surgical risks,* fit to withstand only a minimal amount of surgery. It has the advantage that it may be done under local anesthesia but has the serious drawbacks that (1) it hides the cervix, thus preventing visualization of cervical cancer if it should occur, (2) it makes sexual contact impossible, and (3) it will fail if the patient later becomes very active.

Total Colpocleisis. This is preferable, if the patient can withstand more extensive surgery. The fascia is used for support.

Curettage

This should be looked upon as a *major operation* and be performed by a surgeon with enough experience to deal with any complication that may arise. All too frequently it is turned over to the least experienced man on the service, who, in turn, can get into dire difficulties if confronted with such emergencies as rupture of the uterus with intestinal damage or profuse hemorrhage.

At the present time, far more curettements are being performed than ever before, in the increasingly intensive search for early carcinoma of the uterus. Since even the most experienced surgeon may easily miss some pathologic condition during curettage, how much more frequently will this happen to the inexperienced! Conversely, the more a man has seen, the oftener he can make a correct tentative diagnosis from the gross material. Even so, many times the microscopic diagnosis will contradict these gross findings.

The most efficient method of curettage is the fractional approach—first, material from the portio, then from the cervical canal, followed by that from the endometrial cavity. These are kept separate and will serve to pinpoint the location of any lesion found.

Perforation of the Uterus. Complications can most easily be prevented by keeping constantly in mind the possibility of a perforation, doing the dilation with gentleness and refraining from sudden introduction of the dilators into the canal. Another safeguard is to determine the *length* of the canal with the first dilator, then introduce the subsequent ones no farther than the first; if this were literally observed, there would be less chance of perforating the uterine wall. However, even with every safeguard, anyone doing this operation, at one time or another, under some conditions, can produce damage. The surgeon who boasts that he has never had a perforation during sounding or curettage either has seldom done this procedure or is being careless with the truth!

Management After Mishap. If it seems fairly certain that a perforation has occurred, the procedure should be stopped at once, for there is the possibility of tearing a "knuckle" of bowel that has become pinched in the opening. If the patient is a young woman in whom the uterus should be preserved, it should be gently packed with gauze and the patient kept under observation for 24 to 48 hours. However, if there is pre-existing uterine infection, it is best to do a hysterectomy, followed by large doses of antibiotics.

If material removed from the uterus during curettage resembles fat or serosa, a celiotomy should be done to determine the extent of the damage to the contents of the abdominal cavity and to ascertain the need for corrective procedures. At the same time, the rent in the uterus may be sutured, or, if the damage is beyond repair, a hysterectomy may be done.

Infection. In the uterus, infection renders all instrumentation dangerous, since an active infection may thus be spread or a latent one excited.

Curettage Before Hysterectomy. Most gynecologists now agree that a diagnostic curettage should be done before either a vaginal or an abdominal hysterectomy is to be performed. This is to rule out carcinoma. If malignancy is found to be present, it may be preferable to use radium prior to surgery.

Sequelae of Curettage. If the surgeon uses strong strokes and a sharp curet, he may remove most of the endometrium, with resultant amenorrhea or sterility. He may also weaken the uterine wall to an extent that will induce rupture during subsequent pregnancy. If curettage is done in the presence of a submucous fibroid, hemorrhage or infection may follow. This last may be avoided by stopping the curetting of any area where the instrument meets with an obstruction.

Fibroids and Myomas

When enucleating fibroids, care must be exercised to approximate the uterine bed very accurately so as to eliminate pockets in which blood may collect. Such retention of blood may cause postoperative hemorrhage or invite infection. If possible, avoid entering the uterine cavity during the enucleation; thus, if pregnancy occurs later, there will be less likelihood of rupture of the uterus during the later months of gestation or during labor.

If severe damage has been done to the uterine wall during a myomectomy prior to pregnancy, serious consideration should be given to doing cesarean section before term. This is especially true if the baby is large or if there is disproportion because of a narrow pelvis.

As an added safeguard during myomectomy, an exact seroserous peritonealization should be done at the site of the excised tumor to discourage formation of adhesions.

Submucous Pedunculated Fibroids. In order to prevent a pyometra, submucous pedunculated fibroids protruding from the cervix should be removed, even when other fibroids are also present. It is better to remove the pedunculated fibroid first, so that good drainage from the uterine cavity may be established, followed in 7 to 10 days by the needed additional surgery. This is an essential safeguard, even with the use of chemotherapy.

Hysterectomy for Fibroids. In general, this should be routine when the age of the patient permits. The incidence of malignancy in fibroids is rather low—only about 1 or 2 per cent; still, because of the possibility, usually the entire organ should be removed. An additional reason is the fact that incipient tumors, as yet too small to recognize, may be present, which, if not automatically removed by the radical procedure, may later enlarge to the point of call for further surgery. On the other hand, the conservative approach, i.e., myomectomy, is the method of choice in a young woman desiring children, thus conserving the uterus, even though there will be need for further surgery later. This is borne out by the fact that removal of a fibroid frequently allows pregnancy to take place and to go to full term successfully. This may even be true of women who have had several miscarriages.

Fibroids in the Pregnant Uterus. By no means does this condition always call for surgical intervention. Even in cases that appear to be very precarious, an attitude of "wait and see" will "pay off" far more often than not; in one of my own cases, the uterus extended almost to the ziphoid process at 4 months, yet went to term, when a 10-pound child was delivered by cesarean section. Hysterectomy was also done, the uterus weighing 18 pounds; this patient was a 39-year-old primigravida.

One error that must be avoided is to make a diagnosis of fibroids in a woman of childbearing age from amenorrhea alone. *Fibroids do not cause amenorrhea.* A tragically common error is to operate for fibroids and find a normal, pregnant uterus! Before operating, every resource must be used to rule out pregnancy.

Precaution. Extreme care must be exercised in removing intraligamentary fibroids because of the ureter which may lie contiguous with the capsule. It is best to enucleate the fibroid and leave the capsule intact. Never put a clamp lateral to the fibroid because of the possibility of catching in the ureter.

Also, since fibroids have a poor blood supply, one must be constantly aware of the likelihood of vital adhesions, particularly to the intestines. There may also be attachment to the omentum with very large, dilated veins; when removing such growths, be certain to tie each vessel securely.

When a fibroid is "molded" to the pelvis, care must be taken lest the rectosigmoid be attached and be torn open. This accident could be fatal. The same is true when the bladder is to be separated from the uterus; in some cases, it is better to enucleate the fibroid from beneath the bladder, especially if the latter is distorted, pushed out of place and intimately attached to the growth, as is frequently the case. In some instances it is better to morcellate the central portion of the mass before attempting to raise the uterus, thus avoiding the tearing of other vital structures.

In passing, it might be worthwhile to mention the possibility of mistakenly diagnosing neoplasms in neighboring structures as uterine or ovarian fibroids. Crotti describes a case of small, round-cell sarcoma of Meckel's diverticulum in a postmenopausal virgin that was diagnosed at the beginning of the operation as pedunculated fibroid of the uterus. This patient made an uneventful recovery at the time but died 4 years later of generalized metastases. Similarly, *ovarian fibroids,* being much

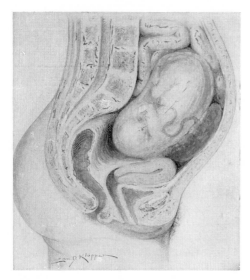

FIG. 449. Abdominal pregnancy; schematic view.

less common, are often referred, preoperatively, to the uterus.

ECTOPIC PREGNANCY

Recognition of the tragedy of ruptured ectopic pregnancy (Fig. 449) is not difficult; the symptoms are classic. The patient of childbearing age has missed 1 or 2 "periods," then is seized by a severe attack of abdominal pain and goes into shock. A diagnosis of ruptured ectopic pregnancy comes at once to mind; nevertheless, it is necessary to think of other possibilities such as acute appendicitis, ureteral stone, a twisted viscus (usually the ovary), pedunculated fibroid or appendiceal epiploicae. However, since surgery is indicated in most of these, exploratory laparotomy does no harm.

The chief problem is to make a correct diagnosis when the classic symptoms are minimal; an axiom well worth following is: "Any woman of childbearing age who has had amenorrhea, together with slight, continuing, one-sided abdominal pain, should be considered suspect (for ectopic pregnancy) until proved otherwise." Unfortunately, there are several other pathologic states which may produce like symptoms: ovarian dyscrasias, corpus luteum cyst (chocolate cyst), simple follicular cyst, small-cyst disease of the ovary and low-grade salpingitis. Because of

the possibility of these other conditions, it is an error to perform a celiotomy on a patient with the cited symptoms without other corroboratory evidence. An attempt should be made at diagnosis via the vagina. Conventional pregnancy tests are of little value, as fully one quarter of ectopic pregnancies give negative results, and, even if the result is "positive," there is no way to distinguish between uterine, ectopic and combined pregnancies. Similarly, blood examination is of little value in minimal cases. In most instances the correct diagnosis can be made only by means of posterior colpocentesis or posterior colpotomy.

TECHNIC

Use a large 18- or 20-bore needle and a 10-cc. syringe. With this, the cul-de-sac may be entered easily and without danger. If no fluid can be procured, tubal abortion or rupture is ruled out. A finding of fluid blood with small clots speaks for ruptured ectopic pregnancy. Straw-colored fluid, hemolyzed fluid or pus indicates the existence of follicular cyst, chocolate cyst or pelvic inflammation.

However, even if no exudate is obtained, *unruptured* ectopic pregnancy is not ruled out. A posterior colpotomy should then be done and the tubes examined from the uterine horn outward, as well as the ovaries from all surfaces. In most cases any pathologic conditions encountered can be removed through the colpotomy incision, thus saving the patient from undergoing a celiotomy, with its greater risk and longer convalescence.

In general, once the suspicion of ectopic pregnancy has been aroused, there must be no temporizing. Many cases of coinciding uterine and tubal pregnancy are encountered —be always on the lookout for this. *The diagnosis must be made before the case becomes one of tragedy!*

An abdominal pregnancy may be recognized by injection of a radiopaque substance into the uterine cavity, followed by the taking of a flat plate. The normal uterine cavity will appear with the fetal structures outside of it. Some surgeons believe that dilatation and curettage are helpful in making the diagnosis of ectopic pregnancy because of the decidual reaction. In some extra-uterine gestations, there is a great amount of material inside the uterine cavity. This proliferation of the endometrium *may* indicate a coinciding intra-uterine pregnancy. I have seen a number of cases where, because curettage produced a large amount of material, normal pregnancy was diagnosed, and nothing further was done for the patient. Several hours later she went into shock, and operation revealed a ruptured ectopic pregnancy. It is a grave error not to await a microscopic study of the tissues to see whether there are any trophoblastic elements present. Occasionally there will be passed a complete decidual cast which resembles the gestation sac in uterine pregnancy. If nothing more is done, the extra-uterine pregnancy then may continue to progress and later result in a tragedy.

When operating for an abdominal pregnancy, the placenta must be removed with great care, as it may be attached to some surface with marked vascularization, from which removal could produce a fatal hemorrhage. Under these conditions it is best to remove only the membranes, cord and part of the placenta, leaving the rest in the abdomen; there is no need to drain, as the retained portion will be absorbed.

Vaginal Bleeding

The amount and the character of vaginal bleeding may be an aid in distinguishing between uterine and ectopic pregnancy. In most instances excessive blood with clots bespeaks a uterine pregnancy; the blood lost will usually be more than the amount of a normal menstruation. However, bleeding may also be excessive in an interstitial ectopic pregnancy which ruptures into the uterine cavity, although more often this variety ruptures into the abdominal cavity or into the broad ligament. If bleeding is slight, dilatation and curettage should not precede a posterior colpotomy, for, if this is done routinely, a normal uterine pregnancy may easily be disturbed. If the blood loss is excessive, curettage may be done before colpotomy.

Operation

A safeguard when undertaking operation for ruptured tubal pregnancy is to precede it by blood transfusions. During the operation extra blood should be at hand. With the profusion of blood banks, it is no longer necessary or advisable to attempt reprocessing of blood removed from the abdomen; fresh blood, properly typed and crossmatched, gives much less chance for contamination.

Any *additional surgery* that might appear to be indicated—removal of normal appendix, myomectomy or contralateral salpingectomy—should be avoided if there is excessive blood in the abdomen or when the patient is in shock.

Precautions and Safeguards

These have been well summarized by Lull as follows:

1. In the management of ectopic pregnancy, there can be no definite rules. Each case is a law unto itself.

2. The advisability of delay, with the idea of obtaining a living child, is questionable. If diagnosis is made only late in the pregnancy, operation should be done between the 36th and 38th weeks; to wait longer decreases chances for a successful outcome.

3. If the fetus dies, defer operation 3 or 4 weeks to allow vascularity of the placenta to decrease and partial separation to take place. The patient should be kept in the hospital under close observation for hemorrhage and infection of the gestational sac. If the fetus is known to have been dead for several weeks, immediate operation is indicated.

4. Before operation is attempted, the patient's blood should be typed and a supply for transfusion provided.

5. The abdominal incision should be made over the *body* of the fetus rather than over the placenta.

6. Careful removal of the fetus without disturbing the placental site is important.

7. In operating when the fetus is known to have been dead for some time, the fact must not be lost sight of that removal of the placenta may still give rise to serious hemorrhage. Although removal can usually be accomplished, in some instances it is necessary to resort to packing to control bleeding. Do not disturb this packing for at least 10 days.

8. Approach the sac carefully and, if possible, without broaching the peritoneum. In these cases, *drain the sac; never remove it.*

9. Packing should be removed only after having been loosened on several successive days, and removal should be attempted only after careful preparation for possible transfusions and the reopening of the abdomen.

10. When a living child is removed, no attempt

at removal or separation of the placenta should be made; close the abdomen without drainage.

11. If the placenta fails to be absorbed, making secondary removal necessary, and if the entire sac cannot be removed, marsupialization and packing of the cavity are indicated.

HYSTERECTOMY

Today, this operation is far less dangerous than formerly. The patient is better prepared for surgery through the use of antibiotics and blood transfusions, attention to fluid balance, improved anesthetics and anesthetic technics and better and broader surgical training. However, complications still will be met with occasionally. Also, it should be borne in mind that the broader the surgeon's experience with this particular type of operation, the less often will he run into trouble; if trouble turns up frequently, the surgeon would be wise to review his technics. Also, the more extensive the operation, the greater

the danger of injury to adjacent organs, especially in surgery for cancer, where more complications will arise than in simpler procedures.

The chief dangers of a hysterectomy are (1) injury to ureters and bladder (Figs. 450 and 451), (2) hemorrhage, (3) slipping of clamps and ligatures, (4) tears into adjacent viscera, (5) shock and (6) secondary ileus and peritonitis.

Hemorrhage (due to increased vascularity) often can be controlled by the use of warm packs, particularly in cases where there have been adhesions which involve no large vessels but leave an oozing bed. If important vessels are double ligated with fixation sutures there will be less chance of *slipping of ligatures* with consequent hemorrhage. Where there is marked *edema* of the tissues, extreme care is necessary in tying vessels. Slipping can also be prevented by tying vessels primarily, or at

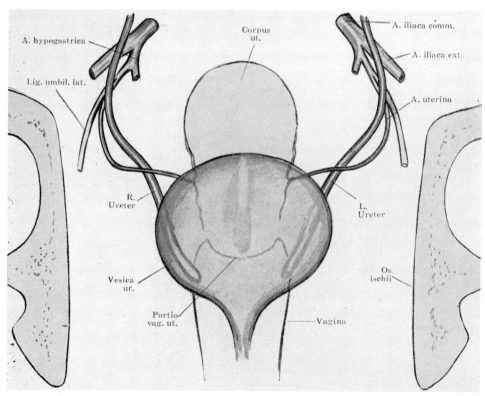

Fig. 450. Topographic relation among uterus, bladder, ureter and uterine artery (normal position of the organs). (Martius, H.: Die Gynäkologischen Operationen, Stuttgart, Thieme)

FIG. 451. The 3 parts of the retinaculum uteri when the uterus is drawn down and the bladder detached and lifted high. (I, II, III) Transfixion of the parametrium in simple vaginal total extirpation of the uterus. (Martius, H.: Die Gynäkologischen Operationen, Stuttgart, Thieme)

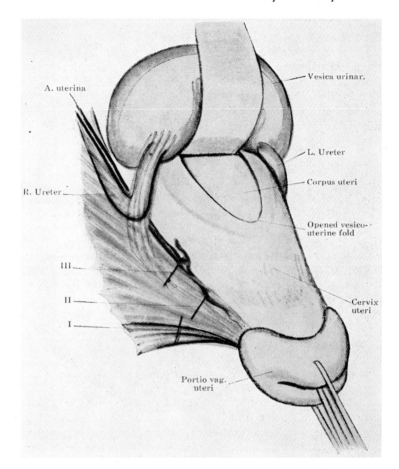

A. uterina

R. Ureter

III

II

I

Vesica urinar.

L. Ureter

Corpus uteri

Opened vesicouterine fold

Cervix uteri

Portio vag. uteri

least by *not* tying them into large pedicles. *Paralytic ileus and bowel obstruction* may be minimized by careful handling of tissues, use of transfusion to cover blood loss and precise peritonealization.

TOTAL VS. SUBTOTAL HYSTERECTOMY

At present there remains little argument against "panhysterectomy." There are only a few conditions in which it is now considered advisable to leave the cervix behind, such as when the patient's status requires terminating the procedure as fast as possible, or when the cervix is infiltrated by endometriosis or adhesions due to some inflammatory condition. Removal under such circumstances could be hazardous.

INDICATIONS

Total hysterectomy is now considered advisable in all situations which make necessary removal of the body of the uterus, whether the patient is nulliparous or multiparous, and regardless of whether the condition found is benign or malignant—*provided* that the surgeon is familiar with the required technic.

PREOPERATIVE PRECAUTIONS

Infections due to organisms originating in the vagina or the cervix should not occur today. Careful preparation of the vagina—cleaning up of any disease condition of the cervix, or of vaginitis, by introduction of a suppository of 100,000 units of penicillin, or bacitracin, for one or several nights prior to surgery—should eliminate this possibility. The vagina should be thoroughly cleansed with green soap immediately before surgery and painted with an antiseptic. However, *make sure that the patient is not sensitive to any drug that is to be used.*

Surgery After Irradiation. Surgery should

not be undertaken for about 3 weeks following the last exposure. In my own experience, surgery after such treatment is not much more difficult than otherwise, provided that one remembers the danger of necrosis when a skin incision is made in an irradiated area.

The best possible anesthetic technic and adequate exposure are essential.

Operative Safeguards

Ligating Uterine Arteries. When ligating the uterine arteries, the surgeon must be ever mindful of their proximity to the ureters in the cardinal ligament area. Other points where the ureters are vulnerable are in the vesicouterine ligament, as they enter the trigone, and in the intraligamentary broad ligament masses. Care must also be used when separating adhesions around the ovaries and the tubes when they lie in the cul-de-sac. It is quite possible to cut or tear the ureters when handling diseased tissues. Especially in *radical procedures,* care must be exercised not to remove all the blood supply of the ureter, otherwise a ureterovaginal fistula may follow.

Many surgeons who specialize in urologic surgery believe that it does more harm than good to introduce a catheter as a safeguard before starting surgery. A ureteritis may develop, followed by an ascending infection.

Operative and Postoperative Complications

Interference with Micturition. This is sometimes thought to follow many gynecologic operations which interfere with the normal physiologic expansion of the bladder —for when the bladder cannot expand, urination is too frequent. However, the bladder is an organ which can accommodate itself to changing situations, as, for example, during pregnancy or when uterine tumors encroach upon it.

Urinary Retention. This may also follow pelvic surgery. This is especially apt to be the case when the surgery has been performed for the repair of cystocele or urinary incontinence. For this reason, the introduction of a Foley catheter for 4 or 5 days may assist the patient to empty her bladder. Antibiotics or chemotherapy must be instituted while the catheter is in the bladder. Even in spite of this routine, there will be some patients who

are unable to void. Many methods have been suggested to help in this situation. Some work for one patient and not for another. For the disturbed or psychoneurotic patient, hot sitz baths and a tranquilizing drug are most helpful.

Damaged Ureter. When no urine is secreted for 24 hours, it does not necessarily mean that the ureters have been ligated, but if there is none for 48 hours, it is time to become very suspicious. Attempts to pass a retrograde catheter rarely meet with success because of the edema and distortion. Two choices are then open: (1) to operate and try to untie the ligature, or (2) to do a nephrostomy. Nephrostomy drainage may save the patient's life, at the same time giving the ligature a chance to loosen. However, if no urine can be obtained from the bladder, a celiotomy *may reveal* the location of the stricture, which can then be released.

If a *ureter is cut* during a procedure, the surgeon may repair it in any one of a number of ways, by a uretero-ureteral, ureterocolic, ureterovesical or ureterocutaneous anastomosis. The choice is governed by the skill of the individual surgeon and the particular situation. Sometimes it is possible to pass a catheter up to the renal pelvis and down into the bladder, where a few fine sutures may be set to approximate the cut ends. Most repairs to the ureter ultimately end up in a stricture, requiring occasional dilatation.

Try not to destroy the ureteral blood supply, keeping in mind that it varies at each level of its course.

Vaginal Urinary Fistulae. At one time these fistulae were usually the result of obstetric accidents. With today's increased use of cesarean section and of antibiotics and chemotherapy, this source has mostly been eliminated. Now they are apt to be the result of gynecologic radiation and operations such as those for malignant disease of the uterus. To prevent their occurrence, the topography of the pelvic ureter must be kept constantly in mind.

The repair of ureterovaginal fistulae depends on the condition of both the affected kidney and the contralateral one, the condition of the portion of the ureter involved and the amount of scar tissue present.

If the ureter has been cut close to the

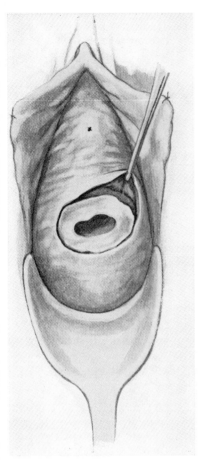 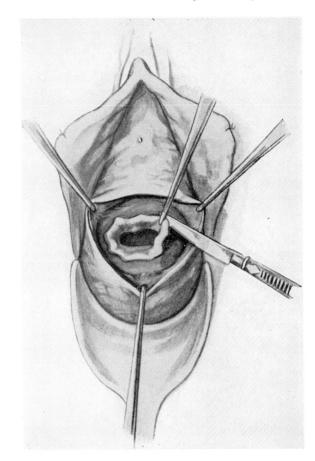

Fig. 452. Operation for a vesicovaginal fistula. (*Left*) First step. Circumcision of the fistulous opening. (*Right*) Second step. The circumcised ring of vaginal mucosa is undermined toward the fistula so that a collar is created. The vaginal mucosa is dissected extensively all around and outward from the bladder. (Martius, H.: Die Gynäkologischen Operationen, Stuttgart, Thieme)

bladder, it is usually impossible to make a uretero-ureteral anastomosis, especially if the lower cut end is imbedded in scar tissue. A ureter cut higher up may sometimes be anastomosed over an olive catheter, or some other of the previously cited anastomoses may be made. Or, if the kidney on the affected side is in poor condition, it should be removed, provided, of course, that the remaining one is in normal health.

Vesicovaginal Fistulae. Attempts to repair this type of fistula (Figs. 452 and 453) frequently fail because certain conditions have not been fulfilled before the surgery is undertaken. The following should be considered:

1. The introduction of *indigo carmine* into the bladder before surgery will aid in finding a fistulous opening. When doing a vaginal or an abdominal hysterectomy, the indigo carmine helps to detect any rent in the bladder—made inadvertently—which might otherwise be missed.

2. Three months should be allowed to elapse before secondary closure is done. Primary closure, of course, should be done if the bladder is opened accidentally during the original operation.

3. If cystitis is present, this must be cleared up before repair is attempted.

4. Any salt crystals collected at the stoma

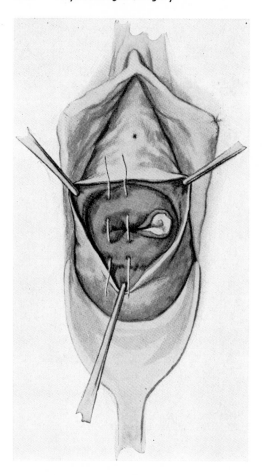

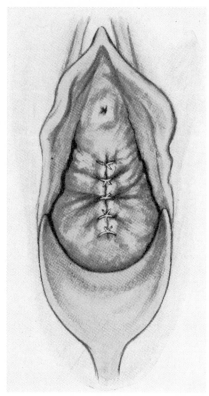

Fig. 453. (*Left*) Third step. The first row of sutures inverts the vaginal mucosa frill (collar). The mucous membrane of the bladder is not touched. (*Right*) Fourth step. Vaginal suture through which the vaginal wall contracts inwardly. (Martius, H.: Die Gynäkologischen Operationen, Stuttgart, Thieme)

should be removed before surgery is carried out.

5. Cystoscopy should be carried out, with particular reference to the relation of the ureters to the fistulous tract.

6. Accessibility is very important; the operator should choose the approach with which he is most familiar, whether transabdominal, transvesical, extraperitoneal or vaginal. Other things being equal, the vaginal approach seems to be best because there is less shock and, in the event of failure, the urine does not enter the abdominal cavity. If the vaginal approach is used, either a midline, a mediolateral or a Schuchardt incision will give plenty of working space.

7. The tissue involved must be so tied that there is no tension on the sutured area.

8. The finest size of catgut should be selected to close the opening, for there must be complete hemostasis. The least amount of

suture material possible should be used in order not to devitalize the tissues.

9. The Latzko method gives the best results. In this technic, the opening is not freshened, and a piece, of vaginal mucous membrane is left attached. This is inverted, so that there are no sutures in the mucosa of the bladder, thus giving less chance for formation of a hematoma, and, in the event that the maneuver is unsuccessful, the hole is no larger than it was originally.

10. An indwelling catheter should be maintained for 8 to 10 days, or the bladder must be catheterized at least every 6 hours. Antibiotics must be given to prevent cystitis.

Rectovaginal Fistulae. Although these are no longer common, they do occur often enough that the modern surgeon must be prepared to handle them. They may occur anywhere between the upper and the lower limits of the area where vagina and rectum are adjacent and may result from (1) surgical procedures, (2) irradiation or (3) some infectious or cancerous process. Those of surgical origin may be due to poor technic and follow such procedures as total abdominal or vaginal hysterectomy or posterior colpotomy. Those due to unskilled use of irradiation therapy are most likely to follow treatment of carcinoma of the cervix, for which reason such treatment should be given only by those specially trained in these technics, not by the average physician. Perirectal abscess or extension of carcinoma of the cervix into the rectovaginal septum are occasional causes.

PREPARATION FOR SURGICAL REPAIR. A course of chemotherapy should be instituted 4 days preoperatively to reduce the colon bacilli in the stool. Just before the patient is to go to surgery, she should be given a cleansing enema. Other preparation is routine.

TECHNIC. If difficulty is experienced in finding the fistulous tract, an injection of methylene blue usually will reveal it.

A *small fistula* may be closed by encircling the fistulous opening with an incision and mobilizing the bowel, then inserting several purse-string sutures.

For a *large fistula,* purse-string sutures are not suitable. The vaginal mucous membrane is dissected back far enough to permit mobilization of the bowel. Interrupted sutures, mattress type, may then be used, or the edges may be inserted into the bowel with a continuous suture. The first layer should be reinforced by a second row of sutures. The mucous membrane should then be trimmed and approximated, leaving no "dead spaces." When a large fistula lies just above the anal sphincter or the perineal bridge, the bridge should be cut. Repair is then done as for a "third-degree tear." Or, when the fistula lies close to the rectal sphincter, external tenotomy of the sphincter, at about "5 o'clock," is the procedure of choice. This will prevent tension on the sutured area from any accumulation of gas or feces.

In fistulae occurring after irradiation or previous surgery, where there is marked scar formation, a colostomy may be necessary before closure is attempted. A colostomy is most likely to be needed when the fistula is located at the top of the vagina. In some cases of this type, if the rent is readily accessible, it may be closed by a technic similar to that of Latzko for vesicovaginal fistula. Two weeks should be allowed to elapse between the making of the colostomy and the repair of the fistula, with 2 months more allowed before closing the colostomy.

SAFEGUARDING THE URETER IN GYNECOLOGIC OPERATIONS

The ureter may be injured where it crosses the brim of the pelvis, particularly when the infundibulopelvic ligament is congenitally short or has been shortened by some inflammatory disease. It may be accidentally tied or cut where it goes through the cardinal ligament area when the uterine artery is being secured. In peritonealization of the pelvis following surgery, the ureter must always be safeguarded against constriction.

In extensive operation for uterine carcinoma, the ureter may be laid bare, removing its blood supply, which (as previously pointed out) changes at each level of its course. Fully 10 per cent of the early Wertheim operations were followed by the formation of ureterovaginal fistulae. Now that surgeons realize that they must not leave the ureter bare, but must permit it to remain in its bed, the ureteral damage in this procedure has dropped to no more than 2 per cent, in skilled hands.

Again, in removing a *fibroid* which extends into the broad ligament, it is easy to injure the ureter. To avoid this error, such a tumor should be enucleated from its capsule. When removing *intraligamentary cysts,* dissect the ureter away from the growth before placing a clamp on the most dependent portion of the cyst. It is a good idea to do an intravenous pyelogram before attempting the removal of all intraligamentary broad ligament masses.

Not infrequently the ureter is injured when removing chronic inflammatory lesions of the tubes and the ovaries, when they are adherent posteriorly to the uterus and the broad ligament. To avoid trouble, it is necessary to be meticulous in the removal of the adherent adnexal masses from their broad ligament attachments, paying particular attention to the cardinal ligament and infundibulopelvic ligament regions. When it is necessary to tie off the ovarian vessel, leave an inch or so of the distal end of the ligament to prevent catastrophe.

In a *presacral neurectomy,* safeguard against tying of the ureters. Identify them on each side before removing the tissues which contain the presacral nerves.

STRESS INCONTINENCE

No operation for this condition should be done until it has been determined that the loss of urine is due to weakness *at the urethrovesical junction.* The following conditions, which may produce incontinence, must be ruled out:

1. Medical affections, such as tabes, multiple sclerosis, pernicious anemia with cord involvement and spina bifida occulta

2. "Paradoxical" incontinence, where the loss of urine is due to overfilling of the bladder

3. Uretheral problems, such as urethral stricture or diverticulae of the urethra (congenital or acquired)

4. Polyps at the urethrovesical junction

5. Psychotic states in which the urine is lost during sleep

6. Atrophy of the anterior vaginal vault, as found late in the menopause and in old age

7. Marked cystitis with vesical spasm causing urgency and inability to hold the urine

Even after all these conditions have been ruled out, surgery is still not indicated until a course of exercises has been tried to strengthen the urethrovesical sphincter. This may be accomplished by the use of the Kegel's perineometer or by having the patient alternately void and stop voiding several times at each emptying of the bladder. Many women will regain full control after a few months of such management.

However, if no relief is obtained by medical management, surgery is indicated. Many operations for the purpose have been devised, some of them so formidable that they are needed only in extreme cases. Most patients can be relieved by tightening the urethrovesical junction. The problem is *to know exactly where this area is located.* This may be determined by inserting a Foley catheter with the collar distended. Then, by dissecting

off the mucous membrane, the area which needs tightening may be felt. The sutures should be placed while the catheter is in the bladder, and it should then be left in for at least 5 days to provide constant drainage. This use of the indwelling catheter has done much to reduce the proportion of failures.

VAGINAL OR ABDOMINAL SURGERY FIRST?

When a woman must have both vaginal and abdominal surgery, the question often arises as to which should be done first. It is the present writer's feeling that vaginal surgery should precede the abdominal. Repair of a lacerated cervix or of cystocele or urethrocele should be accomplished first, if it is relatively certain that the added abdominal operation will not be too strenuous for the patient. If the abdominal procedure is followed by vaginal work, it is possible that tugging on the tissues might pull the ligatures off some major vessel, with resulting fatal hemorrhage.

On the other hand, if the abdominal surgery promises to be difficult, with the probability of much loss of blood, it is wiser to do this first and finish the vaginal work at some later time. In most instances, however, when a blood bank is available, both the abdominal and vaginal operations may safely be completed at one time.

OVARIAN CYSTS

Because of the slow growth and the lack of overt symptoms in ovarian cysts, every opportunity should be taken to inspect the ovaries with this in mind. In most instances the malignant nature of an ovarian growth is not suspected before surgical exposure; sometimes it is recognized only after pathologic study. The following may give valuable opportunities to diagnose ovarian neoplasms:

1. Any abdominal operation near the pelvic area

2. Following vaginal hysterectomy

3. Routinely, during abdominal or vaginal sterilization

4. On the opposite side, when one ovarian tumor is being removed

5. Following removal of any surface tumor (which should always be sent to the laboratory)

6. Periodic pelvic examinations, either vaginal or rectal, particularly during menarche and menopause

7. When postmenopausal bleeding occurs, and dilatation and curettage are negative, a posterior colpotomy should be done.

8. Routinely, during an interposition operation

9. Any ovarian mass larger than a small orange which is present during 3 consecutive examinations 2 weeks apart calls for further investigation.

10. During repair of a prolapsed uterus, whether or not hysterectomy is being done (through an anterior or posterior colpotomy incision)

11. During exploratory operation over an ovarian mass with ascites. Ascites may be a Meigs's syndrome, which, in turn, may be present with a fibroma of the ovary, a Brenner tumor or some other new growth.

SYMPTOMS

1. Most ovarian tumors are "silent," unless they have grown large enough to cause pressure on adjacent viscera (bladder, intestine, ureter).

2. Overt symptoms may result from:

A. a twisted pedicle, inducing peritoneal irritation

B. rupture, with resultant "chemical" peritonitis

C. rupture of a blood vessel into the cyst, producing anemia and pain due to tension on the ovary

D. functional tumors which may produce indirect symptoms

AIDS IN DIAGNOSIS

Twenty per cent of all proliferative ovarian tumors are *hard*, but, of these, only about 1 in 5 will be malignant. The remaining 80 per cent are of the cystic variety, of which about 3 in 8 are malignant. One or 2 per cent of dermoid cysts will be malignant. In attempting to make a diagnosis, peritoneoscopy, culdoscopy, posterior colpocentesis and posterior colpotomy may be of assistance.

REMOVAL OF BOTH OVARIES

When should both be removed as a prophylactic measure? Many gynecologists set an arbitrary age limit, after which this may be done routinely. This limit varies from 37 to 43 years as a minimum. However, it is my own impression that if the ovaries are grossly normal they should not be removed this early because in many instances they continue to function until the age of 55 or even later. That the ovaries have functions other than reproductive has been definitely established. Randall states that the incidence of ovarian carcinoma should be reduced to *only 6 or 7 per thousand* if both ovaries were removed routinely during any pelvic celiotomy in the preclimacteric period. This seems to be an odd conclusion in view of the fact that, at present, malignancy of the ovary develops in *less than one woman in a thousand* and calls into question the advisability of such prophylactic oophorectomy. In support of this is Griffith's statement that because of the ovaries' important role in the body's economy, they should *not* be removed except for the most urgent of reasons. Therefore, it becomes the clinician's problem to balance possible beneficial results of oophorectomy against (1) certain loss to the patient of orderly hormonal interchange and (2) certain loss of the protective action of the ovarian secretion. Rarely do the benefits outweigh the deleterious effects. Save in very exceptional instances, the bad effects on the cardiovascular system alone are important enough to offset any possible beneficial results. Further, it is questionable that prophylactic removal of *one ovary* will materially reduce the incidence of ovarian cancers.

OPERATIONS ON THE OVARIES

OVARIAN CYSTS

Remove Cysts Intact. In general, this is the preferred practice, even if it necessitates a large incision. In many cases evacuation of the contents of a cyst is impossible; this is particularly true of pseudomucinous cysts. When evacuation is necessary, the greatest care must be exercised to avoid implanting the malignant cells elsewhere in the operative field, for it is better to be on the safe side and suspect malignancy until its absence is proved. Wall off the peritoneal cavity thoroughly before doing the puncture. Also, keep in mind that a rupture of a pseudomucinous cyst may lead to pseudomyxomatous peritonitis.

Adhesions. Ovarian cysts of long standing are likely to have formed extensive adhesions to all the structures in their vicinity, i.e., the uterus, the rectum, the bladder, the intestines, the pelvic peritoneum and the abdominal wall. Removal of such adhesions must be done with extreme care. All bleeding must be checked, and careful peritonealization of all surfaces is essential. When the tube stands in the way of such careful removal, or when it is also diseased, it should be removed along with the cyst.

In my personal experience, only twice has a carcinoma of the ovary been encountered following a previous hysterectomy.

Ovarian Tumors

All proliferative tumors should be treated surgically. Operation should be strongly advised when any ovarian tumor larger than a small orange is continuously present at successive examinations 2 weeks apart. When the tumor is hard and nodular, the need for immediate surgery becomes imperative (Fig.

454). In general, treatment can be (1) palliative only or (2) definitely curative. Palliative procedures include:

1. Isotope gold or nitrogen mustard for intraperitoneal implantations
2. Androgen therapy
3. Hemisulfur mustard
4. Triethylene melanine

These do not cure but may prolong life for many months. They may also reduce the necessity of frequent tapping.

Curative procedures are only:

1. Surgery alone
2. Surgery plus irradiation therapy

Value of Pregnancy Tests in Diagnosis of Hydatidiform Mole and Chorio-epithelioma

When the uterus is larger than normal during a period of amenorrhea, and when normal pregnancy, multiple pregnancy and fibroid have been ruled out, the use of the chorionic gonadotropic test may be informative. In most cases of hydatidiform mole there will be an overwhelming production of chorionic gonadotropin; as little as 1.5 cc. of urine

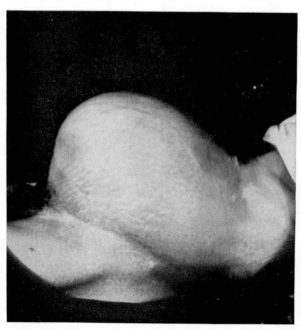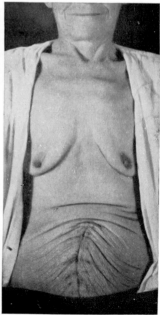

Fig. 454. (*Left*) Stretching of abdominal skin over large ovarian cystoma. (*Right*) Unsightly folding of skin which will result after removal of such growths if not resected at time of operation.

FIG. 455. Proper method of removing tumor from broad ligament.

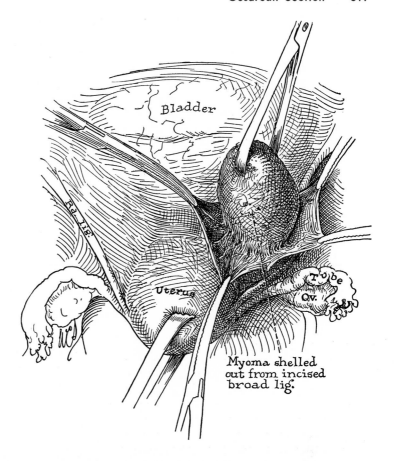

Bladder

Bd lig

Uterus

Tube Ov.

Myoma shelled out from incised broad lig.

may be used to accomplish the test, instead of 15 to 20 cc. If the result is positive with this fractional test, there is a strong likelihood that a mole is present. If the uterus continues to enlarge rapidly, and especially if there is spotting, a flat plate of the abdomen should be taken. When the uterus is at or above the navel and no fetal parts are demonstrated, evacuation is indicated.

Since fully a quarter of chorio-epitheliomata are secondary to hydatidiform mole, observation of the patient should be continued after the uterus is evacuated. This may be done conveniently by repeating the pregnancy test every 2 weeks with the 1.5 cc. of urine. If, after 3 tests at 2-week intervals, the result is still positive, a diagnostic dilatation and curettage should be done. Two weeks after this, another test should be made; if this is also positive with 1.5 cc. of urine, the uterus should be removed. However, if the tests are negative after the curettement (3 tests *with 20 cc. of urine* at 2-week intervals),

the possibility of chorio-epithelioma may be dismissed.

Caution. If, after a few tests with 20 cc. of urine, the test turns positive, the possibility of a new pregnancy must be considered. There are several cases on record of a uterus being removed, only to find that a normal pregnancy was the reason for the increased prolan.

CESAREAN SECTION

This may come within the province of the obstetrician or of the general surgeon. In either event, additional procedures during the section should be restricted to actual necessities, postponing everything else which might increase the risk for the patient.

The *low cervical* or *low fundal* section is preferable to the classic cesarean, except when it is essential to perform other operative procedures at the same time, or in the presence of placenta praevia. There is also the question of performing an extraperitoneal section in the presence of infection or in a long-delayed labor. At present, because of the difficulties of doing the extraperitoneal section, Kobak has had excellent results with the low cervical section, with the use of antibiotics and chemotherapy. The advantages of this approach include reduced chance for future rupture through the scar and better peritonealization.

Safeguards in Cesarean Section

Whereas peritonitis once played an important role in maternal morbidity and mortality, today, following this operation, the chief causes of death are hemorrhage, ileus, embolism and accidents of anesthesia. This last may be prevented by more judicious use and choice of anesthetic to fit the needs of the individual patient. For example, if the patient has recently eaten, in order to avoid pulmonary complications, either her stomach must be pumped out or local or spinal anesthesia should be used.

Hemorrhage. During the operation, hemorrhage is often unpredictable. One unit (500 cc.) of matched blood should be available in the operating room at the time of surgery. If bleeding does not exceed 500 cc., no blood should be given unless hemoglobin and red count were low before the operation. If bleeding is excessive, the blood should be started flowing while another unit is being obtained.

If the uterus fails to contract, oxytocics should be injected either directly into the uterine wall or intravenously. If massage and the use of oxytocics do not stop the bleeding, a hysterectomy may be necessary.

Other Complications. By handling the intra-abdominal contents as little as possible after the section, other complications may be avoided. However, the pelvic viscera should be inspected, though no elective surgery should be done following the section—except sterilization, if required. Needless to add, this is decided upon only after consultation with a disinterested committee.

Repeated Cesarean Sections. Many obstetricians believe that "once a cesarean, always a cesarean." However, this is not necessarily true, although it is an essential safeguard to have the surgeon on hand and the operating room set up during any labor subsequent to a cesarean in case of need. If the indications for the first section remain valid, there should

be no hesitation to perform another, but it must be kept in mind that fatal complications may arise in a second, or even a third, operation when earlier ones went smoothly.

It must also be borne in mind that uterine rupture in such subsequent pregnancies may cause the loss of the child, unless an elective cesarean is done before term. Yet, there again, a nice balance must be struck between this possibility and that of losing the child due to the complications of prematurity.

TUMORS OF THE BROAD LIGAMENT

When removing tumors in this area it is a gross error to remove the ligament with the tumor. Instead, the ligament should be opened, the tumor removed and the layers of the ligament closed again (Fig. 455). Keep a careful watch for the ureter to safeguard it in removing any intraligamentous tumors.

Prognosis

Injuries to the ureter and uncontrollable venous hemorrhage are the chief causes of the high morbidity rate in operations of this type. When working with intraligamentary cysts, this morbidity may be reduced by dissecting the ureter and retracting it away from the cyst before removing the growth. When enucleating fibroids, their capsules should be left intact to avoid ureteral injuries.

BIBLIOGRAPHY

Brunschwig, A., and Daniel, W.: Pelvic exenterations for advanced carcinoma of the vulva, Am. J. Obst. & Gynec. 72:489, 1956.

Frank, R. T.: Formation of artificial vagina without operation (intubation method), New York State J. Med. 40:1669, 1940.

Kanter, A. E.: Congenital absence of the vagina; a simplified operation, Am. J. Surg. 30:314, 1935.

Kanter, A. E., and Klawans, A. H.: Prolapse of the uterus—operation for its relief, J. Internat. Coll. Surgeons 16:37, 1951.

———: Ovarian tumors, S. Clin. North America 33:279, 1953.

Kobak, A. D., Fields, C., and Turow, D. D.: Prophylactic chemo-antibiotic therapy and low cervical cesarean section in potential and actual infections, Am. J. Obst. & Gynec. 60:1129, 1950.

Lull, C. B.: Abdominal pregnancy, Am. J. Obst. & Gynec. 40:194, 1940.

Meigs, J. V.: Cancer of the cervix; an appraisal, Am. J. Obst. & Gynec. **72**:467, 1956.

Mischell, D. R.: Endometrial biopsy in early extrauterine pregnancy, Am. J. Obst. & Gynec. **41**:129, 1941.

Palmer, J. P., and Spratt, D. W.: Pelvic carcinoma following irradiation for benign gynecological diseases, Am. J. Obst. & Gynec. **72**:497, 1956.

Pemberton, F. A.: Carcinoma of ovary, Am. J. Obst. & Gynec. **40**:751, 1940.

Randall, C.: Indication for resection or removal of the ovary, Connecticut M. J. **19**:947, 1955.

Index

Abdomen, "silent," significance, 406
  with perforated peptic ulcer, 367
  wall reconstruction, use of tantalum gauze mesh and
    Fortisan fabric, 351
Abdominal cavity, natural subdivisions, 337
Abdominal surgery, value of pabulum in digestive
    tract during, 332
Abdominoperineal resection, retention of urine after,
    566
ABO system of blood grouping, 53
Abortifacient devices as foreign bodies, 25
Abortion, peritonitis after, 348
  spontaneous, shortening of round ligament for, 603
Abrasion treatment, liability to keloid after, 90
  precautions, 90
  use of face-lifting after, 90
Abruptio placentae, 59
Abscess(s), brain, relation to otitis media and mas-
    toiditis, 148
    symptoms, 148
    treatment, 122
      by craniotomy, 122
  cerebellar, symptoms, 148
  "cold," precautions in treatment, 236
  differentiating from aneurysm, 207
  extradural, headache as symptom, 147
    mastoidectomy for, 147
  formation after acute pancreatitis, 500
  hepatic, 466
  lateral sinus, prognosis, 148
  pelvic, drainage, 594
    procedures for treating, 601
  perinephritic, 582
  perisinus, defined, 148
  peritonsillar ("quinsy sore throat"), 158
    surgery, 158
  psoas, differential diagnosis, 508
  scrotal, after epididymitis, 546
  septal, symptoms, 152
  stitch, precautions, 347
  subaponeurotic, 103
  subphrenic, dangers of chemotherapy in treatment,
    473
    diagnosis, difficulty of, 472
    draining, 474
    locating, 474
    locations in relation to causes, 472
    or perigastric, after perforated gastric ulcer, 367
    surgical approach, 474
    surgical treatment, indications for, 473
A.C.D. Solution, 57
Acetylcholine test, 207
Acidity, gastric, relation to cure of gastric ulcer, 368
Acidosis, postoperative, in children, 334
  respiratory, defined, 41

Acne, danger of surgery with, 11
Acrylic in plastic surgery, 95
"Active patch" defined, 53
"Acute abdomen," 446
Adenocarcinoma, in adenoma of thyroid, 166
  diffuse, of thyroid, 166
  of gallbladder, jaundice, 481
    relation of gallstones, 481
  papillary, of thyroid, 166
Adenoidectomy, control of bleeding after, 160
  nature and special precautions, 160
Adenoma of thyroid, adenocarcinoma, 166
Adenomyoma of biliary tract, 480
Adhesions, avoiding, in gallbladder surgery, 494
  complications caused by, after biliary surgery, 495
  mistaken for peritoneum, 340
  postoperative, causes, 352
    value, 352
  precautions in removing fibroids in presence of, 605
  problems in gastric surgery, 366
    with ovarian cyst, 616
  use of omentum to prevent, 494
Adrenal gland, care during renal surgery, 578
Adrenalectomy, approaches for, 587
  supportive treatment after, 579
  transperitoneal, 583
Adrenalin, special precautions in presence of cyclo-
    propane anesthesia, 66
  use with intravenous saline, 14
    for postoperative oozing after facial-defect re-
    pair, 80
Aerocele, traumatic, 106
Age of patient, relation to operative shock, 9
Aged patient, anesthetic considerations, special, 334
  colonic tumors, removal, 432
  herniorrhaphy, 524
  lumbar position, difficulty, 583
  neoplasms, biologic inactivity, 562
  spinal anesthesia ideal, 43
Aged woman, "stress incontinence," 596
  See also Elderly patient, Geriatrics, etc.
Agglutinins, appearance during pregnancy, 55
Agglutinogens defined, 53
Air, injections of, use in brain tumor diagnosis, 115
  operating-room, how contaminated, 12
  sterilization by ultraviolet radiation, 12
  swallowed, need to remove, 421
Air-conditioning, value in preventing postoperative
    pneumonia, 353
Aird, I., 371
Airway, general requirements, 37
  vital importance, in craniofacial trauma, 70
Albuminuria associated with hemoglobinuria, 61
Alcoholic patient, use of tranquilizers, 34
Alcoholism, relation to anesthesia, 31